Adult Reconstruction & Arthroplasty: Core Knowledge in Orthopaedics

Other Volumes in the *Core Knowledge in Orthopaedics* Series

Foot & Ankle

Hand, Elbow & Shoulder

Pediatric Orthopaedics

Spine

Sports Medicine

Trauma

ADULT RECONSTRUCTION & ARTHROPLASTY: CORE KNOWLEDGE IN ORTHOPAEDICS

JONATHAN P. GARINO, MD
Director
The Joint Reconstruction Center at Penn–Presbyterian Medical Center
Director
The Adult Reconstruction Fellowship
Associate Professor
Department of Orthopaedic Surgery
University of Pennsylvania School of Medicine
Philadelphia, PA

PEDRO K. BEREDJIKLIAN, MD
Assistant Professor
Department of Orthopaedic Surgery
University of Pennsylvania School of Medicine
Philadelphia, PA

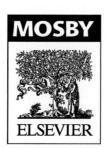

MOSBY

ELSEVIER

MOSBY
ELSEVIER
An Imprint of Elsevier Science

1600 John F. Kennedy Boulevard
Suite 1800
Philadelphia, PA 19103-2899

ADULT RECONSTRUCTION AND ARTHROPLASTY: ISBN-13: 978-0-323-03370-1
CORE KNOWLEDGE IN ORTHOPAEDICS
Copyright © 2007 by Mosby, Inc., an affiliate of Elsevier Inc.

NOTICE

Knowledge and best practice in this field are constantly changing. As new research and experience broaden our knowledge, changes in practice, treatment, and drug therapy may become necessary or appropriate. Readers are advised to check the most current information provided (i) on procedures featured or (ii) by the manufacturer of each product to be administered, to verify the recommended dose or formula, the method and duration of administration, and the contraindications. It is the responsibility of the practitioner, relying on their own experience and knowledge of the patient, to make diagnoses, to determine dosages and the best treatment for each individual patient, and to take all appropriate safety precautions. To the fullest extent of the law, neither the Publisher nor the Editors assumes any liability for any injury and/or damage to persons or property arising out of or related to any use of the material contained in this book.

The Publisher

Library of Congress Cataloging-in-Publication Data
Adult reconstruction and arthroplasty: core knowledge in orthopaedics/
[edited by] Jonathan P. Garino, Pedro K. Beredjiklian. – 1st ed.
    p. ; cm.
    Includes bibliographical references.
    ISBN-13: 978-0-323-03370-1
  1. Arthroplasty. 2. Surgery, Plastic. I. Garino, Jonathan P. II.
Beredjiklian, Pedro K.
    [DNLM: 1. Arthroplasty, Replacement. 2. Adult. WE 312 A244 2007]
RD686.A36 2007
617.4′7059–dc22

                                                              2006035901

Publishing Director: Kim Murphy
Developmental Editor: Pamela Hetherington
Publishing Services Manager: Tina Rebane
Senior Project Manager: Amy L. Cannon
Design Manager: Steven Stave

Printed in the United States of America

Transferred to Digital Printing, 2013

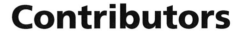

Contributors

JOSEPH A. ABBOUD, MD
Clinical Assistant Professor, Department of Orthopaedics, University of Pennsylvania School of Medicine, Philadelphia, PA

PEDRO K. BEREDJIKLIAN, MD
Assistant Professor, Department of Orthopaedic Surgery, University of Pennsylvania School of Medicine, Philadelphia, PA

DAVID J. BOZENTKA, MD
Chief, Hand Surgery, Penn Orthopaedic Institute; Associate Professor, Department of Orthopaedic Surgery, University of Pennsylvania School of Medicine, Philadelphia, PA

GREGORY F. CAROLAN, MD
Instructor, University of Pennsylvania School of Medicine, Philadelphia, PA

ROBERT B. CARRIGAN, MD
Physician, Premier Orthopaedics and Sports Medicine, Ridley Park, PA

DOUGLAS L. CERYNIK, MD
Research Fellow, Department of Orthopaedic Surgery, Hahnemann University Hospital/Drexel University College of Medicine, Philadelphia, PA

KINGSLEY R. CHIN, MD
Chief, Division of Orthopaedic Spine Surgery and Assistant Professor, Department of Orthopaedic Surgery, University of Pennsylvania School of Medicine, Philadelphia, PA

IAN C. CLARKE, PhD
Professor and Director, Department of Orthopaedics, Orthopaedic Research Center, Loma Linda University and Medical Center, Loma Linda, CA

THOMAS DONALDSON, MD
Assistant Clinical Professor and Co-Director, Department of Orthopaedics, Orthopaedic Research Center, Loma Linda University and Medical Center, Loma Linda, CA

EDWARD EBRAMZADEH, PhD
Director, Implant Performance Biomechanics Laboratory, Los Angeles Orthopaedic Hospital and Adjunct Professor, Department of Orthopaedic Surgery, University of California at Los Angeles, Los Angeles, CA

MARK I. FROIMSON, MD, MBA
Staff Surgeon, Department of Orthopaedic Surgery, Cleveland Clinic Foundation, The Cleveland Clinic, Cleveland, OH

JONATHAN P. GARINO, MD
Director, The Joint Reconstruction Center at Penn-Presbyterian Medical Center; Director, The Adult Reconstruction Fellowship and Associate Professor, Department of Orthopaedic Surgery, University of Pennsylvania School of Medicine, Philadelphia, PA

CHARLES L. GETZ, MD
Assistant Professor, Department of Orthopaedic Surgery, University of Pennsylvania; Assistant Professor, Division of Shoulder and Elbow Surgery, Penn-Presbyterian Medical Center, Philadelphia, PA

DAVID GLASER, MD
Assistant Professor, Department of Orthopaedic Surgery, University of Pennsylvania School of Medicine, Philadelphia, PA

NADIM J. HALLAB, PhD
Associate Professor and Director, Materials Testing Laboratory, Department of Orthopaedic Surgery, Rush University Medical Center, Chicago, IL

WILLIAM G. HAMILTON, MD
Orthopaedic Surgeon, Anderson Orthopaedic Research Institute and Instructor, Anderson Clinic Postgraduate Fellowship, Alexandria, VA

HARISH S. HOSALKAR, MD, MBMS (ORTH), DNB (ORTH)
Clinical Instructor and Resident, Department of Orthopaedic Surgery, University of Pennsylvania School of Medicine, Philadelphia, PA

CRAIG L. ISRAELITE, MD
Co-Director of Knee Service and Assistant Professor, Department of Orthopaedic Surgery, University of Pennsylvania School of Medicine, Philadelphia, PA

JOSHUA J. JACOBS, MD
Crown Family Professor of Orthopaedic Surgery, Rush University Medical Center, Chicago, IL

CHRISTOPHER JOBE, MD
Chairman of Orthopaedic Surgery, Department of Orthopaedics, Orthopaedics Research Center, Loma Linda University and Medical Center, Loma Linda, CA

NORMAN A. JOHANSON, MD
Chairman, Department of Orthopaedic Surgery, Hahnemann University Hospital/Drexel University College of Medicine, Philadelphia, PA

KRISTOFER J. JONES, BA
Medical Student, University of Pennsylvania School of Medicine, Philadelphia, PA

LISA KHOURY, MD
Resident, Department of Orthopaedic Surgery, Hospital of the University of Pennsylvania, Philadelphia, PA

SHARAT K. KUSUMA, MD, MBA
Resident and Clinical Instructor, Department of Orthopaedic Surgery, University of Pennsylvania School of Medicine, Philadelphia, PA

RICHARD D. LACKMAN, MD
Chairman and Professor, Division of Orthopaedic Surgery, Pennsylvania Hospital, Philadelphia, PA

STEVE MASCHKE, MD
Resident Surgeon, Department of Orthopaedic Surgery, Cleveland Clinic Foundation, The Cleveland Clinic, Cleveland, OH

ROBERT MOLLOY, MD
Staff Surgeon, Department of Orthopaedic Surgery, Cleveland Clinic Foundation, The Cleveland Clinic, Cleveland, OH

SANJIV NAIDU, MD
Professor, Orthopaedic Surgery and Rehabilitation, Penn State College of Medicine, Hershey, PA

CHARLES L. NELSON, MD
Assistant Professor, Department of Orthopaedic Surgery, University of Pennsylvania School of Medicine, Philadelphia, PA

ENYI OKEREKE, MD, PHARMD
Associate Professor and Chief, Orthopaedic Foot and Ankle Services, University of Pennsylvania School of Medicine, Philadelphia, PA

BRADFORD PARSONS, MD
Assistant Professor, Department of Orthopaedics, Mt. Sinai School of Medicine, New York, NY

JAVAD PARVIZI, MD, FRCS
Associate Professor, Jefferson Medical College, Rothman Institute, Thomas Jefferson University, Philadelphia, PA

DAVID I. PEDOWITZ, MD, MS
Chief Resident, Department of Orthopedic Surgery, Hospital of the University of Pennsylvania, Philadelphia, PA

MATTHEW L. RAMSEY, MD
Chief, Shoulder Study Group; Director, Shoulder and Elbow Fellowship; Associate Professor, Department of Orthopaedic Surgery; and Chief, Shoulder and Elbow Service, University of Pennsylvania School of Medicine, Philadelphia, PA

SUDHEER REDDY, MD
Instructor, Department of Orthopaedic Surgery, University of Pennsylvania School of Medicine, Philadelphia, PA

JAMES A. SANFILIPPO, MD, MHS
Resident, Department of Orthopaedic Surgery, Thomas Jefferson University Hospital, Philadelphia, PA

SOPHIA N. SANGIORGIO, PHD
Manager, Implant Performance Biomechanics Laboratory, Los Angeles Orthopaedic Hospital, University of California at Los Angeles, Los Angeles, CA

PETER SHARKEY, MD
Professor of Orthopaedic Surgery, Jefferson Medical College, Rothman Institute, Thomas Jefferson University, Philadelphia, PA

NEIL P. SHETH, MD
Resident, Department of Orthopaedic Surgery, Hospital of the University of Pennsylvania, Philadelphia, PA

EHSAN TABARAEE, MS
Medical Student, George Washington University School of Medicine, Washington, DC

VIRAK TAN, MD
Associate Professor, Department of Orthopaedics, University of Medicine and Dentistry of New Jersey, Newark, NJ

BRIAN VANNOZZI, MD
Resident, Department of Orthopaedic Surgery, Hospital of the University of Pennsylvania, Philadelphia, PA

MATTHEW WERGER
Medical Student, Georgetown University Medical Center, Washington, DC

BRENT WIESEL, MD
Resident, Department of Orthopaedic Surgery, Hospital of the University of Pennsylvania, Philadelphia, PA

GERALD R. WILLIAMS, JR., MD
Attending Surgeon, The Rothman Institute of Orthopaedic Surgery, Thomas Jefferson University, Philadelphia, PA

*To my wonderful wife Jennifer and my children, Jonathan Jr., Christopher, and Sophia,
who inspire all aspects of my life.*

–JPG

*To my lovely wife Mary, without whose support, patience, and dedication
none of this work would be possible.*

–PKB

Contents

Preface

The field of reconstructive orthopaedic surgery has grown exponentially over the past several years. Advances in this area have yielded greater insights and knowledge of prosthetic materials and biomechanics, surgical techniques, and the biologic response to prosthetic implants. These advancements have resulted in significant enhancements to patient care.

The ability of the orthopedic surgeon to assimilate this wealth of information and use it effectively has become an overwhelming challenge. This text represents one method of aggregating and organizing the key concepts of adult reconstruction to assist in this knowledge review and assimilation process.

Its concise nature, logical organization, and annotated bibliography make it an ideal reference for everyday use or as a study supplement for residents and practicing orthopedists. It represents an important addition to the Core Knowledge in Orthopaedics series, which together make a valuable addition to any orthopaedic library.

Jonathan P. Garino, MD
and
Pedro K. Beredjiklian, MD
Editors

Total Joint Replacement
Effects of Materials and Designs on Osteolysis

Ian C. Clarke,* Thomas Donaldson,† and Christopher Jobe‡

*PhD, Professor and Director, Department of Orthopaedics,Orthopaedic Research Center,
Loma Linda University and Medical Center, Loma Linda, CA
†MD, Assistant Clinical Professor and Co-Director, Department of Orthopaedics, Orthopaedic
Research Center, Loma Linda University and Medical Center, Loma Linda, CA
‡MD, Chairman of Orthopaedic Surgery, Department of Orthopaedics, Orthopaedics
Research Center, Loma Linda University and Medical Center, Loma Linda, CA

Introduction

- Total joint replacements can fail early for a variety of reasons, including sepsis, inadequate implant positioning, inferior fixation, and poor-quality bone stock. Beyond 6 to 8 years of follow-up, *osteolysis*, a destructive process created by the body's reaction to accumulating wear debris, becomes the major cause of revision.
- The release of submicron particulates elicits a foreign body tissue response that, given enough time, will result in implant loosening, pain, and revision (Amstutz et al. 1992, Charnley et al. 1969, Clarke and Campbell 1989, Hamilton and Gorczyca 1995). Thus to be successful, the total hip replacement (THR) design has to minimize the amount of wear debris released over 1 or more decades of use.
- The history of THR began with metal-on-metal (MOM) bearing concepts (Amstutz and Clarke 1991). Over the decade 1955 to 1965, only the cobalt-chromium (CoCr) metal alloy proved suitable for this purpose. MOM systems were developed in Europe by surgeons McKee, Muller, and Ring using large ball diameters (32, 35, and 41.5 mm).
- In 1963, the late Sir John Charnley introduced the 22.25-mm diameter metal ball with a cemented polyethylene cup (MPE) (Charnley et al. 1969). This approach received widespread acceptance, and the use of MOM bearings quickly dwindled by the early 1970s.
- Starting in 1970, European surgeons such as Boutin, Griss, Mittelmeier, and Salzer saw the opportunity to develop ceramic-on-ceramic (COC) bearings (Boutin 1972,

Clarke and Willmann 1994). This advance also made ceramic-polyethylene (CPE) combinations possible.
- The decade from 1965 to 1975 saw three competing bearing concepts emerge: plastic, metal, and ceramic (MPE or CPE, MOM, COC). In the beginning, the polyethylene (PE)-related osteolysis risk was ameliorated somewhat by the finding that after 20 years, patients' mortality rate frequently exceeded 50% (Sochart 1999).
- Because today's patient populations live longer and are much more active, the goal is to determine what combination of materials and THR design features will consistently minimize risk of osteolysis for more than 20 years of use.

40 Years of Experience With Polyethylene Cups
Risks of Debris-Driven Osteolysis

- Osteolysis has been associated with the formation of a granulomatous, periprosthetic membrane containing abundant PE particles and macrophages (Clarke and Campbell 1989). Osteolysis is more likely when the number of particles exceeds 10 billion/g of tissue (Ingham and Fisher 2000, Ingham and Fisher 2005, Ingram et al. 2004, Kobayashi et al. 1997).
- Multitudes of biochemical mediators of cellular recruitment, inflammation, and bone resorption have been found in these membranes (Box 1–1). Therefore the most

Box 1–1	Cytokines Involved in the Osteolytic Cascade

- Tumor necrosis factor-α
- Interleukin-1β
- Interleukin-6
- Interleukin-8
- Interleukin-11
- Transforming growth factor-β

direct way to combat the implant disease called *osteolysis* is to reduce the accumulation of wear debris.

Complexity of Clinical Wear Issues

- Understanding the significance of various clinical parameters has been complicated by many variables (Box 1–2).
- Thus many design and patient-related factors can add risk to the anticipated clinical success. For example, the metal-backed PE cup adds several confounding variables (Table 1–1) (Hamilton et al. 2005, Kurtz et al. 2005, Oparaugo et al. 2001). Roughening of CoCr balls and other third-body abrasive wear effects also come into play (Box 1–3) (Bauer et al. 1996, Hall et al. 1997).

Charnley's Small Ball Wear Paradigm

- The1960s' pioneering era with polytetrafluoroethylene acetabular cups revealed several design and wear paradigms that remain significant to this day (Box 1–4).
- The surgeon would obviously like to choose a large femoral ball for both stability and range of motion. Thus the late Sir John Charnley began with a ball diameter of 41.5 mm, then downsized in his search to minimize cup-loosening problems (Fig. 1–1).

Box 1–2	Multifactorial Complexity in Clinical Studies

- Implant design
- Fixation concepts
- Ball material and diameter (metal, ceramic)
- Type of cup backing and use of screw-holes
- Locking mechanism for cup liner
- Type of polyethylene used
- Type of polyethylene sterilization (irradiation, ethylene oxide, gas plasma)
- Post-sterilization polyethylene treatments (annealing; remelting)
- Implant positioning
- Third-body abrasive wear encountered in vivo
- Bone quality
- Severity of patient activities
- Duration of clinical studies
- Quality of clinical studies
- Outcome measures used

Table 1–1	Comparison of Parameters That Added Confounding Factors to Clinical Studies of Wear

PARAMETER	COMPLEXITY OF CLINICAL WEAR STUDIES
Large-diameter balls	Higher cup wear
Thin polyethylene cups	Wear studies generally confounded by use of larger balls
Metal-backed cups	Thinner polyethylene liners, with varied capture mechanisms
Backside wear	Design dependent; difficult to quantify
Femoral ball	SS, Ti6Al4V, cobalt chromium: roughening increases polyethylene wear
Femoral stem	Mode of fixation/potential for release of fretting debris
Acetabular cup	Mode of fixation/potential for release of porous coatings
Implant positioning	Impingement, subluxation, and dislocation
Patient	Varied activity levels
Follow-up	Varied duration

SS, 316 stainless steel; Ti6Al4V, titanium alloy.

- Wear was an important criterion for him because the prototypical polytetrafluoroethylene cups simply wore out in 3 years (Charnley et al. 1969).
- During his experimentation with various ball diameters, Charnley and later studies showed that the smallest ball (22 mm) produced the least amount of debris (see Fig. 1–1) (Clarke et al. 1997).
- The *small ball paradigm* has been proved time and time again. Most conspicuous were the disastrous results with large MPE hip resurfacing (Callaghan et al. 2002, Clarke and Campbell 1989, Kabo et al. 1993, Livermore et al. 1990). Thus PE cups had an essential design conflict, namely, a large ball was desired for stability but the small ball was necessary to minimize osteolysis.
- For patients younger than 50 years old at the time of their index operation, follow-up of the Charnley series demonstrated excellent 94% survivorship at 10 years (Fig. 1–2). However, with survivorship plotted to 30 years,

Box 1–3	Confounding Parameters in Metal-Backed Cup Designs

- Metal shell is deformed during insertion
- Added backing reduces thickness of UHMWPE liner
- Design reduces size of femoral ball
- Design introduces backside wear of UHMWPE (fretting)
- Flexible UHMWPE liner introduces debris-pumping action
- Introduction of screw holes gives debris access
- Metal-on-metal impingement creates abrasive third-body wear
- Roughening of cobalt-chromium ball is more likely (higher UHMWPE wear)

UHMWPE, ultrahigh-molecular-weight polyethylene.

Box 1–4	Charnley's Ultrahigh-Molecular-Weight Polyethylene Wear Paradigms

- Volumetric wear rate was the appropriate parameter for assessing the risk of osteolysis.
- Increasing polyethylene volumetric wear rates produced faster and more severe osteolysis.
- The larger ball diameters increased the amount of polyethylene debris by 10% for each added millimeter of ball diameter.
- The smallest ball (22 mm) minimized both frictional torque and the risk of osteolysis with polyethylene cups.

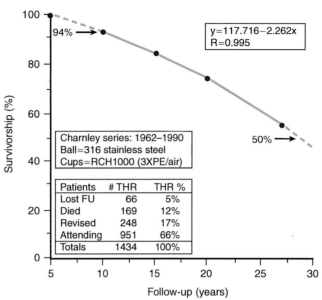

Figure 1–2: Survivorship study.
Survivorship study of 1434 hips followed for 30 years (original Charnley series started in 1962 using 22-mm stainless-steel ball). *FU,* follow-up. (Data from Wroblewski BM, Siney PD, Fleming PA [2002]. Charnley low-frictional torque arthroplasty in patients under the age of 51 years: Follow-up to 33 years. *J Bone Joint Surg Br* 84:540-543.)

the 6% failure at 10 years had increased to 50% because of accumulation of problems with osteolysis and loosening (Sochart 1999, Wroblewski and Siney 1992, Wroblewski et al. 1999, Wroblewski et al. 2002).

- Charnley, the first to measure wear, used migration of the femoral head on radiographs as his surrogate wear assessment (Charnley and Cupic 1973). Linear wear rates ranged up to 0.67 mm/year, with an average of 0.1 mm/year (Box 1–5).
- The corresponding *average* and *maximum* volumetric wear rates were 40 and 260 mm³/year (Fig. 1–3). Thus the

maximum wear rates placing patients at risk were generally five- to sevenfold higher than averages in those series (Wroblewski et al. 1999, Wroblewski et al. 2002).

- The unsuccessful Hylamer cups γ-sterilized in air (GIA) were associate with a much higher risk of osteolysis, averaging wear of 280 mm³/year in elderly patients (see Fig. 1–3) (Donaldson et al. 2004).
- One clinical study suggested that linear wear of 0.2 mm/year with the 32-mm ball was a useful index of

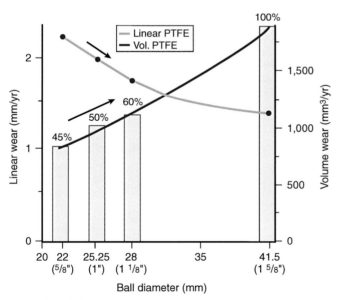

Figure 1–1: Linear wear.
With polytetrafluoroethylene *(PTFE)* cups, Charnley and associates documented that linear wear (ball migration on x-ray studies) decreased with increasing ball diameter. More important, these investigators noted that volumetric wear more than doubled over the same range (notice the very large volumes; for comparison, a 25-cent coin has a volume approximating 600 mm³). (Data from Charnley J, Kamangar A, Longfield MD [1969]. The optimum size of prosthetic heads in relation to the wear of plastic sockets in total replacement of the hip. *Med Biol Eng* 7:31-39.)

Box 1–5	Ultrahigh-Molecular-Weight Polyethylene Wear Performance

- Linear wear in Charnley's series — 0.01–0.67 mm/year (average, 0.1 mm/year)
- Average volumetric wear — 40 mm³/year
- Peak volumetric wear — 260 mm³/year
- Range of averages in studies — 0.07–0.14 mm/year (Callaghan et al. 1995, Schmalzried et al. 1998)
- Osteolysis problems at 10 years — 6%
- Osteolysis problems at 28 years — 50%
- Desirable range of volumetric wear — 25–55 mm³/year (Clarke 1992)
- Threshold for osteolysis — 80 mm³/year (Zichner and Willert 1992)
- Average Hylamer volumetric wear — 280 mm³/year (Donaldson et al. 2004)

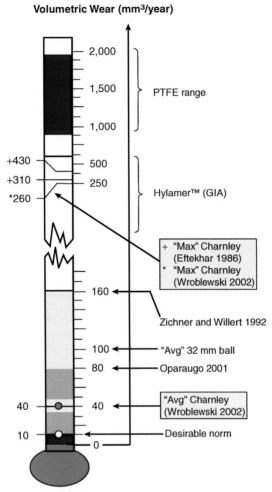

Volumetric Wear (mm³/year)

Figure 1–3: Annual wear rates in total hip replacement *(THR)*. Schematic representation of annual wear rates. Major revisions were experienced with Hyalmer cups (Donaldson et al. 2004) and polytetrafluoroethylene *(PTFE)* cups. Possible wear thresholds for polyethylene cups have been indicated at 80 mm³/year (Oparaugo et al. 2001) and 160 mm³/year (Zichner and Willert 1992). To maintain a low osteolytic threshold, average wear rates less than 10 mm³/year would be desirable. *GIA*, γ-sterilized in air.

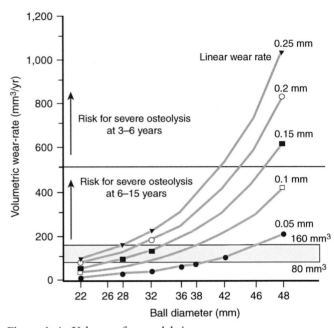

Figure 1–4: Volume of wear debris.
Comparison of linear wear rates (0.05 to 0.25 mm) combined with effect of ball diameter (22 to 48 mm) to create the volume of wear debris. Debris volumes of 160 to 500 mm³/year risked severe osteolysis over a 6- to 15-year period and volumes greater than 500 mm³/year risked catastrophic osteolysis in less than 6 years of follow-up. (Data from Charnley J, Kamangar A, Longfield MD [1969]. The optimum size of prosthetic heads in relation to the wear of plastic sockets in total replacement of the hip. *Med Biol Eng* 7:31-39; and Donaldson T, Williams P, Andrusak L, et al. [2004]. Effect of sterilization on the clinical wear of Hylamer cups. In: *Transactions of the 7th World Biomaterials Congress.* Sydney, Australia, p 815.)

osteolysis risk (corresponding volumetric rate, 160 mm³/year: see Fig. 1–3) (Zichner and Willert 1992). However, wear rates in revised cases were typically double the successful average, that is, 75 mm³/year compared with 35 mm³/year, respectively (Isaac et al. 1992, Sochart 1999).

• Thus a more conservative index for osteolytic threshold would appear to be much less than 80 mm³/year (see Fig. 1–3 and Box 1–5).

• From the foregoing, it is apparent that the 22-mm ball was the safest size to use with PE cups (Fig. 1–4 and Box 1–6). Therefore to minimize future osteolysis risks, the desired average ultrahigh-molecular-weight PE (UHMWPE) wear would be less than 10 mm³/year (see Table 1–1; Table 1–2). This observation has important implications for the success

of contemporary 5XPE and 10XPE liners used with larger ball diameters (Shaju et al. 2005).

Wear Rates of Cross-Linked Polyethylene Cups

• Sterilization of PE cups was traditionally performed by either ethylene oxide gas or GIA. However, γ-irradiation conferred the added benefit of cross-linking (i.e., as the radiation energy created scission of the molecular chains of PE, the chains recombined to form additional cross-links) (Fig. 1–5, type II, 3XPE/air).

Box 1–6	**Ultrahigh-Molecular-Weight Polyethylene Wear Parameters**
• Ball diameter for least risk of wear	22 mm
• Ideal polyethylene wear rate	<10 mm³/year (average in series)
• Maximum acceptable wear rate	50 mm³/year (high-risk cases)

Table 1–2   Comparison of Volumetric Wear Rates Produced With Increasing Linear Wear Rates and Increasing Ball Diameters*

DIAMETER (mm)	LINEAR WEAR RATE (mm/year)				
	0.05	0.1	0.15	0.2	0.25
22.2	19	39	58	**78**	**97**
26	27	53	80	**107**	**134**
28	32	64	**96**	**128**	**160**
32	45	**90**	**135**	**180**	**224**
36	63	**126**	**189**	**251**	**314**
38	75	**151**	**226**	**302**	**377**
42	**106**	**211**	**317**	**422**	**528**
46	**148**	**296**	**443**	**591**	**739**
50	**207**	**414**	**621**	**828**	**1,035**

*High-risk values (>80 mm³/year) are shown in **bold text**.
From Oparaugo PC, Clarke IC, Malchau H, Herberts P (2001). Correlation of wear debris-induced osteolysis and revision with volumetric wear-rates of polyethylene: A survey of 8 reports in the literature. *Acta Orthop Scand* 72:22-28.

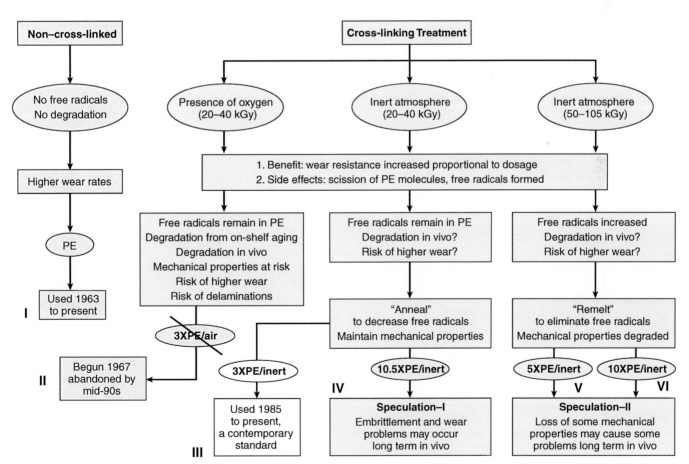

Figure 1–5: Polyethylene *(PE)* cross-linking.
Comparison of polyethylene cross-linking evolution over 40 years with claimed advantages. For the six general types of cross-linking processes (I to VI) that have come to market, only type II has been discontinued (type VI sterilization is by the electron beam method, and the others use γ-irradiation). *XPE,* cross-linked polyethylene.

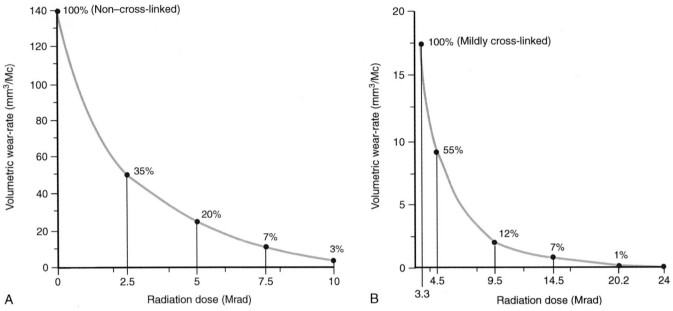

Figure 1–6: Two hip simulator studies showing typical wear trends with increased irradiation for GUR4150 cups run on 32-mm cobalt-chromium balls (percentage values show relative wear decrease from control). **A,** Cups are subjected to annealing after irradiation (0 to 10 Mrad). **B,** Cups are subjected to remelting after irradiation (3 to 24 Mrad). (**A,** Data from Wang A, Essner A, Polineni VK, et al. [1998]. Lubrication and wear of ultra-high molecular weight polyethylene in total joint replacements. *Tribology International* 31(1-3):17-33. **B,** Data from McKellop HA, Shen FW, Campbell P, Ota T [1999]. Effect of molecular weight, calcium stearate, and sterilization methods on the wear of ultra high molecular weight polyethylene acetabular cups in a hip joint simulator. *J Orthop Res* 17:329–339.)

- It was recognized in the early 1970s that this GIA treatment created a beneficial improvement in wear resistance of acetabular cups (Fig. 1–6; Table 1–3) (Oonishi et al. 1996a, 1996b, 2001).
- Three long-term clinical studies of cross-linked PE (XPE) cups, each with unique, highly cross-linked, cemented PE cups, have been conducted. Beginning in 1971, a Japanese series of cups was sterilized by

100 Mrad in air (see Table 1–3), and 28 of the original 71 (39%) cases remained for study beyond 20 years.
- The wear rate established over the first 6 years averaged 0.08 mm/year with 28-mm balls and represented a three- to fourfold reduction compared with a series of T-28 THRs (Oonishi et al. 1996a, Oonishi et al. 1996b, Oonishi et al. 2001).

TYPES	STERILIZATION	CROSS-LINKING	ATMOSPHERE	THERMAL	FREE RADICALS	TRADE NAME
I	Ethylene oxide gas	None	Ethylene oxide gas	None	None	—
II	3 Mrad	Moderate	Air	None	Yes	—
IIIa	3 Mrad	Moderate	Argon	None	Yes	Arcom
IIIa	3 Mrad	Moderate	Nitrogen	None	Yes	Sulzer
IIIb	3 Mrad	Moderate	Nitrogen	Annealed	Some	Duration
IV	10.5 Mrad	High	Nitrogen	Annealed	Some	Crossfire
V	5 Mrad	Moderate	Nitrogen	Melted	None	Marathon
VI	10 Mrad E-beam	High	Nitrogen	Melted	None	Durasul, Longevity
VI	10 Mrad E-beam	High	Nitrogen	Melted	None	XLP
Japan	100 Mrad/air	Very high	Air	None	Yes	Custom
South Africa	13 Mrad /acetylene	High	Acetylene	None	Some	Custom
United Kingdom	Silane	High	NA	NA	NA	Custom

Table 1–3 Summary of Polyethylene Processing (I to VI) Used for Polyethylene Cups in the United States and Alternate Custom Polyethylene Processing Used Clinically in Japan, England, and South Africa

NA, not available in the literature.

Table 1–4	Summary of Radiographic Wear Data on 13XPE/Air Cups Used With 30-mm Balls		
CASE NUMBER	LINEAR WEAR RATE (mm/year)	FOLLOW-UP (years)	VOLUME WEAR (mm³/year)
1: Osteolysis	0.19	16	134
2: Osteolysis	0.14	14	99
3: No osteolysis	0.07	14	49

- In the South African study, the cups were processed with a 10-Mrad dose under acetylene gas to promote cross-linking. These were then sterilized by a further 3-Mrad dose in air. Two revised cases had linear wear rates greater than 0.1 mm/year, and volumetric wear rates were higher than 100 mm³/year (Table 1–4).
- In a unique series of 14 XPE cases from England, cups that were chemically cross-linked with a Silane process showed a 10-year wear average of 0.02 mm/year (Wroblewski et al. 1996). No revisions were reported in this series.
- The competing mechanism to cross-linking was oxidation of the severed PE chains; that is, oxygen molecules could combine with the damaged chains and a detrimental oxidation state was created, leading to PE embrittlement with the potential for higher wear. Such GIA oxidation effects were easily eliminated using γ-irradiation in an inert atmosphere (Streicher 1993). Now all γ-irradiated PE implants are sterilized in inert atmospheres such as argon or nitrogen gas (see Table 1–3; see Fig. 1–5, type III; Box 1–7).

- Sterilization chemically by ethylene oxide or gas plasma processes does not create free radicals and therefore appears immune to oxidation effects (see Fig. 1–5, type I). However, lacking the beneficial cross-linking effects, the ethylene oxide and gas plasma sterilized cups produce higher wear rates (see Fig. 1–6A).
- A secondary concern with radiation increased to 5 Mrad and higher was how to eliminate the additional load of free radicals created without degrading the mechanical properties. One approach was to anneal the XPE after sterilization and thereby maintain mechanical properties but at the expense of retaining some free radicals (see Fig. 1–5, type III).
- Thus the first highly cross-linked (10.5-Mrad) cup on the market used an annealing process to accelerate the cross-linking transformation with partial elimination of free radicals (see Fig. 1–5, type IV).
- A second approach was to remelt the XPE material, which eliminated free radicals but reduced mechanical properties such as resistance to crack propagation, by 40% to 60%. Remelted cups are currently available with a moderate 5-Mrad dose (type V) and a 10-Mrad or slightly higher dose (see Fig. 1–5, type VI).
- Compared with no cross-linking, increased irradiation dosage dramatically reduced the wear rates of XPE cups (see Fig. 1–6A; Box 1–8). Compared with 3XPE cups as contemporary controls, the 10XPE cups showed almost 90% wear reduction in the laboratory (see Fig. 1–6B and Box 1–8).
- Many simulator studies have shown that wear of 10XPE cups decreased to an unmeasurably low value (see Fig. 1–6). However, laboratory predictions must always be interpreted with some caution. Debris recovered from one such study of 10XPE cups revealed that an estimated

Box 1–7	Important Observations of Ultrahigh-Molecular-Weight Polyethylene Wear Performance

- Cross-linking of polyethylene significantly reduces wear rates.
- The γ-irradiation dose is 2.5–4 Mrad (average, 3 Mrad).
- Sterilization by ethylene oxide gas or gas plasma methods does not create cross-linking.
- γ-Sterilized polyethylene has lower wear rates than ethylene oxide or gas plasma sterilization.
- Sterilization in air results in a process whereby free radicals produced could react to create an oxidized polyethylene bearing.
- Oxidation of polyethylene can be detrimental to wear performance.
- Polyethylene bearings are now sterilized in an inert atmosphere and packaged in oxygen-free barrier packs to eliminate risk of oxidation.
- As a precaution, polyethylene implants have a shelf life not to exceed 3 years.

Box 1–8	Beneficial Wear Reductions With Cross-Linked Polyethylenes

- Compared with non–cross-linked cups (ethylene oxide, gas plasma):
  - 2.5XPE cups: 65% wear reduction under ideal laboratory conditions
  - 5.0XPE cups: 80% wear reduction under ideal laboratory conditions
  - 10XLE cups: 97% wear reduction under ideal laboratory conditions
- Annealing causes some reduction of free radicals and some loss of mechanical properties.
- Remelting causes elimination of free radicals and greater loss of mechanical properties.
- The conservative point of view is that new XPE cups have potential to reduce wear rates by factor of 3.
- It is likely that XPE cup wear will increase in vivo as a result of third-body abrasive wear and other effects.

XPE, cross-linked polyethylene.

Table 1–5	Summary Data From Simulator Study Comparing Wear (mm³/Million Cycles) of Non-XPE With 10XPE Cups (GUR1050 Remelted; 32 mm) With Smooth and Roughened Balls					
COBALT-CHROMIUM BALL	PE WEAR	10XPE WEAR	RATIO	PE DEBRIS* (N × 10⁶)	10XPE DEBRIS (N × 10⁶)	DEBRIS RATIO PE/XPE
Smooth	38	0	NA	8	2.2	3.6
Rough	76	15.4	20%	10.5	8.9	1.2
Ratio rough/smooth	2.0	NA	—	1.3	4.0	—

NA, not available in the literature; PE, polyethylene; XPE, cross-linked polyethylene.
*Wear debris frequency = (N × 10⁶) measured per step the patient takes.
From Scott M, Morrison M, Mishra SR, Jani S (2005). Particle analysis for the determination of UHMWPE wear. *J Biomed Mater Res B Appl Biomater* 73:325–337.

2.2 million particles had been produced during each step in the walking cycle (Table 1–5, smooth CoCr balls).

- It is also true that simulator studies with roughened CoCr balls showed that such cups were quite sensitive to abrasive wear conditions; under some conditions, they had higher wear than controls (Table 1–6).
- Taking a conservative point of view, it would be wise to assume there could be a threefold reduction with 5XPE to 10XPE cups in patients, but it will never be zero.
- Short-term clinical studies of contemporary cup designs appeared to show much reduced radiographic wear with 5XPE and 10XPE cups (Digas et al. 2003, Heisel et al. 2004, Krushell et al. 2005, Manning et al. 2005, Martell et al. 2003). In this regard, it is worth remembering (see Box 1–7) that the original Charnley THR with its use of 3XPE/air cups (now superseded) only produced 10% to 30% osteolysis with follow-ups extended over 15 to 20 years (Oparaugo et al. 2001, Sochart 1999, Wroblewski et al. 1999).
- A study of 12 retrieved Crossfire liners (Stryker Orthopaedics, Mahwah, NJ) extending over 4 years of use showed no evidence of severe oxidation, white subsurface banding, or other abnormalities. One retrieval report showed evidence of some surface cracking in XPE cups (Bradford et al. 2004).

- Clearly, it will take studies with 10- to 15-year results before there is any clear statement of clinical improvement with the XPEs that are highly cross-linked (Box 1–9).

Submicron Cross-Linked Polyethylene Debris

- The foreign body reaction depends on many factors (Box 1–10).
- Although the PE particles retrieved from tissues have varied greatly in size and morphology, most appeared to be submicron, globular PE debris with their peak frequency (mode) occurring at less than 0.5 μm (Fig. 1–7).
- More than 50,000 ellipsoidal XPE 0.19-μm particles could be contained within one red blood cell (Box 1–11).
- The extent of the PE wear process can be visualized by calculating the number of wear particles likely to be released with each step the patient makes. With improved data regarding debris morphology (Fig. 1–8), our predictions have increased from 40,000 particles released every step to an astoundingly large number of 12,000,000 particles per step (see Box 1–11).
- In cell culture studies, induction of bone-resorbing activity has been shown to depend on particle size and concentration.

Box 1–9	Clinical History of Cross-Linked Polyethylene Cups
• Cup types I to III	>20 years follow-up
• Cup types IV to VI	<8 years follow-up

Box 1–10	Debris Effects and Osteolysis
• Rate of deposition	
• Rate of transport from the joint	
• Particle type and toxicity	
• Size (shape) distribution	
• Concentration at various tissue sites	
• Interaction of macrophage cells with micron-size particles	
• Interaction of foreign body giant cells with particles >10 μm	

Table 1–6	For GUR1020 Cups, Simulator Wear (mm³/Million Cycles) Varied With Sterilization Either by Ethylene Oxide or 4-Mrad Radiation Dose (Vacuum Foil–Packed Bags) and Whether Run With Smooth Cobalt-Chromium Balls or Balls Roughened by Three Scratches 4-μm Deep		
COBALT-CHROMIUM BALL	ETHYLENE OXIDE	4XPE	RATIO XPE/PE
Smooth	49	35	0.7
Scratched	98	115	1.2
Ratio	2.0	3.3	

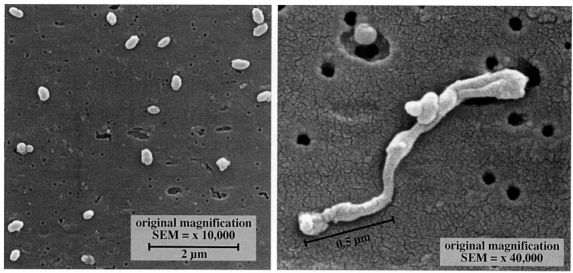

Figure 1–7: Wear debris.
Comparison of globular and fibrillar cross-linked polyethylene wear debris against the background of filter pores (hip simulator studies). *SEM*, scanning electron micrography. (Courtesy of P. Williams, Peterson Tribology Laboratory, Loma Linda University, Loma Linda, CA.)

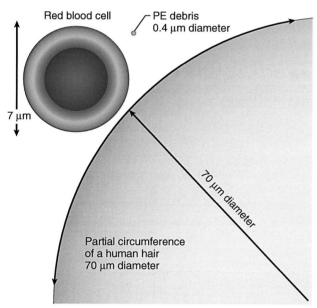

Figure 1–8: Wear particle.
Comparison of cross-linked polyethylene *(PE)* wear particle (0.4 μm) to diameter of a red blood cell (7 μm) and a human hair (70 μm). How many XPE particles would it take to match the volume of one red blood cell with approximate volume 60 μm³? For median diameters of 0.08, 0.11, and 0.19 μm for ellipsoidal particles of PE, 5XPE, and 10XPE, it would require 670,000, 260,000, and 50,000, respectively. (Data from Scott M, Morrison M, Mishra SR, Jani S [2005]. Particle analysis for the determination of UHMWPE wear. *J Biomed Mater Res B Appl Biomater* 73:325-337.)

The critical size creating higher biologic activity appeared to be smaller than 0.5 μm (Box 1–12).

- Thus it is important to consider how many XPE particles are produced in the critical range and their volume when considering osteolytic potential.
- Recent characterization by scanning electron micrography (SEM) and atomic force microscopy provided an ellipsoidal model of the XPE wear particle whose thickness approximated one third of its diameter (Scott et al. 2005).
- For the critical size range (Fig. 1–9 and Box 1–13: <0.2 μm), the 5XPE had the highest volume of particles (40%) followed by the 10XPE (22%).
- Thus overall the 5XPE cups created the highest number of particles (N = 12 million/step) and in the critical size had the highest volume of debris.
- The critical effect of particulate size and volume variations can be illustrated using the debris distributions from published debris models (Ingham et al. 2002; Galvin 2005) (pin-on-flat wear studies; Tables 1–7 and 1–8). In the first example, termed the *PE model*, 90% of the particles were smaller than 0.5 μm diameter with a very small secondary peak at 1.3 μm (Fig. 1–10*A*).
- For an assumed PE wear rate of 50 mm³/year (see Fig. 1–3), the total number of particles generated for

Box 1–11	Debris Estimates Improving With Time
• 1989: Estimate 1	40,000 particles/step (Clarke and Campbell 1989)
• 1996: Estimate 2	0.5–1.1 million particles/step (Fisher et al. 2000, McKellop et al. 1995)
• 2003: Estimate 3	2–12 million particles/step (Good et al. 2003, Scott et al. 2005)

Box 1–12	Ultrahigh-Molecular-Weight Polyethylene Debris Affects Bone Resorption (Cell Cultures)
• Small UHMWPE particles (0.24 μm)	Reacts at debris volume 10 μm³/cell
• Midsize UHMWPE particles (0.45–1.7 μm)	Reacts at debris volume 100 μm³/cell
• Large particles	No effect

UHMWPE, ultrahigh-molecular-weight polyethylene.
Data from Green TR, Fisher J, Matthews JB, et al. (2000). Effect of size and dose on bone resorption activity of macrophages by in vitro clinically relevant ultra high molecular weight polyethylene particles. *J Biomed Mater Res* 53:490-497.

Table 1–7 Pin-on-Flat Wear Studies of Non–Cross-Linked Polyethylene (GUR1120) Showed Particle Distributions by Size and by Volume*

DEBRIS SIZE RANGES	SIZE (N%) DISTRIBUTION	VOLUME (V%) DISTRIBUTION
<0.5 μm	88	60
0.5–1 μm	8	16
>1 μm	4	24

*Polyethylene debris larger than 1 μm accounted for less than 4% of the particles but represented 24% of total debris volume.
From Ingram J, Matthews JB, Tipper J, et al. (2002). Comparison of the biological activity of grade GUR 1120 and GUR 415 HP UHMWPE wear debris. *Biomed Mater Eng* 12:177–188.

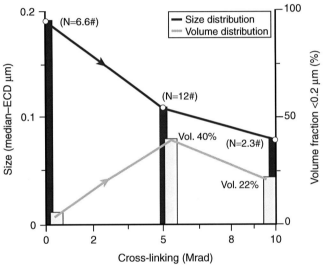

Figure 1–9: Effect of cross-linking on debris size. Median size (ECD μm) of debris decreased with increased cross-linking (32-mm cobalt-chromium balls, GUR1050/remelted, 0XPE, 5XPE, and 10XPE cups). In contrast, volume fraction of particles first increased and then decreased somewhat. The volume fraction of particles smaller than 0.2 μm is indicated by volume percentage values, and the number of particles released per step (N) is indicated in millions. (Data from Scott M, Morrison M, Mishra SR, Jani S [2005]. Particle analysis for the determination of UHMWPE wear. *J Biomed Mater Res B Appl Biomater* 73:325-337.)

each patient step would be 15 million in our model. The corresponding volumetric distribution showed the major peak at 0.5 μm, whereas the second peak at 1.3 μm was now more pronounced due to the geometric effects of the larger-diameter particles (Fig. 1–10*B*). It was noted that fewer than 1% of the particles were smaller than 0.5 μm, and they represented 58% of the total wear volume.

• In the second example, termed the *5XPE model*, 99% of the particles were less than 0.5 μm in diameter, with a very small secondary peak at 0.13 μm (Fig. 1–11*A*). For an assumed 5XPE wear rate of 10 mm³/year (Fig. 1–11*B*), the total number of particles generated for each patient step was 87 million. The particles smaller than 0.5 μm now represented 88% of the total wear volume.

New Polyethylenes

• Production of new PEs designed to improve wear and oxidation resistance while maintaining good mechanical properties includes sequential irradiation and annealing of PE (X3: Stryker, Mahwah, NJ), mechanically enhanced processing (MEP), and vitamin E–doped cups (Biomet, Warsaw, IN).
• The X3 process involves irradiation to 3 Mrad followed by annealing, and this process is repeated three times for a cumulative dose of 9 Mrad.

Table 1–8 Pin-on-Flat Wear Studies of Polyethylene (0-, 5- and 10-Mrad, XPE Remelted) Showed Particle Distributions by Cross-Linking

SIZE RANGE BY DIAMETER	5-MRAD (N%)	10-M RAD (N%)	5-MRAD (VOL%)	10-MRAD (VOL%)
<0.1 μm	61	62	9	12
0.1–1 μm	38	37	80	83
>1 μm	1	1	11	5

From Galvin AL, Tipper JL, Ingham E, et al. (2005). Nanometre size wear debris generated from crosslinked and non-crosslinked ultra high molecular weight polyethylene in artificial joints. *Wear* 259:977-983.

Box 1–13	Median Particle Size (see Fig. 1–9)
• PE	0.19 μm
• 5XPE	0.11 μm
• 10XPE	0.08 μm

PE, polyethylene; XPE, cross-linked polyethylene.

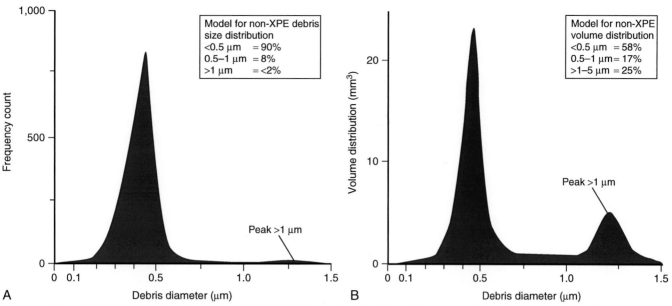

Figure 1–10: Model for polyethylene debris built from data in pin-on-flat wear studies of non–cross-linked GUR1120.

A, Size distribution (assumed continuous 0 to 5 μm) showing a major peak between 0.4 and 0.5 μm and a secondary but insignificant peak at 1.3 μm. **B,** Volume distribution showing the same major peak between 0.4 and 0.5 μm, but now the secondary peak shows a significant geometric size effect (i.e. particles >1 μm account for 25% of total volume). *XPE,* cross-linked polyethylene. (From Ingram J, Matthews JB, Tipper J, et al. [2002]. Comparison of the biological activity of grade GUR 1120 and GUR 415 HP UHMWPE wear debris. *Biomed Mater Eng* 12:177–188.)

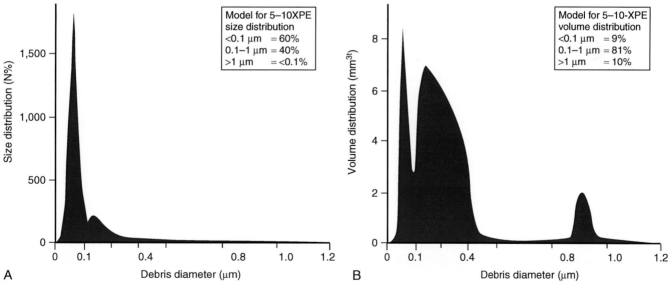

Figure 1–11: Model for cross-linked polyethylene *(XPE)* debris based on data from pin-on-flat wear studies of cross-linked GUR1120.

A, Size distribution (assumed continuous from 0 to 5 μm) showing a major peak at less than 0.1 μm and a significant secondary peak at less than 0.2 μm diameter. **B,** Volume distribution showing same major peaks at less than 0.1 μm and at less than 0.2 μm and also showing a significant geometric size effect at less than 1 μm (particles 0.1 to 1 μm diameter account for 81% of volume). (Data from Galvin AL, Tipper JL, Ingham E, et al. [2005]. Nanometre size wear debris generated from crosslinked and non-crosslinked ultra high molecular weight polyethylene in artificial joints. *Wear* 259:977-983.)

- The cups with mechanically enhanced processing are γ-irradiated at 5 Mrad to induce cross-linking and are then preheated to 130°C and solid-state deformed to remove free radicals. This is followed by annealing and then sterilization by gas plasma. Simulator studies show excellent wear reduction and little difference in debris morphology compared with controls (Bowsher et al. 2006, Schmalzried et al. 1996a).

Newer Ceramic Femoral Heads

- Newer materials have or are becoming available for femoral heads (Box 1–14). The monoblock Zirconia ball introduced into the United States in 1989 (Prozyr; Norton Desmarquest, France) was taken off the market by 2000 because of inconsistencies in manufacture and the resulting instability that the material demonstrated in vivo.
- The Zirconia-surface ball made of zirconium metal (Oxinium, Smith and Nephew, Memphis, IN) represents a different ceramic option and is in use today.
- The only new ceramic approved by the US Food and Drug Administration (FDA) for CPE options is a stronger ceramic composite made of alumina and 24% Zirconia (Biolox delta; CeramTec Inc., Germany).

Consensus Building on Polyethylene and Cross-Linked Polyethylene Cups

- Cross-linked cups provide much improved wear resistance compared with sterilization by ethylene oxide or gas plasma methods (non–cross-linking processes).
- The larger the femoral ball, the more PE debris will be produced.
- Historical results with 22-mm balls and 3XPE/air cups showed 95% survivorship at 10 years but only 50% at 30 years owing to osteolytic effects.
- The patients most at risk for PE wear and osteolysis have five to seven times higher wear rates than the average wear rates given in clinical series.
- It is estimated that 1 to 8 million 3XPE/air particles are released with every step the patient takes.
- Oxidation of XPE bearing surfaces was implicated in some severe wear problems.
- Cup sterilization methods are now performed in oxygen-free atmosphere to reduce the risk of

---

Box 1–14	Alternative Materials for Femoral Heads

- Zirconia (Y-TZP: tetragonal)
- Ceramic-surfaced metal balls (Oxinium; FDA approved for CPE)
- Alumina-Zirconia composite (FDA approved for CPE)
- Silicone nitride (under development)
- Ceramic-surfaced metal ball (under development)
- Diamond-surfaced metal ball (under development)
- Diamond-impregnated metal matrix (under development)

CPE, ceramic-polyethylene combinations; FDA, Food and Drug Administration.

---

oxidation, and cups are given maximum shelf life of 3 years.
- Some portion of debris load may come from backside wear of XPE liners in modular cups.
- Screw holes for cup fixation may promote the distribution of XPE wear debris in modular cups.
- Additional cross-linking (>3 Mrad) markedly improved wear resistance of XPE cups in all laboratory studies.
- The population of free radicals in XPE cups may be partially reduced by annealing techniques or eliminated by remelting techniques. Such processes result in some degradation of mechanical properties.
- Additional cross-linking (5XPE, 10XPE) increases the proportion of debris in the more biologically active size distribution.
- Although laboratory wear studies predicted near zero wear rates for 5XPE and 10XPE cups, the wear seen in vivo will likely average three- to fourfold reduction compared with controls.
- Laboratory studies predicted that 2 to 12 million particles (5XPE, 10XPE) could be released for each step the patient takes.
- The 5XPE and 10XPE cups are more sensitive to effects of roughened CoCr balls than historical controls.
- Three clinical series with long-term experience of unique cemented XPE cups (13XPE-100XPE) claimed superior results, but such cups are not available in the United States.
- Contemporary clinical results in the United States, with 3 to 8 years experience of 5XPE and 10XPE cups, show very low wear.
- Efficacy of the new XPE cups will only be determined with more than 10 years of follow-up.
- The use of large-diameter femoral balls with 5XPE and 10XPE cups has become acceptable. However, only detailed clinical studies will show whether the original Charnley small ball paradigm has been successfully reversed.
- New XPE cups are on the market with sterilization steps that provide enhanced cross-linking effects (5 to 9 Mrad). Claimed benefits are maintained mechanical properties as well as very high resistance to oxidation effects in the body.

40 Years of Experience With Cobalt-Chromium Cups
Introduction to All-Metal Bearings

- MOM systems, going back to the 1940s, represent the grandfather designs of THR (Box 1–15). The high-strength, CoCr alloy demonstrated very low wear rates and facilitated the design of thin acetabular cups, thus permitting larger ball sizes. However, from those pioneering studies we also learned that approximately 40% of cases had to be revised.
- The notable feature of pioneering designs was that they developed femoral heads in 32- to 41.5-mm diameters.

Box 1–15	Development of First-Generation Metal-on-Metal Devices
• 1938	First MOM THR (English surgeon Philip Wiles)
• 1955–1965	MOM 32-mm CoCr (McKee-Farrar, Mueller-Huggler, Ring and Stanmore) (Amstutz and Clarke 1991, Schmalzried et al. 1998)
• 1960	MOM 41.5-mm CoCr ball
• 1966	MOM 35-mm CoCr ball
• 1970	MPE 22-mm Charnley THR accepted worldwide

CoCr, cobalt chromium; MOM, metal-on-metal; MPE, metal-polyethylene combination; THR, total hip replacement.

Box 1–16	Development of Second-Generation Metal-on-Metal Devices
• 1988	Launch of 28- and 32-mm Metasul MOM in Europe
• 1999	FDA approval of 28-mm Metasul MOM
• 2004	FDA approval of 32-mm Metasul MOM
• 2001–2003	FDA approval of 32- to 60-mm MOM (Wright Medical Technology; Biomet Inc.)

FDA, Food and Drug Administration; MOM, metal-on-metal.

- In contrast, the PE cups required, as Charnley's experience showed, a small ball diameter to minimize PE debris (see Figs. 1–1 and 1–3).
- The second-generation, MOM system (Metasul, Sulzer Inc./Zimmer Inc.) departed from historical concepts (Table 1–9) in that it came with small ball diameters (Box 1–16). The CoCr liner was also unconventional; it was a sandwich design with a PE sleeve (see Box 1–13). In addition, these devices were combined with hemispherical CoCr shells incorporating well established, bone-ingrowth features.

Risks of Metal-on-Metal Bearings

- With MOM bearings, given the potential toxicities of Co and Cr ions, the concern has always been the release and distribution of wear products (Jacobs et al. 2003). MOM wear rates are too low to monitor by radiographic means.
- This makes assessment of metal ions in patients' blood, serum, and urine the surrogate wear method. Some metal ions may stay bound to local tissues, and some may bind to protein moieties that are transported to distant organs.
- Thus the question about safety of MOM systems has generally not been about osteolysis but rather about systemic biologic effects. As summarized by Jacobs and colleagues, association of metal ion release with any metabolic, bacteriologic, immunologic, or carcinogenic event currently remains conjectural (Butterfield et al. 2002, Jacobs et al. 2004). Therefore those issues are not belabored here.

Clinical Wear Rates of Metal-on-Metal Bearings

- Worn CoCr surfaces show many features, the most notable of which are arrays of carbides 5 to 20 μm, light polishing scratches, deeper gouges made by third-body particulates, and micropitting (Fig. 1–12; Box 1–17). In discussions of such worn MOM surfaces, the concept of *self-healing* is frequently advanced (Coleman et al. 1973, Wimmer et al. 2001). This term suggests that the CoCr alloy has the ability to render the surface smooth again quickly (Fig. 1–13, see also Box 1–17).
- MOM run-in wear (ball and cup) in the first year typically was less than 50 μm and in subsequent years decreased to less than 10 μm in the steady-state phase (Coleman et al. 1973; Rieker et al. 1998). Comparison of MOM retrieval studies showed good agreement in that wear typically averaged a low 3 to 5 mm^3/year over a 25-year period (Fig. 1–14) (Chang et al. 2005; Milosev 2006; Wagner and Wagner 2000).
- Overall, the tissue reaction to metal particles did not dominate the histologic appearance as was frequently the

Table 1–9	Manufacturing Parameters Known to Influence the Wear Rate and Corrosion of Metal-on-Metal Bearings		
MOM BEARING PARAMETERS	**MOM DETAILS**	**CONTROVERSY**	
Diameter effect	38–60 mm	Yes	
MOM carbon content	High or low	Yes	
Alloy type	Cast or wrought	Yes	
Alloy heat treatments	Solution anneal, chipping	Yes	
Variability in processing unique to MOM bearings	Possible	Yes	
Sphericity of bearings	<10 μm	No	
Surface finish	<30 nm	No	
Diametral mismatch of ball to cup	50–300 μm	Yes	
Dimensional stability of acetabular cup	Variable	Yes	

MOM, metal-on-metal.

Box 1–17	Self-Healing in Metal-on-Metal Devices (see Figs. 1–12 and 1–13)

- Edges of a scratch may undergo plastic flow that camouflages the defect without producing particulates (see Fig. 1–13*B*) (Scott and Lemons 1998).
- Protruding edges of a scratch may be abraded, thereby producing wear debris (see Fig. 1–13*C*).
- Surface scratches may be worn down by normal metal-on-metal wear rates of 5 μm/year.

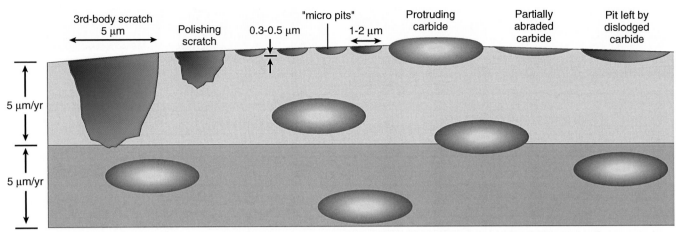

Figure 1–12: Scale model of features found on worn cobalt-chromium surfaces.
Existing polishing scratches and third-body abraded scratches up to 5 μm deep will be polished away by wear
(average erosion = 5 μm/year; Metasul). Micropits are frequently seen on retrievals, as well as arrays of
protruding hard carbides, some of which wear down and leave areas with shallow pits. (Data from Ishida [2006]
ORS; Park [1999]; Rieker CB, Kottig P, Schon R, et al. [1998]. Clinical wear performance of metal-on-metal
hip arthroplasties. In: Jacobs J, Craig TL, eds. *Alternative Bearing Surfaces in Total Joint Replacement*. Special
Technical Publication 1346. Fredericksburg, VA: American Society for Testing and Materials, pp 144-156.)

case with PE debris (Clarke et al. 2005). Microscopically, the MOM debris was usually to be found in mononuclear phagocytes close to the vicinity of blood vessels transitioning between the inner synovial lining and the outer joint capsule (Chang et al. 2005; Milosev 2006).
- Because the CoCr particulate generally has a median size smaller than 50 nm (Fig. 1–15), the resulting surface area of metal exposed to body fluids is quite large (Walker and Erkman 1972).

Peripheral and Polar Wear Scars on Metal-on-Metal Bearings

- Retrieval studies of MOM bearings showed a polar wear scar, offset somewhat from the ball's dome (Fig. 1–16).

- Sometimes a more peripheral wear scar was also identified (Chang et al. 2005, Walker and Gold 1971, Williams et al. 2004), typically referred to as *stripe wear* in ceramic retrievals (Coleman et al. 1973, McKellop et al. 1996, Rieker et al. 1998, Wagner and Wagner 2000). Our retrieved Metasul THRs have also demonstrated stripe wear (Fig. 1–17).
- Simulator studies using microseparation test modes also produced stripe wear. It is therefore interesting that a retrieval study of 22 McKee THRs noted that those with the more "peripheral" wear had an average life span of only 9 years compared with those with polar wear that averaged longer at 13 years (Schmalzried et al. 1996b). Were these higher rates of revision in response to higher stripe wear, or were there concomitant

Table 1–10	Simulator Wear Studies of 28- to 56-mm, High-Carbon Metal-on Metal Bearings With Varied Radial Clearance (Ranked by Ball Diameter)					
STUDY	HEAD DIAMETER (mm)	MEAN RADIAL CLEARANCE (μm)	INITIAL RADIAL CLEARANCE (μm)	VOLUMETRIC WEAR RATE (mm³/million cycles) RUNNING IN	STEADY STATE	RATIO RUNNING IN/STEADY STATE
Bowsher et al. 2004	28	42	~10	4.20	0.92	4.6
Liao et al. 2004	36	70	10	0.25	0.08	3.1
Goldsmith et al. 2000	36	71	6–35	1.20	0.36	3.3
Collins et al. 2004	54	NA	NA	1.91	0.43	4.4
Bowsher et al. 2006	40	119	15	2.20	0.4	5.4
Chan et al. 1996	45	10–300	25–51	5.00	0.6	8.3
Bowsher et al. 2004	56	142	15	7.10	0.32	22.2

NA, not available.

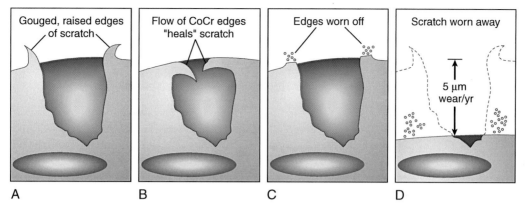

Figure 1–13: Scratching and self-healing wear features on cobalt-chromium (CoCr) surfaces. **A,** Wear by third-body particle scratched the surface, released debris, and created a 5-μm deep gouge with sharp raised edges, thereby roughening the surface. **B,** Flow of thin lips of gouge could obscure the scratch but not create more debris. **C,** Abrasive wear polishes the raised lips and releases CoCr debris. **D,** Linear wear of 5 μm/year eliminated gouge with release of more wear debris.

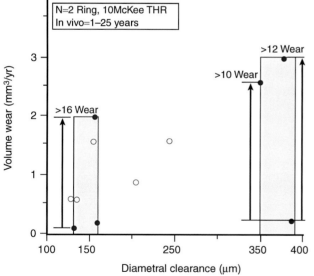

Figure 1–14: Volumetric wear from metal-on-metal retrievals. Volumetric wear from metal-on-metal retrievals shown by minimum, average, and maximum values. Wear rates given for femoral balls were simply doubled to approximate wear rates for total hip replacements *(THR)*. (Data from McKellop H, Park SH, Chiesa R, et al. [1996]. In vivo wear of three types of metal on metal hip prostheses during two decades of use. *Clin Orthop Relat Res* 329[Suppl]:S128-S140; and Rieker CB, Kottig P, Schon R, et al. [1998]. Clinical wear performance of metal-on-metal hip arthroplasties. In: Jacobs J, Craig TL, eds. *Alternative Bearing Surfaces in Total Joint Replacement.* Special Technical Publication 1346. Fredericksburg, VA: American Society for Testing and Materials.)

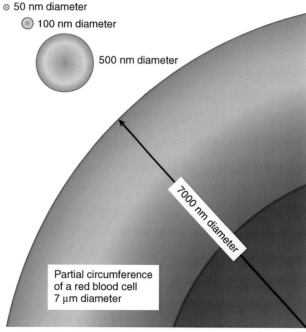

Figure 1–15: Cobalt-chromium (CoCr) particles. Comparison of CoCr particles (0.05, 0.1, and 0.05 μm diameter) to a peripheral segment of a red blood cell. CoCr particles retrieved from metal-on-metal cases had a median size of 95 nm (range, 20 to 960 nm). With an average diameter of 50 nm, approximately 1 million CoCr particles would be required to fill such a cell. (Data from Doorn PF, Campbell PA, Worrall J, et al. [1998]. Metal wear particle characterization from metal-on-metal total hip replacements: Transmission electron microscopy study of periprosthetic tissues and isolated particles. *J Biomed Mater Res* 42:103-111.)

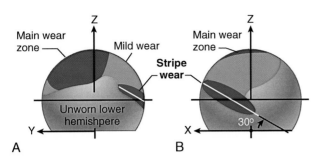

A **B**

Figure 1–16: Wear maps.
A and **B,** Two views of wear maps for a 28-mm Metasul ball retrieved at 9 years (Ishida 2006). Light microscopy and scanning electron microscopy showed the main wear zone (purple), and a large area of mild wear (stippled region) and inclined stripe wear (black/white line), quite similar to ceramic retrievals (Data from Shishido T, Clarke IC, Williams P, et al. [2003]. Clinical and simulator wear study of alumina ceramic THR to 17 years and beyond. *J Biomed Mater Res* 67:638–647.)

impingement problems resulting from suboptimal implant positioning?

Laboratory Wear Rates With Metal-on-Metal Bearings

- MOM cups are rigid, and therefore the area of contact is dictated by the manufacturer's specifications. The diameter of the femoral head has to be somewhat smaller than the acetabular liner (i.e., an intentional mismatch).
- A very small mismatch (radial or diametral clearance) may result in stress concentrations around the cup rim, lubricant starvation, and high frictional torques (Heisel et al. 2004, Manning et al. 2005, Wroblewski et al. 2002).
- Conversely, a high mismatch may result in stress concentrations in the dome with higher wear. Thus the effects of ball diameter, asphericity, and diametral

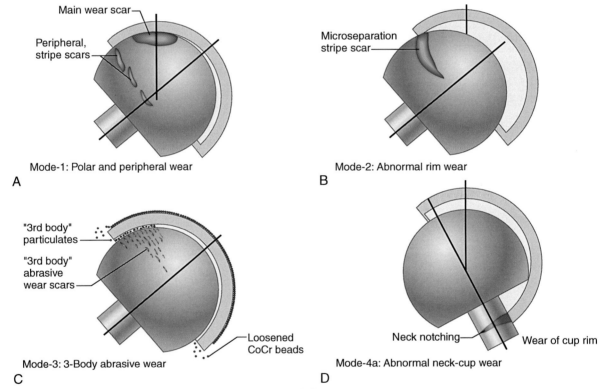

A **B**

C **D**

Figure 1–17: Modes of wear relevant to metal-on-metal designs.
A, Mode-1 wear (McKellop et al. 1995) is defined as habitual wear between bearing surfaces of ball and cup. The cobalt-chromium (CoCr) cup also has the potential in this mode to create a mild stripe scar on the opposing ball surface because of the stress enhancement effect of its rigid rim. **B,** Mode-2 wear occurs when a bearing surface is damaged by a nonbearing part of the implant, such as may occur with impingement of cup rim on femoral ball during microseparation. Stripe may be more severe than in mode 1 because of the additional impact of cup rim and relocation during heel strike. **C,** Mode-3 wear occurs with any third-body, abrasive particle. Examples would include carbides ejected from the CoCr surfaces and any metal fragments released from porous-coated surfaces. **D,** Mode-4 wear occurs when two nonbearing surfaces collide, and here we further classified it as mode-4a wear for metal-on-metal (Clarke et al. 2005). For mode-4b, we refer to backside wear that may be unique to the polyethylene liner in modular THR cups. Backside wear is not an issue for contemporary nonmodular CoCr cups.

mismatch are subject to much interpretation (Box 1–18) (Chang et al. 2005).

- Laboratory studies of MOM wear trends generally showed two discrete wear regimens, namely *run-in and steady-state phases* (Fig. 1–18). Run-in wear is generally accomplished within the first 1 million cycles (1 Mc) as the bearings coadapt. In the laboratory, the serum lubricant may turn gray because of rapidly accumulating metal particulates (Fisher et al. 2000, McKellop et al. 1995). It is apparent that this bedding-in process will become greater as the initial radial mismatch is increased (Manning et al. 2005). It is also apparent that bearings with higher roughness and higher out-of-round features will produce greater volumes of debris during run-in wear (Good et al. 2003, Yamamoto et al. 2001).

- Under the ideal laboratory conditions, the MOM volumetric wear rates (Fig. 1–19) were an order of magnitude less than MPE (see Fig. 1–3). For MOM wear rates of approximately 3 mm³/Mc, calculations showed that particles of mode size 30 nm would be released at

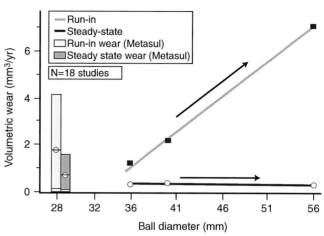

Figure 1–19: Wear phases.
Simulator metal-on-metal wear predictions for run-in and steady-state phase with range of diameters. (Data from Clarke IC, Donaldson T, Bowsher JG, et al. [2005]. Current concepts of metal-on-metal hip resurfacing. *Orthop Clin North Am* 36:143-162, viii.)

rate of 110 million each walking cycle (Fisher et al. 2000).

- Overall, there would appear to be reasonable agreement between laboratory and clinical wear studies. Both have predicted that the highest wear rates occur during the run-in phase (<8 mm³/year) over perhaps 1 to 2 years and then decrease substantially (<1 mm³/year). Thus the volume of MOM debris varies from 10 to 100 times less than with 3XPE/air cups.

40 Years of Cobalt and Chromium Ions

- Co and Cr ion levels provide a surrogate method of MOM wear detection (Jacobs et al. 2003). Only recently have testing protocols become stringent enough to allow discrimination at parts per billion (ppb) (Jacobs et al. 2004). These data will also be of assistance in identifying patient variables relevant to simulator wear models (see Table 1–5).

- However, metal ions can have many sources. Stem burnishing and neck-cup impingement are common examples (Amstutz and Clarke 1991, Walker and Erkman 1972). As another example, studies of MPE bearing systems found three- to sevenfold elevated levels of urine Cr resulting from fretting corrosion at some taper junctions used with modular femoral heads (Fig. 1–20).

Consensus Building on Cobalt-Chromium Cups

- MOM linear wear in retrieval studies is very low, with THR run-in and steady-state wear rates less than 50 and less than 10 µm/year, respectively.

- There appears to be minimal risk of debris-mediated osteolysis with well-functioning MOM bearings.

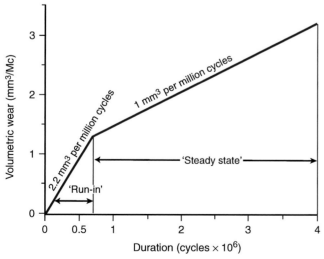

Figure 1–18: Wear phases.
Metal-on-metal simulator study showing the steady-state wear phase reduced 2.2-fold from the run-in phase (28-mm Metasul total hip replacement). (Data from Anissian HL, Stark A, Good V, et al. [2001]. The wear pattern in metal-on-metal hip prostheses. *J Biomed Mater Res* 58:673-678.)

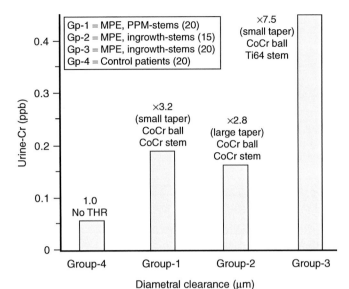

Figure 1–20: Elevated urine chromium (Cr) release. Elevations of urine Cr (three- to sevenfold) release resulting from modular cobalt-Cr *(CoCr)* balls undergoing fretting corrosion on femoral tapers in patients with metal-polyethylene (MPE) bearings (CoCr; Ti6Al4V). *PPM*, parts per million. (Data from Jacobs JJ, Skipor AK, Patterson LM, et al. [1998]. Metal release in patients who have had a primary total hip arthroplasty. A prospective, controlled, longitudinal study. *J Bone Joint Surg Am* 80:1447-1458.)

- Several studies reported that high-wear MOM retrieval cases were greater than 20 mm³/year, thus comparable to wear range of 3XPE/air cups. Such MOM bearings were reputed to have had poor geometric tolerances or may have had mechanical problems of impingement and dislocation. In the laboratory, the MOM bearings showed an initial high-wear during run-in phase that normally decreased two- to threefold around 1 Mc for the steady-state wear phase (see Fig. 1–18).
- Volumetric wear in MOM laboratory studies was very low, with THR run-in and steady-state wear rates less than 8 and less than 1 mm³/Mc, respectively.
- There appeared to be good agreement between laboratory and clinical wear predictions that MOM wear was an order of magnitude less than historical wear rates for 3XPE cups.
- For each walking step, it is estimated that 100 to 200 million CoCr particulates will be released.
- CoCr debris varies over a wide size range, but the typical particle has a diameter smaller than 50 nm. One million such particles approximate the volume of a red blood cell.
- The tissue reaction to MOM debris generally does not dominate the histologic appearance, as seen with the response to PE debris.
- The main concern with MOM debris is the toxic nature of Co and Cr species and their systemic distribution with the risk of adverse biologic reactivity.

- Blood, serum, and urine concentrations of Co and Cr ions can be elevated some four- to sixfold on average with use of MOM bearings.
- On an individual patient basis, some ion levels were elevated 50- to 90-fold during the course of 6 years of study.
- The wide variation in metal ion levels among patients is not well understood.
- Reports showed the higher ion levels at the end of some published studies, thus showing no indication of a reduced steady-state wear response.
- This finding has raised conjecture that the dominance of the debris from the steady-state wear phase may still be contributing ions in the long term.
- The association of metal ion release with any metabolic, bacteriologic, immunologic, or carcinogenic event is currently considered only conjectural.
- The increased prevalence of metal sensitivity in patients with loose MOM implants prompted speculation that immunologic processes may be a factor.
- The low MOM wear rates give the surgeon considerable flexibility in choosing larger ball diameters for greater range of motion and improved stability.
- The CoCr bearing provides the thinnest acetabular cup design and aids the surgeon in the selection of ball diameter.

35 Years of Experience With Alumina Cups

Introduction to Ceramic-on-Ceramic Bearings

- Ceramic THR evolved with the pioneering studies of Boutin in France (Boutin 1972) and Griss and Mittelmeier in Germany (Griss 1984, Mittelmeier and Harms 1979). Over a short period of introduction in the United States, the original design of Mittelmeier's THR showed unacceptably high revisions (Box 1–19). Nevertheless, this unique ceramic experience paved the way for the FDA's 1989 downward classification for 28- and 32-mm CPE combinations.
- Sedel's group (Hospital Saint Louis, Paris) provided a series of clinical studies over a 30-year period (Bizot et al. 2000, Hamadouche et al. 2002, Prudhommeaux et al. 2000,

Box 1–19	Evolution of Ceramic Hip Replacements
• 1970	Introduction of alumina-on-alumina THR
• 1973	Introduction of modular ceramic balls
• 1977	Clinical series of ceramic THR begins in Paris
• 1981–1985	US clinical experience with Mittelmeier's THR
• 1989	FDA marketing approval for 28/32-mm MPE (alumina, zirconia balls)

FDA, Food and Drug Administration; THR, total hip replacement.

Sedel et al. 1994, Sedel 2000). However, the original one-piece alumina cup (Fig. 1–21*A*) never achieved the desired results (Box 1–20). Nevertheless, because of ultralow wear rates experienced with COC, osteolytic complications were exceedingly rare (Bizot et al. 2000). This encouraging French experience set the stage for future development of modular ceramic cups.

- In 1997, orthopaedic companies began the first FDA-monitored, multicenter clinical studies of alumina-on-alumina THR in the United States (Box 1–21).
- In 2000, a new composite ceramic (Biolox delta) was introduced in Europe. This composite ceramic provides superior mechanical properties, almost double the strength of Biolox forte balls. Thus from the point of view of a composite ceramic, the alumina phase provided an ideal bearing surface, whereas the Zirconia phase contributed to strength and toughness.
- As of 2006, the FDA approval is only for 28- and 32-mm Biolox delta balls used with PE cups.

Risks of Ceramic-on-Ceramic Total Hip Replacement

- Any concerns regarding alumina debris and osteolysis have been discounted over the last 30 years of clinical experience (Boehler et al. 1994, Bos and Willmann 2001, Sedel 2000).

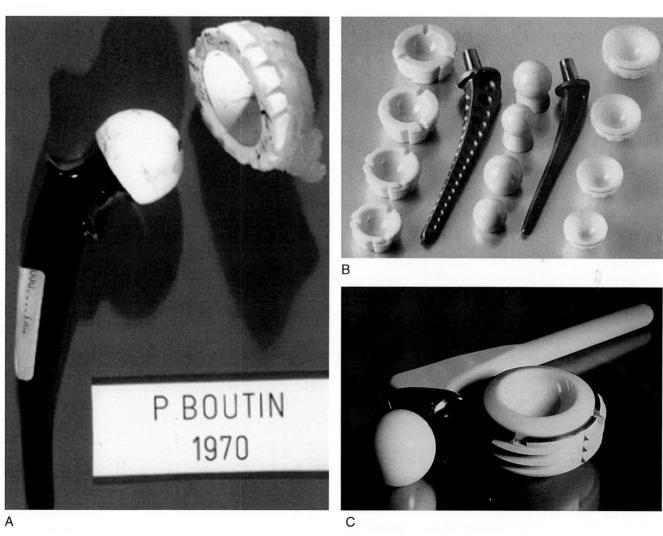

Figure 1–21: Three pioneering ceramic-on-ceramic total hip replacements from 1970 to 1990. **A,** From Boutin, the first ceramic-on-ceramic with cemented monoblock cup combined with cemented Ti6Al4V stem (Ceraver, Inc.). **B,** From Mittelmeier, cemented and press-fit cobalt-chromium stems combined with a range of monoblock, screw-type, alumina cups (Courtesy of Feldmuhle Inc./CeramTec, Inc.). Some alumina balls also had bulky skirts. **C,** The first modular, metal-backed cup (hydroxyapatite-coated, screw-type) for ceramic liners (JRI, Inc). (From Furlong RJ, Osborn JF [1991]. Fixation of hip prostheses by hydroxyapatite ceramic coatings. *J Bone Joint Surg Br* 73:741-745.)

COC wear rates have been so low that retrievals show a very mild periarticular response, the least of any of the biomaterials (Griss et al. 1976, Sedel et al. 1994). Regarding the risk of abnormally high ceramic wear (*avalanche* or gross wear), several retrieval reports are discussed in the next section. Although alumina ceramic is the most rigid biomaterial available, early concerns over stress shielding have faded from view (Willmann 2000).

- Ceramic fractures have been the major discussion point for 30 years. The highest incidence of fractures has been with first-generation alumina and with 28-mm or smaller balls. Historically, fracture rates have varied from as high as 10% to less than 0.03% (Heros and Willmann 1998).
- Contemporary third-generation alumina is reputed to have a worldwide fracture rate lower than 0.004% (Tateiwa et al. 2006).
- In the FDA-monitored experience with modular, metal-backed ceramic cups, more than 2700 cases have been enrolled, and five manufacturers have been involved. With follow-ups now extending over 8 years, no fractures have been reported (D'Antonio et al. 2002, D'Antonio et al. 2005).

Clinical Wear Rates of Ceramic-on-Ceramic Bearings

- The COC bearing has demonstrated ultra low wear over 35 years (Boutin 1972). The average wear was reported to be of the order 2 to 5 μm/year (Griss et al. 1976, Walter and Plitz 1984). In some cases, the original machined marks could still be seen after more than a decade of use.

However, ball wear up to 36 μm/year was reported in cases with one-piece cups that were loosened and tilting with continued patient function (Dorlot 1992, Walter and Plitz 1984).

- Severe ceramic wear has been reported. Pioneering studies have shown the (one hopes) rare occurrence of alumina balls badly misshapen by gross wear (Nevelos et al. 1999).
- One of the more complete COC retrieval studies examined 11 Ceraver and 11 Mittlemeier THRs (Fig. 1–22). However with the exception of noting cup angles, no patient history was presented to explain such severe wear. It may be that such wear reflected the poorer quality alumina with design, fixation, and migration problems unique to one-piece cups.
- The more visible wear scar occurs as a narrow, dull stripe on the femoral ball (Fig. 1–23) and a narrow zone of rim wear on the acetabular cup (Nevelos et al. 1999, Walter et al. 2003). This phenomenon of stripe wear has been recognized from the earliest retrieval studies (Prudhommeaux et al. 2000, Shishido et al. 2003, Walter and Plitz 1984, Walter et al. 2003).
- Stripe wear has been attributed to negative clearance between ball and cup and to vertically inclined or migrating or tilting cups that loosened (Clarke et al. 2005, Dorlot 1992, Yew et al. 2003).

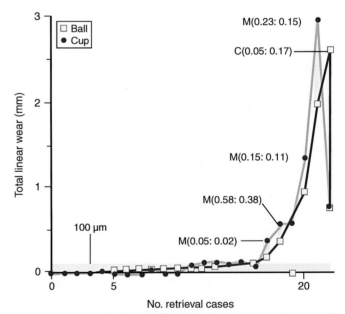

Figure 1–22: Comparison of linear wear measured in retrievals (11 cases each of Ceraver (C) and Mittelmeier (M) total hips). Wear rates (mm/year) indicated for pairings (cup:ball). The *horizontal gray rectangle* indicates the 100-μm wear threshold, and the *vertical gray boxes* indicate cup:ball pairings. (Data from Nevelos JE, Prudhommeaux F, Hamadouche M, et al. [2001]. Comparative analysis of two different types of alumina-alumina hip prosthesis retrieved for aseptic loosening. *J Bone Joint Surg Br* 83:598–603.)

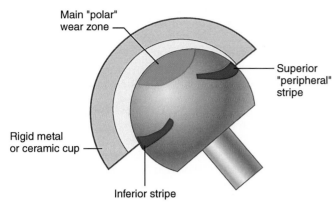

Figure 1–23: Microseparation.
With microseparation, ball impingement on the inferior rim of rigid cup will form stripe wear as the ball rotates. On heel strike, the ball relocates into the cup impinging on the superior rim of rigid cup, thereby creating a second stripe.

- Stripe wear has also been suggested to be a likely natural consequence of using rigid cup materials (Clarke et al. 2005), that is, a stress concentration effect of the rigid cup rim wearing on the femoral ball during normal hip function.
- Volumetric wear was measured in a retrieval study of a modern THR design (Nevelos et al. 2001).
- Macroscopic evidence of narrow stripe wear was seen on a specific site of the femoral head and the beveled rim of the ceramic liner (Box 1–22). Explanation offered was that the stripes formed during repetitively loaded, flexion activities such as stair climbing or rising from a chair.
- These volumetric wear data for COC patients with up to 2 years follow-up are of great interest for validation COC simulator wear studies.
- In our COC implant retrievals at Loma Linda University and Medical Center (Loma Linda, CA), three examples with 16 to 22 years of follow-up showed a superior wear scar and varied peripheral wear stripes. For comparison

between clinical and simulator wear maps, the alumina wear progression was ranked into five grades by SEM observations of surface burnishing and pitting (Shisido et al. 2003).

- The main wear zone was generally grade 4, and the peripheral wear zones showed more damage at grade 5.
- The gray surface discoloration turned out to contain Co and Cr, that is, wear debris contaminants from fretting by the tip of the femoral stem against endosteal bone.
- Thus stripe wear appeared to form early and was also evident after 20 years in vivo. Although not always visually apparent, these wear formations are probably a normal occurrence in most rigid-on-rigid bearings.

Laboratory Wear Rates of Ceramic-on-Ceramic Bearings

- Boutin first described the run-in wear phase of COC with linear wear as low as 10 μm during the first million cycles (Boutin 1972); thereafter, COC wear was undetectable. Later simulator studies using water or saline as the lubricant confirmed this ultralow, linear wear (Kaddick and Pfaff 2000, Kaddick and Pfaff 2002, Oonishi et al. 1996, Saikko and Pfaff 1997, Walter 1997).
- Steady-state wear rates were much more difficult to quantify and thus were simply reported as "undetectable" (Boutin 1972, Kaddick and Pfaff 2000, Kaddick and Pfaff 2002, Plitz et al. 1984, Toni and Affatato 1999).
- Thus, the likely wear reduction from run-in to steady state (Box 1–23) for COC bearings could vary from 3- to 25-fold (Fig. 1–23) (Stewart et al. 2003). Compared with the historic rates of 3XPE, this steady-state phase with alumina cups represented a 1600- to 4000-fold wear reduction.
- The Leeds Groups UK introduced microseparation during simulator swing-phase and successfully demonstrated the peripheral stripe wear seen on retrievals. One study (Iida et al. 1999) examined three 28-mm combinations of Biolox forte and Biolox delta for three ball–cup combinations (i.e., FF, DF, and DD). In their so-called severe MSX mode, run-in wear increased to 4 mm^3/Mc and steady state to 1.3 mm^3/Mc (see Table 1–2). Compared with their prior STD data, the severe MSX mode had increased wear some 26-fold. These results were comparable to the high-wear THR cases from the most recent retrieval study (Nevelos et al. 2001).

Box 1–22	Stripe Wear Analysis on Retrieved Ceramic-on-Ceramic Bearings
Retrievals	= 11 balls, 8 liners
Alumina	= BIOLOX-forte™ (Ceramtec Inc, Germany)
Vendor	= Stryker Inc., Mawah NJ
Follow-up	= up to 2.5 years
Stripes	= posteriorly inclined (average tilt 20 degrees)
Latitudinal site	= 47° above the equator (average for stable implants)
Mild ball wear on balls	= 1 mm^3/year
Maximum ball wear	= 3.5mm^3/year

From Dawihl W, Dorre E, Altmeyer G (1980). [Determination of the service life of a friction locking fixation element for use in ceramic total hips (author's transl)]. *Biomed Tech (Berl)* 25:311-315.

Box 1–23	Ceramic-on-Ceramic Simulator Wear Rates ("Standard" Gait Test)
Run-in range	0.02-1 mm^3/Mc
Run-in average	0.5 mm^3/Mc
Steady-state range	0.02-0.05 mm^3/Mc
Steady-state average	0.04 mm^3/Mc

1. Wear rates in well performing COC are low, with average linear wear rates quoted <5 μm/year in retrieval studies.
2. Volumetric wear in COC clinical studies is low, with THR clinical average wear rates <4 mm^3/Mc.
3. Ceramic debris covers a wide range of sizes from nanometer to several microns. The mode value for the particulate distributions tends to be in the 10-30 nm range, and a high percentage of debris is believed to be <50 nm.
4. In the laboratory, the COC bearings show an initial high wear during run-in phase that normally decreases 4- to 8-fold around 1 million cycles for the steady-state wear phase.
5. There appears to be good agreement between laboratory and clinical wear predictions.
6. There is general agreement that COC wear rates are generally lower than either MOM or MPE.
7. In general, there appears to be minimal risk of a debris-mediated osteolysis with well functioning COC followed over 30 years.
8. However, pioneering COC designs with monoblock cups have also shown gross linear wear >1 mm. The common explanations for this wear are cups too vertical, cup loosening, and migration with the patients continuing to walk on the affected cups for years.
9. Non-modular ceramic cups were used from the 1970s into the 1990s and are now considered obsolete.
10. The modern metal-backed cup with a taper-locked ceramic liner was introduced in 1989, and contemporary ceramic designs all use the hemispherical metal backing with a taper-lock for the ceramic liner.
11. Current clinical studies being monitored by the FDA have accumulated several thousand cases, some followed over 8 years, with satisfactory results to date.
12. Incidence of reported ceramic fractures in the FDA-monitored series is zero.
13. Ceramic liners embedded in polyethylene backing (so-called sandwich cup designs) show a tendency to disassociate in vivo, and some fractures result.
14. Retrieval studies of contemporary designs have shown both normal wear zones and stripe wear zones. The stripes have been documented over the 35-year history of ceramic THRs and created a higher wear response.
15. New ceramics, such as composite alumina-zirconia, appear more resistant to stripe wear than old ceramics.
16. Contemporary design trend is moving toward ceramic ball sizes 32 mm and larger.

Figure 1–23: Consensus building on ceramic cups.

Table 1–11	Summary of Known or Anticipated Risks and Benefits of the Bearing Combinations Used in Total Hip Replacement	
COMBINATIONS	**ANTICIPATED BENEFITS**	**ANTICIPATED RISKS**
Metal-polyethylene	40-year history, best-described system Low frictional torque No squeaking	Always some risk of higher wear, some risk of osteolysis Roughening of CoCr ball could play a role in polyethylene wear Unknown how new polyethylenes will perform over 10 years Unknown how use of balls >32 mm will perform over 10 years Unknown effects of backside wear for polyethylene liner in metal cup
Ceramic-polyethylene	30-year history, well-described system Expected polyethylene wear reduced 50% versus metal ball Alumina bearings will not roughen Frictional effect threefold less than with metal-metal system	Unknown how the new polyethylenes will perform over 10 years Unknown how use of balls >32 mm will perform over 10 years Unknown effects of backside wear for polyethylene liner in metal cup
Metal-metal	40-year history, moderately well-described system Osteolysis anticipated to be nonexistent owing to low wear rates Large balls can be used because of low wear rates Thin CoCr cups offer choices of many sizes of femoral head	Early history problematic resulting from suboptimal designs Biologic effects of the debris and metal ions not well understood Since the early 2000s, >42 mm diameter have no clinical history Use of thin CoCr cups lacking adjunct fixation (screws, fins, etc.) may create additional distortion and fixation problems Friction threefold higher than with other systems
Ceramic-ceramic	30-year history, moderately well-described system Osteolysis anticipated to be nonexistent owing to low wear rates Large balls can be used because of low wear rates No backside wear with taper-locked ceramic liners Metal-backed cups offer standard options for adjunct fixation No backside wear with one-piece or taper-locked CoCr liners Frictional effect threefold less than with metal-metal system	Early history problematic owing to inadequate cup fixation Brittle material with infrequent but troublesome fracture risk Large balls limited in size because of the need for metal backing Squeaking anticipated in some 1% to 4% of cases

CoCr, cobalt chromium.

- We followed the Leeds example and modified our simulators to run microseparation wear studies (Eickmann et al. 2003). We diametrically matched a set of 36-mm Biolox forte and Biolox delta over a range of tolerances. The sets were mounted anatomically on a hip simulator customized for microseparation (MSX).
- All combinations demonstrated stripe wear phenomenon showing clearly that the microseparation test mode made a significant contribution to wear rates and created stripes indicative of those on retrievals. Stripe wear scars were visible within the 100,000 cycles and corresponded to the following:
  - The inferior cup rim impinging on ball surface during distraction phase
  - The superior cup rim impinging on ball during the re-location phase
- Typically, there were two regions of stripe initiation on the balls: a superior stripe at approximately 45 to 60 degrees and another at 75 to 90 degrees (relative to the pole). These scars elongated over the course of the study, forming a complete stripe. The cups showed a narrow scar spanning approximately a 20- to 40-degree arc from the center of the cup along the rim. The peripheral wear scars always showed a more severe grade of wear than the main wear zone.
- The THR sets with Biolox forte balls and cups had the highest wear rate, averaging just over 1.5 mm^3/Mc. In contrast, all Biolox delta combinations averaged wear rates lower than 0.5 mm^3/Mc, with the Biolox delta ball and cup set having the least wear.
- Thus all Biolox delta combinations were more resistant to stripe wear than Biolox forte alone, a finding confirming the results of the previous study.

Concluding Remarks

- It is obvious from the foregoing review that there is no perfect materials combination, and all options offer some risks on close inspection (Table 1–11). PE cups are well understood, widely used, and relatively forgiving in terms of impingement problems.
- However, in relative terms, PE represents the poorest bearing material and therefore has the highest risk of contributing significant amounts of wear particles.
- CPE may be a safer choice for the younger patient because it is immune to third-body abrasive wear and has averaged 50% less wear over decades of clinical study.
- Although the laboratory data are consistent in showing virtually no PE wear at radiation doses from 5 to 10 rad, ample evidence exists to believe that the in vivo environment will be a much harsher judge. There is also the upside risk of moving to larger femoral heads and thereby violating Charnley's original paradigm of the small ball and with the additional risk of thinner liners.

- MOM bearings are the optimal choice in terms of many diameters of femoral heads and a low risk of wear problems.
- The real problem is one of a nonforgiving bearing in the risk situations created by activities typical of daily life. In addition, the clinical history has been with 32-to 41.5-mm balls, so there is little or no prior clinical experience with MOM balls larger than 42 mm in diameter. The long-term risk of metal ions is also not understood and defies definition at this time.
- COC appears to be the optimal bearing because it is inert and has ultralow wear. However, it does have the disadvantage of being a brittle material, and fracture has been a persistent although relatively rare occurrence. In addition, contemporary ceramic THR designs are limited in diameters of femoral heads. The ceramic liner may also be less forgiving than PE in cases with suboptimal cup position carrying an increased risk of rim impingement.
- In terms of lubrication modes, the COC bearing appeared to be the only one capable of operating under fluid film conditions. The metal/UHMWPE and MOM bearings appeared to be operating under the mixed-lubrication mode (i.e., with some metal contact) (Scholes and Unsworth 2006). This frictional risk is also difficult to assess because many other factors are involved, such as the geometry of the MOM implants and any distortion introduced into the acetabular cup at the time of surgical impaction.
- For the first time in history, the orthopaedic surgeon has a choice of femoral heads ranging from 22 to 60 mm in diameter. Some of these MOM devices are interchangeable between resurfacing and THR systems (36- to 60-mm range). With no dominant choice regarding bearing materials, the choice of MPE, CPE, MOM, or COC will depend on the circumstances of the individual patient and the surgeon's preference. It is hoped that this review offers the surgeon a fair perspective of the risks and benefits associated with each bearing material combination as he or she makes that choice.

References

Amstutz HC, Campbell P, Kossovsky N, Clarke IC (1992). Mechanism and clinical significance of wear debris-induced osteolysis. *Clin Orthop Relat Res* 276:7-18.

Amstutz HC, Campbell P, McKellop H, et al. (1996). Metal on metal total hip replacement workshop consensus document. *Clin Orthop Relat Res* 329(Suppl):S297-S303.

Amstutz HC, Clarke IC (1991). Evolution of hip arthroplasty. In: Amstutz HC, ed. *Hip Arthroplasty*, vol. 1-14. New York: Churchill Livingstone.

Anissian HL, Stark A, Good V, et al. (2001). The wear pattern in metal-on-metal hip prostheses. *J Biomed Mater Res* 58:673-678.

Bauer TW, Ming J, D'Antonio JA, Morawa LG (1996). Abrasive three-body wear of polyethylene caused by broken multifilament cables of a total hip prosthesis: A report of these cases. *J Bone Joint Surg Am* 78:1244-1247.

Bizot P, Banallec L, Sedel L, Nizard R (2000). Alumina-on-alumina total hip prostheses in patients 40 years of age or younger. *Clin Orthop Relat Res* 379:68-76.

Boehler M, Knahr K, Plenk H Jr, et al. (1994). Long-term results of uncemented alumina acetabular implants. *J Bone Joint Surg Br* 76:53-59.

Bos I, Willmann G (2001). Morphologic characteristics of periprosthetic tissues from hip prostheses with ceramic-ceramic couples: A comparative histologic investigation of 18 revision and 30 autopsy cases. *Acta Orthop Scand* 72:335-342.

Boutin P (1972). [Total arthroplasty of the hip by fretted aluminum prosthesis: Experimental study and first clinical applications]. *Rev Chir Orthop Reparatrice Appar Mot* 58:229-246.

Bowsher JG, Hussain A, Williams P, et al. (2004). Effect of ion implantation on the tribology of metal-on-metal hip prostheses. *J Arthroplasty* 19(Suppl 3):107-111.

Bowsher JG, Nevelos J, Williams PA, et al. (2006). "Severe" wear challenge to "as-cast" and "double heat-treated" large-diameter metal-on-metal hip bearings. *Proc Inst Mech Eng [H]* 220:135-143.

Bowsher JG, Williams P, Clarke I, Donaldson T (2006). Severe wear challenge to 36mm mechanically enhanced crosslinked polyethylene hip liners. In: *Transactions of the 52nd Meeting of the Orthopaedic Research Society*. Chicago: Orthopaedic Research Society.

Bradford L, Baker DA, Graham J, et al. (2004). Wear and surface cracking in early retrieved highly cross-linked polyethylene acetabular liners. *J Bone Joint Surg Am* 86:1271-1282.

Butterfield M, Stewart T, Williams S, et al. (2002). Wear of metal-metal and ceramic-ceramic hip prostheses with swing phase microseparation. In: *Transactions of the 48th Meeting of the Orthopaedic Research Society*. Dallas, TX: Orthopaedic Research Society, p 129.

Callaghan JJ, Brown TD, Pedersen DR, Johnston RC (2002). Choices and compromises in the use of small head sizes in total hip arthroplasty. *Clin Orthop Relat Res* 405:144-149.

Callaghan JJ, Kim YS, Brown TD, et al. (1995). Concerns and improvements with cementless metal-backed acetabular components. *Clin Orthop Relat Res* 311:76-84.

Chan FW, Bobyn JD, Medley JB, et al. (1996). Engineering issues and wear performance of metal on metal hip implants. *Clin Orthop Relat Res* 333:96-107.

Chang JD, Lee SS, Hur M, et al. (2005). Revision total hip arthroplasty in hip joints with metallosis: A single-center experience with 31 cases. *J Arthroplasty* 20:568-573.

Charnley J, Cupic Z (1973). The nine and ten year results of the low-friction arthroplasty of the hip. *Clin Orthop Relat Res* 95: 9-25.

Charnley J, Kamangar A, Longfield MD (1969). The optimum size of prosthetic heads in relation to the wear of plastic sockets in total replacement of the hip. *Med Biol Eng* 7:31-39.

Clarke IC (1992). Role of ceramic implants: Design and clinical success with total hip prosthetic ceramic-to-ceramic bearings. *Clin Orthop Relat Res* 282:19-30.

Clarke IC, Campbell P (1989). Interface failure dynamics: Osteoclastic and macrophagic bone loss. In: Kenedi RM, Paul JP, eds. *Progress in Bioengineering*. Glasgow: Strathclyde University, pp 104-115.

Clarke IC, Donaldson T, Bowsher JG, et al. (2005). Current concepts of metal-on-metal hip resurfacing. *Orthop Clin North Am* 36: 143-162, viii.

The authors reviewed the design, biomechanics, wear, and clinical results of MOM resurfacing designs. Comparisons are made between laboratory predictions and the clinical results of MOM resurfacing compared with MOM THR. The problems of fixation of the femoral shell and neck fractures identified in the earlier designs of the 1980s remain as a potentially troublesome but fortunately only small risk in the latest designs. Release of metal ions has been measured for both THR and resurfacing, and it was concluded that more studies were needed for clarification of the issues.

Clarke IC, Good V, Anissian L, Gustafson A (1997). Charnley wear model for validation of hip simulators: Ball diameter versus polytetrafluoroethylene and polyethylene wear. *Proc Inst Mech Eng [H]* 211:25-36.

Clarke IC, Willmann G (1994). Structural ceramics in orthopedics. In: Cameron HU, ed. *Bone Implant Interface*. St. Louis: Mosby, pp 203-252.

Coleman RF, Herrington J, Scales JT (1973). Concentration of wear products in hair, blood, and urine after total hip replacement. *BMJ* 1:527-529.

Collins T, Carroll M, et al. (2004). Wear of large diameter metal on metal hip bearings in primary and revision surface replacement. 50th Annual Meeting of the Orthopaedic Research Society, March 7-10, San Francisco, CA.

D'Antonio J, Capello W, Manley M, Bierbaum B (2002). New experience with alumina-on-alumina ceramic bearings for total hip arthroplasty. *J Arthroplasty* 17:390-397.

D'Antonio J, Capello W, Manley M, et al. (2005). Alumina ceramic bearings for total hip arthroplasty: Five-year results of a prospective randomized study. *Clin Orthop Relat Res* 436:164-171.

Digas G, Karrholm J, Thanner J, et al. (2003). Highly cross-linked polyethylene in cemented THA: Randomized study of 61 hips. *Clin Orthop Relat Res* 417:126-138.

Donaldson T, Williams P, Andrusak L, et al. (2004). Effect of sterilization on the clinical wear of Hylamer cups. In: *Transactions of the 7th World Biomaterials Congress*. Sydney, Australia, p 815.

Doorn PF, Campbell PA, Worrall J, et al. (1998). Metal wear particle characterization from metal-on-metal total hip replacements: Transmission electron microscopy study of periprosthetic tissues and isolated particles. *J Biomed Mater Res* 42:103-111.

This well-documented study examined the tissues from 13 patients who had undergone revision of all-metal THRs. Metal particles were recovered only from tissues that were visibly gray or black and varied in size range from 0.006 to 0.74 μm (average, 0.04 to 0.08 μm). This median-sized metal particle was more than a 100 times smaller than a red blood cell. Frequency estimates would place the number of particles at 5 to 250 million particles released for each step the patient takes. The authors noted that the larger number of metal particles and the resulting large surface area they represented did not produce any severe, local tissue reactions.

Dorlot JM (1992). Long-term effects of alumina components in total hip prostheses. *Clin Orthop Relat Res* 282:47-52.

Dumbleton JH, Manley MT (2005). Metal-on-metal total hip replacement: What does the literature say? *J Arthroplasty* 20:174-188.
> For surgeons using all-metal implants, the ever-present caution with such materials is the risk of biologic issues resulting from elevated metal ions. This very detailed review of all-metal hip systems compares results of the first-generation and second-generation designs with respect to clinical results, survivorship data, release of metal ions, retrieval data, wear, metal debris, tissue reactions, carcinogenicity, mutagenicity, and hypersensitivity issues. The authors concluded that prospective, randomized clinical studies were required with follow-ups of 15 years or more to evaluate the role of all-metal implants properly.

Eickmann T, Manaka M, Clarke IC, Gustafson A (2002). Squeaking and neck-socket impingement in a ceramic total hip arthroplasty. In: Ben-Nissan B, Sher D, Walsh W, eds. *Bioceramics-15*. Enfield, NH: Trans Tech Publications, pp 849-852.

Essner A, Schmidig G, Herrera L, et al. (2005). Hip wear performance of a next generation cross-linked and annealed polyethylene. In: *Transactions of the 51st Annual Meeting of the Orthopaedic Research Society*. Washington, DC: Orthopaedic Research Society, p 830.

Firkins PJ, Tipper JL, Ingham E, et al. (2001). Influence of simulator kinematics on the wear of metal-on-metal hip prostheses. *Proc Inst Mech Eng [H]* 215:119-121.

Fisher J, Besong AA, Firkins P, et al. (2000). Comparative wear and debris generation in UHMWPE on ceramic, metal on metal, and ceramic on ceramic hip prosthesis. In: *Transactions of the 46th Annual Meeting of the Orthopaedic Research Society*. Orlando, FL: Orthopaedic Research Society, p 587.

Galvin AL, Tipper JL, Ingham E, et al. (2005). Nanometre size wear debris generated from crosslinked and non-crosslinked ultra high molecular weight polyethylene in artificial joints. *Wear* 259: 977-983.

Garino JP (2000). Modern ceramic-on-ceramic total hip systems in the United States: Early results. *Clin Orthop Relat Res* 379:41-47.

Goldsmith AA, Dowson D, Isaac GH, Lancaster JG (2000). A comparative joint simulator study of the wear of metal-on-metal and alternative material combinations in hip replacements. *Proc Inst Mech Eng [H]* 214:39-47.

Good V, Ries M, Barrack RL, et al. (2003). Reduced wear with oxidized zirconium femoral heads. *J Bone Joint Surg Am* 85(Suppl 4): 105-110.

Green TR, Fisher J, Matthews JB, et al. (2000). Effect of size and dose on bone resorption activity of macrophages by in vitro clinically relevant ultra high molecular weight polyethylene particles. *J Biomed Mater Res* 53:490-497.

Griss P (1984). Four- to eight-year postoperative results of the partially uncemented Lindenhof-type ceramic hip endoprosthesis. In: Morscher E, ed. *The Cementless Fixation of Hip Endoprostheses*. New York: Springer-Verlag, pp 220-224.

Griss P, Silber R, Merkle B, et al. (1976). Biomechanically induced tissue reactions after Al2O3-ceramic hip joint replacement: Experimental and early clinical results. *J Biomed Mater Res* 10:519-528.

Gustafson A, Shishido T, Clarke IC, et al. (2003). Consolidation of clinical and experimental experiences with all-alumina total hip replacements. In: *70th Annual Meeting of the American Academy of Orthopaedic Surgeons*. New Orleans: American Academy of Orthopaedic Surgeons, p SE211.

Hall RM, Siney P, Unsworth A, Wroblewski BM (1997). The effect of surface topography of retrieved femoral heads on the wear of UHMWPE sockets. *Med Eng Phys* 19:711-719.

Hamadouche M, Boutin P, Daussange J, et al. (2002). Alumina-on-alumina total hip arthroplasty: A minimum 18.5-year follow-up study. *J Bone Joint Surg Am* 84:69-77.

Hamilton HW, Gorczyca J (1995). Low friction arthroplasty at 10 to 20 years. Consequences of plastic wear. *Clin Orthop Relat Res* 318:160-166.

Hamilton WG, Hopper RH Jr, Ginn SD, et al. (2005). The effect of total hip arthroplasty cup design on polyethylene wear rate. *J Arthroplasty* 20(Suppl 3):63-72.

Heisel C, Silva M, dela Rosa MA, Schmalzried TP (2004). Short-term in vivo wear of cross-linked polyethylene. *J Bone Joint Surg Am* 86:748-751.

Heros RJ, Willmann G (1998). Ceramic in total hip arthroplasty: History, mechanical properties, clinical results, and current manufacturing state of the art. *Semin Arthroplasty* 9:114-122.

Ingram J, Matthews JB, Tipper J, et al. (2002). Comparison of the biological activity of grade GUR 1120 and GUR 415HP UHMWPE wear debris. *Biomed Mater Eng* 12:177-188.

Ingham E, Fisher J (2000). Biological reactions to wear debris in total joint replacement. *Proc Inst Mech Eng [H]* 214:21-37.

Ingham E, Fisher J (2005). The role of macrophages in osteolysis of total joint replacement. *Biomaterials* 26:1271-1286.
> This review provides the latest concepts of stimulation of macrophage cells by UHMWPE wear debris, an important part of the osteolytic cascade. UHMWPE-driven osteolysis is associated with inflamed periprosthetic membranes rich in macrophages, cytokines, and wear debris. UHMWPE particles smaller than 1 μm appear to be the most reactive, with stimulation of cytokine tumor necrosis factor-α as a key activator. This review gives a complete description of how macrophages react to the debris and current knowledge on the role of the macrophages in osteoclast differentiation from monocyte/macrophage precursors and osteoclastogenesis in arthroplasty-derived tissue macrophages.

Ingram JH, Stone M, Fisher J, Ingham E (2004). The influence of molecular weight, crosslinking and counterface roughness on TNF-alpha production by macrophages in response to ultra high molecular weight polyethylene particles. *Biomaterials* 25:3511-3522.

Isaac GH, Wroblewski BM, Atkinson JR, Dowson D (1992). A tribological study of retrieved hip prostheses. *Clin Orthop Relat Res* 276: 115-125.

Jacobs JJ, Skipor AK, Patterson LM, et al. (1998). Metal release in patients who have had a primary total hip arthroplasty. A prospective, controlled, longitudinal study. *J Bone Joint Surg Am* 80:1447-1458.

Jacobs JJ, Hallab NJ, Skipor AK, Urban RM (2003). Metal degradation products: A cause for concern in metal-metal bearings? *Clin Orthop Relat Res* 417:139-147.

Jacobs JJ, Skipor AK, Campbell PA, et al. (2004). Can metal levels be used to monitor metal-on-metal hip arthroplasties? *J Arthroplasty* 19(Suppl 3):59-65.

Kabo JM, Gebhard JS, Loren G, Amstutz HC (1993). In vivo wear of polyethylene acetabular components. *J Bone Joint Surg Br* 75:254-258.

Kaddick C, Pfaff HG (2000). Wear study in the alumina-Zirconia system. In: Willmann G, Zweymuller K, eds. *Bioceramics in Hip Joint Replacement (Proceedings of the Fifth International CeramTec Symposium)*. New York: Georg Thieme Verlag, pp 146-150.

Kaddick C, Pfaff HG (2002). Results of hip simulator testing with various wear couples. In: Garino J, Willmann G, eds. *Proceedings of the Seventh International Biolox Symposium*, pp 16-20.

Kobayashi A, Bonfield W, Kadoya Y, et al. (1997). The size and shape of particulate polyethylene wear debris in total joint replacements. *Proc Inst Mech Eng [H]* 211:11-15.

Krushell RJ, Fingeroth RJ, Cushing MC (2005). Early femoral head penetration of a highly cross-linked polyethylene liner vs a conventional polyethylene liner: A case-controlled study. *J Arthroplasty* 20(Suppl 3):73-76.

Kurtz SM, Harrigan TP, Herr M, Manley MT (2005). An in vitro model for fluid pressurization of screw holes in metal-backed total joint components. *J Arthroplasty* 20:932-938.

Liao YS, Fryman C, et al. (2004). Effects of clearance, head size, and start-stop protocol on wear of metal-on-metal hip joint bearings in a physiological anatomical hip joint simulator. 50th Annual Meeting of the Orthopaedic Research Society, San Francisco, CA.

Livermore J, Ilstrup D, Morrey B (1990). Effect of femoral head size on wear of the polyethylene acetabular component. *J Bone Joint Surg Am* 72:518-528.

Manaka M, Clarke IC, Yamamoto K, et al. (2004). Stripe wear rates in alumina THR: Comparison of microseparation simulator study with retrieved implants. *J Biomed Mater Res* 69:149-157.

Manning DW, Chiang PP, Martell JM, et al. (2005). In vivo comparative wear study of traditional and highly cross-linked polyethylene in total hip arthroplasty. *J Arthroplasty* 20:880-886.

Martell JM, Berkson E, Berger R, Jacobs J (2003). Comparison of two and three-dimensional computerized polyethylene wear analysis after total hip arthroplasty. *J Bone Joint Surg Am* 85:1111-1117.

McKee GK, Chen SC (1973). The statistics of the McKee-Farrar method of total hip replacement. *Clin Orthop Relat Res* 95:26-33.

McKellop H, Campbell P, Park SH, et al. (1995). The origin of submicron polyethylene wear debris in total hip arthroplasty. *Clin Orthop Relat Res* 311:3-20.

McKellop H, Park SH, Chiesa R, et al. (1996). In vivo wear of three types of metal on metal hip prostheses during two decades of use. *Clin Orthop Relat Res* 329(Suppl):S128-S140.

Milosev I, Trebse R, Kovac S, et al. (2006). Survivorship and retrieval analysis of Sikomet metal-on-metal total hip replacements at a mean of seven years. *J Bone Joint Surg Am* 88(6): 1173-82.

Mittelmeier H, Harms J (1979). [Treatment of post-traumatic hip joint disease by total replacement with a ceramic endoprosthesis]. *Unfallheilkunde* 82:67-75.

Mittelmeier H, Heisel J (1992). Sixteen-years' experience with ceramic hip prostheses. *Clin Orthop Relat Res* 282:64-72.

Muller ME (1995). The benefits of metal-on-metal total hip replacements. *Clin Orthop Relat Res* 311:54-59.

Nevelos JE, Ingham E, Doyle C, et al. (1999). Analysis of retrieved alumina ceramic components from Mittelmeier total hip prostheses. *Biomaterials* 20:1833-1840.

Nevelos JE, Ingham E, Doyle C, et al. (2001a). The influence of acetabular cup angle on the wear of "Biolox forte" alumina ceramic bearing couples in a hip joint simulator. *J Mater Sci Mater Med* 12:141-144.

Nevelos JE, Prudhommeaux F, Hamadouche M, et al. (2001b). Comparative analysis of two different types of alumina-alumina hip prosthesis retrieved for aseptic loosening. *J Bone Joint Surg Br* 83: 598-603.

This study is one of the more complete retrieval studies of COC hip replacement with 1 to 18 years of follow-up. Eleven cases were from the United Kingdom and represented the Mittelmeier device from 1974 era. Another 11 cases were from France and represented the Ceraver-Osteal device from the 1977 era. These were classified into three groups: no measurable wear, stripe wear on the ball and cup, and severe macroscopic wear with loss of sphericity. Linear wear rates varied from less than 0.001 mm/year to more than 0.5 mm/year, with a mean value of 0.056 mm/year. The cases with severe wear appeared related to risk factors such as more vertical cup angles with cup tilting and loosening. Thus it was inferred that inferior, one-piece cup designs were the major problem.

Oonishi H, Ishimaru H, Kato A (1996a). Effect of cross-linkage by gamma radiation in heavy doses to low wear polyethylene in total hip prostheses. *J Mater Sci Mater Med* 7:753-763.

Oonishi H, Kadoya Y, Masuda S (2001). Gamma-irradiated cross-linked polyethylene in total hip replacements: Analysis of retrieved sockets after long-term implantation. *J Biomed Mater Res* 58:167-171.

Oonishi H, Kuno M, Tsuji E, Fujisawa A (1996b). The optimum dose of gamma radiation-heavy doses to low wear polyethylene in total hip prostheses. *J Mater Sci Mater Med* 8:11-18.

Oonishi H, Ueno M, Okimatsu H, Amino H (1996c). Investigation of the wear behavior of ceramic on ceramic combinations in total hip prosthesis. In: Kokubo T, Nakamura T, Miyaji F, eds. *Bioceramics-9*. Otsu, Japan: Pergamon Press, pp 503-506.

Oparaugo PC, Clarke IC, Malchau H, Herberts P (2001). Correlation of wear debris-induced osteolysis and revision with volumetric wear-rates of polyethylene: A survey of 8 reports in the literature. *Acta Orthop Scand* 72:22-28.

This survey examined the clinical incidence of UHMWPE wear and its relationship with osteolysis and revision in clinical series from 1983 to 1987. Clinical follow-ups over 10 years revealed design differences that were not evident with shorter follow-up. Osteolysis was found to be rare for UHMWPE with wear rates less than 80 mm³/year, it was up to 31% incidence with wear rates up to 140 mm³/year, and it occurred in 100% of cases with wear rates greater than 140 mm³/year. With regard to design, the cemented UHMWPE cups with small femoral heads did best, the medium-risk group had the metal-backed UHMWPE cup, and the highest-risk group had the 32-mm diameter, noncemented, metal-backed, UHMWPE cup.

Plitz W, Walter A, Jager M (1984). [Material-specific wear of ceramic/ceramic sliding surfaces in revised hip endoprostheses: Clinical and technological considerations.] *Z Orthop Ihre Grenzgeb* 122:299-303.

Prudhommeaux F, Hamadouche M, Nevelos J, et al. (2000). Wear of alumina-on-alumina total hip arthroplasties at a mean 11-year followup. *Clin Orthop Relat Res* 379:113-122.

Rieker CB, Kottig P, Schon R, et al. (1998). Clinical wear performance of metal-on-metal hip arthroplasties. In: Jacobs J, Craig TL, eds. *Alternative Bearing Surfaces in Total Joint Replacement*. Special Technical Publication 1346. Fredericksburg, VA: American Society for Testing and Materials, pp 144-156.

Saikko V, Pfaff HG (1997). Wear of alumina-alumina total replacement hip joints studied with a hip joint simulator. In: *Proceedings of the Second Symposium on Performance of the Wear Couple Biolox-Forte in Hip Arthroplasty*. Stuttgart: CeramTec, pp 117-122.

Schmalzried TP (2005). Metal-on-metal resurfacing arthroplasty. *J Arthroplasty* 20(Suppl 2):70-71.

Schmalzried TP, Clarke IC, McKellop H (1998). Bearing surfaces. In: Callaghan JJ, Rosenberg A, Rubash H, eds. *The Adult Hip*. Philadelphia: Lippincott-Raven, pp 247-265.

Schmalzried TP, Fowble VA, Ure KJ, Amstutz HC (1996a). Metal on metal surface replacement of the hip: Technique, fixation, and early results. *Clin Orthop Relat Res* 329(Suppl):S106-S114.

Schmalzried TP, Peters PC, Maurer BT, et al. (1996b). Long-duration metal-on-metal total hip arthroplasties with low wear of the articulating surfaces. *J Arthroplasty* 11:322-331.

Schmalzried TP, Shepherd EF, Dorey FJ, et al. (2000). The John Charnley award: Wear is a function of use, not time. *Clin Orthop Relat Res* 381:36-46.

Scholes SC, Unsworth A (2006). The effects of proteins on the friction and lubrication of artificial joints. *Proc Inst Mech Eng [H]* 220: 687-693.

> This detailed analysis of friction in hip and knee joint replacements used a variety of lubricant types to compare 28-mm diameter metal/UHMWPE, COC, and MOM bearing performance. In bovine serum and synovial fluid, MOM averaged three- to fourfold higher friction than the metal/UHMWPE and COC combinations. In terms of lubrication modes, COC appeared to be the only one capable of operating under fluid film conditions. The metal/UHMWPE and MOM bearings appeared to be operating under the mixed-lubrication mode (i.e., partial metal contact and partial fluid-film support).

Scott M, Morrison M, Mishra SR, Jani S (2005). Particle analysis for the determination of UHMWPE wear. *J Biomed Mater Res B Appl Biomater* 73:325-337.

Scott ML, Lemons J (1998). The wear characteristics of Sivash SRN Co-Cr-Mo THA articulating surfaces. In: Jacobs J, Craig TL, eds. *Alternative Bearing Surfaces in Total Joint Replacement*. Special Technical Publication 1346. Fredericksburg, VA: American Society for Testing and Materials, pp 159-172.

Sedel L (2000). Evolution of alumina-on-alumina implants: A review. *Clin Orthop Relat Res* 379:48-54.

> This review was compiled by one the leading European ceramic groups with 30 years of experience and many publications. This overview explains the pitfalls encountered in ceramic hip designs of the 1970s and 1980s. Much of the development entailed improving the quality of the alumina ceramic and developing test methods to satisfy the safety of the ceramic implants. Cemented or press-fit, one-piece ceramic cups were bulky and had inadequate fixation. Nevertheless, despite loosening problems, osteolysis was documented to be less than 1% overall. By 1989, better ceramic designs were available using the improved fixation concepts of metal-backed cups designed for bone ingrowth. The major long-term benefit alumina-on-alumina implants has been easy revision with good bone stock preserved because of the absence of osteolysis.

Sedel L, Nizard RS, Kerboull L, Witvoet J (1994). Alumina-alumina hip replacement in patients younger than 50 years old. *Clin Orthop Relat Res* 298:175-183.

Sedel L, Nizard R, Bizot P (2000). Osteolysis and ceramic bearing surfaces. *J Bone Joint Surg Am* 82:1519; author reply 1520-1521.

Semlitsch M, Lehmann M, Weber H, et al. (1977). New prospects for a prolonged functional life-span of artificial hip joints by using the material combination polyethylene/aluminium oxide ceramin/metal. *J Biomed Mater Res* 11:537-552.

Shaju KA, Hasan ST, D'Souza LG, et al. (2005). The 22-mm vs the 32-mm femoral head in cemented primary hip arthroplasty: Long-term clinical and radiological follow-up study. *J Arthroplasty* 20:903-908.

Shishido T, Clarke IC, Williams P, et al. (2001). Clinical wear and simulator study of ceramic-ceramic THR to 20 years and beyond. In: *Transactions of the 47th Meeting of the Orthopaedic Research Society*. Dallas, TX: Orthopaedic Research Society, p 1019.

Shishido T, Clarke IC, Williams P, et al. (2003). Clinical and simulator wear study of alumina ceramic THR to 17 years and beyond. *J Biomed Mater Res* 67:638-647.

Sochart DH (1999). Relationship of acetabular wear to osteolysis and loosening in total hip arthroplasty. *Clin Orthop Relat Res* 363:135-150.

Streicher RM (1993). [UHMW-polyethylene as the substance for articulating components of joint prostheses]. *Biomed Tech (Berl)* 38:303-313.

Tateiwa T, Clarke IC, Garino J, et al. (year?). Use of ceramics in hip replacements: Safety and risks revisited. ???.

Toni A, Affatato S (1999). New wear couples for THR-simulator testing. In: Sedel L, Willmann G, eds. *Reliability and Long-term Results of Ceramics in Orthopaedics*. New York: Georg Thieme Verlag, pp 2191-2197.

Wagner M, Wagner H (2000). Medium-term results of a modern metal-on-metal system in total hip replacement. *Clin Orthop Relat Res* 379:123-133.

Walker PS, Erkman MJ (1972). Metal-on-metal lubrication in artificial human joints. *Wear* 21:377-392.

Walker PS, Gold BL (1971). The tribology (friction, lubrication and wear) of all-metal artificial hip joints. *Wear* 17:285-299.

Walter A (1997). Investigations on the wear couple Biolox forte/Biolox forte and earlier alumina materials. In: *Bioceramics in Joint Arthroplasty: Proceedings of the Second International Biolox Symposium.* Stuttgart: Georg Thieme Verlag, pp 123-135.

Walter WL, Insley G, Walter WK, Tuke M (2003). The mechanics of Stripe Wear formation in a modern ceramic on ceramic bearing. In: *70th Annual Meeting of the American Academy of Orthopaedic Surgeons.* New Orleans, p 278.

Walter A, Plitz W (1984). Wear mechanism of alumina-ceramic bearing surfaces of hip-joint protheses. In: Ducheyne P, Van der Perre G, Aubert AE, eds. *Biomaterials and Biomechanics.* Amsterdam: Elsevier Science, pp 55-61.

Wasielewski RC, Jacobs JJ, Arthurs B, Rubash HE (2005). The acetabular insert-metal backing interface: An additional source of polyethylene wear debris. *J Arthroplasty* 20:914-922.

Williams S, Stewart TD, Ingham E, et al. (2004). Metal-on-metal bearing wear with different swing phase loads. *J Biomed Mater Res B Appl Biomater* 70:233-239.

Willmann G (2000). Ceramic femoral head retrieval data. *Clin Orthop Relat Res* 379:22-28.

Wimmer MA, Loos J, Nassutt R, et al. (2001). The acting wear mechanisms on metal-on-metal hip joint bearings: In vitro results. *Wear* 250:129-139.

Wroblewski BM, Siney PD (1992). Charnley low-friction arthroplasty in the young patient. *Clin Orthop Relat Res* 285:45-47.

Wroblewski BM, Siney PD, Dowson D, Collins SN (1996). Prospective clinical and joint simulator studies of a new total hip arthroplasty using alumina ceramic heads and cross-linked polyethylene cups. *J Bone Joint Surg Br* 78:280-285.

Wroblewski BM, Siney PD, Fleming PA (1999). Low-friction arthroplasty of the hip using alumina ceramic and cross-linked polyethylene: A ten-year follow-up report. *J Bone Joint Surg Br* 81: 54-55.

Wroblewski BM, Siney PD, Fleming PA (2002). Charnley low-frictional torque arthroplasty in patients under the age of 51 years: Follow-up to 33 years. *J Bone Joint Surg Br* 84:540-543.

Yamamoto K, Clarke IC, Masaoka T, et al. (2001). Microwear phenomena of ultrahigh molecular weight polyethylene cups and debris morphology related to gamma radiation dose in simulator study. *J Biomed Mater Res* 56:65-73.

Yew A, Jagatia M, Ensaff H, Jin ZM (2003). Analysis of contact mechanics in McKee-Farrar metal-on-metal hip implants. *Proc Inst Mech Eng [H]* 217:333-340.

Zichner LP, Willert HG (1992). Comparison of alumina-polyethylene and metal-polyethylene in clinical trials. *Clin Orthop Relat Res* 282: 86-94.

Greater Expectations and Greater Loads: Implications for Biomechanics

Edward Ebramzadeh,* Sophia N. Sangiorgio,† and Ian C. Clarke‡

*PhD, Director, Implant Performance Biomechanics Laboratory, Los Angeles Orthopaedic
Hospital, and Adjunct Professor, Department of Orthopaedic Surgery, University of
California at Los Angeles, Los Angeles, CA
†PhD, Manager, Implant Performance Biomechanics Laboratory, Los Angeles Orthopaedic
Hospital, University of California at Los Angeles, Los Angeles, CA
‡PhD, Professor and Director, Department of Orthopaedics, Orthopaedic Research Center,
Loma Linda University and Medical Center, Loma Linda, CA

Introduction

- This chapter addresses some of the challenges of meeting the needs of the increasingly younger, more active, and heavier patients who undergo total hip replacement (THR).
- The established guidelines and criteria for preclinical testing of joint replacements are by and large based on loads and activity levels for patients of the "ideal" age and weight, engaging in routine activities such as walking and stair climbing, but not on activities such as long-distance running or extreme sports.
- To optimize the clinical outcome of total hip arthroplasty, it is imperative to gain a thorough understanding of all the major biomechanical aspects of total joint surgery, especially the maximum loads an artificial joint can withstand without exceeding the functional limits.
- This chapter contains a review of the loads on the hip joint during a variety of daily activities, contrasts these to loads during selected sports and extreme activities, and summarizes the most recent clinical studies on the incidence of acute implant failures, including implant fracture, fracture of the periprosthetic bone, and fracture of the femoral neck in the case of surface replacements.
- The findings of these studies must be taken into consideration collectively before sound recommendations can be made from a biomechanical point of view for each candidate for total joint replacement.

Patient Expectations

Charnley's Expectations

- When Charnley first popularized total hip arthroplasty, he recommended strongly against using THR in patients who were overweight or in those younger than 65 years old (Charnley 1979) (Box 1–24).
- The basis of Charnley's selection criteria was from clinical experience with younger and overweight patients and in vitro studies. In one study, Charnley described the correlation between increased weight and implant fracture, particularly in male patients. In fact, Charnley designed the "extra heavy" prosthesis to accommodate these "over average weight and most certainly patients of 168 lbs (75 kg) and over"(Charnley 1979).
- A study by Griffith and associates (1978) found that patients with femoral stem subsidence greater than 2.0 mm, on average, weighed 9 kg more than those with less than 2 mm subsidence.
- With regard to age and activity level, Charnley was adamant that patients should be older than 65 (Charnley 1979), that they should not be employed in manual labor, and that the "principal motivation should not be to engage in sports" (Eftekhar 1993). This is clearly in stark contrast to many of today's opinions.

Activity Level

- In contrast to Charnley's original point of view about patient selection, THRs today are perceived by many patients and surgeons alike to be not only acceptable in heavier and younger patients but also, in some cases, even beneficial, as a means to continue to participate in sports and activities, particularly after total joint resurfacing. Some consider even extreme and high-impact sports acceptable (Bren 2004) (Box 1–25).
- The primary goal of total joint arthroplasty is to reestablish normal physiologic function in the patient. However, because the practice of engaging in extreme activities is

relatively new to joint replacement patients, its effects on long-term outcome are still unknown. Clearly, extreme activities such as running multiple marathons may represent major biomechanical risks to the stability and longevity of an artificial joint.

- Although case reports and anecdotal data have permeated the scientific and marketing literature, few studies have addressed the effects of extreme sports on outcome in large numbers of patients.
- In contrast to extreme sports, the effects of moderate activities have been the subject of several studies.
- Dubs and associates (1983) compared the clinical outcome of patients who underwent hip replacement and who actively participated in sports with the outcome in patients who did not. These investigators reported that after a mean of 6 years of follow-up, 1.6% of the active patients and 14.3% of the less active patients had undergone revision procedures for loosening.
- Ritter and Meding (1987) reported that low-impact sports, such as golfing and bowling, did not have a negative outcome after 3 years of follow-up. Such studies indicate that a certain amount of activity is not only acceptable but even necessary for optimum outcome in patients with joint replacement.

Weight

- According to the Centers for Disease Control and Prevention, approximately 30% of the adult population in the United States today is obese, a figure that has tripled since 1980.
- Crowninshield and associates (2006) reported that, compared with several decades ago, candidates for total joint replacement are nearly 20% heavier (Fig. 1–24).
- More important, for the general population, the body mass index (BMI) reaches a peak at 60 to 69 years of age, which is the most common age for total joint replacement.

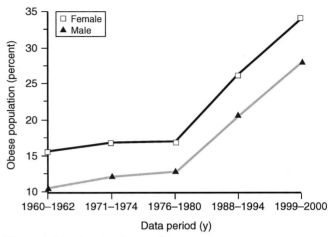

Figure 1–24: America is growing.
Changing demographics of patients with total joint replacement. (From Crowninshield RD, Rosenberg AG, Sporer SM. [2006]. Changing demographics of patients with total joint replacement. *Clin Orthop Relat Res* 443:266-272.

- Although most surgeons would agree that the risk of intraoperative complications is higher in heavier patients, the number of obese and overweight patients receiving total joint replacements, particularly total knee replacements (Wendelboe et al. 2003), continues to rise.
- Some surgeons believe, in agreement with Charnley, that total joint replacements should not be done in obese patients, not only because of the increased surgical risks but also because of the well-known greater risk of revision associated with obesity.
- A counterpoint view is that performing total joint replacement surgery allows the obese or overweight patient to return to a more active lifestyle, hence increasing the probability of losing weight and consequently reducing all the additional health risks associated with obesity. In practice, however, one study reported that only 18% of obese patients lose weight following total joint replacement surgery (Booth 2002), whereas other investigators reported that, by and large, patients gain weight following surgery, regardless of BMI (Heisel et al. 2005, Jain et al. 2003) (Box 1–26).
- The mechanism of failure of total joint replacements appears to vary depending on the patient's weight. Specifically, patients who are not overweight tend to be more active and therefore wear out the polyethylene components faster than overweight or obese patients (Foran et al. 2004).
- In contrast, obese patients are more sedentary, yet their increased weight produces higher stresses at the implant fixation interfaces, and within the polymethylmethacrylate cement in the case of cemented implants, thus leading to greater risk of aseptic loosening. Therefore, in these

patients, a common reason for revision is aseptic loosening (Foran et al. 2004).

Femoral Loads
Calculation of Loads on the Hip Joint: A Historical Review

- Numerous investigators have studied the loads and moments on the hip and knee joints under different activities.
- One of the earliest estimates of loads on the femur was made in 1935 by Pauwels, who, using dimensions he measured from patient radiographs, constructed a simplified free body diagram for single- and dual-legged stance, and the stance phase of gait, and, by applying static equilibrium, estimated forces on the proximal femur.
- In 1947, Inman introduced electromyography to address the separate contributions of the tensor fasciae femoris, gluteus medius, and gluteus minimus during a single-legged stance. Because the action potentials were generated in response to abducting muscles acting to maintain static equilibrium, Inman reasoned that these action potentials were proportional to the rotary force, or torque, about the axis of rotation, of the femoral head.
- Using the torque values converted from his electromyographic measurements in 35 patients, Inman estimated the joint reaction force during single-legged stance to be 2.4 to 2.6 times body weight, and at 19 to 30 degrees to the femoral axis, with a 1.4 to 1.9 times body weight abducting force.
- Additionally, Inman identified the ratio of muscle action during hip abduction for the gluteus medius (57%), gluteus minimus (29%), and tensor fasciae femoris (14%), according to muscle masses.
- The introduction of low-friction arthroplasty in 1959 by John Charnley made it more important than ever to advance the understanding of forces on the hip joint. In 1970, McLeish and Charnley used simultaneous radiography and muscle positions obtained from cadaver

dissections to improve on previous calculations by Inman.
- McLeish and Charnley (1970) stated that moments and forces in the hip are "subject to considerable variation due to spinal and limb movements which are, to quite a large extent, under voluntary control." Specifically, a difference in pelvic tilt (in the coronal plane) of 13.5 degrees could magnify (or divide) the moment about the hip by as much as three times.
- Paul's measurements of double-peak profiles of load on the hip and knee during each step of walking, with the first peak corresponding to heel strike and the second to toe-down, is commonly known as a *Paul curve.*
- Rydell measured the femoral head loads during a single-legged stance to be 2.3 to 2.8 times body weight

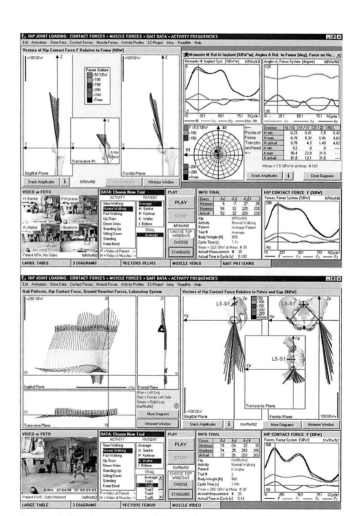

Figure 1–25: Instrumented femoral component data.
Data collected from instrumented femoral component indicating three directions of joint load reaction on the femoral ball, direction of the resultant vector as a function of stride, and its magnitude, and the laboratory setup for gait data collection. BW, body weight. (From Bergmann G, Deuretzbacher G, Heller M, et al. [2001]. Hip contact forces and gait patterns from routine activities. *J Biomech* 34:859-871.)

and approximately 3.0 times body weight during slow gait.

- Bergmann and associates (1993) conducted extensive studies to directly measure the reaction loads in the hip and other joints. They have widely published both hip and spine load profiles under various conditions and have an extensive biomechanics Web site to provide and share their data with the orthopaedic community (*http://www.medizin.fu-berlin.de/biomechanik/*) (Fig. 1–25).

Estimates of Joint Loads and Moments During Different Activities

- Table 1–12 summarizes measurements of hip joint reaction forces, and moments in the hip joint when reported, for a variety of activities. Direct measurements involve the use of an implant instrumented with a device such as a three-dimensional load cell in the femoral ball and perhaps a telemetry unit.

Table 1–12 Hip Joint Reaction Forces and Moments for Various Activities

AUTHORS	ACTIVITY	PEAK JOINT REACTION FORCE	PEAK JOINT MOMENT	NOTES
Pauwels 1935	Single-legged stance	4.0 × BW		
Inman 1947	Single-legged stance	2.4–2.6 × BW		
Rydell 1966	Single-legged stance	2.3–2.8 × BW		
	Slow walking	3.0 × BW		
Paul 1970	Slow walking	4.9 × BW		
	Normal walking	4.9 × BW		
	Fast walking	7.6 × BW		
	Stair climbing	7.2 × BW		
	Stair descent	7.1 × BW		
	Walking up ramp	5.9 × BW		
	Walking down ramp	5.1 × BW		
McLeish and Charnley 1970	Single-legged stance	1.8–2.7 × BW		
Bergmann et al. 1993	Walking, 1 km/hour	2.8 × BW		Measured directly using an instrumented, telemeterized, cemented THR
	Walking, 5 km/hour	4.8 × BW		
	Jogging	5.5 × BW		
	Stumbling	8.7 × BW		
Bergmann et al. 2001	Walking, 4 km/hour	2.4 × BW		
	Stair climbing	2.5 × BW		
	Stair descent	2.6 × BW		
Van den Bogert et al. 1999	Walking	2.5 × BW		
	Running	5.2 × BW		
	Skiing: long turn, flat	4.1 × BW		
	Skiing: short turn, steep	7.8 × BW		
	Skiing: cross-country, classic	4.0 × BW		
	Skiing: cross-country, skating	4.6 × BW		
	Skiing: mogul	8.3–12.4 × BW		
Stansfield et al. 2003	Slow walking	2.0 × BW		
	Fast walking	4.0 × BW		
	Single-legged stance	2.5–3.5 × BW		
	Rising from chair	2.0 × BW		
Stansfield et al. 2002	Walking: men with THR	3–7.5 × BW		
	Walking: men without THR	4.6–10.5 × BW		
	Walking: women without THR	4.3–10.2 × BW		
	Stair descent: men with THR	2.6–6.8 × BW		
	Stair descent: men without THR	3–9.7 × BW		
Nemeth et al. 1984	Lifting, straight knee	2.7 × BW	124 Nm	
	Lifting, flexed knee	3.2 × BW	82 Nm	
Ericson et al. 1986	Cycling: during flexion		34.3 Nm	
	Cycling: during extension		8.9 Nm	
Wretenberg et al. 1996	Deep-squat barbell power lift		324 Nm	4700 N knee F
Shelley et al. 1996	Stair climbing	6.0 × BW	60 Nm	34 degrees of flexion
Simonsen et al. 1995	Walking with 20-kg load	8.0 × BW		>14 × BW in two patients
Andriacchi et al. 1980	Stair climbing		124 Nm	
	Stair descent		113 Nm	

BW, body weight; Nm, newton-meter; THR, total hip replacement.

Figure 1–26: Walking speed. The effect of walking speed on the hip joint. ISO, International Standard Organization. (From Paul JP [1999]. Strength requirements for internal and external prostheses. *J Biomech* 32:381-393.)

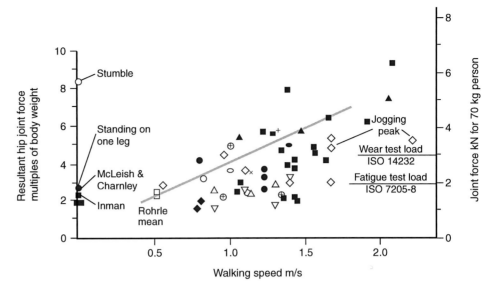

- By far, the more common methods are indirect, that is, three-dimensional motion analysis by high-speed cameras and the use of force plates. Table 1–12 includes data from studies using both methods.
- Considerable variation exists among the reported values, even for the same type of activities, such as walking. Despite the variation, some patterns come into view. For example, fast walking typically increases the peak load on the hip joint, as compared with loads during slow or normal walking. This increase is approximately twofold, increasing the peak joint reaction load in the hip to as much as 7.5 times body weight (Fig. 1–26).
- In some studies, climbing up stairs is associated with greater peak hip joint reaction loads and moments than level walking.
- Specifically, during level walking, peak torque about the shaft of the femur has been estimated at 10 to 15 Nm. In contrast, during stair climbing, the peak torque has been estimated at approximately 30 Nm or greater. The same joint reaction force, when acting at a greater angle from the coronal plane as a result of greater flexion, can produce greater axial torque on the femoral shaft.
- In many activities, as well as stair climbing, axial torques and flexion/extension and abduction/adduction moments have a greater role in producing high stresses than do joint reaction loads on the femoral head.
- In another study, the peak hip joint moment during deep-squat barbell power lifting was estimated at 324 Nm, two to three times greater than the high end of estimated joint moments during stair climbing (see Table 1–12).
- Perhaps the best example that highlights the importance of torque or moments is cycling. A healthy level of torque (34.3 Nm), although not excessive, is estimated in the hip joint during the flexion phase of cycling, when the pedal is being pushed, with lower torques during extension (8.9 Nm). Engaging the shoe with the pedal, either with cages or clips or with clipless attachments, will no doubt increase the torque during the extension phase of pedaling as well, thus providing a more efficient mechanism for the cyclist.
- With regard to the patient with a total joint replacement, even if extreme activity and sports are avoided following surgery, simple situations can apply great joint reaction loads and moments of the hip. For example, stumbling can apply loads as high as 8.7 times body weight on the hip. For a 100-kg man, 8.7 times body weight is equivalent to 8700 N, that is, nearly 2000 lb. Similarly, walking while carrying a 20-kg load is estimated to produce hip joint reaction loads as great as eight times body weight. To put these numbers into context, consider that loads of approximately 9000 N have been reported to cause femoral neck fracture, and loads of 10,000 N can cause implant failure.
- Extreme sports can involve unusual positions of the joint and high forces that place it at especially great risk of dislocation (Fig. 1–27).

Established Preclinical Testing Parameters
Fatigue Failure

- Engineering structures are designed such that anticipated loads on the structure never produce stresses that exceed the yield strength of the material from which the components of the structure are made because a single application of stress above the yield strength can cause failure.

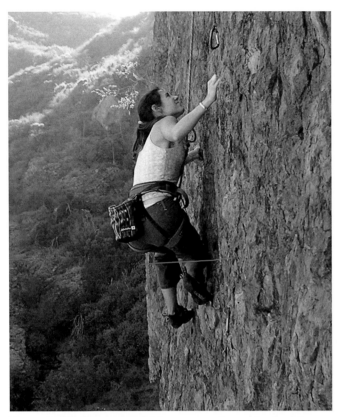

Figure 1–27: Extreme activities may produce risks for joint arthroplasty components.
The rock climber in this photograph would not be applying great joint reaction loads on the hip. However, the position of the legs would place a joint replacement at great risk of dislocation.

- Stresses below the yield strength, however, are still capable of producing material failure if they are applied with great enough frequency. This type of failure is called *fatigue failure*.
- Increasing the amplitude or peak stress closer to the failure strength of the material reduces the number of cycles before failure. In Figure 1–28, a small change in stress is associated with a great difference in cycles to failure because the horizontal axis is on a logarithmic scale (Box 1–27).
- Orthopaedic implants, by design, are at higher risk of fatigue failure than most engineering structures. This is because, in designing most implants, the goal is not only to minimize stresses in the implant but also to make the implant as flexible as possible such that stress shielding is minimized.
- Typically, although not always, making an implant stronger goes hand in hand with making it stiffer. Therefore, in making implants as flexible as possible, the designer accepts relatively large stresses in the implant.

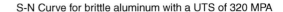

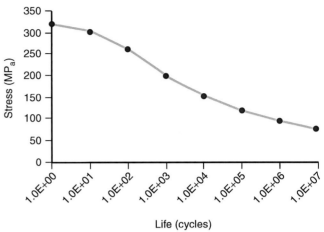

Figure 1–28: Fatigue failure.
Fatigue failure as a function of number of cycles (shown on the *x*-axis) and stress (shown on the *y*-axis), for aluminum with an ultimate tensile strength (UTS) of 320 MPa. As the peak stress of the cyclic loads is decreased, the number of cycles before fatigue failure increases. The *x*-axis is logarithmic.

In Vitro Testing

- Mechanical tests that are conducted to assess the safety and performance of a particular prosthesis before clinical use can be divided into two categories. First, the inherent strength of each implant needs to be tested to ensure that it is capable of withstanding the applied stresses without failure, that is, without fracture or plastic deformation.
- In the United States, the American Society for Testing Materials specifies the details of test methods to determine implant fatigue strength and other mechanical and material properties. Additionally, the International Standard Organization specifies such tests.
- The second type of in vitro mechanical testing of orthopaedic implants concerns measurement of stability of the implant within bone, under simulated physiological load (Ebramzadeh et al. 2004, Sangiorgio et al. 2004). It has long been established that mechanical stability of the total joint arthroplasty components is a major prerequisite for their successful long-term outcome (Ebramzadeh et al. 2003).

Box 1–27	Engineering of a Structure

- Assess the expected loads and moments.
- Calculate the stresses and strains within structure.
- Design for maximum strength or such that maximum stress is substantially below the yield strength of the material, or as follows:
$$\sigma_{max} << \sigma_y$$

- For both types of in vitro testing, most simulations have applied loads characteristic of a slender, elderly patient during routine activities such as slow walking or stair-climbing.
- In fact, the peak of the cyclic load of testing the inherent fatigue strength of femoral stems specified by both ASTM and ISO is in the range of 2300 to 3000 N. A load of 2300 N correspondends to less than three times body weight of an 80 kg person.
- By comparison, in the patient, most implants are subjected to much higher loads during other routine activities and exercises (see Table 1–12). Therefore, these tests may not be adequate to meet the expectations of patients today (see Box 1–25).
- More recently, some in vitro simulators have been designed to apply loads that are more representative of the current heavier, younger, and more active THR population (Sangiorgio et al. 2007).

Hip Implant Failure Modes and Reports

Loosening

- For more than 3 decades, aseptic loosening has been the leading reason for revision in THR, particularly for cemented components (Ebramzadeh et al. 2003).
- The National Swedish Hip Registry, published in 2002, reported that for the THRs performed in Sweden between 1979 and 2000, 75.3% of revisions were attributed to aseptic loosening (Malchau et al. 2002).
- *Loosening* is generally agreed to be a gradual process by which gaps open up between the stem and the cement, the cement and the bone, or the stem and the bone in the case of noncemented arthroplasty.
- Although it is generally accepted that aseptic loosening is the most common reason for implant failure, its causes remain subject to controversy. In the past, loosening was attributed to many factors, including the rigidity or flexibility of the femoral stem alloy, the presence or quality of the cement mantle, the lack of rotational stem stability, and stress risers created by sharp edges intended to improve rotational stability, as well as, of course, wear debris, that is, cement, metal, and polyethylene wear debris leading to osteolysis.
- Currently, most investigators accept that loosening is a multifactorial problem, which can be attributed to a combination of the following: (1) clinical factors, such as patient demographics (e.g., age, weight, gender, and activity level) and surgical technique and experience; (2) mechanical factors, such as femoral stem design (e.g., implant geometry, alloy, metal stiffness and strength, and surface finish), and cement mantle thickness; and (3) biologic factors, particularly osteolysis, as an immunologic response to polyethylene, metal, and cement wear debris, or as bone remodeling in response to stress shielding.

Periprosthetic Bone Fractures

- Although periprosthetic bone fractures form a relatively small percentage of failures in total joint replacements, they present the patient and clinician with serious and unique challenges and are therefore of great clinical significance.
- These fractures occur as a result of trauma and require extensive reconstructive surgery for repair. They may or may not involve implant fracture or failure (Box 1–28).
- In 2002, the Swedish National Hip Registry reported that 5.1% of revisions of THRs were for periprosthetic bone fractures. In contrast, in 2005, the Australian Orthopaedic Association National Joint Replacement Registry reported that 8.4% of revisions between 1999 and 2004 were for periprosthetic bone fractures, approximately double the rate by some northern European registries.

Implant Fractures

- In the 1970s and early 1980s, implant fractures were considered a major cause for concern with the original Charnley and other femoral stem designs. These fractures were reported after medium to long-term follow-up and were therefore clearly fatigue failures. Some resulted from poor alloys and inadequate quality control or manufacturing, whereas others could be attributed to design issues such as sharp corners that acted as stress risers.
- Today, with the advent of better manufacturing technology and quality control, many consider the problem of implant fracture a thing of the past. The Danish National Registry report of 2000 indicates that 4% of revisions were for implant fractures, whereas the Australian, Finnish, and Swedish national registries report slightly lower incidence, at 3%, 2%, and 1.5%, of all revisions, respectively (Box 1–29).
- In the United States, although there is no national registry, a 1995 multicenter study, in which 47% of the membership of the American Association of Hip and Knee Surgeons responded to an implant- and device-related failure survey, reported that 172 of 64,483 femoral stems included in the study had fractured (0.27%) (Heck et al. 1995).

Box 1–28	Periprosthetic Bone Fractures
• Swedish registry	5.1% of failures
• Australian registry	8.4%
• Finnish registry	4.0%
• Norwegian registry	3.9%
• Danish registry	4.6%
• Greater incidence with noncemented stems than with cemented stems	
• Aggressive reaming? Stiffness mismatch?	

Box 1–29	Implant Fracture Failures	
• Danish registry		4.0% of failures
• Australian registry		3.0%
• Finnish registry		2.0%
• Swedish registry		1.5%
• United States		?
• Heck et al. 1995 AAHKS survey		
• 64,483 femoral stems included in study		
• 27/10,000 stem fractures		
• 3.2% of failures from implant fracture		

- The most common device-related failure was failure of the polyethylene, defined as wear through or fracture of the polyethylene component, observed in 0.29% of metal-backed acetabular components and in 2.39% of all-polyethylene components, and an additional 0.15% of polyethylene liner disassociations in modular acetabular components. Ceramic ball fractures were seen in 0.22% of cases. In all, 3.2% of revisions were for implant failure.

Total Surface Replacements

- Designs of total surface replacements in the 1970s and 1980s produced poor outcomes, which were attributed predominantly to polyethylene wear.
- Excessive polyethylene wear and its fatigue failure were common with these designs because, to accommodate the larger femoral ball and to minimize bone removal from the acetabulum, the acetabular components were thin.
- Modern total surface replacements have metal-on-metal bearing surfaces. Compared with MOM articulations

from the 1960s, and based on decades of advances in materials and manufacturing technology and quality control, these implants have improved mechanical properties, including better sphericity, controlled clearance, and smoother, more highly polished surface finishes. Early clinical results with metal-on-metal surface replacements have been reported by Amstutz and colleagues (2004).

- In laboratory joint simulator studies, these improvements have been shown to reduce wear compared with older designs.
- Additionally, these improvements allow the use of larger balls, which offer greater range of motion and a lower risk of dislocation, while still using smaller acetabular components because there is no need to accommodate the extra thickness of a polyethylene liner.
- Total surface replacements with hybrid fixation, that is, a cemented femoral component and a porous ingrowth metal acetabular component, have provided more promising results in early to midterm follow-up. With these implants, the most commonly reported modes of failure are femoral neck fracture and aseptic loosening of the femoral component (Beaulé et al. 2004).
- The largest study to report contemporary total surface replacement outcome is, by far, the Australian Orthopaedic Association National Joint Replacement Registry. In the 2005 report, surface replacements were separated from conventional joint replacements because of their increasing popularity.
- Of the 5379 surface replacements implanted in Australia between 1999 and 2005, the overall rate of revision was 2.2%, as compared with 1.9% for the 65,992 conventional THRs performed during the same time period. Of the

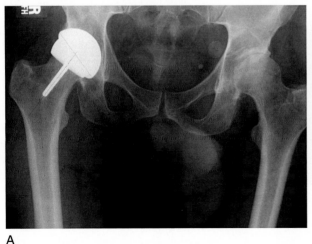

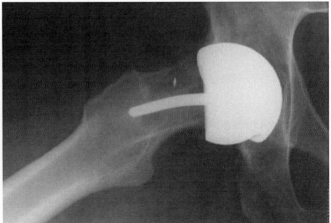

A   B

Figure 1–29: Femoral neck fracture.
The patient was a 53-year-old man with osteoarthritis. **A,** Postoperative view at 3 months. **B,** Femoral neck fracture 5 months after resurfacing. The patient had been doing single knee bends for exercise.

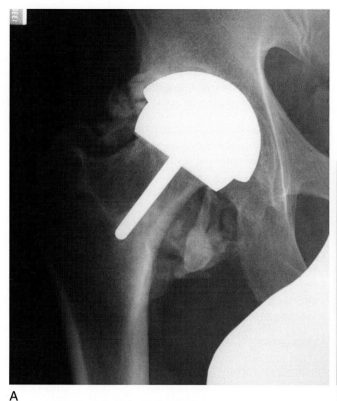

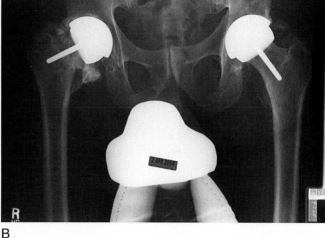

A   B

Figure 1–30: Femoral component loosening.
This 66-year-old man with osteoarthritis weighed 68 kg and was a half-marathon runner. The femoral component loosened 65 months after resurfacing. The patient had a femoral metaphyseal stem radiolucency 38 months after surgery. **A,** Early postoperative view (13 months). **B,** Loose femoral component on the right hip.

surface replacements that were revised, more than half (59%) failed because of catastrophic femoral neck fracture.

- Figures 1–29 and 1–30 demonstrate examples of femoral neck fracture and femoral component loosening, respectively, in two highly active patients with surface replacements.
- Today, it is clear that, as with conventional THRs, fixation of the acetabular component by noncemented porous ingrowth provides successful outcome. However, with total surface replacements, the fixation of the femoral component and the risk of femoral neck fracture need to be addressed further.
- In the Australian Orthopaedic Association National Joint Replacement Registry, although 70% of the patients who had surface replacements were male, the risk of failure for women was twice that for men.
- Additionally, for women older than 55 years and for men older than 65 years, the risk of revision is more than double that of men younger than 65 years old. This trend is not consistent with conventional THR, in which women typically have better outcomes than men, and 65 years is considered to be an optimal age for the patient. Beaulé et al. (2004) also reported that, contrary to conventional THR patients, heavier patients have a more successful outcome than lighter patients when surface replacements are used.

References

Amstutz HC, Beaule PE, Dorey FJ, et al. (2004). Metal-on-metal hybrid surface arthroplasty: Two to six-year follow-up study. *J Bone Joint Surg* 86:28-39.

> This is a clinical follow-up study of 400 metal-on-metal surface arthroplasties with cemented femoral components and uncemented acetabular components. Most of the patients in the study were highly active; their average age was 48 years. The authors drew attention to the importance of patient selection and reported that women and patients with femoral head cysts had less successful results.

Andriacchi TP, Andersson GB, Fermier RW, et al. (1980). A study of lower-limb mechanics during stair-climbing. *J Bone Joint Surg Am* 62:749-757.

Beaulé PE, Dorey FJ, LeDuff M, et al. (2004). Risk factors affecting outcome of metal-on-metal surface arthroplasty of the hip. *Clin Orthop Relat Res* 418:87-93.

> This is a follow-up of 119 patients younger than 40 years of age (mean, 34 years) with hybrid metal-on-metal surface arthroplasty. This article introduced a surface arthroplasty risk index and compared it with a conventional THR risk index for younger patients. Specifically, although patients who weighed more than 82 kg were at greater risk of failure using conventional THR, patients who weighed less than 82 kg were at twice the risk of failure using surface arthroplasty.

Bergmann GF, Deuretzbacher G, Heller M, et al. (2001). Hip contact forces and gait patterns from routine activities. *J Biomech* 34:859-871.

The authors described the design of the instrumented prosthesis for in vivo measurement of loads on the hip joint of patients during various activities. They also reported the magnitudes and directions of typical walking and stair-climbing loads, representative of the predominant daily physiologic loading conditions.

Bergmann G, Graichen F, Rohlmann A (1993). Hip joint loading during walking and running, measured in two patients. *J Biomech* 26:969-990.

Booth RE Jr (2002). Total knee arthroplasty in the obese patient: Tips and quips. *J Arthroplasty* 17(4 Suppl 1):69-70.

18% of obese patients were reported to achieve or maintain a significant weight reduction after total knee arthroplasty. However, the author reported that obese patients were the "least complaining and most satisfied" of total knee replacement patients.

Bren L (March-April 2004). *Joint Replacement: An Inside Look.* FDA Consumer Magazine, Pub No. FDA 04-1335C.

The author provides an overview of total hip and knee replacement as well as total surface replacement for the lay reader. Some of the key concerns in total joint replacement are outlined. Additionally, the patient's demands to return to high-impact activities after joint replacement are described.

Charnley J (1979). *Low Friction Arthroplasty of the Hip Theory of Practice.* New York: Springer-Verlag.

Many of Charnley's original articles are now available online, but this book is an excellent summary of his work with low friction arthroplasty. His clinical observations, surgical techniques, implant design rationale, and in vitro studies are summarized. Although some may regard this as outdated, Charnley's vision, insight, and conclusions are still very relevant today.

Crowninshield RD, Rosenberg AG, Sporer SM (2006). Changing demographics of patients with total joint replacement. *Clin Orthop Relat Res* 443:266-272.

This is a summary of the changes in the demographics of the population in the United States over the past 40 years. The authors reported that total joint replacement patients today are 20% heavier, more physically active, and live 25% longer than patients 40 years ago. The authors also reported that the number of TKRs performed annually is increasing at a faster rate than the number of THRs, which is likely due to the stronger correlation between obesity and knee arthritis and the increasing number of obese patients. The authors also reported that more women (60%) have total joint replacement annually than men (40%).

Dubs L, Gschwend N, Munzinger U (1983). Sport after total hip arthroplasty. *Arch Orthop Trauma Surg* 101:161-169.

This is a clinical study that examines the effect of sports on the outcome of cemented total hip arthroplasty at a mean follow-up of 5.8 years. There were 110 patients in the study, 78% of whom were active in sports. Of that active group, there was a 1.6% revision rate, compared with a 14% revision rate for the inactive group. Based on their findings, the authors recommended that non-contact sports be allowed following THR. Specifically, the authors recommended swimming, cycling, rowing, and walking in the first 6 postoperative months, allowing tennis, jogging, cross-country skiing, and hiking after that, but no contact sports.

Ebramzadeh E, Sangiorgio SN, Longjohn DB, et al. (2004). Initial stability of cemented femoral stems as a function of surface finish, collar, and stem size. *J Bone Joint Surg* 86:106-115.

The initial stability of eight otherwise identical stem-types, differing systematically in surface finish, size (small or large), and the presence or lack of a cement collar, were compared using an in vitro proximal femoral load simulator. The authors applied an alternating walking and stair-climbing load profile with a peak load of 1500 N during walking cycles and a peak torque about the femoral shaft of 23 Nm during stair-climbing cycles. Motions were quantified three ways: (1) per-cycle motion, (2) total motion throughout loading (in migration), and (3) rate of migration. These values were determined for the stem-cement interface and the bone-cement interface and compared for each of the eight stem-types to determine the relative importance of each of the three design parameters. Overall, surface roughness had the greatest influence on stability, followed by stem size, with the presence or lack of a collar having the smallest relative effect.

Ebramzadeh E, Normand PL, Sangiorgio SN, et al. (2003). Long-term radiographic changes in cemented total hip arthroplasty with six designs of femoral components. *Biomaterials* 24:3351-3363.

This study reported strong correlations between femoral stem stiffness and radiographic outcome over 30 years of follow-up. The radiographic parameters of looseness were assessed for more than 800 patients, each with one of six stem-types (three stainless steel and three titanium alloy designs) varying in cross-sectional rigidity. The relationships between stem stiffness (due to metal alloy and cross-sectional area) and aseptic loosening, stem–cement radiolucency, bone–cement radiolucency, and calcar resorption, for example, were depicted using survivorship analysis.

Eftekhar N (1993). *Total Hip Arthroplasty.* St. Louis: Mosby-Year Book.

This two-volume book is a collection of information on many aspects of total hip arthroplasty. The author covers history, biomechanics, surgical approaches and techniques, and clinical outcome data and examples collected over many years.

Ericson MO, Bratt A, Nisell R, et al. (1986). Load moments about the hip and knee joints during ergometer cycling. *Scand J Rehabil Med* 18:165-172.

Foran JR, Mont MA, Etienne G, et al. (2004). The outcome of total knee arthroplasty in obese patients. *J Bone Joint Surg Am* 86:1609-1615.

This is a clinical follow-up study that compared the 15-year TKA outcome for matched groups of obese versus non-obese patients. The authors reported that the rate of revision for the obese group was three times higher than that of the non-obese group but that the modes of loosening varied. Specifically, the obese group had a higher rate of aseptic loosening and the non-obese group had a greater risk of accelerated polyethylene liner wear.

Griffiths WE, Swanson SA, Freeman MA (1971). Experimental fatigue of the human cadaveric femoral neck. *J Bone Joint Surg Br* 53:136-143.

Heck DA, Partridge CM, Ruben JD, et al. (1995). Prosthetic component failures in hip arthroplasty surgery. *J Arthrop* 10:575-580.

This article is the result of a survey conducted by the American Association of Hip and Knee Surgeons to determine the members' experience with device failures; 47% of the members participated and reported their results for more than 60,000 arthroplasties in a 5-year period. Complete polyethylene failure for metal-backed shells was reported for 0.29%, and failure of all-polyethylene components had a higher risk of failure of 2.39%. Stem fractures occurred at a rate of 0.27%, and cement ball fractures occurred at a rate of 0.22%. Because no national joint registry exists in the United States, this survey provides the best indication of the risks of device failures in the United States in contemporary THR.

Heisel C, Silva M, dela Rosa MA, et al. (2005). The effects of lower-extremity total joint replacement for arthritis on obesity. *Orthopedics* 28:157-159.

This prospective study investigated the weight change in 100 total joint replacement patients at a minimum of 1-year postoperatively. The patients received total knee replacements ($N = 45$), conventional THRs ($N = 36$), or surface replacement of the hip ($N = 19$). The surface replacement patients were younger (mean, 13 years) than the conventional THR patients. The results indicated that younger patients gained a significant amount of weight after surgery (mean, 3.2 kg), while the older, conventional THR patients did not. Further, the patients who had "normal" or "obese" BMI classifications preoperatively did not lose weight, but those classified as "overweight" before surgery gained a significant amount of weight postoperatively (mean, 3.6 kg). Overall, the authors suggested that the rationale that the weight was a result of the pain, and pain loss would result in weight loss, may not be true.

Inman V (1947). Functional aspects of the abductor muscles of the hip. *J Bone Joint Surg* 29:607-619.

Jain SA, Roach RT, Travlos J (2003). Changes in body mass index following primary elective total hip arthroplasty. Correlation with outcome at 2 years. *Acta Orthop Belg* 69:421-425.

The authors conducted a retrospective clinical study to determine if BMI increased after THR. They compared the preoperative BMI to the BMI at a minimum of 2 years postoperatively. They concluded that there was an average weight gain of 2.5% and BMI increase of 2.1% but that no correlation existed between weight gain and patient satisfaction.

Malchau H, Herberts P, Eisler T, et al. (2002). The Swedish Total Hip Replacement Register. *J Bone Joint Surg Am* 84(Suppl 2):2-20.

This is the Swedish national joint registry, one of the largest and most thorough total joint replacement registries in the literature. The multicenter clinical outcome is presented in many ways, including by stem-type, cemented versus uncemented, hospital type (e.g., rural versus university), and age. The number of implants and the percentage of patients with unrevised replacements at given intervals of follow-up are presented for the most common implants. Additionally, the most common reasons for revision are presented. In addition to this registry, the Finnish, Danish, Norwegian, and Australian registries, for example, can also be found in the literature or online for comparison.

McLeish R, Charnley J (1970). Abduction forces in the one-legged stance. *J Biomech* 3:191-209.

Nemeth G, Ekholm J, Arborelius UP (1984). Hip load moments and muscular activity during lifting. *Scand J Rehabil Med* 16:103-111.

Paul JP (1970). The effect of walking speed on the force actions transmitted at the hip and knee joints. *Proc R Soc Med* 63:200-202.

Paul JP (1999). Strength requirements for internal and external prostheses. *J Biomech* 32:381-393.

The author has numerous publications on gait analysis and joint reaction forces, but this is an excellent review of both his work and the work of others, with regard to load measurements and calculations at the hip and knee. The author provides summary charts of loads reported by himself and others for walking at various speeds, joint load as a function of stride length, and different versions of the Paul curve. Additionally, current implant testing standards are described.

Pauwels F, ed. (1935). *Der Schenkelhalsbruck, ein Mechanisches Problem.* Stuttgart, Germany, Perdinand Enke.

Ritter MA, Meding JB (1987). Total hip arthroplasty. Can the patient play sports again? *Orthopedics* 10:1447-1452.

In this study, a questionnaire was sent to patients with a minimum of 3 years of follow-up, to list the type, degree, and frequency of sports participation before and after surgery and any problems encountered upon returning to a sport after surgery. The authors concluded that there was a significant decrease in all forms of activity after surgery except bicycling, but most patients who were active preoperatively remained active afterward. These investigators reported that activities such as walking, golfing, and bowling had no influence (good or bad) on the outcome of the surgery.

Rydell N (1966). Forces acting on the femoral head-prosthesis. *Acta Orthop Scand* 88(Suppl):1-132.

Sangiorgio SN, Ebramzadeh E, Longjohn DB, et al. (2004). Effects of dorsal flanges on fixation of a cemented total hip replacement femoral stem. *J Bone Joint Surg Am* 86:813-820.

In this study, the authors compared the in vitro stability of otherwise identical straight cemented femoral stems with and without flanges, in two stem sizes, under dynamic physiological loading simulating walking and stair-climbing activities. The authors reported that flanges increased the stability within the cement mantle, but decreased the stability at the bone-cement interface. That is, non-flanged stems were less stable at the stem-cement interface, but more stable at the bone-cement interface than flanged stems.

Sangiorgio SN, Longjohn DB, Dorr LD, et al. (In press). Simulations of loads on the proximal femur: The introduction of a new simulator. *J Appl Biomat Biomech.*

This article provides a review of the literature and current controversies and issues in femoral stem stability testing. Additionally, a new in vitro femoral load simulator that applies higher loads (peak loads: joint reaction: 3500 N; torque: 24 Nm: abductor muscle: 1500 N) through a dynamic alternating walking and stair-climbing load profile is described in detail. Results of preliminary studies comparing the stability measurements using this simulator to that of a previously published simulator, for an identical stem-type are provided.

Shelley FJ, Anderson DD, Kolar MJ, et al. (1996). Physical modelling of hip joint forces in stair climbing. *Proc Inst Mech Eng* [H] 210:65-68.

Simonsen EB, Dyhre-Poulsen P, Voigt M, et al. (1995). Bone-on-bone forces during loaded and unloaded walking. *Acta Anat* (Basel) 152:133-142.

Stansfield BW, Nicol AC (2002). Hip joint contact forces in normal subjects and subjects with total hip prostheses: Walking and stair and ramp negotiation. *Clin Biomech* (Bristol, Avon) 17:130-139.

Stansfield BW, Nicol AC, Paul JP, et al. (2003). Direct comparison of calculated hip joint contact forces with those measured using instrumented implants. An evaluation of a three-dimensional mathematical model of the lower limb. *J Biomech* 36:929-936.

van den Bogert AJ, Read L, Nigg BM (1999). An analysis of hip joint loading during walking, running, and skiing. *Med Sci Sports Exerc* 31:131-142.

Wendelboe A, Hegmann K, Biggs JJ, et al. (2003). Relationships between body mass indices and surgical replacements of knee and hip joints. *Am J Prev Med* 25:290-295.

This frequency-matched case-control study compared 1751 patients who underwent total joint replacement between the ages of 55 and 74 with randomly matched patients who were enrolled in a cancer screening trial. The results indicated that for men, a BMI of 37.5–40 made them 9 times more likely to have a THR and 16 times more likely to have a total knee replacement. For women, a BMI = 40 made them 4 times more likely to have a THR, but 19 times more likely to have a total knee replacement. The authors concluded that while they found links between total joint replacement and obesity, they could not conclude that obesity conferred an independent risk for total joint replacement.

Wretenberg P, Nemeth G, Lamontagne M, et al. (1996). Passive knee muscle moment arms measured in vivo with MRI. *Clin Biomech* (Bristol, Avon) 11:439-446.

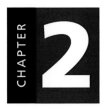

Joint Kinematics and Biomechanics of the Hip and Knee

Craig L. Israelite,* Brian Vannozzi,† Brent Wiesel,‡ and Lisa Khoury§

*MD, Co-Director of Knee Service and Assistant Professor, Department of Orthopaedic Surgery, University of Pennsylvania School of Medicine, Philadelphia, PA
†MD, Resident, Department of Orthopaedic Surgery, Hospital of the University of Pennsylvania, Philadelphia, PA
‡MD, Resident, Department of Orthopaedic Surgery, Hospital of the University of Pennsylvania, Philadelphia, PA
§MD, Resident, Department of Orthopaedic Surgery, Hospital of the University of Pennsylvania, Philadelphia, PA

Definitions

- *Kinematics:* The study of motion without regard to the cause of the motion
- *Kinesiology:* The study of human motion
- *Biomechanics:* The science of the action of forces on the living body
- *Degrees of freedom:* Joint motion described based on rotation and translation in the *x, y,* and *z* planes; therefore *six* positions, or degrees of freedom, used to describe motion
- *Joint reaction force (JRF):* The force generated within a joint in response to external forces

Hip Biomechanics

Hip Joint

- The hip joint is one of the largest and most stable joints in the body. Unlike the knee, the hip has intrinsic stability, largely based on the rigid constraint of the deep-seated ball-and-socket design.
- The extensive mobility about the hip (Table 2–1) allows for the performance of daily activities, such as walking, sitting, squatting, and stair climbing (Table 2–2).
- Large amounts of force, sometimes several times body weight, cross the hip joint repeatedly during everyday activities, and this "wear and tear" can lead to derangements of the hip and, ultimately, degenerative arthritis.

- An understanding of the anatomy and biomechanics of the native hip provides insight into the rational design and placement of a total hip arthroplasty (THA) that can be expected to function in a manner similar to that of the native joint for a sustained period of time.
- Abnormal anatomic relationships result in increased rates of degenerative joint destruction, for example, developmental dysplasia of the hip, limb-length inequalities, and neuromuscular disorders.

Anatomy

- The *acetabulum,* the concave component of the ball-and-socket joint, is covered with articular cartilage that

Table 2–1	Average Hip Range of Motion (From Physical Examination)	
MOTION	**AVERAGE RANGE (DEGREES)**
Flexion	140
Extension	30
Abduction	50
Adduction	25
Internal rotation	70
External rotation	90

From Nordin M, Frankel VH (2001). Biomechanics of the hip. In: Nordin M, Frankel VH, eds. *Basic Biomechanics of the Musculoskeletal System,* 2nd ed. Philadelphia: Lippincott Williams & Wilkins, pp 202-221.

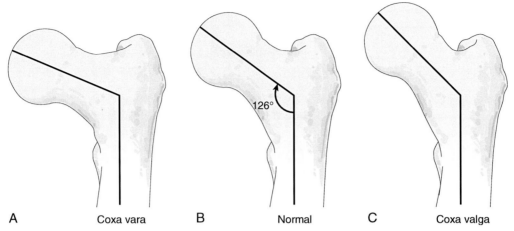

Figure 2–1: Femoral neck-shaft angle.
This angle is formed by the intersection of lines parallel to the femoral neck and femoral shaft. **A,** Coxa vara. **B,** Normal angle. **C,** Coxa valga.

thickens peripherally and predominately laterally and is deepened by a flat rim of fibrocartilage called the *labrum*.

- The labrum allows for increased stability and range of motion (ROM), and if pathologic, it can be a source of pain.
- The *femoral head* is the convex component of the hip, forms two thirds of a sphere, and is covered by articular cartilage that is thickest at the central and medial surface and extends beyond the confines of the acetabular socket.
- The *femoral neck* has two crucial angular relationships with the femoral shaft (Radin 1980):

  1. The neck-shaft angle (normally ~126 degrees)
  2. The angle of anteversion (normally ~15 degrees) (Figs. 2–1 and 2–2)

Motion

- The hip is a spheroidal, or ball-and-socket–type, diarthrodial joint. Motion about the hip occurs in several planes, including flexion/extension, abduction/adduction, and internal/external rotation (Fig. 2–3).

Joint Forces

- Muscle contractions about a joint are the major contributing factors to the JRF. High JRFs correspond with a predisposition to degenerative changes.

Table 2–2	Mean Values for Maximum Hip Motion in Three Planes During Common Activities	
ACTIVITY	**PLANE OF MOTION**	**RECORDED VALUE (DEGREES)**
Tying shoe with foot on floor	Sagittal	124
	Frontal	19
	transverse	15
Tying shoe with foot across opposite thigh	Sagittal	110
	Frontal	23
	transverse	33
Sitting down on chair and rising from sitting	Sagittal	104
	Frontal	20
	transverse	17
Stopping to obtain object from floor	Sagittal	117
	Frontal	21
	transverse	18
Squatting	Sagittal	122
	Frontal	28
	transverse	26
Ascending stairs	Sagittal	67
	Frontal	16
	transverse	18
Descending stairs	Sagittal	36

From Johnson RC, Smidt GL (1970). Hip motion measurements for selected activities of daily living. *Clin Orthop Relat Res* 72:205-215.

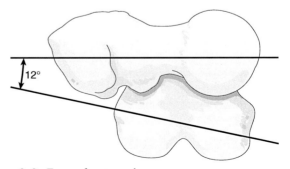

Figure 2–2: Femoral anteversion.
This angle is formed by the intersection of the long axis of the femoral head and the transverse axis of the femoral condyles.

Figure 2–3: Planes of motion about the hip.

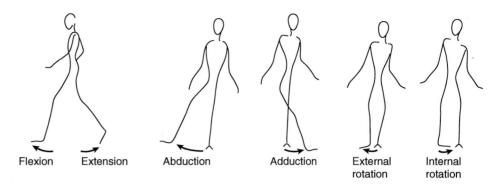

| Flexion | Extension | Abduction | Adduction | External rotation | Internal rotation |

- Based on their primary actions, muscles of the hip joint can be divided into several groups:
  - *Hip flexors:* Psoas, iliacus, rectus femoris, tensor fasciae latae
  - *Hip extensor:* Biceps femoris, semitendinosus, semimembranosus, gluteus maximus
  - *Hip abductors/internal rotators:* Gluteus medius and gluteus minimus
  - *Hip adductors:* Adductors longus, brevis, and magnus and gracilis
  - *Hip external rotators:* Piriformis, quadratus femoris, superior/inferior gemelli, and obturator internus/externus
- Because the hip is stable, when one is standing on two legs an erect posture can be achieved without muscle contraction through the stabilizing effect of the joint capsule and ligaments. Assuming no muscle contraction to maintain an upright position or to prevent swaying, the JRF at the hip can be easily estimated. Each leg is approximately one sixth of the body weight, leaving two thirds of body weight crossing the hips, which when divided equally between both legs leaves a *JRF force at the hip of one-third body weight when one is in a quiet standing position.*
- When a person changes from a two-leg to a one-leg stance, the center of gravity shifts, thus producing moments around the hip joint that must be counteracted by muscle contraction and therefore greatly increasing the JRF. This JRF in the hip can reach three to six times body weight, primarily because of contraction of the abductor muscles that cross the hip (Nordin and Frankel 2001). This effect can be demonstrated with a free body diagram (Fig. 2–4).
- The center of rotation of the hip joint, and therefore the moment arms of the abductors (A) and body weight (B), is an important determinant of JRFs. It can be shown that *decreasing the ratio of A to B would decrease the JRF.* Examples of decreasing this ratio include medialization of the acetabulum during a THA, use of a long-neck prosthesis during a THA, and lateralization of the greater trochanter.
- People with weak hip abductors or a painful hip usually lean toward the affected side, a gait called an *abductor gait*

or *Trendelenburg's gait.* This lean toward the affected side shifts the center of gravity of the body closer to the hip joint and therefore reduces the rotational force exerted by body weight by decreasing its moment arm. This change, in turn, decreases the abductor forces needed to stabilize the pelvis and thus reduces the JRFs across the hip. *Therefore, Trendelenburg's gait reduces both the JRF and abductor moment when one leans over the affected side.*
- The abductor gait or *Trendelenburg's gait secondary to hip pain can be corrected more effectively with a walking stick held in*

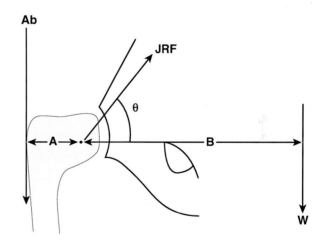

Assume A = 5 and B = 12.5

ΣM = 0 (Sum of moments = 0)
−5 Ab(y) + 12.5W = 0
Ab(y) = 2.5

ΣF(y) = 0 (Sum of forces = 0)
−Ab(y)− W + JRF(y) = 0
JRF(y) = 3.5W
JRF = JRF(y)/(cos 30 deg)
JRF = 4W (approx)

Therefore, the joint reaction force across the hip during one leg stance is approx 4x body weight.

Figure 2–4: Joint reaction force for single-leg stance. *A,* abductor moment arm; *Ab,* abductor force; *B,* moment arm of body weight; *JRF,* magnitude joint reaction force; *W,* body weight; *θ,* direction.

the contralateral hand because it is desirable to increase the moment arm of the aiding force, which decreases the JRFs across the painful hip (Fig. 2–5).

- *Trendelenburg's sign is positive* (i.e., weakness of the ipsilateral abductors) when the patient is unable to maintain a level pelvis while lifting the contralateral leg during standing.
- Weakness of the hip abductors may be a source of instability during hip replacement surgery.
- Injury to the superior gluteal nerve (~5 cm above the greater trochanter) can be an iatrogenic cause for abductor weakness or instability.

Total Hip Arthroplasty

- The femoral stem component rigidity is directly related to stem length and diameter: using a longer stem or increasing the stem diameter increases the *rigidity* of the femoral component.
- *Rigidity of a three-dimensional structure* is defined as the slope of the load–deformation curve, constructed similarly to a stress–strain curve, and for a *cylinder is proportional to the radius to the fourth* (r^4).

- The slope of the stress-strain curve, known as *Young's modulus of elasticity (E)*, is a measure of the stiffness of a material, or its ability to resist deformation.
- All current femoral components have higher Young's modulus than the corresponding bone and therefore lead to stress shielding (stainless steel > cobalt-chromium alloy > titanium > cortical bone > polymethylmethacrylate [bone cement] > cancellous bone > cartilage).
- *The femoral component should be in neutral or slight valgus to* decrease moment arm, cement stress (if cemented), and abductor length (Fig. 2–6).
- Increasing femoral component offset increases the abductor attachment moment arm, and this decreases the magnitude of abductor force necessary for normal gait and thereby decreases the JRF (Fig. 2–7).
- The mechanical ability of the abductors is affected by the neck-shaft angle, the neck length, and the joint center position, all of which are frequently altered during a THA.
- *Decreasing the neck-shaft angle (varus hip) enhances the mechanical advantage of the abductors* by increasing the moment arm and therefore decreasing the JRF.

Using a walking stick: how it reduces JRF

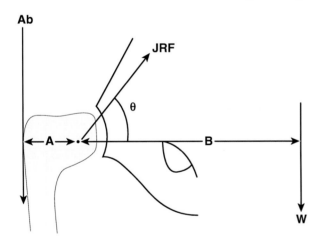 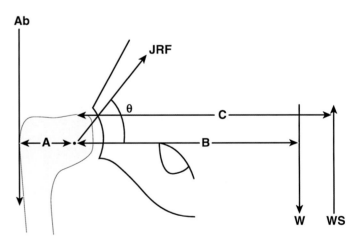

Simplistically
In equilibrium sum of moments = 0

Without Stick	With Stick
Ab!A=W!B	(Ab!A)+(WS!C)=W!B
Ab=(W!B) / A	Ab=[(W!B)-(WS!C)] / A

(WS x C) is a positive number, therefore numerator will be smaller, therefore Ab (the force required by the abductors) is smaller if a stick is used.

As C (the walking stick's moment arm) becomes larger, Ab, (the force required by the abductors) becomes smaller, **therefore a walking stick in the hand furthest away from the hip is most effective.**

In equilibrium, the sum of the forces in the Y plane=0

Without Stick	With Stick
JRF sin θ=Ab+W	JRF sin θ+WS=Ab+W
	JRF sin θ=Ab+W-WS

Therefore JRF is less when a walking stick is used. Not only is Abductor force smaller, but the upward force exerted by the stick reduces the joint reaction forces further.

Figure 2–5: On which side should you use a walking stick?
A, abductor moment arm; *Ab,* abductor force; *B,* moment arm of body weight; *C,* moment arm for walking stick; *JRF,* magnitude joint reaction force; *W,* body weight; *WS,* walking stick force; *θ,* direction.

Figure 2–6: Positions for a total hip arthroplasty. **A,** Varus position. **B,** Neutral position. **C,** Valgus position.

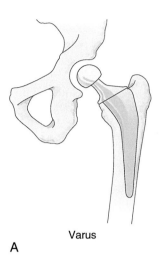
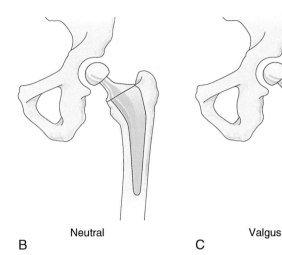

Varus

A

Neutral

B

Valgus

C

- Restoration of the hip center to as near normal as possible is paramount. Otherwise, joint instability, increased JRFs, and limb-length inequalities may result.
- Alteration in the hip center can have large effects on muscular moments around the hip and on the resultant hip reaction forces. With experimental and analytical models, *predicted joint forces were minimized when the joint center was moved medially, inferiorly, and anteriorly* (Doehring et al. 1996). This maximized the moment-generating capacity of the abductors and moved the hip center close to the line of action of the foot-floor reaction force.
- Large joint forces are predicted for hip centers that are superior, lateral, and posterior compared with the native location.
- *Medializing* the acetabular component, while decreasing the JRF, may increase hip instability if the center of hip rotation is not maintained.
- Conversely, *lateralizing* the acetabular component may increase joint stability but at the expense of increasing the JRF (Blaha 1993).

Hip Arthrodesis (Beaule et al. 2002)

- The basis for the positioning of the limb during hip arthrodesis is ultimately the ability of the contiguous joints to accommodate for the motion necessary for daily activities.
- Positioning can have a profound effect on energy expenditure, early satisfaction, and ultimate durability of the hip fusion.
- Investigators have reported that the optimal position for hip fusion is between 20 and 30 degrees of hip flexion, 5 and 7 degrees of adduction, and 5 and 10 degrees of external rotation.

Knee Biomechanics
Introduction

- Unlike in the hip, the bony surfaces of the knee are relatively incongruent. The soft tissue structures therefore play a crucial role in maintaining stability by resisting the complex forces acting across the joint.
- It is imperative that the surgeon be aware of the normal alignment of the lower extremity, the forces acting across

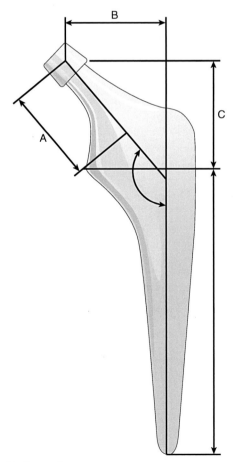

Figure 2–7: Femoral component measurement. Neck length *(A)*, stem offset *(B)*, and neck height *(C)*.

Table 2–3	Range of Tibiofemoral Joint Motion in the Sagittal Plane During Common Activities
ACTIVITY	**RANGE OF MOTION FROM KNEE EXTENSION TO FLEXION (DEGREES)**
Walking	0–67
Climbing stairs	0–83
Descending stairs	0–90
Sitting down	0–93
Tying a shoe	0–106
Lifting an object	0–117

From Kettelkamp DB, Johnson RJ, Smidt GL, et al (1970). An electrogoniometric study of knee motion in normal gait. *J Bone Joint Surg Am* 52:775-790.

the knee joint, and the restraints that govern motion of the joint.

- An understanding of these factors allows for the rational design and placement of a total knee arthroplasty (TKA) that can be expected to function in a manner similar to that of the native joint for a sustained period of time.

Motion

- The knee is not a simple hinge joint. Motion about the knee is complex and involves a combination of flexion/extension, internal/external rotation, and abduction/adduction.
- Failure to account for this complex motion is responsible for the accelerated failure of highly constrained total knee prostheses. This was especially true of highly constrained early "hinged" designs that permitted motion only in the sagittal plane.
- The primary ROM of the knee is from 0 to 20 degrees of extension (recurvatum) to 125 to 165 degrees of flexion (Arnoczky and McDevitt 2000). The functional ROM is from 0 to 115 degrees. Normal gait requires an ROM of 0 to 70 degrees (Table 2–3).
- Flexion and extension of the knee involve a combination of rolling and sliding with the instant center of rotation

shifting posteriorly on the femoral condyles with increasing flexion. The *instant center of rotation* is defined as the contact point between the femur and the tibia. This posterior shift of the instant center of rotation is known as *posterior femoral rollback* and allows for increased flexion of the knee by preventing impingement of the tibia on the femur. It also increases the moment arm of the extensor mechanism, which increases the amount of force that can be generated by the quadriceps muscle (Fig. 2–8).

- In the native knee, femoral rollback is regulated by the four-bar linkage system. The anterior cruciate ligament (ACL) and the posterior cruciate ligament (PCL) form the ligamentous links in this system, and the bony bridges between their attachments on the tibia and femur form the remaining two links. The instant center of rotation of the knee is the point where the ACL and PCL cross (Fu et al. 1993) (Fig. 2–9).
- In PCL-sparing TKAs, the retained PCL regulates posterior femoral rollback; however, because of the absence of the ACL and the disruption of the four-bar linkage system, this rollback has not been shown to reproduce normal knee kinematics (Dennis et al. 1998).
- In posteriorly stabilized TKAs in which the PCL is sacrificed, femoral rollback is regulated by an interaction between a cam on the femoral component and a tibial post. This leads to more predictable rollback, although still less than in the native knee. The cam-post interface also creates another possible source of wear particles and increased constraint (Mont et al. 2003).
- External rotation of approximately 5 degrees of the tibia on the femur occurring during the final 15 degrees of extension is known as the "screw home" mechanism. This is regulated by the size and shape of the medial femoral condyle and the muscle and soft tissue structures about the knee (Arnoczky and McDevitt 2000).
- The primary restraint to varus forces about the knee is the lateral collateral ligament, whereas the superficial portion of the medial collateral ligament is the primary restraint to

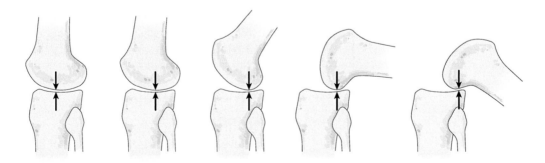

Figure 2–8: Femoral rollback.
As the knee flexes, the femoral contact point translates posteriorly on the tibia. This allows for greater flexion, increases the quadriceps lever arm, and thus increases the quadriceps force.

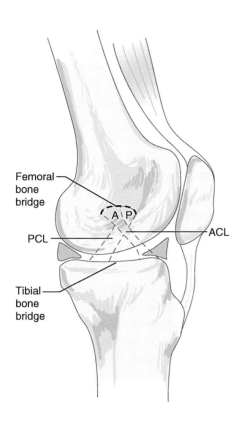

Figure 2–9: Four-bar linkage system.
The four-bar linkage system consists of the anterior cruciate ligament *(ACL)*, the posterior cruciate ligament *(PCL)*, and the bony bridges between their attachments on the femur and tibia. In the native knee, the linkage system regulates femoral rollback. *A,* ACL; *P,* PCL.

valgus stress. During revision knee arthroplasty, these ligaments may be attenuated or absent, so the use of components that are more constrained in the coronal plane may be required.

Mechanical Alignment

- The mechanical axis of the lower extremity is a vertical line from the center of the femoral head to the center of the ankle (Fig. 2–10).
- In a normal lower extremity, this line passes through or slightly medial to the center of the knee joint. With a varus deformity of the knee, the line passes medial to the center of the knee joint and causes an increased load in the medial compartment. This increased load creates a vicious cycle that leads to a progressively worsening deformity. As the deformity becomes more severe, the patient may experience a lateral thrust to the knee with weight bearing. With a valgus knee deformity, the line passes lateral to the knee joint with an increased load passing through the lateral side and stretching/attenuation of the medial support structures.

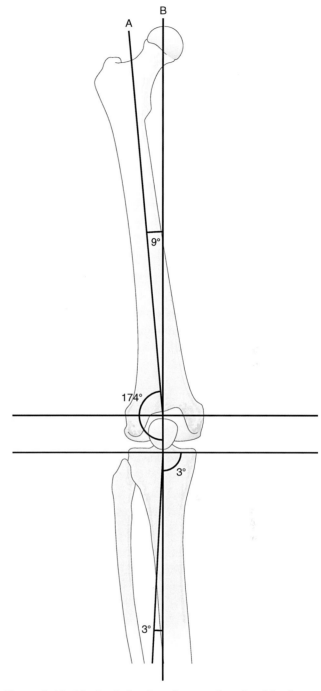

Figure 2–10: Mechanical axis and anatomic axis of the knee. Anatomic axis *(A)* and mechanical axis *(B)*.

- The anatomic axis of the femur is a line down the center of the femoral shaft. This axis subtends an angle of 5 to 9 degrees of valgus with a line drawn perpendicular to the distal femoral articular surface. In shorter individuals, this angle is increased, whereas it is decreased in taller individuals.
- The anatomic axis of the tibia is a line drawn down the center of the tibial shaft. This axis subtends an angle of

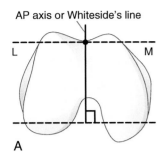 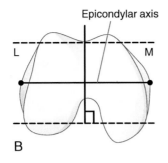 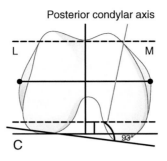

Figure 2–11: Femoral component of external rotation. **A,** Anteroposterior *(AP)* axis of the femur. **B,** Epicondylar axis. **C,** Posterior condylar axis. *L,* lateral; *M,* medial.

3 degrees of varus with a line drawn perpendicular to the proximal tibial articular surface. In the lateral plane, the proximal tibial articular surface has a posterior slope of 5 to 7 degrees compared with a line drawn perpendicular to the anatomic axis of the tibia.

- The normal angle between the anatomic axis of the femur and the tibia is 174 degrees if it is measured on the outside of the leg (6 degrees of valgus).
- To create a reproducible cut with even distribution of forces across the tibial component, the proximal tibia is typically cut at 90 degrees to the anatomic axis of the femur during TKA.
- To recreate the normal angle of 174 degrees between the mechanical axes in extension, the distal femur is cut at 6 degrees of valgus relative to its mechanical axis.
- To balance the knee in flexion, the femoral component is externally rotated 3 degrees, thus compensating for the 3 degrees of varus that is removed from the proximal tibia by cutting it in neutral. This also aids in improving the tracking of the patellofemoral joint.
- Landmarks to reproduce the 3 degrees of external rotation include the epicondylar axis, Whiteside's line or AP axis, and the posterior femoral condyles. Can also parallel the cut tibia if cutting the tibia before the femoral cuts (Fig. 2–11).

Joint Forces

- Knee joint (tibial-femoral) surface loads are three times body weight during normal walking and four times body weight when climbing stairs. Sixty percent of the force is transmitted through the medial compartment, whereas 40% passes through the lateral compartment.
- In the native knee, the menisci serve to increase the conformity between the femoral condyles and the tibial plateau. This increased conformity increases the surface area over which the JRFs are distributed and thereby decreases the force applied to each specific point on the joint surface (Shrive et al. 1978). Consequently, meniscectomy leads to an increase of up to 400% in the force experienced by the articular cartilage.
- During normal flexion of the knee from 0 to 120 degrees, there is 5 mm of excursion of the medial meniscus and 11 mm of excursion of the lateral meniscus (Arnoczky and McDevitt 2000).

- For TKAs, greater conformity between the femoral and the tibial components leads to a larger joint surface area with lower contact stress and less wear. However, this increased conformity reduces freedom of motion, which may lead to decreased joint ROM and increased stress within the polyethylene and at the bone-cement interface.
- The conflict between increased conformity and decreased motion in TKAs is known as the *kinematic conflict.*
- One possible solution to the kinematic conflict is mobile-bearing knee prostheses. The polyethylene component in these prostheses is highly conforming with the femoral component because a second articulation between the polyethylene component and the tibial tray allows for rotational or anterior/posterior motion. Although these designs are theoretically attractive, clinical results to date have been no better than traditional fixed-bearing designs (Callaghan et al. 2000).
- In the coronal plane, it is important that the edges of the femoral component be rounded. Otherwise, an adduction force across the knee with weight bearing and a sharp edge on the femoral component would lead to point loading at the medial corner with extremely high JRFs.

Patellofemoral Joint

- The patellofemoral joint is a sliding articulation, with the patella moving 7 cm caudally during full flexion.
- As the patella moves in the caudal direction (knee flexion), it becomes centered in the trochlear groove, and the area of contact between the patella and the femur shifts from the inferior end of the patella toward the superior pole.
- The purpose of the patella is to increase extensor strength by increasing the moment arm of the extensor mechanism on the tibia. It also helps to distribute the contact stress between the extensor mechanism and the distal femur and provides a sesamoid bone for the attachments of the quadriceps and patellar tendons.
- The patella has the thickest cartilage in the body because it is exposed to some of the greatest loads. The force across the patella ranges from one half of body weight during normal walking to seven times body weight during deep knee bends or running (Arnoczky and McDevitt 2000).

Table 2–4	Biomechanical Interventions to Improve Patellar Tracking
INTERVENTION	**EFFECT**
External rotation of the femoral component	Decreases the height of the lateral ridge of the trochlea and decreases the medially directed force this ridge places on the patella
Lateralization of the femoral component on the distal femur	Shifts the trochlear groove laterally which decreases the Q angle by shifting the apex laterally
Medialization of the patellar component on the patella	Decreases the tension on the lateral patellar retinaculum by shifting the remaining native patella laterally when it is reduced in the trochlear groove
External rotation of the tibial component on the tibia	Rotates the tibial tubercle medially when the tibial component is reduced on the femoral component and thus decreases the Q angle
Lateral release of the extensor retinaculum	Decreases the laterally directed forces on the patella and thus allows the patella to shift medially, decreasing the Q angle

From Scuderi GR, Insall JN, Scott WN (1994). Patellofemoral pain after total knee arthroplasty. *J Am Acad Orthop Surg* 2:239-246.

- Removal of the patella following trauma or complications associated with TKA decreases the moment arm of the extensor mechanism by the width of the patella and increases the force the quadriceps must generate to extend the knee by 15% to 30% during terminal extension (Arnoczky and McDevitt 2000). For TKA following patellectomy, the surgeon generally chooses a posterior stabilized design because these prostheses have more reliable femoral rollback, which increases the quadriceps moment arm.
- Patellar tracking following TKA can be enhanced by external rotation of the femoral component, lateralization of the femoral component on the distal femur, medialization of the patellar component on the patella, external rotation of the tibial component, or lateral release of the extensor retinaculum (Scuderi et al. 1994) (Table 2–4).
- The average patella is 25 mm thick. During resurfacing of the patella, it is important to retain at least 10 mm of native patella to decrease the rate of subsequent fracture. Metal-backed patellar components have had poor results secondary to high contact stress across a thin polyethylene component.
- To preserve the normal patellofemoral relationship, it is important that the joint line not be raised or lowered more that 8 mm during TKA. This is especially true during revision arthroplasty because extensive bone loss can make accurate placement of the native joint line difficult. Excessive elevation of the joint line causes patella baja, which leads to impingement of the patella on the tibial polyethylene with flexion.

References

Arnoczky SP, McDevitt CA (2000). The meniscus: Structure, function, repair and replacement. In: Buchwalter JA, Einhorn TA, Simon SR, eds. *Orthopaedic Basic Science*, 2nd ed. Rosemont, IL: American Academy of Orthopaedic Surgeons, pp 531-545.

This chapter provides a detailed explanation of the anatomy, structure and function of the meniscus.

Beaule PE, Matta JM, Mast JW (2002). Hip arthrodesis: Current indications and techniques. *J Am Acad Orthop Surg* 10:240-258.

This article provides an in-depth analysis and an explanation of clinical decision making as well as operative considerations of hip arthrodesis.

Blaha JD (1993). Principles of joint prostheses. In: Wright V, Radin EC, eds. *Mechanics of Human Joints: Physiology, Pathophysiology, and Treatment*. New York: Marcel Dekker, pp 373-390.

This chapter is an excellent introduction to the rationale behind joint replacement, an overview of the mechanical considerations including the materials involved, and an explanation of force transmission between prostheses and native skeleton.

Callaghan JJ, Isnall JN, Greenwald AS, et al. (2000). Mobile-bearing knee replacements. *J Bone Joint Surg Am* 82:1020-1041.

This article reviews the rationale and results of mobile-bearing knee replacements. It includes a thorough discussion of the kinematic conflict and how mobile bearings may provide a solution.

Dennis DA, Komistek RD, Colwell CE, et al. (1998). In vivo antero-posterior femorotibial translation of total knee arthroplasty: A multi-center analysis. *Clin Orthop Relat Res* 356:47-57.

In this classic article, the authors performed a fluoroscopic in vivo weight-bearing analysis of posterior femoral rollback in PCL-retaining and PCL-substituting TKAs. They found that PCL-retaining TKAs actually undergo paradoxical anterior translation of the femur on the tibia with knee flexion. The PCL-substituting designs did experience posterior femoral rollback, although it was less than occurs in native knees.

Doehring TC, Rubash HE, Shelley FJ, et al. (1996). The effect of superior and superolateral relocations of the hip center on hip joint forces: An experimental and analytical analysis. *J Arthroplasty* 11:693-703.

This article attempts to evaluate the effect of location of hip center on hip JRFs by using both experimental measurements and theoretical calculations.

Fu FH, Harner CD, Johnson DL, et al. (1993). Biomechanics of knee ligaments. *J Bone Joint Surg Am* 75:1716-1727.

This review article explores the role of the four main knee ligaments in the biomechanics and kinetics of the knee.

Mont MA, Booth RE Jr, Laskin RS, et al. (2003). The spectrum of prosthesis design for primary total knee arthroplasty. *AAOS Instr Course Lect* 52:397-407.

This article provides an in-depth review of the six types of total knee prosthesis currently used in the United States.

Nordin M, Frankel VH (2001). Biomechanics of the hip. In: Nordin M, Frankel VH, eds. *Basic Biomechanics of the Musculoskeletal System*, 2nd ed. Philadelphia: Lippincott Williams & Wilkins, pp 202-221.

This excellent in-depth textbook on the biomechanics of the musculoskeletal system includes specific chapters on hip and knee biomechanics, as well as an introductory chapter on the engineering perspective.

Pauwels F (1980). *Biomechanics of the Locomotor Apparatus*. New York: Springer-Verlag, pp 1-228.

This classic monograph attempts to describe the entire lower extremity from a biomechanical perspective and includes an excellent description of the complexity of locomotion.

Radin EL (1980). Biomechanics of the human hip. *Clin Orthop Relat Res* 152:28-34.

This article explains in detail the relationship between hip structure and function and provides an excellent overview of the anatomic considerations of native hip biomechanics.

Scuderi GR, Insall JN, Scott WN (1994). Patellofemoral pain after total knee arthroplasty. *J Am Acad Orthop Surg* 2:239-246.

The review article discusses the various causes of patellofemoral pain following TKA. The authors outline the intraoperative adjustments that can be used to reduce patellofemoral pain.

Shrive NG, O'Connor JJ, Goodfellow JW (1978). Load-bearing in the knee joint. *Clin Orthop Relat Res* 131:279-287.

This article explores the role of the meniscus in the transmission of force across the knee joint. It also describes the increase in JRFs following removal of the meniscus.

Simon SR, ed. (1994). *Orthopaedic Basic Science*. Rosemont, IL: American Academy of Orthopaedic Surgeons, pp 405-407.

This book is an excellent review of the kinesiology of all the major joints in the body. The knee section specifically addresses the static and dynamic restraints to motion in each plane, with an emphasis on the role of the cruciate ligaments.

CHAPTER

3

Joint Biology

David Glaser

MD, Assistant Professor, Department of Orthopaedic Surgery, University of Pennsylvania School of Medicine, Philadelphia, PA

Introduction

- The diarthrodial joint depends on finely balanced interactions between soft and hard tissues, including cartilage, synovial fluid (SF), synovial membrane, bone, supporting ligaments, and surrounding muscles (Buckwalter et al. 2000).
- Diseases manifested primarily in one structure can affect the others.
- The ultimate measure of the health of a joint is clinical function.
- Joint function can be assessed by the ability to perform activities of daily living, range of motion, and strength and by somewhat more disease-specific abnormalities such as swelling, tenderness, crepitus, and instability.
- Specific radiographic, histopathologic, biochemical, immunologic, or molecular changes are often disease specific and involve individual tissues.

Articular Cartilage (Hyaline Cartilage)

- *Articular cartilage* is composed of both solid and fluid phases.
- The primary components of cartilage are water (~65%), proteoglycans(~15%), collagens(~15%, type II), and chondrocytes (~5%) (Ulrich-Vinther et al. 2003).

Water

- *Water* is the most abundant component of normal articular cartilage. It decreases in concentration from approximately 80% at the surface to 65% in the deep zone.
- Weight bearing pushes water through the extracellular membrane by compressing the solid matrix. A cartilage cushioning effect occurs through resistance against the flow of water through the extracellular membrane.

Collagen

- Type II *collagen* represents 90% to 95% of the total collagen. Collagen is a triple-helix protein. Collagen represents more than 50% dry weight of articular cartilage.

Proteoglycans

- *Proteoglycans* consist of a protein core with covalently bound glycosaminoglycan chains.
- *Glycosaminoglycans* consist of long-chain, unbranched, repeating disaccharide units.
- Three major types of glycosaminoglycans have been found in cartilage:
  - Chondroitin sulfate (found in two isomeric forms, chondroitin 4-sulfate and chondroitin 6-sulfate)
    - Most prevalent glycosaminoglycans in cartilage
    - Accounting for 55% to 90% of the glycosaminoglycans (percentage decreases with the age of the subject)
  - Keratan sulfate
  - Dermatan sulfate
- Hyaluronate is also a glycosaminoglycan, but unlike those described earlier, it is not sulfated. Hyaluronate is not bound to a protein core.

Microarchitecture of Hyaline Cartilage

- The structure and composition of the articular cartilage vary throughout its depth, from the articular surface to the subchondral bone. These differences include cell shape and volume, collagen fibril diameter and orientation, proteoglycan concentration, and water content.
- Articular cartilage has four zones:
  - The superficial tangential zone
    - This zone has a smooth, nearly frictionless gliding surface.
    - Thin collagen fibrils are arranged parallel to the surface.

- Chondrocytes are elongated, with the long axis parallel to the surface.
  - Proteoglycan content is at its lowest concentration.
  - Water content is at its highest.
- The middle or transitional zone
  - Collagen fibers with less apparent organization, and the chondrocytes have a more rounded appearance.
- The deep zone
  - Collagen fibers are vertical to the joint surface.
  - Chondrocytes are arranged in a columnar fashion.
  - Proteoglycan concentration is highest.
  - Water content is lowest.
- The calcified zone
  - This is the deepest layer.
  - It separates hyaline cartilage from the subchondral bone.

Synovial Fluid

- Grossly normal SF is viscous and clear, containing fewer than 200 cells/mm^3.
- Cells are predominantly monocytes.
- Cartilage is nourished from synovium via the SF. Hyaluronic acid, lubricin, and phospholipids in SF provide lubrication.
- Altered production of SF can impair cartilage nourishment. Inflammatory mediators in the SF can destroy cartilage. Effusion and swelling of tissues can produce gelling. Diseased SF loses its lubricating effects.
- Different types of effusions display disease-specific characteristics (Table 3–1).

Synovial Membrane

- The synovial membrane makes up the inner lining of diarthrodial joints. It is important for many aspects of normal function of the joint.
- Major known functions of the synovial membrane are related to its production of the SF and the many components of fluid that are important in function of the entire joint complex:
  - Nourishment of the avascular cartilage through the SF
  - Maintaining fluid and small molecule homeostasis via osmotic effects and synovial lymphatics
  - Removing particulates via the macrophage-like synovial lining cells
- Synovial membrane consists of one to two cell layers of surface cells and underlying tissue of various depths but not including the fibrous capsule. This vascular tissue has a thin lining that includes the following:
  - Type A cells, which are monocyte-derived phagocytic cells that produce interleukin-1 and tumor necrosis factor and are responsible for removal of debris
  - Type B cells, which are synthetic secretory cells producing the hyaluronate that makes SF viscous as well as prostaglandins and metalloproteinases that can be increased in disease
- The surface has villous folds and undulations that increase the surface area (Fig. 3–1).
- Synovium can be any of the following:

  1. Loose or areolar with some collagen and fat cells (see Fig. 3–1)
  2. Almost purely fatty as in the infrapatellar fat pad
  3. Fibrous

- The areolar tissue appears better adapted for movement, whereas the fibrous synovium is present at sites where support is more critical. The fibrous synovium normally tends to be less vascular.

Ligaments

Composition and Organization

- *Ligaments* consist of highly organized, anisotropic tissue (tissue property changes with load).

Table 3–1 General Characteristics of Synovial Fluid in Different Types of Effusions

CHARACTERISTICS	NORMAL	INFLAMMATORY CONDITIONS	NONINFLAMMATORY CONDITIONS	SEPTIC CONDITIONS
Volume	1–4 mL	Increased	Increased	Increased
Color	Clear to pale yellow	Cloudy, yellow/green	Straw	White/yellow
Clarity	Transparent	Opaque	Transparent	Opaque
Viscosity	Very high	Low	High	Very low
White blood cell count (per mm^3)	Few	10,000–20,000	500	≥ 50,000
Predominant white blood cell type	Monocytes	Neutrophils	Monocytes	Neutrophils
Glucose (relative to serum)	Equal	Low	Equal	0 to low
Crystals	Negative	Positive in gout and calcium pyrophosphate deposition disease	Negative	Negative
Cultures	Negative	Negative	Negative	Positive

From Carpenter CA, Rosenberg AE, Freiberg AA (2002). Synovial conditions of the knee. In: Callaghan J, Rosenberg A, Rubash H, et al., eds. *The Adult Knee*. Philadelphia: Lippincott Williams & Wilkins.

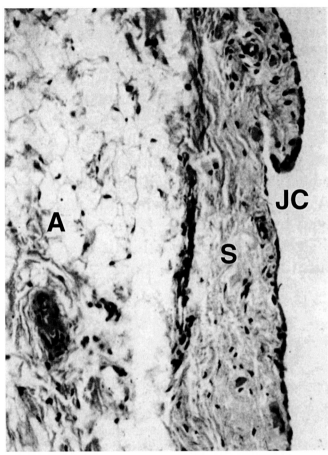

Figure 3–1: Synovium.
The inner surface of a diarthrodial joint is lined by synovium *(S)*, with its one to two cell layers of surface cells and underlying loose connective tissues including a rich vascular network. Synovial folds may extend into the joint cavity *(JC)*. The synovial connective tissue contains numerous blood and lymphatic vessels, nerves, and a variable number of adipocytes *(A)*. (From Wheater PR, Burkitt HG, Daniels VG [1987]. Skeletal tissues. In: Wheater P, Burkitt G, eds. *Functional Histology*, 2nd ed. Cambridge, UK: Churchill Livingstone.)

- They are composed of longitudinally oriented collagen fibers.
- More than 90% of collagen is type I, with type III making up a majority of the remainder.

- Increased stiffness occurs with increased load.
- Ligament collagen is arranged in a longitudinal pattern with crimp.
- *Crimp* is a waveform pattern of ligament fascicles that allows for elongation without tearing of the fascicles. This permits increased stiffness with increased load. These crimped fascicles are arranged like a spring that can elongate under load.
- Ligament insertion
  - Direct attachment pattern: The four zones are ligament, nonmineralized fibrocartilage, mineralized fibrocartilage, and bone.
  - Indirect attachment: Fibers blend with the bone periosteal layer.

Ligament Injury

- Ligament injury can be classified into three grades:
  - Grade I: Strain of fibers occurs, with pain but with no instability or laxity of ligaments.
  - Grade II: Partial tearing of the ligament occurs, with failure of fascicles. Laxity is present.
  - Grade III: Complete tear. The healing potential varies depending on the ligament. The location of the ligament influences the healing rate. For example, an intra-articular anterior cruciate ligament has a lower healing rate than a proximal (extra-articular) medial collateral ligament.

References

Buckwalter JA, Einhorn TA, Simon SR, eds. (2000). *Orthopaedic Basic Science: Biology and Biomechanics of the Musculoskeletal System.* Rosemont, IL: American Academy of Orthopaedic Surgeons.
  A comprehensive reference devoted to the basic science of the musculoskeletal system.

Ulrich-Vinther M, Maloney MD, Schwarz EM, et al. (2003). Articular cartilage biology. *J Am Acad Orthop Surg* 11:421-430.
  An overview article focused on articular cartilage biology. Its focus is the biologic processes involved with tissue maintenance and repair, highlighting several steps targeted by therapeutic applications.

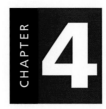

CHAPTER 4

Biology of Bone Graft

Gregory F. Carolan,* Kingsley R. Chin,† and Matthew Werger‡

*MD, Instructor, University of Pennsylvania School of Medicine, Philadelphia, PA
†MD, Chief, Division of Orthopaedic Spine Surgery and Assistant Professor, Department of
Orthopaedic Surgery, University of Pennsylvania School of Medicine, Philadelphia, PA
‡MD, Medical Student, Georgetown University Medical Center, Washington, DC

Introduction

- Over the past 3 decades, the science of bone grafting has advanced dramatically, and accordingly, the clinical use of bone grafts has increased.
- As of 2002, an estimated 500,000 to 600,000 bone grafting procedures were performed annually in the United States (Buckolz 2002).
- Most bone grafting procedures are undertaken by orthopaedic surgeons.
- Bone grafts are often used by spine, joint reconstruction, tumor, and sports subspecialists to augment fusion of or to reconstruct bone defects.
- Synthetic bone graft substitutes make up approximately 10% of the bone graft market (Buckolz 2002).

Classification

- Transplanted biomaterials are classified based on origin (Day et al. 2000):
  - *Autograft:* Tissue transplanted from one location to another within the same individual (e.g., autologous bone marrow, vascularized grafts)
  - *Allograft:* Tissue transplanted from genetically nonidentical individuals of the same species
  - *Xenograft:* Tissue transplanted from one species to another
  - *Synthetic:* Nonbiologic tissue (demineralized bone matrix [DBM], collagen, ceramics, cements, silicones and other polymers) serves as a structure on which host bone can grow

- Bone grafts are further subclassified by their predominant structural makeup (i.e., cancellous, cortical, or corticocancellous).
- In some instances, bone marrow may be transplanted to aid healing of a graft or bone defect.
- In orthopaedics, cancellous and cortical autografts and allografts are the most commonly used bone graft types.
- Xenograft is rarely used in humans because of the massive immune response to this material and its subsequent high failure rate (Bauer and Muschler 2000).
- Limited supply, donor site morbidity from harvesting autografts, and concerns regarding the safety and efficacy of allografts have made synthetic graft substitutes a more desirable alternative.

Principles

- The incorporation of bone graft into a host is the result of three distinct biologic processes (Goldberg and Stevenson 1987):
  - *Osteogenesis:* The ability of graft or host cells to synthesize new bone
    - Graft cells from properly handled, fresh cortical and cancellous grafts survive transplant to the host site and synthesize the new bone that is critical for early graft success.
    - This process is facilitated by the use of cancellous grafts with a larger surface area of trabeculae lined with osteoblasts and by the presence of decorticated host bone with exposed marrow elements containing

osteoinductive proteins, osteoprogenitor cells, and a local blood supply (Bauer and Muschler 2000).
  - Osteogenesis is responsible for initiating incorporation of the graft into host bone on the time scale of weeks after transplantation.
- *Osteoconduction:* The process by which host blood vessels and osteoprogenitor cells invade the three-dimensional lattice network of the graft
  - It results in the ordered formation of new bone.
  - It facilitates the union of graft with host bone.
  - The process depends on the structure of the graft into which the host cells and blood vessels can invade and repopulate.
  - Although it is an inherent property of all successful bone grafts and substitutes, cancellous grafts are considered to be the most osteoconductive.
- *Osteoinduction:* The process by which osteoprogenitor cells and mesenchymal stem cells are recruited into the graft and are stimulated to differentiate into chondroblasts and osteoblasts necessary for bone formation; influenced by the following:
  - Bone morphogenetic proteins (BMPs)
  - Mitogens, such as platelet-derived growth factor, insulin-like growth factor, and granulocyte-macrophage colony-stimulating factor
  - Angiogenic factors, such as vascular endothelial-derived growth factor

Bone Morphogenetic Proteins

- These are proteins with strong osteoconductive and osteogenic properties from DBM (Urist 1965).
- Since their discovery in 1965, BMP-1 through BMP-8 have been isolated and molecularly cloned.
- BMPs are found in all fresh autograft as well as in allograft that has been prepared without ionizing radiation or autoclaving (Goldberg 2003).
- BMP concentrations are somewhat less in allograft.
- BMP-2 and BMP-7 (BMP-7 is also known as osteogenic protein-1 or OP-1) are both commercially available in recombinant preparations (Burkus et al. 2004).
- These preparations contain much higher BMP concentrations than those found in normal bone.
- Their clinical use is currently under investigation for promotion of spinal fusion.
- BMPs have been shown to be normally expressed in bone during embryonic development and repair (Issack and DiCesare 2003).
- BMP-2 through BMP-8 have been found to be the largest members of the transforming growth factor-β family (Hahn et al. 1992).
- Each BMP (except BMP-1) is by itself sufficient for the initiation of new bone formation (Wozney 2002).

Incorporation

- Incorporation of bone graft can be separated into two phases: a predominantly inflammatory early phase and a later, bone-forming phase.
- The process of incorporation proceeds in a stepwise fashion from the moment the graft enters the host (Bauer and Muschler 2000, Day et al. 2000, Goldberg 2003, Goldberg and Stevenson 1987, Kahn et al. 2005).
- The primary bone healing phase (hemorrhage, inflammation, revascularization, and osteoinduction) results in active bone formation and resorption by 4 weeks for cancellous autografts.
- Osteoconduction predominates in the secondary phase, which begins when osteoblasts line the endosteal surfaces of the graft and lay down a seam of osteoid that eventually surrounds a core of graft bone.
- Osteoclasts begin to resorb the necrotic graft while host marrow cells reconstitute the graft.
- Incorporation concludes with normal remodeling of the new bone according to the biomechanical forces to which it is exposed.
- The temporal relationship of each stage varies with the type of graft used, the size of the area grafted, and a variety of host factors (Box 4–1).
- Steroids and anti-inflammatory drugs are contraindicated during these early stages because they inhibit differentiation of the following:
  - Osteoblastic cells (steroids)
  - Prostaglandin-mediated inflammation (anti-inflammatory drugs)
- Smoking tobacco has long been attributed to failure of bone graft incorporation as a result of its vasoconstrictive effects.
  - Avoid smoking in the early postgrafting period (the amount of time to when smoking can be allowed is controversial but is probably no earlier than 3 months from grafting).

Autograft

- Autologous bone marrow has been found to contain mesenchymal stem cells that can be stimulated to differentiate into osteoblasts and produce bone.
- It is most commonly used in tibial fractures that have either gone on to nonunion or are at high risk for this complication.
- Autologous bone marrow is aspirated from the patient's iliac crest and is injected into the fracture or nonunion site (Kahn et al. 2005).
- Use of autograft is limited by the following:
  - The amount of graft material available to harvest (especially in smaller individuals and elderly patients). It is estimated that bone marrow contains 1 stem cell per 50,000 nucleated stem cells in young adults and approximately 1 per 1 million nucleated cells in the elderly.

Box 4–1	Stages of Graft Incorporation

1. Hemorrhage and Inflammation

- This stage begins immediately after transplantation and forms a hematoma rich in inflammatory cells (e.g., osteoclasts, neutrophils, lymphocytes, monocytes).
- At 2 weeks, the inflammation results in abundant granulation tissue in the region of the graft and provides an environment conducive to the beginning of the subsequent vascularization stage.

2. Vascularization

- The length of the vascularization stage varies according to the type of graft used (autograft cancellous is the shortest and allograft cortical is the longest).
- Vascularization may begin as early as 2 days after implantation.
- As the vascularization of the graft continues, the host is exposed to the graft's antigenicity for the first time (important in allografts).

3. Osteoinduction

- Marrow spaces are repopulated with primitive mesenchymal stem cells of the host.
- These cells differentiate into osteogenic cells to begin the process of new bone formation and graft resorption.
- Osteogenic cells from the graft survive in significant concentrations only in fresh cancellous autograft.
- It is in these grafts that early success of graft-based osteogenesis is observed.
- The length of the osteoinduction stage varies with the type of graft.
- Some large cortical allografts are never fully revascularized and therefore are never fully incorporated.

Box 4–2	Common Neurovascular Associations and Complications With Autograft Harvest

Posterior Iliac Crest Harvest

- Superior cluneal nerves and superior gluteal vessels
  - Avoid transverse incisions beyond 7 cm lateral of the posterior iliac spine
  - Direct bone graft harvesting parallel to the iliac crest

Anterior Iliac Crest Harvest

- Lateral femoral cutaneous nerve
  - Supplies skin sensation to the anterolateral thigh and has variable positions relative to the anterior superior iliac spine
  - Can be avoided in most patients by harvesting graft beyond 3 cm posteriorly from the anterior superior iliac spine

Fibular Graft Harvest

- Peroneal nerves and vessels
  - Nerves at risk from harvest in the proximal third of the fibula
  - Peroneal vessels at risk in the middle third of the fibula

- The potential for significant donor site morbidity
  - Complications from the harvest of these grafts include blood loss, infection, neurovascular damage (Box 4–2), pain, and formation of additional scars (Younger and Chapman 1989, Vail and Urbaniak 1996).
- The prolonged operative time needed for harvest and microvascular repair (Vail and Urbaniak 1996)
- Inability to concentrate the marrow at the site of interest. Centrifugation or ex vivo cell cultures have been studied as ways to improve concentration (Lindholm et al. 1982).
- Vascularized autografts are cortical bone harvested with an intact vascular pedicle and transplanted with anastomosis of the vascular supply, such as fibular autograft for avascular necrosis of the femoral head (Chin et al. 1999, Urbaniak and Harvey 1998).
  - Benefits (Box 4–3)
- Cancellous grafts are the most common form of autograft and can be obtained from the wing of the ilium, the proximal tibia, and the proximal humerus.
  - Timing of incorporation of cancellous grafts (Box 4–4)
- Cortical autograft is usually taken from the fibula or rib.

- The incorporation of cortical autograft is similar to that of cancellous autograft, but the process takes much longer.
- The inflammatory stage is basically the same as is seen in cancellous grafts; however, effective revascularization takes up to 2 to 3 months to begin (as opposed to 4 weeks in cancellous grafts).
- Some larger grafts may only be 50% revascularized by 1 year.
- Vascular penetration of the cortical graft occurs by peripheral osteoclastic resorption and vascular infiltration of the haversian canals of the graft (Goldberg and Stevenson 1987).
- Osteoconduction and osteoinduction progress at a slower rate, and in some large grafts, this process never truly finishes; the result is a conglomerate of new host bone and necrotic graft bone.
- Most of the osteoblasts do not survive transplantation, a feature that makes osteogenesis in cortical grafts deficient.
- Because of this predominately resorptive process of incorporation, cortical autografts are weaker than normal bone in the early stages (6 weeks to 6 months).

Box 4–3	Benefits of Vascularized Bone Grafts

- Host bone causes no immunologic response.
- Most of the graft's osteoblasts should survive the transplant and begin the process of osteogenesis shortly after transplant (Bauer and Muschler 2000).
- With adequately stable fixation, the graft can act as a sound structural support immediately.

Box 4–4	Stages of Cancellous Graft Incorporation Following Autologous Transplantation

Less Than 2 Weeks (Inflammatory Stage)
- Transplanted marrow in graft is replaced by granulation tissue.
- Some of the graft osteoblasts survive the transplant and begin the process of osteogenesis.

First 4 Weeks
- The graft is revascularized and the host osteoprogenitor cells are recruited to the graft by the bone morphogenetic proteins in the graft.

First 2 to 3 Months
- Osteoprogenitor cells differentiate into osteoblasts and osteoclasts, and the dynamic process of new bone formation and old bone resorption continues for 2 to 3 months.
- Osteoinduction is complete.
- Osteoconduction continues with neovascularization, establishment of viable bone marrow, and resorption of the necrotic graft remnants.
- This is visualized radiographically by areas of increased density in the graft reflecting the entrapment of the necrotic bone by new host bone.

At 6 Months
- The entire graft has been replaced by new bone.
- The process of remodeling of the newly formed bone in response to mechanical stresses is well under way.

Within 1 Year
- The graft has been fully incorporated into the host.

- By 1 year after transplantation, a cortical autograft has recovered to approximately 50% of normal strength as a result of appositional new bone formation and remodeling.
- The process of cortical autograft incorporation may continue for years to life in some large grafts.

Allograft

- All allografts incorporate more slowly than autografts and have higher failure rates, likely secondary to the immunogenic response of the host toward the foreign tissue.
- Modification of the immunogenicity of the allograft and assurance of sterilization is achieved by low-dose irradiation (<20 kGy), ultrasonic or pulsatile washes, ethanol treatment, antibiotic soaking (4°C for at least 1 hour), freeze-drying (lyophilizing), or freezing the fresh graft.
- The modification and sterilization techniques seem to decrease the host immune response while still preserving some important osteoinductive mediators (e.g., BMPs).
  - These treatments may adversely affect the mechanical strength of the graft in a dose-dependent manner.

- Freezing minimally affects the graft's mechanical properties, but freeze-drying can cause microfractures along the collagen fibers in the matrix that render the graft susceptible to mechanical failure.
- Some form of rehydration is required before the use of grafts treated by freeze-drying.
- Irradiating and autoclaving the grafts alter the immunogenicity; however, these techniques also result in destruction of the BMPs in the graft and further retard the process of incorporation.
- Skeletal allografts are harvested from organ donors in a process regulated by the American Association of Tissue Banks.
  - Donors are routinely screened for risky behavior or exposure to potentially infectious diseases (via serology).
  - Before process regulation, viral infections such as hepatitis C and B and human immunodeficiency virus (HIV) posed the most concern (Kahn et al. 2005).
  - Since the institution of donor screening protocols in 1980, only two cases of HIV transmission have been reported in more than 3 million cases of allograft transplantation (Centers for Disease Control and Prevention 1988; Gazdag et al. 1995).
  - No cases of HIV transmission occurred in more than 2 million cases of allograft bone grafting from 1998 to 2002 (Gamradt and Lieberman 2003).
  - Currently, the largest infection risk with bone grafts is the transmission of bacterial contaminants (specifically spore-forming bacteria such as clostridia) as a result of faulty sterilization techniques.
    - Sterilization now includes the addition of sporicidal techniques to address this risk.
    - The allografts are either harvested in a sterile condition (e.g., in the operating room after the removal of a donor's other soft tissue organs) or are harvested in a nonsterile condition and are secondarily sterilized.
- The incorporation of cancellous and cortical allografts occurs through a process similar to that observed in autograft incorporation, although progress is slower.
  - In some circumstances, the graft never becomes incorporated and eventually results in resorption by the host.
- Revascularization (inflammatory stage), which occurs so efficiently in cancellous autograft, initially fails in cancellous allograft because of the immune response of the host to the foreign antigens on the graft.
  - In cortical allografts, incorporation usually succeeds if adequate stability of fixation is achieved at the graft-host junction.
  - The host may resorb and replace a cortical allograft by creeping substitution, or the graft may become a mixture of necrotic graft bone and new host bone.
  - This leads to necrosis of the graft and resorption by the host to predominate over new bone formation.

- Osteoinduction is delayed by the lower concentration of osteoinductive molecules in allograft (or the complete lack of these in grafts prepared by irradiation or autoclaving).
- Remodeling of cancellous allografts begins at 1 year, as opposed to 3 to 6 months in cancellous autografts.
- At 1 to 2 years following transplantation, a successfully incorporated cortical allograft may be structurally and mechanically similar to a matching cortical autograft, that is, 50% of normal bone strength (Goldberg and Stevenson 1987).

Bone Graft Substitutes

- Nonallograft structural bone graft substitutes have become more popular in recent years.
  - The advantages of bone graft substitutes are shown in Box 4–5.
- Bone graft substitutes are osteoconductive, but they do not provide structural support as a result of their brittle, crystalline nature (Buckolz 2002).
- Bone graft substitutes are used primarily as void fillers in conjunction with internal fixation and as graft extenders, and they are being investigated as carriers for prolonged delivery of pharmaceuticals such as antibiotics.
  - These grafts are resorbed at varying rates.
- Some of these substitutes are now being combined with osteoinductive agents (e.g., DBM or recombinant BMPs) in the hopes of expanding their current use.
- Interporous hydroxyapatite is a coral-derived bone graft substitute marketed under the name of Pro-Osteon (Interpore Cross International, Irvine, CA).
  - The calcium carbonate coral is replaced by hydroxyapatite producing a structure that is very similar to trabecular bone.
  - It does not provide significant structural support.
  - The purposes of this substitute are to fill bone voids in non–load-bearing areas and to serve as a bone graft expander.
  - It has been shown to be osteoconductive and is used mainly to aid autograft or allograft procedures (e.g., in spinal fusion and trauma).
- β-Tricalcium phosphate (marketed as Vitoss, Orthovita, Inc., Malvern, PA) is a bone graft substitute that is similar to interporous hydroxyapatite.
  - It mimics trabecular bone, and like interporous hydroxyapatite, is osteoconductive only.

Box 4–5   Advantage of Bone Graft Substitutes

- Endless supply
- Ease of sterilization and storage
- Limitation of infectious disease transfer
- Diminished host immune response toward graft

- The difference between interporous hydroxyapatite and β-tricalcium phosphate is that the latter has a smaller pore size that allows enhanced fluid flow through the graft matrix.
  - This property ideally improves dissolution and cell-mediated resorption during bone remodeling and allows the graft to match the natural course of bone healing after implantation more closely (Buckolz 2002).
- Calcium sulfate (Osteoset, Wright Medical, Arlington, TN, and Bone Plast, Interpore Cross International, Irvine, CA) is a third type of bone graft substitute.
  - It is osteoconductive only and is used for the same indications as the products mentioned earlier.
  - Its mechanism of action is not known; however, consistent resorption and rapid regeneration of bone defects filled with calcium sulfate are reported (Buckolz 2002).

Osteoinductive Agents (e.g., Demineralized Bone Matrix and Recombinant Bone Morphogenetic Proteins)

- These materials are osteoinductive only and are used mainly in conjunction with autograft, allograft, and structural bone graft substitutes.
- DBM is the product of the acid extraction of bone and is technically allograft.
- Osteoinductive properties result from the component proteins (BMPs).
- Many different preparations of DBM are available commercially, and the differences observed in the effectiveness of these products are likely related to the method by which they are processed, such as being demineralized and morcelized (Bauer and Daisuke 2003).

Summary

- Given recent advances in the science of bone grafting, it has become increasingly important for the orthopaedic surgeon to understand the basic science behind the technique.
- With increased experience using bone graft substitutes and osteoinductive agents, the future surgeon may be able to perform successful bone graft procedures by avoiding the following:
  - Morbidity of harvesting autograft
  - Potential infectious disease transmission of allograft

References

Bauer TW, Daisuke T (2003). Bone graft substitutes: Towards a more perfect union. *Orthopedics* 26:925-926.

A brief update on new advances in bone graft substitutes including hydroxyapatite (corals), calcium-based products, and injectable cements.

Bauer TW, Muschler GF (2000). Bone graft materials. *Clin Orthop Relat Res* 371:12-14.

This article presents a thorough overview of the basic science behind the clinical use of various bone graft materials. Included in the discussion are autografts, allografts, and synthetics. A very nice and concise explanation of the various stages of bone graft incorporation is included.

Buckolz RW (2002). Nonallograft osteoconductive bone graft substitutes. *Clin Orthop Relat Res* 395:44-52.

This is the most comprehensive review of the biology behind the clinically available bone graft substitutes. For each substitute, the author describes the relevant histology, the pertinent clinical experience to date, the clinical indications, and future development potential.

Burkus JK, Heim SE, Gornet MF, Zdeblick TA. (2004). The effectiveness if rhBMP-2 in replacing autograft: An integrated analysis of three human spine studies. *Orthopedics* 27:723-728.

This is a pooled analysis of three studies comparing commercially available recombinant BMP-2 (rhBMP-2) with iliac crest autograft in anterior lumbar diskectomy and interbody fusion. The rhBMP-2 group was shown to have a shorter hospital stay, fewer graft harvest complications, a higher fusion rate, and a higher rate of return to work than the autograft group.

Centers for Disease Control and Prevention (1988). Transmission of HIV through bone transplantation: Case report and public health recommendations. *MMWR Morb Mortal Wkly Rep* 37: 597-599.

This report by the Centers for Disease Control and Prevention describes the last two cases of HIV transmission linked to allograft in the United States from 1980 to 1988.

Chin KR, Spak JI, Jupiter JB (1999). Septic arthritis and osteomyelitis of the wrist: reconstruction with a vascularized fibula graft. *J Hand Surg Am* 24:243-248.

This article is a case report describing a novel use of vascularized fibular autograft to reconstruct a large bone defect in the distal radius and carpus. No donor site morbidity was reported, and incorporation of the graft was achieved.

Day SM, Ostrum RF, Chao EYS, et al. (2000). Bone injury, regeneration and repair. In: Buckwalter JA, Einhorn TA, Simon SR, eds. *Orthopaedic Basic Science*, 2nd ed. Rosemont, IL: American Academy of Orthopaedic Surgeons.

This textbook chapter explains the basic science behind the incorporation of bone graft into host bone as well as the biologic and mechanical properties of bone healing. This book is the definitive resource for all orthopaedic basic science topics.

Gamradt SC, Lieberman JR (2003). Bone graft for revision hip arthroplasty: Biology and future applications. *Clin Orthop Relat Res* 417:183-194.

This is a brief but excellent review of the biology and applications of the various bone graft materials used in revision total hip arthroplasty. Autograft, allograft, DBM, ceramics, growth factors (i.e., BMPs), and even genetic engineering are mentioned.

Gazdag AR, Lane JM, Glaser D, Forster RA. (1995). Alternatives to autogenous bone graft: Efficacy and indications. *J Am Acad Orthop Surg* 3:1-8.

This thorough review of bone grafts and bone graft substitutes includes an excellent discussion of the biologic properties of bone graft, osteogenesis, osteoconduction, and osteoinduction. It also includes sections on autografts, allografts, ceramics, DBM, bone marrow, and composite grafts.

Goldberg VM, Stevenson S (1987). Natural history of autografts and allografts. *Clin Orthop Relat Res* 225:8-9.

This is a classic article describing the biology of autografts and allografts. The sequence of events leading to the incorporation of bone graft is explained starting from implantation through remodeling of both autograft and allograft, with the clinically relevant differences highlighted.

Goldberg VM (2003). The biology of bone grafts. *Orthopedics* 26: 923-924.

This is a short update on the biology of bone grafting by one of the experts in the field.

Hahn GV, Cohen RB, Wozney JM, et al. (1992). A bone morphogenic protein subfamily: Chromosomal localization of human genes for BMP 5, BMP 6, and BMP 7. *Genomics* 14:759-762.

Although this technical article describes the localization of BMP-5 and BMP-6 to human chromosome 6 and BMP-7 human chromosome 20, it also provides an excellent review of the characterization of the clinically relevant BMPs.

Issack PS, DiCesare PE (2003). Recent advances toward the clinical application of BMP in bone and cartilage repair. *Am J Orthop* 32:429-436.

This article is a nice review of the basic science behind the BMPs and includes a discussion of clinical applications that are currently being studied, both in humans and animals. Applications in all fields of orthopaedics are discussed.

Khan SN, Cammisa FP Jr, Sandhu HS, et al. (2005). The biology of bone grafting. *J Am Acad Orthop Surg* 13:77-86.

The most complete and up-to-date review of the biology of bone grafts in the literature, this is an excellent source for anyone interested in learning more about the topic.

Lindholm TS, Nilsson OS, Lindholm TC (1982). Extraskeletal and intraskeletal new bone formation induced by demineralized bone matrix combined with bone marrow cells. *Clin Orthop Relat Res* 171:251-255.

This article is a basic science examination of the enhanced bone forming potential of DBM when centrifuged autogenous bone marrow cells are added.

Urbaniak JR, Harvey EJ (1998). Revascularization of the femoral head in osteonecrosis. *J Am Acad Orthop Surg* 6:44-54.

This article is a review of current treatments options for osteonecrosis of the femoral head. A retrospective review of 646 hips with various stages of osteonecrosis treated with extracapsular placement of a vascularized fibular graft in the subchondral region of the femoral head with a 1- to 17-year follow-up is also presented. The authors report a 10-year survival rate of more than 80%, a finding suggesting that this procedure is successful in delaying progression to total hip arthroplasty.

Urist MR (1965). Bone formation by autoinduction. *Science* 150:893-899.

This classic and groundbreaking article describes the protein (BMP) found in DBM extract capable of inducing ossification in rats when it is placed in extraskeletal tissue.

Vail TP, Urbaniak JR (1996). Donor-site morbidity with use of vascularized autogenous fibular grafts. *J Bone Joint Surg Am* 78:204-211.

This article is a retrospective review of 247 vascularized fibular autografts preformed in 198 consecutive patients for osteonecrosis of the femoral head. The authors found that 19% had at least one of the following symptoms in the harvested extremity: ankle or generalized leg pain, objective motor weakness, or sensory abnormalities. Although motor weakness was found to decrease with time, the ankle pain, leg pain, and sensory deficits *were found to increase with time from the procedure.*

Wozney JM (2002). Overview of bone morphogenic proteins. *Spine* 27(Suppl):S2-S8.

This article is a review of the history of the BMPs and their current and possible futur*e clinical use, with an emphasis on spine surgery.*

Younger EM, Chapman MW (1989). Morbidity at bone graft donor sites. *J Orthop Trauma* 3:192-195.

This article is a retrospective review of the complication rate of autograft harvest in 239 patients. An overall major complication rate of 8.6% and a minor complication rate of 20% were reported.

Joint Anatomy

Mark I. Froimson,* Robert Molloy,† and Steve Maschke,‡

*MD, MBA, Staff Surgeon, Department of Orthopaedic Surgery, Cleveland Clinic
Foundation, The Cleveland Clinic, Cleveland, OH
†MD, Staff Surgeon, Department of Orthopaedic Surgery, Cleveland Clinic Foundation,
The Cleveland Clinic, Cleveland, OH
‡MD, Resident Surgeon, Department of Orthopaedic Surgery, Cleveland Clinic Foundation,
The Cleveland Clinic, Cleveland, OH

Introduction

- Successful surgical interventions of the hip and knee depend on a thorough and accurate understanding of the relevant surgical anatomy of these regions.
- Restoration of function generally follows correction of anatomic pathology derived from degenerative, traumatic, and inflammatory processes.
- Avoidance of complications requires comprehensive understanding of the location and proximity of vital neurovascular structures (Schmalzreid et al. 1991, Wasielewski et al. 1990).
- Principles that apply to any approach to the hip or knee include the following:
  - Visualization of relevant anatomy
  - Understanding of the spatial relationship of anatomic structures
  - Preservation of functional tissue
    - Muscle function is preserved through protection of innervation by dissecting through internervous planes
    - Protection of vascular structures
    - Protection of nerves (particular nerves susceptible to injury)
    - Protection of tendinous insertion sites
  - Restoration of soft tissue balance
  - Restoration of joint kinematics
  - Access to bony surfaces for prosthetic joint implantation and removal of excess cement or osteophytes
  - Appropriate alignment of implants and correction of deformity through soft tissue balancing
  - Removal of osteophytes, release of restrictive capsular elements
- Surgeons should be familiar with a variety of surgical approaches so that access to the relevant structures can be optimized to address and correct the specific anatomy and pathologic features present (Hoppenfeld and DeBoer 1994).
- Any approach should allow for extensile maneuvers to facilitate completion of the procedure in the event of adverse or unexpected findings.
- Anatomic variations are known to exist, and the most common forms should be familiar to the operative surgeon (Gray and Goss 1973).
- When both hip and knee reconstruction are being considered in the ipsilateral extremity, several anatomic and alignment considerations determine whether the hip or knee should be addressed first.
  - The hip should be addressed first in the following circumstances:
    - The center of rotation of the hip is likely to be corrected by hip reconstruction, thus affecting the alignment target of the knee (Fig. 5–1).
    - A stiff hip with limited flexion may interfere with the ability to obtain knee flexion postoperatively, whereas a hip flexion contracture predisposes to a postoperative knee flexion contracture.
  - The knee should be addressed first when extensive knee valgus will predispose to hip adduction, thus increasing risk of postoperative hip dislocation.

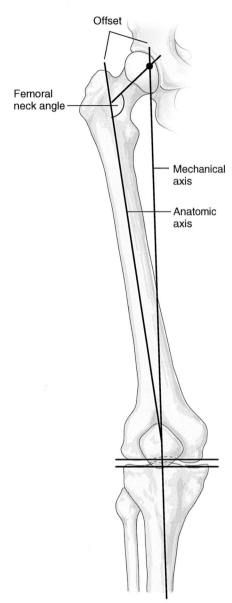

Figure 5–1: Anatomic and mechanical axes of the lower extremity.
Femoral offset is the distance between the center of hip rotation and the anatomic axis of the femur. The femoral neck angle is shown.

Surgical Approaches to the Hip
Overview

- A detailed understanding of hip anatomy, including the bony, neurovascular, and soft tissue anatomy, is essential for safe and effective surgical exposure (Fig. 5–2).
- The surgical principles necessary for successful total hip arthroplasty include a thorough understanding of the anatomy, meticulous exposure and hemostasis, proper patient positioning, and adequate and precise skin incisions (especially with the increasing demand for minimally invasive surgery).

- Intimate knowledge of the relationship of the bony pelvis to the spine and the status of the contralateral hip should be emphasized. The presence and nature of any preexisting pelvic obliquity should be known, with the causes understood and the impact on postsurgical leg-length equalization assessed.
- Severe deformity and revision surgery demand careful preoperative planning and selection of the optimum surgical approach to maximize visualization of the hip joint while minimizing surgical trauma (Hoppenfeld and DeBoer 1994).
- Preoperative assessment should determine the status and quality of bone available for reconstruction, with specific defects and deficiencies documented and potential solutions available.

Basic Anatomy
Bony Anatomy

Hip Joint

- The *hip joint* is a simple ball-and-socket joint, formed by the articulation of the acetabulum with the femur.
- It is intrinsically stable because of the large contact area afforded by the bony architecture. This stability is further augmented by a substantial rim of fibrous tissue, the acetabular labrum.
- The hip capsule is more robust and well defined anteriorly, where it also extends further distally along the femoral neck to the intertrochanteric line.
- The strongest, most clearly defined ligament in the anterior capsule is the *Y ligament of Bigelow*, also known as the *iliofemoral ligament*, originating from the anterior iliac spine.
- Other named ligaments contributing to the hip capsule include the pubofemoral and ischiofemoral, but they are not as strong.

Femur

- The *proximal femur* includes the head, neck, lesser and greater trochanters, and proximal femoral diaphysis. The internal architecture of the proximal femur is complex, with a series of tension trabeculae, running horizontally, and compression trabeculae, running more vertically (Singh et al. 1970).
- The *femoral head* averages 46 mm in diameter, and the *head-neck angle* averages 130 degrees. *Femoral anteversion* averages 10 to 15 degrees. The size and relationship of these elements vary considerably and affect the kinematics of the hip. The femoral head diameter is normally at least 1.2 times the neck diameter. Lesser ratios, prominences of the femoral neck, or posterior angulation of the femoral head can result in anterior impingement and degeneration of the hip (Miller and Gomez 2000, Noble et al. 1988).

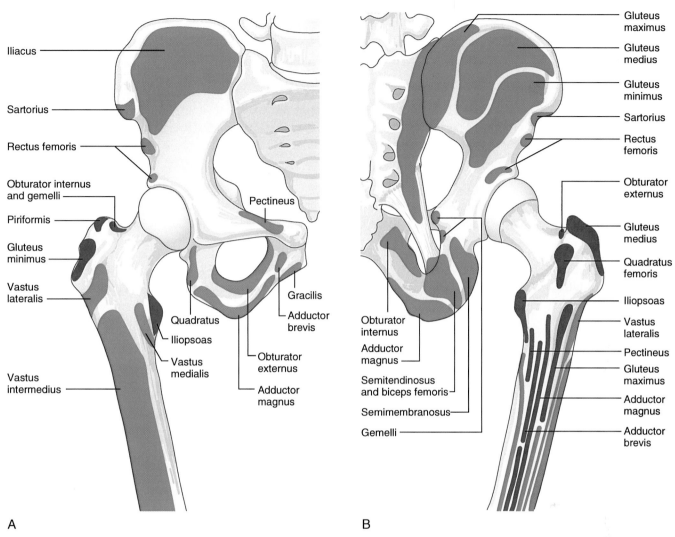

Figure 5–2: The bony pelvis and femur with the location of the muscular attachments.
A, Anterior view. B, Posterior view.

- The femoral neck is not coplanar with the plane of the femoral condyles. *Femoral neck version* is defined as the angle of the femoral neck with respect to the condylar plane (Fig. 5–3).
- *Femoral offset* is defined as the distance from the midline of the longitudinal axis of the femur and the center of rotation of the femoral head. *Hip joint contribution* to lower limb length is defined as the vertical distance from the center of the femoral head to a fixed point on the proximal femur, usually measured from the lesser trochanter (see Fig. 5–1).
- Variations in the head-neck angle and femoral anteversion give rise to changes in femoral offset and hip joint contribution to limb length (Noble et al. 1988).
  - Patients with *hip dysplasia* tend to have increasing valgus and increasing femoral anteversion, with resultant decrease in offset and increase in limb length.
  - In *coxa vara* hips, the femoral neck angle is reduced to 125 degrees or less, leading to greater offset and a tendency to shortening.

- Laterally, the *greater trochanter* provides an extensive area for musculotendinous insertion. The relationship between the medial aspect of the greater trochanter and the center of the femoral shaft varies. Failure to appreciate overhang of the trochanter during hip reconstruction can lead to errors

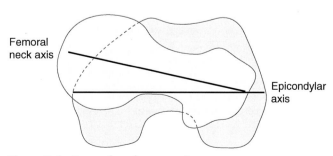

Figure 5–3: Femoral neck anteversion.
The angle between the epicondylar axis and the femoral neck axis defines femoral neck anteversion.

in femoral positioning secondary to improper choice of entry point. In addition, deformity of the greater trochanter can be a source of impingement following hip reconstruction, and consequently it should be assessed and corrected.

- The *piriformis fossa* sits at the junction of the base of the neck and greater trochanter and serves as a reliable entry point for femoral preparation.
- The *lesser trochanter* lies posteromedially and provides for insertion of the iliopsoas tendon. It provides a stable reference point for the location of the proximomedial aspect of the prosthesis during hip reconstruction that has been determined by preoperative templating. An alternative reference, when the lesser trochanter is not well visualized, is the location of the lateral shoulder of the implant to the tip of the greater trochanter.
- The *proximal femoral diaphysis* is funnel shaped.
  - Three types of femoral shape are suggested, based on the relationship between the metaphyseal and diaphyseal anatomy.
    - Champagne flute femora (type A) have wide metaphyses and a narrow diaphysis and may pose challenges to prosthetic fit.
    - Normal (type B) femora have a smooth transition from proximal to distal.
    - Stove pipe (type C) femora, usually found in osteoporotic individuals, have a wide diaphysis that often nearly matches the breadth of the metaphysis.

Acetabulum

- The *acetabulum* is formed by the fusion of the ilium, ischium, and pubis.
- The acetabulum faces anteriorly and caudally. It averages 15 degrees of anteversion and 45 degrees of abduction. The *abduction angle* is defined by the relationship of the line extending from the inferomedial to the superolateral extents of the acetabulum with the horizontal. *Anteversion* is the amount of forward flexion of the acetabulum, as measured from lateral to medial with reference to the sagittal plane.
- The *sourcil* is the weight-bearing dome of the acetabulum. It should comprise an arc of 135 degrees.
- Inadequate acetabular anteversion may result in decreased range of motion secondary to anterior impingement, and may predispose to degenerative changes. Inadequate prosthetic anteversion is a primary source of hip instability following hip replacement.
- Hip dysplasia results in a relatively shallow acetabulum, with increased abduction. With increasing degrees of severity of dysplasia, an increasing amount of femoral head is left uncovered by acetabular bone. Corrective osteotomies have been designed to reorient the retroverted or dysplastic acetabulum in an attempt to restore normal relationships.
- *Protrusio* denotes an acetabulum whose depth is increased by medial displacement or migration of the femoral head.

This results in significant impairment of range of motion and adduction contracture.

- The acetabulum is deepened by the *labrum*. The inferior continuation of the labrum comprises the *transverse acetabular ligament*. This consistent structure is a reliable landmark for restoration of acetabular height when significant deformity or proximal migration is present.
- The *cotyloid notch* lies at the base of the acetabulum. Within the notch lies a fat pad, the *ligamentum teres*, and the artery of the ligamentum teres, which enters the hip by coursing beneath the transverse acetabular ligament.

Vascular Anatomy

- Seven arteries supply the region of the hip joint, and they arise from the *common iliac artery*. The common iliac artery branches into the internal and external iliac arteries, with the bifurcation occurring around the level of S1 (Gray and Goss 1973, Hoppenfeld and DeBoer 1994, Netter 1987).
- Relevant branches of the internal iliac are the obturator, superior gluteal, and inferior gluteal.
- The external iliac artery becomes the femoral artery as it passes under the inguinal ligament, and then it gives rise to the profunda femoris, medial and lateral femoral circumflex, and perforating and nutrient vessels.
- Damage to one of the major vessels around the hip is rare, with an incidence of approximately 0.25%
  - Damage can occur through the use of retractors; an anterior acetabular retractor places the femoral vessels at risk, and an inferior retractor places a branch of the obturator at risk.
  - Damage may occur when using screws to secure the acetabular component; the iliac vessels are at risk in the anterosuperior zone, and the obturator vessels are at risk from anteroinferior screws. Wasielewski and colleagues devised an acetabular quadrant system based on cadaver studies to minimize this risk, with the safe zone considered the posterior superior and posterior inferior quadrants (Keating et al. 1990, Wasielewski et al. 1990) (Fig. 5–4).
- Lateral femoral circumflex artery
  - Branch of the profunda femoris
  - Supplies the iliopsoas, vastus lateralis, vastus intermedius, and tensor fasciae lata
- Medial femoral circumflex artery
  - Branch of femoral artery
  - Courses posteriorly between the iliopsoas and the pectineus.
  - Is a common source of bleeding around the quadratus muscle in the distal extent of the posterior approach to the hip
  - Supplies the adductor muscles, gracilis, and obturator externus
  - Is the major blood supply to the femoral head in adults, with compromise of this vessel during surgical

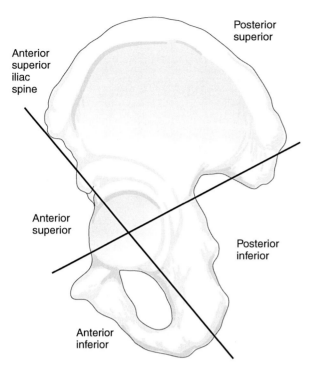

Anterior superior iliac spine

Posterior superior

Anterior superior

Posterior inferior

Anterior inferior

Figure 5–4: Quadrant system of the acetabulum. The posterior two quadrants are safest for screw placement, with the superior quadrant offering the most robust bone.

exposure leading to avascular necrosis (AVN) of the femoral head
- Often anastomoses with the obturator artery
- Obturator artery
  - Branch of internal iliac artery
  - Sends a branch, the acetabular artery, beneath the transverse acetabular ligament and is at risk of damage from placement of retractors or by dissection here. Appropriate medialization of the acetabular component often results in bleeding and necessitates cautery of this vessel.
  - Supplies obturator externus and internus and portions of adductor brevis and magnus
- Superior gluteal artery
  - Branch of internal iliac artery, exiting the pelvis posteriorly
  - Courses above the piriformis muscle and divides into superficial and deep branches
  - Supplies the gluteus medius and portions of the gluteus minimus
  - Supplies the superior and posterior portion of the acetabulum
- Inferior gluteal artery
  - Branch of external iliac artery
  - Supplies the bulk of the gluteus maximus
  - Supplies the short external rotators: piriformis, portion of obturator internus, superior and inferior gemellus, and quadratus femoris
  - Provides blood supply to the sciatic nerve via a transverse branch

- First perforating artery
  - Branch of femoral artery
  - Supplies the adductor brevis
- Nutrient artery
  - Branch of profunda femoris
  - Supplies the major blood supply to the femoral diaphysis

Nerves

- The hip joint has an abundant nervous supply. The most important nerves during hip arthroplasty are the lateral femoral cutaneous nerve, the femoral nerve, the sciatic nerve, and the superior gluteal nerve (Gray and Goss 1973, Hoppenfeld and DeBoer 1994, Netter 1987).
- Lateral femoral cutaneous nerve (L2-L3)
  - Branch of lumbar plexus
  - No motor function, provides sensation to the lateral thigh
  - Enters the deep fascia 2 to 3 inches below the anterior superior iliac spine in the interval between the tensor fasciae lata and sartorius
  - Most at risk during an anterior (Smith-Peterson) approach. Avoidance of the nerve is best accomplished by moving the incision laterally into the fascia of the tensor (Light and Keggi 1980, Smith-Peterson 1949).
- Femoral nerve (L2-L4)
  - Branch of lumbar plexus
  - Runs lateral to the femoral artery, as the most lateral structure in the femoral sheath
  - Separated from the hip capsule by the iliopsoas
  - Rarely encountered during hip arthroplasty, although can be damaged by improperly placed retractors over the anterior acetabular rim
  - Supplies the pectineus, sartorius, and quadriceps femoris muscles.
- Superior gluteal nerve (L4-S1)
  - Branch of sacral plexus
  - Courses from posterior to anterior between the gluteus medius and minimus, accompanying superior gluteal artery
  - Provides innervation to the gluteus medius, gluteus minimus, and tensor fasciae lata
  - Is most at risk during a lateral approach to the hip while splitting the abductors
    - A "safe zone" has been described that suggests staying within 5 cm of the tip of the greater trochanter when utilizing this approach.
- Sciatic nerve (L4-S3)
  - Branch of sacral plexus
  - Two divisions: tibial, L4-S3, and common peroneal, L4-S2
  - Although bifurcation usually occurring distally at the apex of the popliteal fossa, can bifurcate proximally around the piriformis

- In most cases, passes out of the greater sciatic foramen and courses anterior to, and then descends below, the piriformis muscle; in 2% of cases, pierces the piriformis. It is at greatest risk from posterior surgical retractors during the posterior approach (Marcy and Fletcher 1954).
- Supplies the semimembranosus, semitendinosus, long head of the biceps femoris, and posterior adductor magnus

Surgical Approaches

Anterior Approach

- Classically described by Smith-Peterson, this approach had fallen out of favor, but it is having a resurgence in minimally invasive hip arthroplasty either alone or as part of a two- or three-incision approach, as a result of the preservation of the posterior stabilizers (Light and Keggi 1980, Smith-Peterson 1949).
- The patient is positioned in the supine or lateral position.
- This approach utilizes a true internervous plane between the sartorius (femoral nerve) and the tensor fasciae lata (superior gluteal nerve) (Fig. 5–5).

Technique

- Superficial dissection
  - Classically, the skin incision begins along the anterior half of the ilium to the anterior superior iliac spine (ASIS) and then is carried distally for 10-12 cm
  - For the minimally invasive approach, only 8 to 10 cm of the distal limb is utilized.
  - Modifications of the skin incision have been proposed to allow for elevation of the femur out of the wound when this is the only incision utilized.
- The interval between the tensor fasciae lata and the sartorius is developed.
  - Alternatively, the tensor fasciae lata can be incised longitudinally. This is thought to reduce the incidence of lateral femoral cutaneous nerve injury.
- The ascending branch of the lateral femoral circumflex artery is reliably found just lateral to the rectus and should be identified and ligated.
- The tensor fasciae lata is retracted posteriorly, and the sartorius and rectus femoris are retracted anteriorly.

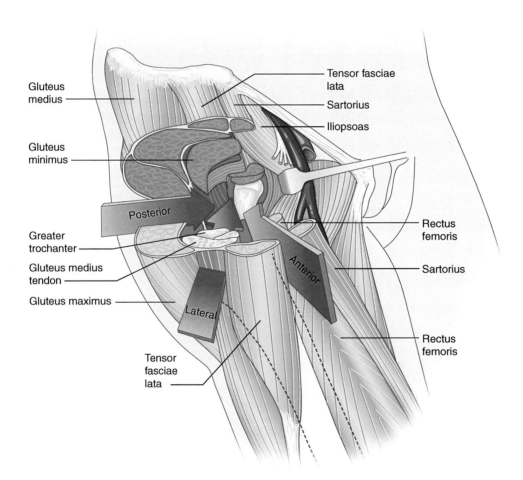

Figure 5–5: Surgical approaches to the hip.
Diagram of surgical approaches to the hip, including muscular intervals for the posterior, lateral, and anterior approaches.

The rectus has two origins; the direct head with origin on the anterior inferior iliac spine is retracted medially. The femoral neurovascular bundle courses medial to the rectus and iliopsoas and is protected by this maneuver.

- Deep dissection
  - The indirect head of the rectus femoris and gluteus medius is now visualized.
  - Elevate the indirect head of the rectus femoris off the anterior capsule and retract it medially. Retract the gluteus medius laterally.
  - The anterior capsule is then visualized and excised to expose the hip joint. Retention with later closure of the anterior capsule is another alternative.
  - External rotation, extension, and adduction of the femur facilitate placement of the femoral prosthesis. In stiff hips, the posterior capsule may need to be released.
- Structures at risk
  - Lateral femoral cutaneous nerve
    - This reaches the thigh by passing over the sartorius approximately 2.5 cm below the anterior superior iliac spine.
  - Ascending branch of lateral femoral circumflex artery
    - This runs between the tensor fasciae lata and the sartorius.
- Advantages to this approach include minimal blood loss and minimal soft tissue trauma, as well as preservation of a large portion of the posterior soft tissue envelope and abductor mechanism. Visualization of the acetabulum and accurate placement of the prosthesis are facilitated.
- Disadvantages include poor visualization of posterior acetabular wall and column and difficult access for femoral preparation in some patients. Care must be taken to ensure adequate visualization of the posterior aspect of the femoral neck to guard against improper femoral placement.

Anterolateral Approach

- This approach uses the interval between the tensor fasciae lata and the gluteus medius (Hoppenfeld and DeBoer 1994, Miller and Gomez 2000).
- Supine or lateral positioning is indicated.
- No true internervous plane exists, but the superior gluteal nerve enters the tensor fasciae lata near its origin and is therefore well protected (see Fig. 5–5).

Technique

- Superficial dissection
  - The skin incision can be a straight lateral incision centered over the greater trochanter or may be curved slightly posteriorly at the proximal extent.
  - The iliotibial band is next incised in line with the skin incision.
  - A retractor is placed deep to the gluteus medius and minimus, and these muscles are retracted proximally and laterally away from the joint capsule

- Deep dissection
  - This consists of detaching the anterior part of the abductor mechanism.
  - It can be accomplished by trochanteric osteotomy or by abductor muscle detachment.
    1. Trochanteric osteotomy
       - Begin at the base of the vastus lateralis ridge.
       - Osteotomize the trochanter and reflect the abductors superiorly.
       - Although rarely used in primary arthroplasty, it can be helpful in revision cases.
    2. Abductor detachment
       - Dissect the distal and anterior gluteus medius tendon off the femur subperiosteally.
       - Continue this proximally to the tip of the greater trochanter then continue proximally in line with the gluteus medius.
       - Secure reattachment of the abductors at closure is essential to prevent Trendelenburg's gait.
       - Retract the gluteus medius proximally and identify the gluteus minimus.
       - Separate the minimus from the anterior capsule, release it, and retract it superiorly with the medius.
       - Elevate the reflected head of the rectus femoris off the anterior capsule.
       - The capsule can now be excised or incised in a T shape for later repair.
- Structures at risk
  - Superior gluteal neurovascular bundle
    - Proximal extension puts these structures at risk.
  - Femoral nerve
    - This lies most laterally in the femoral triangle and is closest to the operative field.
    - It can rarely be injured by overexuberant retraction or compression by a poorly placed retractor. Retractors must be kept lateral to the rectus and iliopsoas.
  - Femoral artery and vein
    - These vessels lie on the surface of the iliopsoas.
    - Incorrectly placed retractors that pierce the iliopsoas can damage these vessels.

Lateral (Transgluteal) Approach

- No true internervous plane exists (Frndak et al. 1993, Hardinge 1982).
- Lateral patient positioning is indicated.
- The gluteus medius is split in line with its fibers distal to where the superior gluteal nerve supplies the muscle (see Fig. 5–5).

Technique

- Superficial dissection
  - The skin incision can either be a straight lateral incision centered over the greater trochanter or may be curved slightly posteriorly at the proximal extent.

- Incise the iliotibial band in line with the incision.
- Deep dissection
  - Beginning near the tip of the trochanter, incise the gluteus medius in line with its fibers no more than 5 cm above the tip of the greater trochanter to avoid injury to the superior gluteal nerve.
  - Continue distally incising the gluteus medius and vastus lateralis off the femur.
  - Develop an anterior flap consisting of the gluteus medius, the underlying gluteus minimus, and the anterior portion of the vastus lateralis.
  - Continue anteriorly until the anterior hip capsule is exposed. The anterior portion of insertion of the gluteus minimus will need to be released off the greater trochanter.
  - The capsule can now be excised or incised in a T shape for later repair.
- Structures at risk
  - Superior gluteal nerve
    - This runs between the gluteus medius and minimus approximately 5 cm above the upper border of the greater trochanter.
    - More proximal dissection may injure the nerve.
  - Femoral nerve
    - This lies most laterally in the femoral triangle and is closest to the operative field.
    - It can rarely be injured by overexuberant retraction or compression by a poorly placed retractor.
  - Femoral artery and vein
    - These vessels lie on the surface of the iliopsoas.
    - Incorrectly placed retractors that pierce the iliopsoas can damage these vessels.
  - Lateral circumflex artery
    - This must be cauterized as the vastus lateralis is mobilized.

Posterior Approach

- This is the most common approach to the hip because it allows safe, reproducible, and wide exposure without violating the abductor mechanism. Also, it is easy to extend using extensile maneuvers both proximally and distally (Hoppenfeld and DeBoer 1994, Marcy and Fletcher 1954).
- The patient is in the lateral decubitus position, and the pelvis must be stable to allow acetabular exposure and positioning. The weight of the leg anteriorly tends to pull the patient forward.
- There is no internervous plane, but the gluteus maximus is split in line with its fibers and is not significantly denervated (see Fig. 5–5).

Technique

- Superficial dissection
  - The skin incision can be varied, but generally it curves posteriorly from the center or posterior aspect of the greater trochanter.

- The less invasive posterior approach requires the incision to be moved to the posterior edge of the gluteus medius and greater trochanter and to be placed with precision.
- Incise the fascia in line with the skin incision distally. Proximally, split the gluteus maximus in line with its fibers.
- Deep dissection
  - Identify the approximate location of the sciatic nerve before placing a self-retaining retractor into the fascia anteriorly and posteriorly, approximately at the level of the greater trochanter.
  - The posterolateral aspect of the femur is now visualized.
  - The sciatic nerve passes under the piriformis and runs on top of the short external rotators and can now be identified, but it should not be exposed.
  - Internally rotate the femur to put the short external rotators on stretch, and establish and place a retractor in the interval between the piriformis and gluteus medius.
  - Detach the piriformis, superior and inferior gemellus, and obturator internus from their femoral insertion and reflect them posteriorly. A branch of the inferior gluteal artery routinely runs with the piriformis and should be coagulated.
    - This exposes the hip capsule and protects the sciatic nerve.
    - The piriformis is commonly tagged with a heavy suture for later reattachment.
    - Alternatively, the external rotators and hip capsule can be raised as a single flap.
  - A portion of the quadratus femoris may also have to be released. Care should be taken to avoid injury to the medial femoral circumflex as it courses in the distal extent of the quadratus. Control of this vessel is important to avoid significant hemorrhage.
  - The capsule can now be excised, or a flap can be made for later repair.
    - Repair of the hip capsule with or without repair of the short external rotators significantly decreases the risk of postoperative hip dislocation.
  - The femur must be subluxed anteriorly to allow for acetabular preparation. Release of the anterior capsule off of the anterior rim and release of the reflected head of the rectus facilitate this exposure.
- Structures at risk
  - Sciatic nerve
    - Care must be taken when placing retractors, especially a self-retaining retractor on the fascia, so as to not compress the nerve.
    - Be aware of occasional, known anatomic anomalies.
    - The peroneal trunk is proximal to tibial trunk within the nerve, and when there is an early bifurcation, the peroneal trunk exits first.
  - Inferior gluteal neurovascular bundle

- This can be injured by aggressive division of the gluteus maximus.

Surgical Approaches to the Knee

Overview

- A detailed understanding of knee osteology, as well as neurovascular and soft tissue anatomy, facilitates safe and effective surgical exposures for knee arthroplasty (Andriacchi 2000).
- All surgical exposures involve three distinct steps: (1) skin incision, (2) arthrotomy, and (3) mobilization of the extensor mechanism (Younger et al. 1998).
- With the increasing demand for smaller incisions and expeditious return to vocational and recreational activities, a higher priority arises for precise surgical exposures and meticulous soft tissue management.
- Several "alternative" surgical exposures have evolved from the advances gained in minimally invasive surgery and the appreciation for preserving the extensor mechanism. These approaches all have the common goals of (1) reducing patellofemoral complications, (2) expediting the return of quadriceps function, and (3) improving both short-term and long-term outcomes of total knee arthroplasty (TKA). Minimally invasive surgery should never be performed at the expense of safe and accurate component positioning.
- Severe deformity, previous operative interventions, and revision arthroplasty all demand careful preoperative planning with the implementation of specialized exposures to optimize visualization and avoid severe complications (Keblish 1991, Younger et al. 1998).
- Specific postoperative complications may be directly related to the operative approach and must be understood and anticipated; early diagnosis of these complications will facilitate treatment and optimize outcomes.
- Surgeons cannot rely on one single or standard operative approach for every patient undergoing knee arthroplasty. Familiarity with several specialized techniques allows for preoperative and intraoperative adaptation to the encountered pathologic features.

Basic Anatomy

Bony Anatomy

- The *knee joint* consists of the distal femur, the proximal tibia, proximal fibula, and the patella.
- The articular surfaces of these bony structures are covered by hyaline cartilage and are arranged into three distinct compartments: the medial compartment, the lateral compartment, and the patellofemoral compartment (Gray and Goss 1973, Miller and Gomez 2000, Netter 1987).
- Degenerative arthritis can involve a single compartment (unicompartmental) or all three compartments (tricompartmental), each to a different extent.

Femur

- The *distal femur* is composed of medial and lateral condyles that converge anteriorly as the *femoral trochlea*. The coronal plane alignment averages 5 to 7 degrees of valgus. Each condyle is directed posteriorly with diminishing radii of curvature from anterior to posterior. Viewed axially, the *lateral condyle* is taller, with an overall straight alignment. Conversely, the *medial condyle* is larger, with a more uniform radius of curvature. These anatomic points account for the "screw home mechanism of the knee."
- *Screw home mechanism:* As the knee is brought into full extension, the tibia externally rotates on the femur with the medial tibial plateau riding along the curvature of the medial condyle. This mechanism "locks" the knee in terminal extension.
- The strongest bone is found posteriorly on both condyles with relatively weak central areas. Trabecular bone strength increases as one moves further proximally from the subchondral plate.

Tibia

- The articular surface of the *tibia* is aligned perpendicular to its long axis, but it can exhibit a varus slope of up to 3 to 5 degrees. This surface slopes from anterior to posterior, averaging 10 degrees. The medial tibial plateau is concave, whereas the lateral plateau is convex; the intervening menisci increase conformity with the femoral condyles.
- The *trabecular bone* of the tibial epiphysis and metaphysis is responsible for load transmission. The trabecular bone strength significantly declines at a distance 5 mm or greater from the articular surface. This point is critical when planning bony resection because removing more than 10 mm of bone equates to diminished support for the prosthesis and a potential for an increased risk of component loosening, subsidence, and eventual failure. At increasing levels of tibial resection, load sharing with the cortical rim becomes more important.

Patella

- The *patella*, the largest sesamoid bone in the human body, is enclosed entirely within the quadriceps tendon. The patella articulates with the femoral trochlea from 35 to 135 degrees of knee flexion. Functionally, the patella imparts mechanical advantage to the quadriceps myotendinous unit by increasing the moment arm, and it provides protection to the anterior knee. The *median ridge* divides the bone into medial and lateral facets, and a second *vertical ridge* near the medial border creates the "odd" facet.
- The average thickness of the patella is 23 to 25 mm. Resurfacing the patella has become standard practice in TKA, and bony thickness after resection must be a minimum of 12 to 15 mm to decrease the risk of fracture. In addition, excessive thickness after resection can increase stress

in the patella and is also a risk factor for patellar fracture as well as knee stiffness.

- Improper patellar component positioning or improper soft tissue balancing may lead to poor *patellar tracking,* a common cause of postoperative anterior knee pain and disability.
- The complex blood supply to the patella is at risk during operative exposure for knee arthroplasty and can lead to AVN and fracture (see later).

Alignment

- The goal of any knee arthroplasty is to restore the mechanical axis through bony cuts, soft tissue balancing, and accurate component implantation.
- Most TKA systems utilize either intramedullary or extramedullary cutting guides to approximate the anatomic axes. The guides allow precise changes in rotation and angulation for both the femoral and tibial bone cuts, with the goal of using the anatomic axis to restore the mechanical axis (cut the femur in 5 to 7 degrees of valgus to its anatomic axis, and cut the tibia perpendicular to the shaft; see Fig. 5–1).

Mechanical Axis

- The *mechanical axis* is defined by a line extending from the center of the femoral head to the center of the tibial plafond and extending to the center of the ankle.
- The normal mechanical axis distributes 60% of the load to the medial compartment and 40% to the lateral compartment.
- Congenital, arthritic, and traumatic conditions can alter the mechanical axis, thus shifting the load disproportionately to one compartment and leading to progressive degeneration.

Anatomic Axis

- The *anatomic axis* is the angle created at the tibiofemoral joint by the intersection of lines drawn parallel to the femoral and tibial intramedullary canals.
- The *femoral anatomic axis* averages 5 to 7 degrees of valgus.
- The *tibial anatomic axis* parallels the mechanical axis and is perpendicular to the articular surface.

Q Angle

- The *Q angle* is the angle formed by the intersection of a line parallel to the pull of the quadriceps tendon with a line parallel to the pull of the patellar tendon (angles >20 degrees considered abnormal).
- The Q angle must be restored during knee arthroplasty by appropriate component rotation, medialization of the patellar button, and soft tissue balancing (e.g., lateral release) as necessary.
- *Patellar maltracking* is a common source of anterior knee pain following TKA, and several alternative surgical approaches have been described attempting to diminish this common complication.

Patella Height

- *Patella alta:* High riding
- *Patella baja:* Low riding
- Patella baja frequently encountered in TKA (especially following high tibial osteotomy)
- Measures
  - *Insall-Salvati index:* Ratio of patellar tendon length to patellar height (normal = 1.0, alta >1.2, baja <0.8)
  - *Blumensaat's line:* With knee in 30 degrees of flexion, inferior pole of the patella should lie on a line extended from the intercondylar notch
  - *Blackburne-Peel index:* Ratio of line drawn from tibial plateau to the inferior articular surface of the patella to the length of the patellar articular surface (normal, 0.8; alta, >1.0)

Vascular Anatomy

- The blood supply to the knee arises from several named branches forming a rich vascular anastomotic ring.
- Proximally, the *superficial femoral artery* courses along the medial thigh, giving rise to the descending genicular artery before entering the adductor hiatus.
- The *descending genicular artery* travels through the vastus medialis and anastomoses with the superior medial and lateral genicular arteries.
- Distally, the *anterior tibial recurrent artery* branches anterolaterally from the anterior tibial artery. The anterior tibial recurrent artery courses proximally to anastomose with the inferior medial and lateral genicular arteries.
- The remaining branches all arise from the *popliteal artery,* which is the terminal branch of the superficial femoral artery (name change occurs as the artery courses through the adductor hiatus).
- Understanding this complex blood supply allows safe surgical exposures.

Skin

- The vascular supply to the skin overlying the anterior knee must be clearly understood.
- The arterial plexus described earlier sends perforators through the deep fascia, thus creating a superficial anastomosis of vessels responsible for the blood supply to the skin. Most of these deep perforators arise medially, and the entire anastomosis lies just superficial to the deep fascia (Netter 1987, Scapinelli 1967).
- These points are critical for understanding:
  - *Superficial dissection:* Wide dissections superficial to the deep fascia compromise the skin overlying the anterior knee. Thus, all flaps must be created deep to the deep fascia.
  - *Skin incisions:* When that patient has multiple, previous, longitudinal skin incisions, the most lateral of these incisions should be utilized when feasible.
    - The majority of the blood supply to the anterior skin of the knee arises medially.

- Previous, single transverse anterior skin incisions can be crossed at 90 degrees with little concern.
- Any prior longitudinal skin incision should be utilized when feasible.
- If a parallel longitudinal incision must be created, be careful to maintain at least a 5- to 7-cm skin bridge.

Patella

- Six arteries supply both the extraosseous and intraosseous blood supply to the patella (Scapinelli 1967). These vessels form branches along the anterior surface of the patella and provide an intraosseous blood supply via perforating vessels that penetrate the middle third of the anterior patella with a smaller contribution entering the distal pole (Fig. 5–6).
  - The medial superior and inferior genicular arteries along with the descending genicular artery course from medial to lateral contributing to the patellar vascular ring. All three vessels are divided during standard medial parapatellar arthrotomy.
  - The lateral superior and inferior genicular arteries along with the anterior tibial recurrent artery course from lateral to medial contributing to the patellar vascular ring. The lateral inferior genicular artery is compromised during excision of the lateral meniscus. The anterior tibial recurrent artery is at risk with excision of the infrapatellar fat pad, whereas the lateral superior genicular artery is at risk during lateral release.

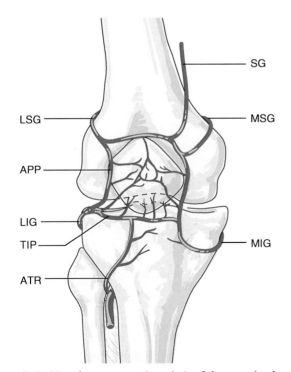

Figure 5–6: Vascular anatomy (arteries) of the anterior knee. *APP*, ascending parapatellar; *ATR*, anterior tibial recurrent; *LIG*, lateral inferior genicular; *LSG*, lateral superior genicular; *MIG*, medial inferior genicular; *MSG*, medial superior genicular; *SG*, supreme genicular; *TIP*, transverse infrapatellar.

- Preserving the lateral superior genicular artery has been shown to preserve the patellar blood supply. This vessel runs horizontally just inferior to the vastus lateralis and with careful dissection can be protected.
- Numerous studies have shown an increased risk for patellar AVN during standard medial parapatellar arthrotomy and concurrent lateral release. Previous concern that excision of the infrapatellar fat pad will also compromise patellar viability has not been proven in the literature.

Nerves

- The peripheral nerve pathways about the knee have been described in detail elsewhere (Gray and Goss 1973, Netter 1987).
- Inadvertent sectioning of these sensory nerves can lead to bothersome sensory disturbances, painful neuromas, chronic regional pain syndrome (type II), and continued pain following lateral release.
- *Medially*, three constant nerves have been identified:
  - The *terminal branch of the medial femoral cutaneous nerve* courses 1 cm distal to the adductor tubercle and crosses laterally to form a prepatellar plexus and continues to the lateral aspect of the knee (crosses the midline).
  - The *infrapatellar branch of the saphenous nerve* exits Hunter's canal near the joint line and courses medially and distally toward the tibial tubercle. It supplies the medial and anterolateral skin below the patella, as well as the anteroinferior joint capsule. It crosses the midline, and its division is a source of postoperative numbness following knee arthroplasty.
  - The *medial retinacular nerve* is the terminal branch of the nerve to the vastus medialis. It supplies sensory innervation to the medial retinaculum. It does *not* cross the midline.
- *Laterally*, two consistent lateral retinacular nerves have been identified with variable sensory innervation to the skin.
  - Lateral sensory innervation to the skin is provided by the *lateral femoral cutaneous nerve* and by branches from the *femoral nerve*.
  - The *lateral retinacular nerves* arise from the sciatic nerve proximal to the popliteal fossa. They are at risk during lateral release. Inadvertent sectioning may potentially lead to a painful neuroma. This fact may explain the infrequent patient whose condition worsens following a lateral release.

Soft Tissue

- The knee joint depends on its numerous *soft tissue restraints* for stability and function.
- These structures may become contracted or attenuated as part of the arthritic process.
- Operative dissection must respect these soft tissues to maintain appropriate balance, stability, and function.

Before operative closure, the knee must be taken through a full range of motion to ensure stability and integrity of all soft tissue restraints.

- Understanding this complex anatomy is enhanced by compartmentalizing the knee.

Medial: Divided Into Three Distinct Layers

- *Layer 1:* The most superficial layer, consisting of the sartorius and fascia
  - The tendons of the gracilis and semitendinosus lie between layers 1 and 2.
- *Layer 2:* Consisting of the superficial medial collateral ligament (MCL)
  - The MCL, which is the primary restraint to valgus stress, travels from the medial epicondyle to insert broadly 5 to 7 cm distal to the joint line immediately deep to the pes anserinus.
  - The superficial MCL must be protected with appropriate retractor placement throughout the entire operative procedure. Unrecognized iatrogenic injury to the superficial MCL can lead to medial instability and rapid failure following TKA.
- *Layer 3:* Consisting of the deep MCL and the joint capsule
  - The deep MCL is intimately associated with the medial meniscus.
  - This layer is dissected subperiosteally from the proximal or medial tibia during all surgical exposures that incorporate a medial arthrotomy (the dissection must stay directly on bone to avoid inadvertent transection of the superficial MCL).

Lateral: Divided Into Three Distinct Layers

- *Layer 1:* The most superficial layer, composed of the iliotibial band, biceps femoris, and fascia
- *Layer 2:* Consisting of the lateral retinaculum and patellofemoral ligament
- *Layer 3:* Consisting of the arcuate ligament, the lateral collateral ligament (LCL), and the joint capsule
  - The LCL arises from the lateral epicondyle and inserts onto the fibular head.
  - The LCL is less intimately involved with the lateral meniscus and joint capsule compared with its medial counterpart; the popliteus tendon intervenes between the LCL and lateral meniscus.
  - The inferior lateral geniculate artery is deep to the LCL and may be encountered during lateral meniscectomy.

Posterior

- The posterior aspect of the knee rarely, if ever, requires exposure during TKA. However, several posterior structures and osteophytes may require surgical release or resection to restore full range of motion in knees with significant preoperative flexion contractures. Safely addressing these structures requires knowledge and avoidance of the popliteal neurovascular contents.

- The *popliteal artery* runs centrally and distally in the popliteal fossa just posterior to the joint capsule. The nerve and vein are more superficial and less at risk.
- The *posterior joint capsule* inserts on the femur proximal to the condyles and deep to the medial and lateral heads of the gastrocnemius. The posterior capsule can be subperiosteally stripped off the posterior femoral condyles to aid in soft tissue balancing and release. Transection of the posterior capsule is not recommended and can jeopardize the popliteal contents.
- The *posterior cruciate ligament* (PCL) lies in the midline just anterior to the posterior joint capsule. Care must be taken during operative excision of the PCL because penetration of the joint capsule at this level places the popliteal contents at risk.
- *Popliteus muscle:* This arises from the posteromedial surface of the tibia and inserts on the lateral femoral condyle. It intervenes between the LCL and the lateral meniscus and can be easily visualized posterolaterally during knee arthroplasty. It may require division in selected patients for appropriate soft tissue balancing.

Cruciate Ligaments

- The anterior cruciate ligament (ACL) is excised during TKA, whereas the PCL is either retained or resected based on surgeon preference and patient considerations.
- *ACL:* This originates on the posteromedial aspect of the lateral femoral condyle and inserts on the anterior intercondylar tibia. It resists anterior translation of the tibia.
- *PCL:* The stronger of the two cruciate ligaments, the PCL originates on the anteromedial femoral condyle and inserts on the posterior tibial sulcus, distal to the articular surface. It resists posterior translation of the tibia.

Extensor Mechanism

- The *extensor mechanism* is the most critical soft tissue component during TKA. Insufficiency is a contraindication to proceeding with TKA. Adequate surgical exposure requires mobilization of the extensor mechanism to ensure minimal tension on the tibial insertion. Iatrogenic injury to the patellar tendon insertion by avulsion or transection is a devastating complication of TKA and must be avoided. Thus several special techniques have been developed to aid in knee exposure while protecting the integrity of the extensor mechanism (see later).
- The *quadriceps mechanism* consists of four muscles (rectus femoris, vastus lateralis, vastus medialis, and vastus intermedius) that join distally as a common tendon, the *quadriceps tendon.* The quadriceps tendon inserts into the patella. Distally, the *patellar tendon* arises from the distal pole of the patella and inserts into the tibial tubercle. The *vastus medialis obliquus* (VMO), a component of the vastus medialis, is the primary restraint to lateral subluxation of the patella during active knee extension and may be

preserved during alternative surgical approaches to knee arthroplasty.

Surgical Approaches

Medial Parapatellar

Indications

- The gold standard surgical approach for both primary and revision TKA (Insall 1993) (Fig. 5–7)
- Can be applied to almost any knee arthroplasty operation

Contraindications

- Absolute: Preexisting skin incisions preventing safe exposure of the medial side
- Relative: Severe valgus deformity or the need for lateral ligament reconstruction

Advantages

- Utilitarian approach familiar to all orthopaedic surgeons
- Provides wide exposure and clear visualization
- Respects neurovascular anatomy

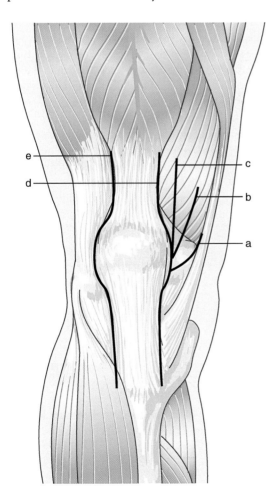

Figure 5–7: Incisions for primary total knee arthroplasty. Subvastus *(a)*, midvastus *(b)*, trivector *(c)*, medial parapatellar *(d)*, and lateral *(e)*.

- Can be extended to a quadriceps snip or V-Y quadricepsplasty if mobilization of extensor mechanism difficult

Disadvantages

- Reports of patellar AVN when combined with lateral release
- Aggressive incision through the quadriceps tendon with acute postoperative inhibition of the quadriceps possibly leading to increased rates of patellar maltracking or chronic quadriceps atrophy

Technique

- Skin incision
  - Use a marking pen to outline the superior, inferior, medial, and lateral borders of the patella. Identify and mark the tibial tubercle.
  - With the knee in flexion, draw a straight, midline, longitudinal incision starting 4 fingerbreadths above the superior pole of the patella and extending just beyond the tibial tubercle. The incision should course medial to the tibial tubercle and not directly over it.
  - With the knee in flexion, incise the skin and subcutaneous tissue down to the fascia.
  - Develop medial and lateral full-thickness flaps, thus exposing the extensor mechanism proximally and distally.
- Arthrotomy
  - With the knee in flexion, identify the quadriceps tendon in the proximal extent of the wound.
  - Longitudinally split the tendon and leave at least two thirds laterally and no more than one third medially.
  - Continue the arthrotomy either medially around the patella (leaving a small cuff of tendon for repair) or directly over the anterior midline of the patella.
  - Distally, continue the arthrotomy just medial to the patellar tendon and slightly beyond and medial to the tibial tubercle.
- Mobilization of extensor mechanism
  - With the knee in full extension, subperiosteally dissect the medial capsule and deep MCL from the proximal tibia. The extent of medial release depends on the preoperative deformity, with greater medial release required in severe varus deformity. Strict adherence to subperiosteal dissection will avoid iatrogenic division of the superficial MCL.
  - Attempt to evert the patella in extension and slowly flex the knee. Critically evaluate the distal insertion of the patellar tendon as the knee is flexed, and stop at any sign of excessive strain. *Patellar tendon avulsion must be avoided.*
  - If the patella cannot safely be everted:
    - Remove all medial and lateral osteophytes from the femur and tibia.
    - Mobilize the lateral quadriceps from the distal femur.
    - Release along the proximal lateral tibia while respecting the insertion of the patellar tendon.

- Perform a quadriceps snip, V-Y quadriceps advancement, tibial tubercle osteotomy, or femoral peel as needed, to ensure safe and adequate mobilization and patellar eversion.
  - Early resection of the patella, protection with a metallic wafer, and lateral subluxation, rather than eversion, have gained popularity during less invasive approaches to the knee.
- Excise the medial and lateral menisci and ACL, with or without the PCL, and any remaining osteophytes.
- Complete the TKA.
- The standard medial parapatellar approach can be modified to fulfill the requirement for minimally invasive TKA.
  - The skin incision extends from the superior pole of the patella to the tibial tubercle.
  - The arthrotomy extends only 2 to 3 cm into the quadriceps tendon, to allow lateral patellar subluxation but not eversion.
  - This procedure is an excellent transition to more advanced minimally invasive surgical approaches.
  - It can easily be converted to standard medial parapatellar arthrotomy.

Subvastus

- Originally described as an alternative quadriceps-sparing approach to TKA (Hofmann et al. 1991)

Indications

- Effective surgical approach to primary knee arthroplasty, both standard and minimally invasive, in the appropriately selected patient

Contraindications

- Absolute: Large flexion contractures, revision TKA, previous knee arthrotomy, severe valgus deformity, and potential skin necrosis
- Relative: Obesity, short femur, and muscular thighs

Advantages

- Only approach to preserve the entire quadriceps mechanism
- Decreased postoperative pain and improved early quadriceps function
- Diminished rates of lateral release and improved patellar tracking
- Improved patient satisfaction with faster recovery and return to function

Disadvantages

- Technically demanding
- Cannot evert patella
- Cannot extend the approach with quadriceps snip or V-Y quadriceps advancement
- Less visualization, especially lateral compartment
- Risk of injury to saphenous nerve and descending genicular artery and of damage to vastus medialis function

Technique

- Incision
  - Standard midline or medialized skin incision
  - Minimally invasive surgery: Anteromedial incision starting just medial to superior pole of the patella and extending to the medial side of the tibial tubercle
- Arthrotomy
  - Identify the medial border of the patella, patellar tendon, tibial tubercle, and VMO.
  - Transverse arthrotomy begins at medial border of the patella just distal to the inferior border of the VMO. This occurs reliably about halfway down the patella. A robust tendinous portion defines the distal extent.
  - Distally, the arthrotomy extends longitudinally just medial to the patellar tendon and ends at the inferior extent of the tibial tubercle.
- Mobilization of extensor mechanism
  - Perform a complete synovial release in the suprapatellar pouch.
  - Bluntly dissect the VMO muscle belly off the intermuscular septum.
  - With the knee in extension, laterally subluxate the patella and slowly flex the knee. Always observe the patellar tendon insertion and avoid avulsion. You may prefer to cut the patella before subluxation; in this circumstance, do not place retractors against the patella because of the increased risk for iatrogenic fracture.
- Midvastus approach
  - This is an alternative to the subvastus approach with the same surgical goals of minimizing trauma to the quadriceps mechanism.
  - The arthrotomy is extended more proximally and divides the VMO muscle belly in line with its muscle fibers.
  - Advantage: It is technically less demanding than the subvastus approach, with improved exposure.
  - Disadvantage: It violates the VMO and is not completely quadriceps sparing. However, significantly less trauma occurs to the quadriceps than with the medial parapatellar approach, with less acute quadriceps inhibition postoperatively.

Lateral

Indications

- The lateral approach has been shown to improve patellar tracking and stability in the severely valgus knee (common deformity seen in rheumatoid arthritis).
- May also be utilized in the multiply operated knee in which undermining the medial side may risk skin necrosis (Keblish 1991).

Contraindications

- Absolute: Previous knee surgery compromising a safe lateral approach and risking skin necrosis
- Relative: Fixed varus deformity, unfamiliarity with operative approach

Advantages

- Directly exposes the pathologic features in fixed valgus deformity
- Facilitates lateral soft tissue management
- Preserves the entire VMO and thus improves patellar tracking
- Poses no risk of patellar AVN

Disadvantages

- Unfamiliar surgical approach to most orthopaedic surgeons
- Difficult exposure of proximal tibia secondary to prominent tibial tubercle (normal anatomy, tibial tubercle 7 mm lateral to midline) may require tibial tubercle osteotomy for adequate exposure
- Difficulty in addressing medial pathologic processes

Technique

- Skin incision: Centered over the lateral patella, extending proximally in line with the vastus lateralis and distally between the tibial tubercle and Gerdy's tubercle
- Arthrotomy and extensor mechanism mobilization

Extensile Exposures

- Approximately 110 degrees of knee flexion are required for component extraction, bony preparation, and knee implantation.
- Obesity and extensive extensor mechanism scarring increase the tensile forces at the tibial tubercle, thus precluding safe and adequate exposure when utilizing the standard medial parapatellar approach. Therefore, proximal and distal extensor mechanism–reflecting techniques have been developed to enhance surgical exposure and protect the integrity of the extensor mechanism.
- All techniques have the common goal of minimizing the risk of iatrogenic patellar tendon avulsion (see Fig. 5–7).

Quadriceps (Rectus) Snip

Indications

- The *quadriceps snip* is an excellent extension of the standard medial parapatellar approach when a moderate amount of additional joint exposure is required (Garvin et al. 1995, Younger et al. 1998) (Fig. 5–8).

Contraindications

- The quadriceps snip does not provide adequate exposure in severe extensor mechanism contracture and scarring.
- Poor-quality proximal soft tissues preclude the use of any proximal extensor mechanism–reflecting technique.

Advantages

- Easy extension of the standard medial parapatellar approach
- No need for postoperative immobilization or alteration of the routine postoperative rehabilitation

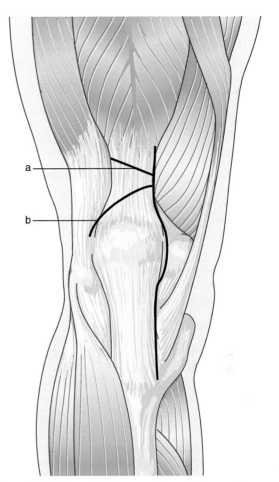

Figure 5–8: Extensile exposure for revision total knee arthroplasty.
Quadriceps snip *(a)* **and modified V-Y quadricepsplasty** *(b)*.

- No evidence of extensor lag or quadriceps weakness compared with contralateral TKA utilizing the standard approach

Disadvantages

- Does not provide the wide exposures seen with V-Y quadriceps advancement or tibial tubercle osteotomy

Technique

- Extend the standard arthrotomy in a proximal and lateral direction.
- The plane of dissection is at an angle of 45 degrees extending into the rectus femoris muscle belly.
- Attempt to evert the patella and slowly flex the knee; if there is continued tension at the tibial tubercle, consider a concomitant tibial tubercle osteotomy.

V-Y Quadriceps Advancement

Indications

- This is utilized as a proximal reflection in cases of severe extensor mechanism contracture and scarring (Trousdale et al. 1993) (see Fig. 5–8).

Contraindications

- Poor-quality proximal soft tissues and limited contractility of the quadriceps mechanism are contraindications to V-Y quadriceps advancement.

Advantages

- Excellent approach in patients with severe extensor mechanism contracture or scarring and contraindications to distal osteotomy.
- Enhanced exposure compared with quadriceps snip

Disadvantages

- Invariably weakens the extensor mechanism, with a persistent extensor lag common
- Requires alteration of the standard rehabilitation program: partial weight bearing, bracing, and limited flexion
- Potential for devascularization of the patella if arthrotomy inadvertently transects the inferior lateral geniculate artery

Technique

- Perform a standard medial parapatellar approach.
- Extend the proximal arthrotomy in a distal and lateral direction at an angle of 45 degrees. The dissection courses through the vastus lateralis and lateral retinaculum, stopping short of the inferior lateral geniculate artery and its branches.
- The "V" can be converted to a "Y" thus lengthening the quadriceps tendon.
- The lateral extent of the exposure can be left open to function as a lateral release and improve patellar tracking.

Tibial Tubercle Osteotomy

Indications

- Affords excellent exposure in the patient with severe extensor mechanism contracture and scarring
- Can be utilized in patients undergoing quadriceps snip and still requiring more mobilization for exposure (Younger et al. 1998)

Contraindications

- Previous operative procedures that have compromised the tibial tubercle
- Poor-quality proximal tibial bone including large tibial defects and osteoporosis
- Lengthening of extensor mechanism required; proximal turndown procedures more efficacious

Advantages

- Improved exposure compared with proximal turndown techniques
- Excellent exposure of the proximal tibia for extraction of well-fixed tibial stems
- Realignment of the extensor mechanism possible
- Early range of motion and full weight bearing encouraged postoperatively

Disadvantages

- Technically demanding
- Risk of nonunion or tendon rupture
- Additional dissection increasing the risk of poor distal wound healing, prolonged drainage, and deep infection

Technique

- Perform a standard medial parapatellar approach.
- Extend the distal dissection along the medial tibial shaft an additional 10 cm.
- Perform the osteotomy in a medial to lateral direction with an oscillating saw or with multiple drill holes and osteotome. The dimensions of the osteotomy are: 8 cm long × 2 cm wide × 1 cm deep (increasing the length of the osteotomy has decreased the rate of nonunion and failure).
- Leave the lateral attachments intact, and hinge open the osteotomy.
- On completion of the TKA, reattach the bone fragment with either two to three cerclage wires angled distally or a screw and washer.

Femoral Peel

Indications

- Utilized in knees when the pathologic process is too great for adequate exposure using the foregoing mentioned techniques (Younger et al. 1998)

Contraindications

- Surgeon not experienced in the technique

Advantages

- Provides wide exposure even in the most ankylosed and scarred knees
- Allows immediate full weight bearing and range of motion

Disadvantages

- Extensive dissection with theoretical risk of devascularizing the entire distal femur

Technique

- Perform a standard medial parapatellar approach.
- Subperiosteally elevate the origins of the MCL and LCL from the distal femur.
- Strip the posterior capsule from the posterior aspect of the femur and release the medial and lateral heads of the gastrocnemius, as necessary.
- Alternatively, a medial or lateral epicondylar osteotomy can be performed and achieves the same goals as the femoral peel.

References

Andriacchi TP (2000). Knee joint: Anatomy and biomechanics. In: Fitzgerald R, ed. *Orthopaedic Knowledge Update*. Park Ridge, Ill: AAOS, section 3, pp 239-248.

  This chapter describes anatomy and mechanical characteristics.

Frndak PA, Mallory TH, Lombardi AV (1993). Translateral approach to the hip: The abductor muscle split. *Clin Orthop Relat Res* 295: 131-141.

This report describes the modified translateral approach to the hip, "the abductor muscle split," in primary total hip arthroplasty. The results of this surgical approach in 50 patients with an average follow-up period of 2.8 years showed excellent restoration of abductor muscle function and gait without compromising surgical exposure.

Garvin K, Scuderi T, Insall J (1995). Evolution of the quadriceps snip. *Clin Orthop Relat Res* 321:131-137.

The results of the quadriceps snip is described in 16 patients (4 women and 12 men) who underwent knee surgery at the average age of 65 years (range, 50 to 73 years). The surgical exposure was done in the treatment of aseptic loosening of a total knee prosthesis in 8 patients, septic loosening in 2 patients, and primary knee arthroplasty in 6 patients with fibrous ankylosis. The authors found no difference compared with the opposite knee that had been replaced and concluded that the surgical technique is safe and simple, did not require special equipment, and did not cause the patient's physical therapy to be altered postoperatively.

Gray H, Goss CM (1973). *Gray's Anatomy.* Philadelphia: Lea & Febiger.

This classic text describes gross anatomy with superb illustrations of anatomic relationships.

Hardinge K (1982). The direct lateral approach to the hip. *J Bone Joint Surg Br* 64:17-19.

This is the original description of the direct lateral approach, with an emphasis on surgical technique, including clear illustrations and early results.

Hofmann AA, Plaster RL, Murdock LE (1991). Subvastus (Southern) approach for primary total knee arthroplasty. *Clin Orthop Relat Res* 269:70-77.

The subvastus technique and rationale including vascular and innervation around the knee are reviewed, and the advantages of this approach to TKA are described.

Hoppenfeld S, DeBoer P (1994). *Surgical Exposures in Orthopaedics: The Anatomic Approach,* 2nd ed. Philadelphia: JB Lippincott.

This classic text describes surgical exposures with superb illustrations, identification of landmarks, and vulnerable structures.

Insall JN (1993). Surgical approaches. In: Insall JN, Windsor RE, Scott WN, et al., eds. *Surgery of the Knee.* New York: Churchill Livingstone, pp 135-148.

Keating EM, Ritter MA, Faris PM (1990). Structures at risk from medially placed acetabular screws. *J Bone Joint Surg Am* 72:509-511.

This study examines anatomic structures at risk from acetabular screws. Medially placed screws either penetrated or came dangerously close to the following: the external iliac vein; the obturator artery, nerve, and vein; and tributaries of the internal iliac vein. To avoid injury to the medial vascular structures, screws should not be placed in the anterosuperior quadrant of the acetabulum.

Keblish PA (1991). The lateral approach to the valgus knee: Surgical technique and analysis of 53 cases with over two year follow-up evaluation. *Clin Orthop Relat Res* 271:52-62.

This article describes the technique for and results of the lateral approach to the valgus knee in 53 cases with a more than 2-year follow-up evaluation. Surgical technique is direct, anatomic, and more physiologic, and it maintains soft tissue integrity. The "lateral release" is performed as part of the approach. The author suggests that the approach is more aesthetic and results are objectively superior for fixed valgus deformity in TKA.

Light TR, Keggi KJ (1980). Anterior approach to hip arthroplasty. *Clin Orthop Relat Res* 152:255-260.

The direct anterior approach to the hip joint is described. Excellent visualization of the acetabulum is afforded by this approach. Modified femoral rasps of varying lengths are employed to rasp the femur with the leg in external rotation. The anterior approach provides a safe and effective approach to total hip arthroplasty with limited morbidity.

Marcy GH, Fletcher RS (1954). Modification of the posterolateral approach to the hip for insertion of femoral head prosthesis. *J Bone Joint Surg Am* 36:142-143.

This is a classic early description of the most commonly employed approach to hip arthroplasty used today, with key anatomic descriptions and techniques.

Miller MD, Gomez BA (2000). *Review of Orthopaedics,* 3rd ed. Philadelphia: WB Saunders, pp 556-577.

This widely used resource provides tabular data and information encapsulated for easy recollection and retention.

Netter FH (1987). *Musculoskeletal System. Part I: Anatomy, Physiology and Metabolic Disorders. CIBA Collection of Medical Illustrations,* vol. 8. Summit, NJ: CIBA-Geigy, pp 77-98.

These highly acclaimed illustrations show normal and pathologic anatomy with attention to key relationships and the interplay of the musculoskeletal and neurovascular anatomy.

Noble PC, Alexander JW, Lindahl LJ (1988). The anatomic basis of femoral component design. *Clin Orthop Relat Res* 235:148-165.

The anatomic variants of the femur were evaluated and described through the detailed study of more than 200 cadavers. Key relationships with normal and ranges of femoral dimensions are clearly catalogued. This is a valuable resource for a basic understanding of femoral anatomy. The authors noted that the dimensions of the femoral canal are variable. These data help to inform choices made in designing contemporary implants.

Scapinelli R (1967). Blood supply of the human patella: Its relation to ischaemic necrosis after fracture. *J Bone Joint Surg Br* 49:563-570.

This is the original description of the blood supply around the anterior knee with injection techniques used to identify details of anastomoses.

Schmalzreid TP, Amstutz HD, Dorey FJ (1991). Nerve palsy associated with total hip replacement. *J Bone Joint Surg Am* 73:1074-1080.

These authors reviewed the results of 3126 consecutive total hip replacements and identified postoperative neuropathy in the ipsilateral lower extremity after 53 (1.7%) overall and after 1.3% of the primary arthroplasties. Congenital dislocation or dysplasia of the hip and the revision carried higher complication rates. The nerves at risk were described, with the sciatic nerve involved in all but five extremities. The cause of the palsy was unclear or unknown in 30 (57%) of the extremities.

Singh M, Nagrath AR, Maini PS (1970). Changes in the trabecular pattern of the upper end of the femur as an index of osteoporosis. *J Bone Joint Surg Am* 52:457-467.

This article offers the systematic radiographic evaluation of the bony trabeculae of the proximal femur and a description of their changing patterns with progressive bone loss.

Smith-Peterson MN (1949). Approach to and exposure of the hip joint for mold arthroplasty. *J Bone Joint Surg Am* 31:40.
This is a classic description of the extensile version of the anterior approach to the hip for arthroplasty.

Trousdale R, Hanssen A, Rand J, Cahalan T (1993). V-Y quadricepsplasty in total knee arthroplasty. *Clin Orthop Relat Res* 286: 48-55.
This article describes the functional results of a V-Y quadricepsplasty in 14 consecutive patients (16 knees) who underwent TKA. Using the Cybex-II system and the knee rating score of the Hospital for Special Surgery, results at a mean of 3 years postoperatively were as follows: 2 excellent, 10 good, 2 fair, and 2 poor. Comparing patients who underwent V-Y quadricepsplasty with those who had normal medial parapatellar TKA, the extensor mechanism was weaker in the V-Y group, but not to a significant degree. These investigators concluded that with a V-Y quadricepsplasty during TKA, one can expect nearly normal active extension and moderate weakness in extension.

Wasielewski RC, Cooperstein LA, Kruger MP, Rubash HE (1990). Acetabular anatomy and the transacetabular fixation of screws in total hip arthroplasty. *J Bone Joint Surg Am* 72:501-508.

These authors describe four clinically useful acetabular quadrants when considering screw placement in total hip arthroplasty. The quadrants are formed first by drawing a line from the anterior superior iliac spine through the center of the acetabulum to the posterior fovea, to form acetabular halves. A second line is then drawn perpendicular to the first at the midpoint of the acetabulum, to form four quadrants. The posterior superior and posterior inferior acetabular quadrants contain the best available bone stock and are relatively safe for the transacetabular placement of screws. The anterior superior and anterior inferior quadrants should be avoided whenever possible because screws placed improperly in these quadrants may endanger the external iliac artery and vein, as well as the obturator nerve, artery, and vein.

Younger AS, Duncan CP, Masri BA (1998). Surgical exposures in revision total knee arthroplasty. *J Am Acad Orthop Surg* 6:55-64.
This nice review describes various approaches useful in revision knee arthroplasty, with emphasis on preoperative planning of the operative approach and wide exposure. Basic principles are emphasized, including careful component removal, soft tissue balancing, management of bone loss, and reimplantation without damaging important structures. Skin necrosis can be avoided by selecting the appropriate incision and dissecting deep to the fascia. Extensile exposure by dissection of scar, quadriceps snip or turndown, tibial tubercle osteotomy, medial epicondylar osteotomy, or femoral peel should be performed early to prevent patellar tendon disruption.

Arthritis

Neil P. Sheth[*] and Charles L. Nelson[†]

[*]MD, Resident, Department of Orthopaedic Surgery, Hospital of the University of
Pennsylvania, Philadelphia, PA
[†]MD, Assistant Professor, Department of Orthopaedic Surgery, University of Pennsylvania
School of Medicine, Philadelphia, PA

Introduction

- *Arthritis* is defined as intra-articular inflammation, which may be a result of several different etiologic factors. Arthritis comprises a diverse group of disorders that are primarily caused by pathology of the synovium, articular cartilage, and supporting subcomponent structures. A majority of diseases, regardless of origin, will lead to destructive degenerative joint disease in untreated cases. End-stage arthritis is often associated with severe pain and disability.
- Patients diagnosed with arthritis commonly have joint pain of the affected joint, decreased range of motion, and potential deformity and instability. The mainstay of therapy is generally nonoperative, with a focus on patient education, activity modification, and treatment with anti-inflammatory medications. Surgical management may be necessary for severe symptoms, and pain relief is the most predictable outcome and indication for joint reconstruction.
- The causes of arthritis can be categorized based on the underlying basis for the disease, which includes the following subgroups: noninflammatory, inflammatory, hemorrhagic, osteonecrotic, and infectious.

Noninflammatory Arthritides (Fries et al. 2003)

Osteoarthritis

- *Osteoarthritis* (OA) is the most common form of arthritis leading to eventual degenerative joint destruction, and it is the leading cause of disability in the developed world. The prevalence of clinically apparent OA is 30% in patients older than 75 years; OA of at least one joint is seen in 80% of this age population. The prevalence increases with age.

- The true cause of the disease is yet unknown, but it is speculated that OA results from the inability of chondrocytes to repair damaged cartilage. OA can be classified as idiopathic or secondary as a result of abnormal forces across the joint in cases such as post-traumatic arthritis or arthritis secondary to congenital deformity or internal joint derangement. Other causes of secondary arthritis include osteonecrosis, inflammatory arthritides, crystalline arthropathies, hemorrhagic arthropathies, and septic arthritis.
- Osteoarthritic cartilage has been shown to have an increased water content, altered proteoglycan concentration, collagen abnormalities, and binding of proteoglycans directly to hyaluronic acid without intervening link proteins. An increase in metalloproteinases and up-regulation of interleukin-1 may have a catabolic effect leading to further cartilage degeneration, which is encouraged by shear stresses and protected by normal compressive loads.
- Pathologic changes that occur in OA commence with deterioration of the bearing surface, followed by osteophyte formation and breakdown at the osteochondral junction. As the disease progresses, cartilaginous disintegration and subchondral microfracture lead to exposure of the subchondral bone.
- The physical examination classically shows a decrease in range of motion, crepitus on passive range of motion, and a possible joint effusion. The knee is the most common joint affected by OA. Patients typically complain of pain on ambulation, especially while climbing stairs, when the knee is the predominant joint involved. Patients with OA of the hip typically report difficulty putting on their shoes and socks as well as pain while descending stairs. OA may also lead to night pain, which is persistent pain from painful ambulation earlier during the day.

- Radiographic imaging requires good weight-bearing views of the involved joints. For OA of the knee, weight-bearing anteroposterior and lateral views are obtained as well as a sunrise or Merchant view for assessment of the patellofemoral joint. A posteroanterior view with the knee flexed 45 degrees and with 10 degrees of caudal tilt to allow the radiograph to be perpendicular to the tibial plateau allows detection of joint space narrowing when cartilage loss is limited to the posterior aspects of the femoral condyles. OA of the hip requires a good anteroposterior view of the pelvis as well as anteroposterior and lateral views of the affected hip. Radiographically, one sees evidence of asymmetric joint space narrowing, osteophyte formation, subchondral cysts on both sides of the joint, and subchondral sclerosis (Fig. 6–1).
- Treatment begins with supportive measures for pain control and efforts to decrease the rate of disease advancement. Initial conservative therapy includes activity modification with a focus on non–weight-bearing or non-impact activities such as swimming, weight loss, and the use of acetaminophen or nonsteroidal anti-inflammatory drugs as anti-inflammatory pain control agents. Because of the increased incidence of gastrointestinal side effects, cyclooxygenase-2 selective inhibitors have been advocated for anti-inflammatory medical treatment of OA, particularly for older patients and for patients at high risk of developing gastrointestinal ulcers.
- Physical therapy is not routinely prescribed for patients with OA because of the possibility of exacerbating the patient's symptoms. Aquatic therapy may be helpful, given that it helps to maintain range of motion without excessive joint impact.
- Over the past decade, viscosupplementation has become increasingly popular for the treatment of mild to

moderate OA. Three to five treatments are injected into the affected joint 1 week apart in an effort to increase the viscosity of the synovial fluid. Response to the treatment is variable, but for some patients, viscosupplementation may be an effective option. Intra-articular corticosteroid injections have been used for a very long time as a temporizing measure for control of pain and inflammation related to OA. However, many people believe that the only definitive treatment for OA is total joint arthroplasty for patients in whom nonoperative conservative therapies have failed.

Neuropathic Arthropathy (Charcot's Arthropathy) (Alpert et al. 1996)

- *Neuropathic arthropathy* or *Charcot's arthropathy* can be considered a severe form of OA that results from dysfunctional sensory innervation within the affected joint and leads to destructive arthropathy secondary to minimal trauma. The diagnosis of neuropathic arthropathy can be made only in patients with an underlying neurologic disorder.
- Causes of neuropathic arthropathy (and the most commonly affected sites) include diabetes (foot), tabes dorsalis or late sequelae of syphilis infection (lower extremity), syringomyelia (most common cause in the upper extremity, typically affecting the shoulder and the elbow), Hansen's disease (second most common cause in the upper extremity), myelomeningocele (foot and ankle), congenital pain insensitivity (foot and ankle), and other neurologic injuries such as spinal cord injuries.
- Neuropathic arthropathy typically progresses through three distinct phases. Phase I is the *destructive phase,* characterized by hyperemia, swelling, and increased osteoclastic activity. Phase II is named the *reparative phase* and starts once the involved joint is immobilized and is protected from further trauma. This stage results in intra-articular dense fibrous tissue deposition as well as osteophyte formation and heterotopic ossificans. Phase III is known as the *quiescent phase* and signifies decreased vascularity and significant sclerosis.
- Charcot's joints develop in 25% of patients with syringomyelia, and 80% of the time they affect the upper extremity. Typically, the patient presents with an unstable, painless, joint effusion, which may result from a hemarthrosis.
- Two radiographic patterns have been described in neuropathic arthropathy, the atrophic and the hypertrophic forms. The *atrophic form* presents with significant bone resorption and nearly complete joint disintegration. This form is prominent in the shoulder, hip, and foot. The *hypertrophic form* is characterized by severe joint destruction, juxta-articular new bone formation, and osseous debris. This pattern is commonly seen in the elbow, knee, and ankle (Fig. 6–2).
- Charcot's arthropathy can be easily confused with osteomyelitis based solely on physical examination and

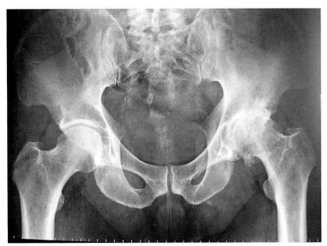

Figure 6–1: End-stage osteoarthritis.
Anteroposterior radiograph of the pelvis of a patient with end-stage osteoarthritis. Note the complete joint space narrowing of the left hip joint with the large inferior osteophyte and periarticular sclerosis.

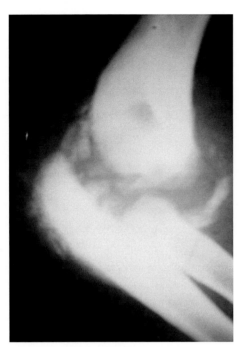

Figure 6–2: Charcot's arthropathy.
Evidence of complete joint destruction of the elbow secondary to Charcot's arthropathy. This is the hypertrophic form, which is characterized by severe joint destruction, juxta-articular new bone formation, and intra-articular osseous debris. This form is commonly seen in the elbow.

radiographic analysis. Symptoms common to both conditions include swelling, warmth to touch, erythema, minimal pain, and an elevated white blood cell count and erythrocyte sedimentation rate. The prevalence of both entities is greater in the diabetic patient population.
- Physical examination is helpful in distinguishing Charcot's arthropathy from osteomyelitis. Elevation of the lower extremity above the level of the heart is typically associated with a decrease in swelling and erythema. In the setting of osteomyelitis, elevation of the leg is usually not associated with a decrease in swelling and erythema. Additional imaging may be required to differentiate Charcot's arthropathy from osteomyelitis. Technetium-99m bone scans show increased tracer uptake in both disorders and are therefore of little use in determining the diagnosis. Indium white cell–tagged scans usually show increased uptake in osteomyelitis and normal uptake in Charcot's arthropathy.
- The goals of treatment of Charcot's arthropathy are focused on limitation of activity and appropriate bracing. Once the skin temperature equalizes to that of the contralateral, unaffected side, bracing or total contact casting may be discontinued. Both total joint arthroplasty and internal fixation are associated with very high complication and failure rates in patients with neuropathic arthropathy.

Other Disorders
Acute Rheumatic Fever
- *Acute rheumatic fever* was previously known as the most common cause of childhood arthritis worldwide before the advent of antibiotics. Now it is rarely seen. Patients diagnosed with a streptococcal throat infection can avoid the late sequelae of acute rheumatic fever with adequate treatment with penicillin.
- Arthritis and arthralgias can be musculoskeletal manifestations of untreated group A β-hemolytic streptococci (*Streptococcus pyogenes*) infections. Patients present with an acute onset of erythematous and extremely painful joint effusions. The arthritis is typically migratory and involves multiple large joints.
- Extraskeletal systemic manifestations include carditis, erythema marginatum (painless red macules on the abdomen but sparing the face), subcutaneous nodules (extensor surfaces of the upper extremities), and choreiform movements. These manifestations in addition to arthritis comprise the major clinical features of the disorder.
- The diagnosis of acute rheumatic fever is based on the *Jones criteria*: a previous history of a streptococcal infection and two major clinical manifestations (listed earlier) or one major clinical manifestation in addition to one minor symptom (fever, arthralgias, prior rheumatic fever, elevated erythrocyte sedimentation rate, or prolonged PR interval on electrocardiogram).
- Serum antistreptolysin O titers are elevated in 80% of affected individuals and assist in confirming the diagnosis.
- Treatment is pharmacologic with the use of penicillin and salicylates.

Ochronosis
- *Ochronosis* is a degenerative arthritis resulting from the rare autosomal recessive disorder *alkaptonuria*. The pathogenesis is based on the inborn defect in the homogentisic acid oxidase enzyme pathway leading to intra-articular deposition of excess homogentisic acid, which eventually polymerizes and turns black.
- Patients in the fourth decade of life may also experience ochronotic spondylitis, progressive degenerative changes, and disk space narrowing and calcifications of the spine. Radiographically, one sees the formation of syndesmophytes, which are small bridges of bone that extend from one vertebral body to another.
- End-stage degenerative arthritis is treated in the same manner as in patients with OA.

Inflammatory Arthritides (Buchanan 1978)
Rheumatoid Arthritis
- *Rheumatoid arthritis* (RA), the most common form of inflammatory arthritis, affects 3% of girls and women and 1% of boys and men. It is a chronic, waxing and waning

symmetric polyarthritis that leads to erosions and eventual joint deformity. RA has also been seen to have an association with an HLA (human leukocyte antigen) focus, either HLA-DR4 or HLA-DW4.

- The etiology of RA is unclear, but it is known that a cell-mediated immune response toward the host soft tissues, cartilage, and bone results in joint destruction. Mononuclear cells are the primary cellular mediators of tissue destruction in RA.

- Patients typically present with long periods of morning stiffness of insidious onset along with fatigue and polyarthritis. Eventually, joint inflammation becomes persistent with warmth, tenderness, effusion, and loss of joint function. Early hand (ulnar deviation and metacarpophalangeal joint subluxation) and foot (metatarsophalangeal joint subluxation, claw toes, and hallux valgus) involvement is seen with RA patients.

- Subcutaneous nodules are seen in 20% of patients affected with RA and are strongly associated with the presence of rheumatoid factor (RF). Elevated erythrocyte sedimentation rate, C-reactive protein, and RF are seen in 80% of patients.

- Patients with RA may present with several systemic manifestations including vasculitis, pericarditis, and pulmonary involvement.

- The diagnostic criteria determined by the American Rheumatism Association include morning stiffness, swelling, subcutaneous nodules, seropositivity for RF, and radiographic evidence of destruction on both sides of the joint.

- Typical RA radiographic characteristics include periarticular erosions and osteopenia. Commonly affected joints include the metacarpophalangeal, proximal interphalangeal, carpal, and the cervical spine. Knee involvement may show tricompartmental osteoporosis and bony erosions (Fig. 6–3). Protrusio acetabuli is commonly seen in patients with RA who have medial translation of the femoral head into the pelvis.

- The goals of treatment in RA are to control synovitis and pain, to maintain joint function, and to prevent deformities. Traditionally, patients with RA were treated conservatively with analgesics and anti-inflammatory agents for symptomatic relief. Disease-modifying antirheumatic drugs (DMARDs) were thought of as second-line agents for refractory or severe cases. However, the thinking has changed based on the philosophy that early aggressive treatment with DMARDs can slow the progression to irreversible joint destruction. As a result, DMARDs have now become the mainstay of pharmacologic therapy in RA.

- Methotrexate is the most common DMARD used in North America. Recent data have shown that combination therapy is more effective than treatment with a single agent. Established combination regimens with methotrexate include hydrochloroquine, sulfasalazine, gold, cyclosporine, or newer anti–tumor necrosis factor-α agents such as etanercept, infliximab, and adalimumab.

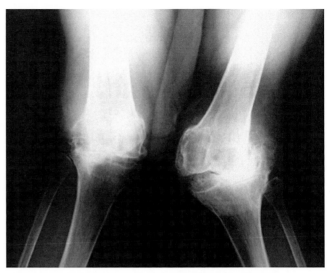

Figure 6–3: Rheumatoid arthritis (RA). Standing anteroposterior radiographs of bilateral knees in patient with long-standing RA. There is joint destruction of both knees with severe valgus deformities, and periarticular osteopenia more commonly seen with RA.

- The anti–tumor necrosis factor-α agents are effective and have minimal adverse effects. However, immunosuppression and the risk of infection are important concerns. As a result, in the perioperative period, it is suggested that surgery be performed when anticytokine drug levels are at their lowest. As a temporizing measure, glucocorticoids are used to prevent acute exacerbations of synovitis in the perioperative period. Glucocorticoids are also used initially when DMARDs are started as a bridging agent until the DMARD becomes effective.

- Surgical intervention in patients with RA requires a multidisciplinary approach to achieve optimal outcomes. Because upper extremity joints such as the shoulder, elbow, and wrist can also commonly be in involved, maximizing upper extremity treatment before lower extremity joint reconstructive procedures may be helpful in the postoperative rehabilitation period with regard to the use of a walker for ambulation. Cervical spine involvement should be evaluated with a flexion and extension lateral radiograph to determine the presence of atlantoaxial instability, which may compromise routine intubation.

- The use of DMARDs as primary pharmacologic therapy along with traditional conservative therapy is in line with treating patients with RA symptomatically and trying to prevent end-stage joint destruction. The progression of the disease is modified with the advent of newer agents, but there is no evidence of complete prevention of joint deterioration. Total joint arthroplasty maintains its place in the spectrum of RA treatment as a last line. Total joint replacement in conjunction with pharmacologic therapy has proven effective in treating pain and in maintaining joint function for patients with severe end-stage RA.

Juvenile Idiopathic Arthritis (Petty 2004)

- *Juvenile idiopathic arthritis* (JIA) is a term that has replaced *juvenile RA* (JRA). This newer classification includes any form of arthritis whose onset is in patients younger than 16 years old, lasts 6 weeks or longer, and specifically excludes any juvenile form of arthritis that has a specific cause, such as juvenile reactive arthritis.
- The former JRA was classified into three major groups: systemic (20%), polyarticular (50%), and pauciarticular (30%). Each group can be further subclassified into patients who are seropositive or seronegative based on the presence of RF. The incidence of seropositivity is less than 15%, and its presence typically indicates the chronic, active, and progressive form of the disease.
- *Systemic JIA* (formerly systemic JRA or Still's disease) includes patients who present with rash, daily febrile episodes, and any number of inflamed joints. These children appear sick and have an elevated white blood cell count, decreased hemoglobin values, hepatosplenomegaly, and lymphadenopathy. It is essential to rule out infection or a malignant process before making the diagnosis of systemic JIA. This affected population has the highest probability of systemic complications and internal organ involvement.
- With the classic terminology, *pauciarticular* referred to involvement of fewer than four joints, and *polyarticular* referred to involvement of four or more joints.
- *Childhood polyarticular arthritis* is divided into RF-positive and RF-negative disease groups. Polyarticular arthritis involves more than four joints in the first 6 months of the disease process. Both large and small joints are involved. Seropositive polyarticular JIA is more common in female patients, results in destructive degenerative joint disease, and frequently has characteristics of adult RA.
- *Childhood oligoarthritis* (formerly pauciarticular JRA) is the most common form and affects approximately 50% of patients with JIA. This form of arthritis typically involves up to four joints in the first 6 months of the disease process. It is more common in female patients, typically involves large joints excluding the hip, and manifests with a limp that improves during the day. Uveitis is present in 20% of affected patients and is associated with a positive antinuclear antibody (ANA) titer. Children who are ANA positive should undergo ophthalmologic screening every 4 months, whereas ANA-negative patients should undergo screening every 6 months to prevent long-term ocular damage.
- The knee (flexion contracture and valgus deformity) is the most common joint affected in JIA, followed by the fingers (extended, swollen, radially deviated), the wrist (flexed and ulnarly deviated), the ankle (dorsiflexion contracture), the hip (flexion contracture and protrusio acetabuli), and the cervical spine (kyphosis, facet ankylosis, and atlantoaxial subluxation). Radiographs may show rarefaction of juxta-articular bone.
- Treatment includes night splinting, high-dose salicylates, and, rarely, gold for refractory polyarticular disease. Synovectomy can also be performed for cases refractory to medical management. Joint arthrodesis or arthroplasty may be necessary for severe end-stage joint destruction.

Spondyloarthropathies (Ahearn et al. 1998)

- The *seronegative spondyloarthropathies* are a group of four disorders: ankylosing spondylitis, reactive arthritis or Reiter's syndrome, psoriatic arthritis, and enteropathic arthritis.
- They all commonly have an association with HLA-B27 positivity and RF negativity. Only 5% to 8% of the general population is HLA-B27 positive, but 50% to 80% of those patients diagnosed with a seronegative spondyloarthropathy are HLA-B27 positive.
- The four spondyloarthropathies often have overlapping symptoms with axial skeletal inflammation including sacroiliitis and enthesitis (inflammation of tendinous attachments to bone). *Enthesitis* is a characteristic finding of this group of disorders.

Ankylosing Spondylitis

- The clinical diagnosis of *ankylosing spondylitis* is confirmed in a male patient who is HLA-B27 positive and RF negative and who has bilateral sacroiliitis with or without acute anterior uveitis.
- Patients typically present with morning stiffness (longer than 1 hour) with an insidious onset of back pain and hip pain in the third to fourth decade of life that eventually leads to progressive loss of spine motion.
- A clinical feature of ankylosing spondylitis is that patients classically complain of back pain that awakens them from sleep and often improves with light exercise. This information from the patient's history may help to differentiate standard mechanical back pain from back pain associated with ankylosing spondylitis.
- Other clinical manifestations include asymmetric peripheral joint inflammation, unilateral anterior uveitis, and rarely, cardiac and pulmonary involvement.
- Radiographic features of ankylosing spondylitis include squaring of the vertebrae, marginal syndesmophyte formation, obliteration of the sacroiliac joints, and ascending ankylosis of the spine, usually starting in the thoracolumbar spine (Fig. 6–4).
- It is not uncommon for patients to present with neck pain resulting from spinal fractures associated with an ankylosed cervical vertebra. A computed tomographic scan of the cervical spine is an essential part of the workup of any patient with ankylosing spondylitis who presents with neck pain, to rule out cervical spinal fractures.
- As the disease progresses, patients are left with complete ankylosis of the spine, also known as *bamboo spine*. This large, brittle block of bone is susceptible to fractures, usually occurring at the cervicothoracic junction. A discontinuity at any level of the spinal column renders that

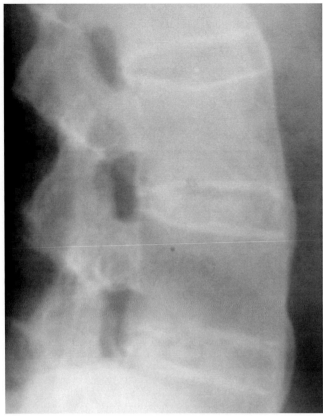

Figure 6–4: Ankylosing spondylitis.
Lateral radiograph of the lumbar spine of a patient diagnosed with ankylosing spondylitis. The marginal syndesmophytes bridging the disk spaces between the anterior margins of the vertebral bodies are characteristic of ankylosing spondylitis.

point a fulcrum at which point the two remaining fused segments of the spine can rotate and cause myelopathy and possible severing of the spinal cord.
- Conservative therapy for this patient population includes physical therapy and nonsteroidal anti-inflammatory medications.
- Surgical treatment includes posterior closing wedge osteotomies for severe kyphosis of the cervical spine as well as bilateral total hip arthroplasty for hip joint ankylosis.

Reactive Arthritis (Reiter's Syndrome)

- The classic clinical presentation is a young male patient with the triad of conjunctivitis, urethritis, and peripheral arthritis. Patients may also present with painless oral or penile lesions as well as pustular lesions on the palms of the hands and soles of the feet (keratoderma blennorrhagicum).
- Nearly 80% to 90% of affected individuals are HLA-B27 positive, and 60% of patients with chronic disease have sacroiliitis.

- Reactive arthritis is typically triggered by a sexually transmitted nongonococcal infection (*Chlamydia*) or a lower gastrointestinal infection (*Yersinia, Salmonella, Campylobacter,* or *Shigella*).
- Arthritis usually causes asymmetric swelling and pain in weight-bearing joints. Recurrent exacerbations are common and may lead to metatarsal head erosions and calcaneal periostitis.
- Conservative therapy is all that is usually required and includes physical therapy and nonsteroidal anti-inflammatory medications.

Psoriatic Arthritis

- Arthritis affects approximately 5% to 10% of patients with psoriasis. Many HLA foci have been identified, but 50% of patients with psoriatic arthritis are HLA-B27 positive.
- The five subtypes of psoriatic arthritis follow:

  1. Oligoarticular and asymmetric
  2. Polyarticular and symmetric
  3. Axial involvement similar to that seen in ankylosing spondylitis
  4. Distal interphalangeal involvement pattern
  5. Arthritis mutilans with telescoping digits

- Most patients have oligoarticular asymmetric arthritis, which affects the small joints of the hand, with pathognomonic involvement of the distal interphalangeal joint.
- Nail pitting and so-called sausage digits are common, and the pencil-in-cup deformity is classic with distal interphalangeal joint involvement (Fig. 6–5).
- Treatment is similar to that mentioned earlier for RA.

Enteropathic (Inflammatory Bowel Disease–Associated) Arthritis

- Approximately 10% to 20% of patients diagnosed with ulcerative colitis or Crohn's disease also suffer from peripheral joint arthritis and 5% are affected by axial arthritis.
- Enteropathic arthritis is nondeforming and typically involves large, weight-bearing joints. The usual presentation is of acute monoarticular synovitis, which may precede bowel symptom exacerbation.
- Nearly 50% of patients with enteropathic arthritis are HLA-B27 positive, and 10% to 15% have associated ankylosing spondylitis.
- Treatment of musculoskeletal manifestations consists of physical therapy and nonsteroidal anti-inflammatory medications.

Crystalline-Induced Arthropathies (Fries et al. 2003)
Gout

- *Gout* is a result of a nucleic acid metabolism disorder that leads to hyperuricemia and monosodium urate crystal

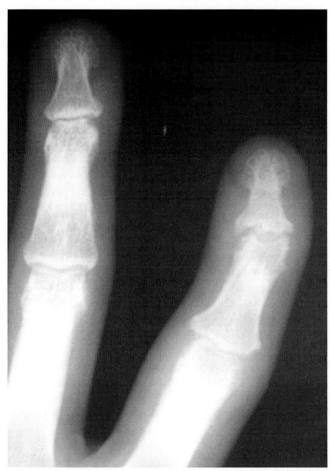

Figure 6–5: Psoriatic arthritis.
Anteroposterior radiograph of the left index finger and long finger of a patient diagnosed with psoriatic arthritis. Note the pathognomonic pencil-in-cup deformity of the distal interphalangeal joint of the index finger.

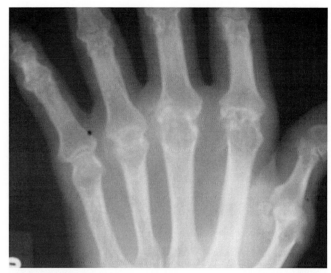

Figure 6–6: Gout.
Anteroposterior radiograph of the left hand of a patient diagnosed with gout. Note the periarticular erosions surrounding the metacarpophalangeal joints.

chronic gout, allopurinol, a xanthine oxidase inhibitor, is the drug of choice. Colchicine is also used for chronic gout. Other agents, such as probenecid, a renal uric acid uptake inhibitor, may also be effective in certain patients.

Chondrocalcinosis

- This disorder has many causes, including calcium pyrophosphate (dihydrate) deposition disease (CPPD or pseudogout), ochronosis, hyperthyroidism, hypothyroidism, and hemochromatosis.
- CPPD is a common cause of chondrocalcinosis. *CPPD is a disorder of pyrophosphate metabolism yielding acute attacks of the lower extremity joints (typically the knee) in the middle-aged and older patient population. Acute CPPD attacks can commonly be mistaken for septic arthritis.
- Patients typically present with a swollen, warm to touch, erythematous knee held in a position that maximizes the intracapsular volume of the joint. The one clinical finding that helps to separate acute CPPD exacerbations from acute septic arthritis is the absence of pain on that micromotion. Patients are reluctant to move the joint through an arc of active range of motion, but they are not as sensitive to micromotion arcs that are done passively as are patients with a septic joint.
- Radiographic evidence of chondrocalcinosis in the knee often appears as linear calcification of hyaline cartilage and more diffuse calcification of the meniscus and other fibrocartilage. Lateral meniscus calcification on a radiograph is pathognomonic for chondrocalcinosis of the knee (Fig. 6–7).
- Diagnosis is made by identification of rhomboidal, positively birefringent crystals in the synovial fluid aspirate.

deposition in the joints. This deposition of crystals yields an inflammatory response, which increases the intra-articular concentrations of proteases, prostaglandins, leukotriene B_4, and oxygen free radicals.
- Recurrent arthritis is seen in the lower extremity, especially the first metatarsophalangeal joint *(podagra)*. The disease typically affects men in the fifth through seventh decades of life, and exacerbations occur with increases in dietary intake of protein and alcohol.
- Classic radiographic evidence of gout includes soft tissue changes and "punched-out" periarticular erosions with sclerotic overhanging borders (Fig. 6–6).
- Diagnosis is made by joint aspiration and microscopic identification of strongly negative birefringent crystals in the synovial fluid.
- Initial therapy is started with indomethacin as an anti-inflammatory agent. Acute treatment with medications such as colchicine, an inhibitor of anti-inflammatory mediators, may exacerbate symptoms. For patients with

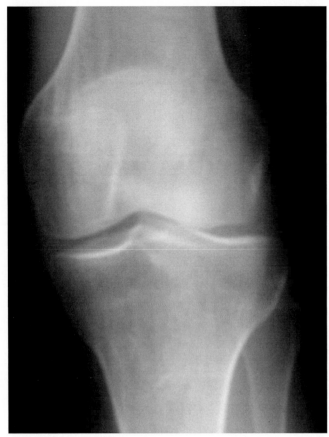

Figure 6–7: Chondrocalcinosis.
Anteroposterior radiograph of the left knee of a patient diagnosed with chondrocalcinosis. Note the pathognomonic lateral meniscal calcification seen between the lateral femoral condyle and the lateral tibial plateau.

- Nonsteroidal anti-inflammatory drug therapy is usually the mainstay for treatment of this disorder.

Calcium Hydroxyapatite Crystal Deposition

- *Calcium hydroxyapatite crystal deposition* can also be associated with chondrocalcinosis and degenerative joint disease.
- End-stage destructive arthropathy is typically found involving the shoulder and the knee.
- The term *Milwaukee shoulder* refers to calcium phosphate deposition in the shoulder associated with cuff tear arthropathy.
- Treatment for this disorder is often supportive and consists of nonsteroidal anti-inflammatory drug therapy.

Hemorrhagic Arthropathies

Hemophilic Arthropathy (Luck et al. 2004)

- *Hemophilia* is a sex-linked recessive trait yielding either a factor VIII deficiency *(hemophilia A)* or a factor IX deficiency *(hemophilia B)*.

- The prevalence of hemophilia A is 1 in 5000 live male births and of hemophilia B is 1 in 30,000 live male births.
- It is necessary to obtain a bleeding history for all preoperative assessments. Patients may have a history of bleeding complications with previous surgical procedures that yields hemophilia among the possible disorders on the differential diagnosis.
- The knee, elbow, and ankle are the most commonly involved joints, but patients may have secondary involvement of the hip, shoulder, and subtalar joints.
- Because of the bleeding tendency, patients have recurrent hemarthroses, which lead to chronic juxtacortical erosions and eventual end-stage arthropathy (Fig. 6–8).
- Goals of treatment include cessation of intra-articular hemorrhage, pain control, resumption and maintenance of function, and prevention of chronic arthropathy.
- Conservative therapy involves factor VIII or IX replacement (depending on deficiency and baseline levels) as soon as prodromal symptoms are present, brief immobilization and splinting for pain, decompression through joint aspiration, and early physical therapy to maintain strength and joint motion.
- Synovectomy (chemical, radioisotope, arthroscopic, or open) is indicated for patients with chronic synovitis (swelling and inflammation present for 3 consecutive months) unresponsive to conservative measures. Synovectomy is not indicated in patients who have end-stage arthropathy.

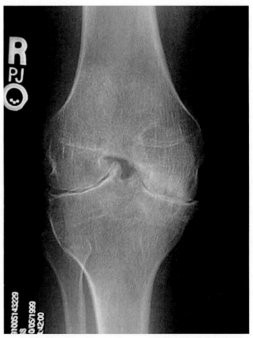

Figure 6–8: End-stage hemophilic arthropathy.
Anteroposterior radiograph of the knee in a patient with end-stage hemophilic arthropathy. Note the loss of the cartilage interval, squaring of the femoral condyles, and flexion contracture resulting in a notch view of the knee.

- Definitive surgical treatment involves total joint arthroplasty or arthrodesis and requires a multidisciplinary approach with collaboration among an orthopaedic surgeon, an anesthesiologist, and a hematologist to minimize the intraoperative and postoperative risk of bleeding.

Pigmented Villonodular Synovitis

- *Pigmented villonodular synovitis* affects the synovial membrane of young adults secondary to extensive hemosiderin deposition within the synovium.
- Patients typically present with pain, swelling, synovitis, and a bloody or rust-colored effusion on aspiration.
- The knee is the most commonly affected joint, but the hip and ankle may also be involved.
- Chronic hemosiderin deposition within the synovium leads to juxtacortical erosions and sclerotic margins of the intra-articular segments of the adjacent bones.
- Surgical treatment requires total synovectomy.
- In patients with end-stage secondary arthritis, concomitant joint arthroplasty may be necessary.
- Residual disease may be treated with intra-articular radioisotope therapy.

Osteonecrosis (Steinberg and Mont 2000)

- *Osteonecrosis*, also known as *avascular necrosis* (AVN), is defined as death of juxta-articular bone tissue from a cause other than infection. Typically, AVN is a result of a disrupted blood supply secondary to trauma or other causes, including steroid use, heavy alcohol use, blood dyscrasias such as sickle cell disease, coagulopathies (protein C or S deficiency or low levels of lipoprotein a), caisson disease, excessive radiation therapy, and Gaucher's disease. Idiopathic osteonecrosis of the hip in the pediatric population is known as *Legg-Calvé-Perthes disease*.
- The hip joint is most commonly affected. The disorder leads to eventual collapse and flattening of the femoral head, typically in the anterolateral portion of the head. An estimated 15,000 to 20,000 new cases of osteonecrosis of the femoral head occur in the Untied States each year, and approximately 10% of total hip arthroplasties are done each year for the treatment of late-stage AVN.
- The pathogenesis of the disease leads to grossly necrotic bone, the presence of fibrous tissue, and subchondral collapse. The characteristic histopathology shows autolytic changes of the osteocytes and necrotic marrow followed by other changes:

1. Inflammation with invasion of primitive mesenchymal tissue and capillaries
2. New lamellar bone deposition on dead or necrotic trabecular bone
3. Dead trabecular bone that undergoes resorption and remodeling by *creeping substitution*; bone is weakest during this phase, and collapse *(crescent sign)* as well as fragmentation can occur

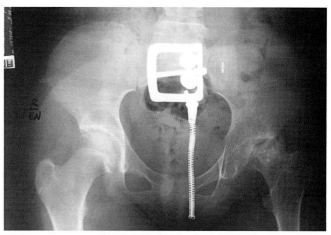

Figure 6–9: Avascular necrosis.
Collapse of the left femoral head resulting from avascular necrosis with secondary degenerative changes.

- The physical examination must include an adequate assessment of the contralateral hip. The typical clinical presentation includes a decrease in hip abduction and internal rotation as well as a limp. Approximately 50% of patients with idiopathic cases and 80% of patients with steroid-induced AVN have bilateral hip involvement.
- Imaging should commence with plain radiographs of the pelvis as well as two views of the affected hip (Fig. 6–9). Early diagnosis can be made using magnetic resonance imaging with very high sensitivity and specificity. Bone scans can also be used for early diagnosis with evidence of increased uptake in the areas of bone remodeling in response to necrotic bone.
- Several classifications have been historically used for defining the severity of a lesion and the patient's prognosis. The University of Pennsylvania System for Staging Avascular Necrosis assesses both the radiologic appearance and the lesion size (Table 6–1). This system is useful in determining prognosis of joint-preserving procedures such as core decompression.
- Treatments range from a spectrum of conservative symptomatic therapy to joint-preserving alternatives for early AVN and hemiarthroplasty and total joint arthroplasty for later-stage AVN. Popular joint-preserving alternatives include core decompression, vascularized fibular grafting, and proximal femoral osteotomy. Total hip replacement does have an increased failure rate in the young patient population.

Infectious Arthritides

Pyogenic (Septic) Arthritis

- *Septic arthritis* is defined as an acute or chronic infection within the capsular confines of a joint. The presence of intra-articular bacteria yields a strong inflammatory response by the host's immune system with an influx of

STAGE	CRITERIA
Table 6-1	**University of Pennsylvania System for Staging Avascular Necrosis**
0	Normal or nondiagnostic radiograph, bone scan, and magnetic resonance image
I	Normal radiograph; abnormal bone scan and/or magnetic resonance image Mild (<15% femoral head involved) Moderate (15%–30%) Severe (>30%)
II	"Cystic" and sclerotic changes in femoral head Mild (<15% femoral head involved) Moderate (15%–30%) Severe (>30%)
III	Subchondral collapse (crescent sign) without flattening Mild (<15% femoral head involved) Moderate (15%–30%) Severe (>30%)
IV	Flattening of the femoral head Mild (<15% femoral head involved) Moderate (15%–30%) Severe (>30%)
V	Joint narrowing and/or acetabular changes Mild (<15% femoral head involved) Moderate (15%–30%) Severe (>30%)
VI	Advanced degenerative changes

From Steinberg ME, BrigthonCT, Corces A (1989). Osteonecrosis of the femoral head: Results of core decompression and grafting with electrical stimulation. Clin Orthop Relat Res 249:199.

cytokines, proteolytic enzymes, and other inflammatory mediators. In addition, having increased intra-articular pressure secondary to the presence of purulent material decreases the ability of the synovium to deliver nutrients adequately to the cartilage. The immune system's defense toward the bacteria as well as decreased nutrition, if allowed to continue for more than 24 to 36 hours, may lead to irreversible hyaline and fibrocartilage damage and eventual joint surface destruction.

- Infections can gain access to an intra-articular space by the hematogenous route from a distant focus, through direct extension from an overlying cellulitis, or by way of direct inoculation. Septic arthritis in the pediatric population may also spread from adjacent metaphyseal osteomyelitis, especially in the shoulder, elbow, proximal femur, and distal tibia, where the metaphysis is intracapsular.

- The most common pathogen is *Staphylococcus aureus*, both in pediatric and adult populations. Specific patient populations based on age as well as associated comorbidities are susceptible to other microorganisms as possible causes of septic arthritis. In neonates with a prolonged neonatal intensive care unit course, line sepsis may lead to hematogenous fungal arthritis secondary to systemic *Candida albicans* infection. Newborns are susceptible to systemic infection with *Streptococcus agalactiae*, transmitted while passing through the birth canal. Young, sexually active patients are at increased risk for gonococcal arthritis caused by *Neisseria gonorrhoeae*. Intravenous drug abusers are highly susceptible to fungal septic arthritis as well as infection, which target the sternoclavicular and the sacroiliac joints. In general, diabetic patients are also at greater risk for septic joints resulting from immune system dysfunction and the high prevalence of associated peripheral vascular disease.

- Metacarpophalangeal joint infections are common after human bites involving the hand (especially fight-related bites). *S. aureus* is considered to be the most common organism seen; however, treatment must also target *Eikenella*, a common oral flora. Most patients undergo formal irrigation and débridement with postoperative intravenous antibiotic therapy such as Unasyn (ampicillin in combination with sulbactam). The wound is typically packed open to allow any purulent drainage to exit the wound. The packing is typically removed 48 hours postoperatively, and soaks in soap and warm water are started three times daily if there is no evidence of persistent infection. Patients can then transition to an oral antibiotic regimen such as Augmentin (amoxicillin and clavulanate), once there has been an adequate response to surgery and intravenous antibiotics.

- Diagnosis is based on clinical presentation as well as on analysis of intra-articular synovial fluid aspirate. Patients typically present with an erythematous, warm to touch, painful joint with a tense effusion. The joint is usually kept in a position to maximize the intra-articular space. The most sensitive physical examination finding is pain on micromotion (Fig. 6–10).

- The diagnosis of a septic joint is confirmed with joint aspiration and assessment of the fluid for cell count, Gram stain, culture and sensitivity, crystal analysis, protein, and glucose concentrations. Typically, septic joint fluid from a native joint has a cell count of more than 100,000 white blood cells and more than 75% polymorphonuclear leukocytes, a positive Gram stain and culture, negative crystal analysis, and increased protein and decreased glucose concentration when compared with serum protein and glucose levels. Because acute attacks secondary to crystal-induced arthropathy may mimic septic arthritis, it is imperative to send the synovial fluid for crystal analysis to rule out acute crystalline arthropathy exacerbations.

- When possible, obtaining joint aspirations for analysis before antibiotic administration will allow for the highest likelihood of identifying a microorganism. A single joint aspiration has a 50% probability of a positive Gram stain and culture. A repeat aspiration increases the likelihood of identifying a microorganism to more than 80%.

- Treatment requires both extended systemic antibiotic administration and either serial aspiration or formal irrigation and débridement, either arthroscopically or as an open procedure. Multiple irrigation and débridement procedures are sometimes required to decompress the

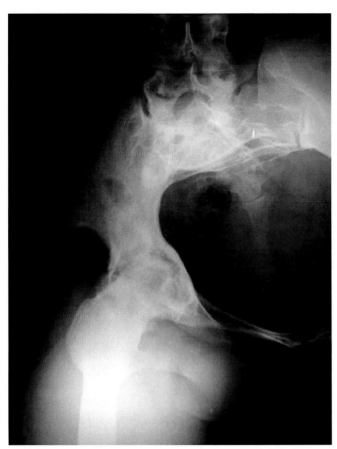

Figure 6–10: Hip sepsis.
Degenerative changes after hip sepsis demonstrated on this anteroposterior radiograph.

infection adequately. The typical postoperative course calls for at least 6 weeks of intravenous antibiotic therapy with an infectious disease expert closely following the patient's case.

Tuberculous Arthritis

- Intra-articular chronic granulomatous infections are typically caused by *Mycobacterium tuberculosis*, secondary to hematogenous spread from a distant focus, usually pulmonary in origin.
- The most common musculoskeletal regions for manifestations of *tuberculosis* are the spine and the lower extremities.
- Mexicans and Asians are most susceptible to atypical bacterial infections, and in more than 80% of cases, a single joint is involved.
- Radiographic evidence of tuberculous activity portrays changes in the articular surface on both sides of the joint. Characteristic changes include subchondral osteoporosis, cystic changes, notchlike bony destruction at the joint edge with joint space narrowing, and osteophyte formation on both sides of the joint.
- Diagnosis of tuberculosis is confirmed with a positive purified protein derivative test along with the presence of acid-fast bacilli and "rice bodies" (fibrin globules) in the synovial fluid.

- Histologic diagnosis is confirmed with characteristic granuloma formation with Langhans giant cells.
- Treatment requires formal irrigation and débridement followed by pharmacologic treatment with isoniazid, rifampin, pyrazinamide, and pyridoxine.

Fungal Arthritis

- Intra-articular *fungal infections* are most commonly seen in neonates in the neonatal intensive care unit setting or in immunocompromised patients with human immunodeficiency virus infection or acquired immunodeficiency syndrome and in intravenous drug abusers.
- The most common fungal pathogen responsible for infections in these patient populations is *Candida albicans*.
- Synovial fluid aspirates should be prepared with potassium hydroxide for identifying intra-articular fungal pathogens.
- Fungal arthritis can be treated pharmacologically with 5-flucytosine.
- Amphotericin B has better efficacy in treating blastomycosis and cryptococcal infections, as well as other fungal infections. Amphotericin B can be administered intra-articularly to minimize the systemic side effects of the drug.

Lyme Arthritis

- *Lyme arthritis* is a late sequela of a primary systemic infection by the spirochete *Borrelia burgdorferi*, transmitted by the *Ixodes* tick.
- Approximately 10% of tick bites yield transmission of the microorganism. The disease typically occurs in three stages: stage I, characterized by a bull's eye rash *(erythema chronicum migrans)* at the site of the bite; stage II, characterized by neurologic symptoms; and stage III, characterized by joint involvement with eventual arthritis in undiagnosed and untreated cases.
- Musculoskeletal manifestations typically present as a self-limiting, monoarticular joint effusion, usually involving the shoulder or the knee. Radiographs are typically negative other than evidence of a radiographic effusion.
- The pathophysiology is based on the intra-articular deposition of immune complexes and cryoglobulins. Diagnosis is confirmed by enzyme-linked immunosorbent assay testing of the synovial fluid aspirate once Gram stain and culture are negative for identifying a microorganism.
- The condition is treated with doxycycline. Treatment may also be conducted with amoxicillin, cefuroxime, or erythromycin in patients with tetracycline allergy or in pediatric patients, in whom the use of doxycycline is not recommended for those less than 8 years of age because of the danger of tendon rupture and cartilage damage.

References

Ahearn JM, Hochberg MC (1998). Epidemiology and genetics of ankylosing spondylitis. *J Rheumatol (Suppl)* 26:22-28.

This article provides a review of the clinical manifestations of ankylosing spondylitis and defines the genetic and epidemiologic basis for the disease.

Alpert SW, Koval KJ, Zuckerman JD (1996). Neuropathic arthropathy: Review of current knowledge. *J Am Acad Orthop Surg* 4:100-108.

This review article is gives an overview and current knowledge of the pathophysiology, risk factors, and natural history of neuropathic arthropathy or Charcot's joints.

Buchanan WW (1978). Clinical features of rheumatoid arthritis. In: Scott JT, ed. *Copeman's Textbook of the Rheumatoid Diseases*, 5th ed. Edinburgh: Churchill Livingstone, pp 318-364.

This chapter is an excellent review of RA and delineates the pathophysiology, clinical presentation, diagnostic criteria, and pharmacologic management of the disorder.

Fries JF, Lorig K, Holman HR (2003). Patient self-management in arthritis: Yes! *J Rheumatol* 30:1130-1132.

This review article provides an excellent overview of current concepts behind conservative therapy for the treatment of OA based on new and existing theories of the pathophysiology of the disease.

Luck J, Silva M, Rodriguez-Merchan EC, et al. (2004). Hemophilic arthropathy. *J Am Acad Orthop Surg* 4:234-245.

This review article is great overview of the pathophysiology of hemophilic arthropathy and how to minimize the probability that a patient will experience end-stage joint destruction.

Petty RE, Southwood TR, Manners P, et al. (2004). International League of Associations for Rheumatology classification of juvenile idiopathic arthritis: Second revision, Edmonton, 2001. *J Rheumatol* 31:390-392.

This article depicts the new classification according to which JRA has become a subset of JIA.

Steinberg ME, Mont MA (2000). Osteonecrosis. In: Chapman MW, Szabo RM, Harder RA, et al. *Chapman's Textbook of Orthopaedic Surgery*. Philadelphia: LWW, pp 3263-3308.

This chapter is an excellent review of AVN with an emphasis on AVN of the hip. It clearly explains the pathophysiology and reviews the classification and predicted prognosis of patients with osteonecrosis of the hip.

CHAPTER 7

Preoperative Assessment

William G. Hamilton* and Ehsan Tabaraee†

*MD, Orthopaedic Surgeon, Anderson Orthopaedic Research Institute and Instructor,
Anderson Clinic Postgraduate Fellowship, Alexandria, VA
†MS, Medical Student, George Washington University School of Medicine, Washington, DC

Introduction

- The preoperative assessment of a patient for arthroplasty is a comprehensive evaluation that includes several components. Each aspect of this evaluation requires careful attention to detail to assist in patient selection, to improve patient outcomes, and to minimize complications.
- As in all fields of medicine, the history and physical examination are the most important parts of the preoperative assessment. The diagnosis and treatment course are primarily based on these portions of the examination.
- Appropriate diagnostic tests should be used to complement the history and the physical examination.

History
General Principles

- A complete examination should begin with a thorough history. Documentation of the onset, location, severity, frequency, factors that improve or worsen the symptoms, associated symptoms, and previous treatment are critical.
- Pain from arthritis is generally exacerbated by activity and relieved with rest. Although advanced arthritis can cause constant pain and can awaken patients at night, if pain persists despite rest, then inflammatory, neoplastic, or infectious processes should be considered.
- All prior treatments should be documented including nutritional supplements, over-the-counter and prescription medications, injections, physical therapy, activity modification, and assistive devices (cane, crutches, walker). Response to each of these treatments should be noted.

Hip

- Information important when examining a hip includes the following:
  - Childhood hip disorders including developmental dysplasia, Perthes' disease, slipped capital femoral epiphysis, polio, sepsis, and trauma
  - Prior trauma to the hip
  - Prior hip surgeries
  - Recent increase in activity level (may raise concern for stress fractures)
  - Risk factors for avascular necrosis (Box 7–1)
- Symptoms related to intra-articular hip joint disease need to be distinguished from extra-articular causes of hip pain (Box 7–2).
- Acute-onset hip pain is more concerning for fracture, dislocation, and sepsis.
- Insidious and chronic hip pain is more commonly associated with inflammatory and degenerative processes.
- True hip pain is most commonly located in the groin and radiates to the knee. It is not uncommon for patients with hip disease to present with a primary complaint of knee pain. Hip pain rarely radiates below the knee.
- Lateral hip pain often results from trochanteric bursitis. Buttock pain and pain that radiates below the knee are likely caused by lumbar spine disease.
- Patients who describe a painful click or "locking" of the hip should be evaluated for loose bodies or labral disorders.
- As hip pain progresses, patients are increasingly limited in their ability to walk, climb stairs, sit comfortably in low chairs, get in and out of a car, and put on their shoes and socks.
- Several different rating scales assessing hip function can be used to evaluate the severity of disease as well as responses to treatment.

Box 7–1	**Historical Factors Associated With Avascular Necrosis of the Hip**

- Steroid use
- Alcohol use
- Trauma, most commonly femoral neck fractures and dislocations
- Scuba diving (caisson disease)
- Avascular necrosis in the contralateral hip
- Gaucher's disease
- Sickle cell anemia
- Previous organ transplant (likely from steroid use)

- The *Harris hip score* is the most widely used and accepted and is scored by the physician. The score is simple to administer and stresses pain, range of motion, and function.
- The *Western Ontario and McMaster University Osteoarthritis index* (WOMAC) is disease specific for hip or knees and is scored by the patient. It stresses pain, stiffness, and function.
- The *36-item Short Form (SF-36)* evaluates the patient's physical and emotional health and is completed by a family member.

Knee

- Similar to the hip, examination of the knee should include any history of old or recent trauma, surgery, contralateral knee pain, and recent activity change.
- The character and location of pain are important in confirming the diagnosis and ruling out referred sources of pain.
- Pain from arthritis is more commonly diffusely localized to the anterior knee, whereas meniscal disease frequently causes focal, posterior joint line pain.
- Pain associated only with bent knee activities such as climbing stairs, prolonged sitting, and kneeling may indicate isolated patellofemoral arthritis. Patients with tricompartmental arthritis have similar symptoms, but they also have pain while walking on a level surface (Outerbridge 1961).
- Complaints of locking are most commonly the result of a torn meniscus that prevents full excursion of the knee,

Box 7–2	**Extra-articular Causes of Hip Pain**

- Lumbosacral disease
- Ovarian cyst/pelvic inflammatory disease
- Inguinal hernia
- Ischemic vascular disease
- Prostatitis/epididymitis/urethritis/hydrocele
- Tumor
- Femoral pseudoaneurysm
- Nephrolithiasis
- Urinary tract infection

but they can also be secondary to loose bodies or an osteochondral defect.
- It is also important to elicit symptoms of instability. Although "giving way" of the knee is most commonly associated with the pain reflex rather than with instability, an underlying ligamentous deficiency (cruciate, collateral, or patellar) may influence surgical decision making. Most surgeons consider a knee with degenerative arthritis and an anterior cruciate ligament (ACL) deficiency a relative contraindication for a high tibial osteotomy or unicompartmental arthroplasty and instead favor concomitant ligament reconstruction or total knee arthroplasty.
- The presence of swelling in the knee commonly accompanies many conditions and is not particularly helpful in determining the diagnosis. However, acute swelling following an injury should raise the suspicion of bony, ligamentous, or meniscal injury. Atraumatic acute knee swelling may be indicative of gout or a septic knee.
- All prior treatments should be reviewed along with the patients' response to these treatments. Patient education, weight loss, medications, physical therapy, bracing or heel wedges, injections (steroid and lubricant), and prior surgical procedures should be documented.

Physical Examination
General Principles

- The physical examination starts from the point the patient walks into the office, observing posture, overall gait and function, and ability to rise from a chair and position himself or herself on the examination table. An overall level of disability should be assessed.
- All patients should be in gowns or shorts to allow full inspection and palpation of the following:
  - Posture
  - Previous surgical scars
  - Muscular atrophy
  - Spinal range of motion
  - Skin lesions, venous insufficiency ulcers, ischemic foot ulcers
  - Neurocirculatory status
  - Muscle strength testing (Table 7–1)
  - Assessment of sensation (Table 7–2)
  - Palpation of pulses:
    - Posterior tibial and dorsalis pedis
  - Test deep tendon reflexes bilaterally
    - Patellar
    - Achilles

Hip

Examination With the Patient Standing

- Palpation should include bony landmarks such as the iliac crest, iliac tubercles, greater trochanter, posterior superior

Table 7–1 Muscle Strength Testing	
ISOMETRIC MOVEMENTS	GRADE (POINTS)
Normal strength against gravity and some resistance	5
Full motion against gravity and against some resistance	4
Fair motion against gravity with resistance eliminated	3
Movement only with gravity eliminated	2
Muscle contractility but no joint motion	1
No evidence of contractility	0

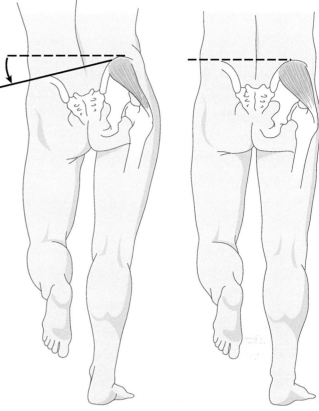

Figure 7–1: Trendelenburg's test.
A positive result of Trendelenburg's test *(left)* indicates weakness of the gluteus medius on the supporting side. (Redrawn from Amstutz H, ed. [1991]. *Hip Arthroplasty.* New York: Churchill Livingstone.)

iliac spine, and ischial tuberosity. Point tenderness over the greater trochanter is suggestive of trochanteric bursitis.

- Pelvic obliquity should be assessed by placing one's fingers just above the iliac crests.
- *Trendelenburg's test* is performed with the examiner behind the patient. The patient performs a single-leg stance on the affected side. A positive test is seen when the opposite side of the pelvis drops and the patient is unable to support the weight, a finding indicating weakness of the gluteus medius on the supporting side (Fig. 7–1).
- Gait should be assessed for the following types of limp (Murray et al. 1971):
  - *Antalgic gait:* Shorter stance phase and stride length are noted on the involved side.
  - *Trendelenburg's test:* The patient leans over affected hip in stance phase to shift the body's center of gravity toward the hip and to compensate for a weakened abductor muscle.

Examination With the Patient Lying Supine

- Position the hip: In the presence of hip disease, patients position the hip to decrease intra-articular pressure. Typically, you will see hip flexion, slight abduction, and external rotation.
- Range of motion (ROM)
  - Always measure both active ROM and passive ROM, as well as the contralateral side for comparison.
  - Internal rotation and abduction are the first motions affected by arthritis.
  - The following are the motions that should be tested in each hip, with range and normal limit in parentheses:

Table 7–2 Dermatomal Distribution	
AREA	NERVE ROOT
Anterior groin and suprapubic	L1
Anterior thigh	L2
Lower anterior thigh and knee	L3
Medial calf	L4
Lateral calf	L5

- Flexion (0 to 135 degrees)
- Extension (0 to 30 degrees): Perform *Thomas' test* to assess for flexion contracture (Fig. 7–2).
- Abduction (0 to 50 degrees)
- Adduction (0 to 30 degrees)
- Internal rotation (0 to 40 degrees): Commonly diminished and painful in arthritis
- External rotation (0 to 60 degrees)
- Ability to perform active straight leg raises; pain in groin with this motion helps to isolate hip disease
- Popping or clicking with range of motion; sources include the following:
  - Iliotibial band popping over greater trochanter
  - Iliopsoas tendon popping over the iliopectineal eminence
  - Iliofemoral ligament rubbing over the femoral head
  - Long head of biceps femoris sliding over ischial tuberosity
  - Loose bodies
  - Synovial chondromatosis
  - Osteocartilaginous exostoses
  - Labral tear

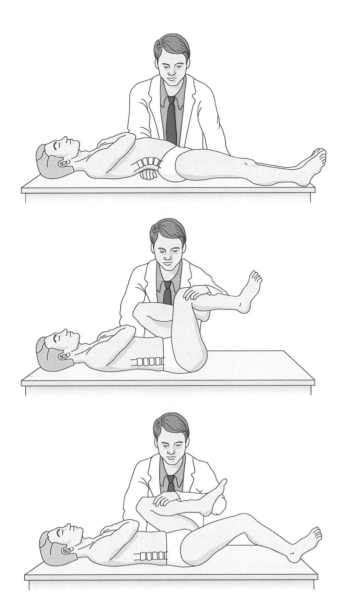

Figure 7–2: Thomas' test.
Thomas' test is used to assess flexion contracture. (Redrawn from Amstutz H, ed. [1991]. *Hip Arthroplasty.* New York: Churchill Livingstone.)

- *McCarthy's sign:* With the opposite hip fully flexed, the affected hip is extended, first in external rotation then in internal rotation. Reproduction of a painful click is consistent with a labral tear.
- *Anterior disease:* The click is reproduced when the hip is moved from a flexed, externally rotated, and abducted position to an extended, internally rotated, and adducted position.
- *Posterior disease:* The click is reproduced when the hip is moved from a flexed, internally rotated, adducted position to an extended, abducted, and externally rotated position.
- Straight leg raise test
  - Radiating pain below the knee suggests nerve root irritation.

- Leg-length measurements should be made with the patient both standing and supine. It is critical to distinguish between a true and an apparent leg-length discrepancy. These conditions can coexist and should be distinguished before any surgical procedure is performed.
  - Apparent leg-length discrepancy
    - The measurements between the anterior superior iliac spine and the medial malleolus are equal despite the apparent leg-length discrepancy (Fig. 7–3*A*).
    - This can be caused by soft tissue contractures involving the diseased hip or from a lumbosacral curvature causing pelvic obliquity. These conditions can be distinguished by observing a sitting patient from behind and determining flexibility of the lumbosacral spine.
    - Flexibility to lateral bending indicates that the spine is likely not involved in the overall leg-length discrepancy.
    - Stiffness to lateral bending indicates that the fixed pelvic obliquity is likely the result of a spinal curvature and not hip disease.

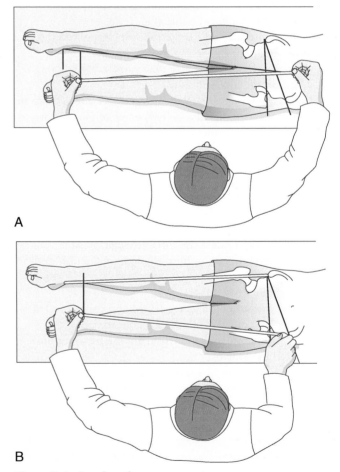

A

B

Figure 7–3: Leg-length measurement.
A, An apparent leg-length measurement is taken from the umbilicus to the medial malleolus. **B,** True leg-length measurements made from the anterior superior iliac spine to the medial malleolus are equal despite the apparent leg-length discrepancy. (Redrawn from Garvin KL, McKillip T [1998]. *The Adult Hip.* Philadelphia: Lippincott Williams & Wilkins, p 327.)

- Soft tissue contractures of the hip can cause apparent leg-length discrepancies and should be carefully examined in the office.
  - Flexion contractures of the involved hip shorten the hip on examination and can be identified with Thomas' test.
  - Abduction contractures cause the involved pelvis to tilt downward, leading to an apparent lengthening of the leg.
  - Adduction contractures cause the involved pelvis to tilt upward, leading to an apparent shortening of the leg.
  - For each 5 degrees of abduction or adduction contracture, the leg will seem 1.6 cm shorter or longer (Ireland and Kessel 1980).
- True leg-length discrepancy
  - This can be caused by a preexisting condition distal to the hip (i.e., femur fracture, congenital condition, and disease of knee or ankle) or from shortening caused by hip disease.
  - Measurements should be made between fixed bony landmarks such as the anterior superior iliac spine and the medial malleolus. A difference in this measurement is indicative of a true discrepancy (Fig. 7–3B).
  - With the patient standing, sequential blocks should be placed under the shorter leg until the pelvis is level to palpation and the patient feels level.

Relevance to Surgical Decision-Making in Total Hip Arthroplasty

- Regardless of situation, pre- and postoperative leg length discrepancies need to be discussed with the patient, including the possibility of a postoperative discrepancy.
- True leg length discrepancies can be corrected intraoperatively by altering implant position.
- Apparent leg length discrepancies caused by soft tissue contractures, in combination with a flexible spine examination, should *not* be corrected by changing implant position or significant postoperative discrepancies may result.

Knee

Examination With the Patient Standing

- The examination should begin with observation of the standing patient in shorts or a gown.
- The anatomic alignment of the extremity should be measured with a goniometer with the patient relaxed and standing. Normal alignment is approximately 6 degrees of tibiofemoral valgus. Deviation from this into varus or valgus should be noted.
- The patient's gait is then carefully observed for the following:
  - *Antalgia:* Shortened stance phase of gait
  - Valgus thrust (Fig. 7–4A)
    - This can be caused by progressive lateral compartment degeneration or laxity of the medial collateral ligament and posteromedial capsule.
  - Varus thrust (Fig. 7–4B)

- This can be caused by progressive medial compartment degeneration or laxity of the lateral collateral ligament and posterolateral capsule.
- Difficulty in performing a deep squat can be informative as well.
- Patients with meniscal disease have great difficulty and localize pain to the posterior aspect of the knee.
- Patients with patellofemoral arthritis will complain of anterior knee pain.

Examination With the Patient Supine

- Start with uninvolved knee for control and examine both knees at the same angle of flexion.
- Quadriceps atrophy can be assessed by measuring the circumference of the thigh at a set distance above the superior pole of the patella.
- Check skin integrity around the injured knee, and note the presence of previous surgical scars.
  - In general, when there are multiple previous vertical incisions, the most lateral incision should be used for an arthroplasty procedure. This is because the major blood supply to the anterior skin of the knee comes from the medial side, and reusing the medial scar may compromise the blood supply in between the two incisions (Callaghan et al. 1998).
- The presence of effusion is seen as fullness in the suprapatellar pouch as well as the ability to ballotte the patella into the femoral trochlea (Fig. 7–5).
- Active ROM and passive ROM is then assessed using a goniometer.
- Normal ROM is 0 to 140 degrees.
  - Loss of both active ROM and passive ROM signifies a chronic problem with contractures or mechanical block.
  - When the active full extension is less than passive extension, this is referred to as an *extensor lag* and may indicate a compromise in the extensor mechanism or weakness of the quadriceps mechanism.
- Palpate the knee in a systematic fashion for focal areas of tenderness. Arthritis tends to cause diffuse pain anteriorly in the knee, whereas meniscal disease causes focal tenderness along the posterior margin of the joint line. Tenderness along the collateral ligaments, extensor mechanism, and pes bursa will help to identify disease in these areas.
- Patellar tracking should also be assessed, as well as the presence of patella alta or baja. Tests that isolate pain to the patellofemoral joint include:
  - *Patellar grind test:* A positive test is seen when pain is elicited with axial compression of the patella against the trochlea.
  - *Patellar inhibition test:* The examiner holds pressure against the superior pole of the patella with the patient's knee in full extension and relaxed and asks the patient to lift the leg off the table. A positive test is seen when pain is elicited and patient cannot tighten the quadriceps muscle.

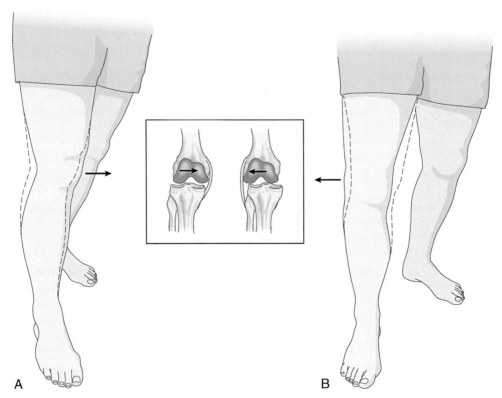

Figure 7–4: Valgus and varus thrust.
A, Valgus thrust can result from lateral compartment degeneration or from medial collateral ligament and posteromedial laxity. **B,** Varus thrust can result from medial compartment degeneration or lateral collateral ligament and posterolateral laxity. (Redrawn from Scott WN [1991]. *Ligament and Extensor Mechanism Injuries of the Knee: Diagnosis and Treatment.* St. Louis: Mosby.)

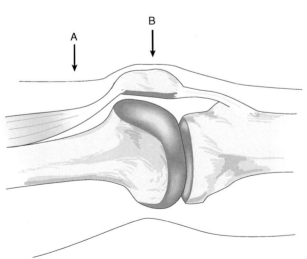

Figure 7–5: Examining for knee effusion.
Apply manual pressure here *(A)* to displace knee fluid into the space behind the patella. Briskly push here *(B)* to thrust the patella against the femur. (Redrawn from Bickley LS, Szilagyi PG [2005]. *Bates' Guide to Physical Examination and History Taking,* 9th ed. Philadelphia: Lippincott Williams & Wilkins.)

- Examination of the collateral ligaments should be performed next, to assess for both integrity and contractures. The knee should be examined in both full extension and at 30 degrees of flexion. At full extension, the posterior capsule and cruciate ligaments contribute to mediolateral stability, whereas at 30 degrees of flexion, the collateral ligaments are isolated.
  - A solid end point to stress examination at 30 degrees of flexion is indicative of intact collateral ligament.
  - Note the degree of correction achieved with the stress examination. Patients who fail to correct to anatomic alignment are more likely to require an intraoperative ligament release at the time of an arthroplasty procedure.
- The cruciate ligaments should also be examined. Before an arthroplasty procedure, the attenuation or absence of one or both of the cruciate ligaments will influence surgical decision making and choice of prosthesis.
  - ACL (Butler et al. 1980)
    - *Lachman's examination:* This is the most sensitive test for integrity of the ACL. In this examination, the tibia is stressed anteriorly on the femur with knee in 30 degrees of flexion.
    A firm end point indicates integrity of ACL.

- *Anterior drawer test:* With the patient's knee flexed to 90 degrees, subluxate the tibia forward and assess the degree of anterior subluxation of tibia compared with the uninvolved side.
- Posterior cruciate ligament (PCL)
  - *Posterior drawer test:* With the patient's knee flexed to 90 degrees, measure the amount of posterior translation of the tibia on the femur with a posteriorly directed force.
  - *Posterior sag test:* With the patient's knee flexed to 90 degrees and the patient relaxed, observe for any posterior subluxation of the tibia on the femur. When results are positive, one notices the loss of normal prominence of tibial tubercle and medial tibial step-off.
  - *Quadriceps active test:* With the patient's knee at 60 degrees of flexion, the patient is asked to extend the knee. If the PCL is torn, the tibia will start subluxated posteriorly on the femur, and attempted active extension will reduce the subluxated tibia into its normal position (Daniel et al. 1988) (Fig. 7–6).

- Meniscal disease can be detected with *McMurray's test.*
  - With the patient supine and the knee and hip both flexed to 90 degrees, internally and externally rotate the patient's foot. A positive test is seen when a click or pop is heard or felt under the examiner's fingers (Fig. 7–7).

  - The *flexion McMurray test* can be more provocative. To test for a medial meniscus tear, the patient's knee is flexed and the foot is externally rotated. The knee is then brought into extension, and a positive test occurs when the patient has pain over the posterior joint line.

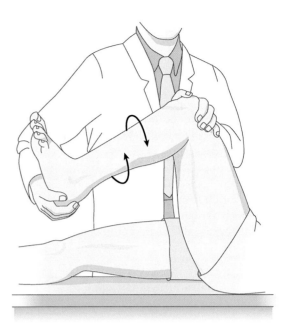

Figure 7–7: McMurray's test.
A click or pop is heard or felt under the examiner's fingers during McMurray's test. (Redrawn from Insall JA, ed. [1984]. *Surgery of the Knee.* New York: Churchill Livingstone.)

The same is done for a lateral meniscus tear, except the foot is held in internal rotation.

Medical Evaluation
General Principles

- The preoperative medical assessment of the arthroplasty patient is important to characterize operative risk and to minimize perioperative complications. The evaluation is similar to the basic principles used for patients undergoing anesthesia and noncardiac surgery.
- Routine preoperative laboratory testing is commonly used but is not of significant value in a majority of patients. Therefore selective use of preoperative studies is now recommended.
  - A complete blood count should be obtained in all patients undergoing arthroplasty because of expected blood loss. This count can also help to guide the use of preoperative autologous transfusions. Patients taking preoperative steroids may have leukocytosis.
  - Routine chemistry studies are of little value except in selected cases indicated by the patient's history, as follows:
    - Renal function can be affected in patients with congestive heart failure and diabetes mellitus, as well as in those taking nonsteroidal anti-inflammatory agents.
    - Liver enzyme elevation is seen in patients with history of hepatitis or significant alcohol use.
  - Coagulation studies are generally not very helpful in identifying asymptomatic patients with bleeding

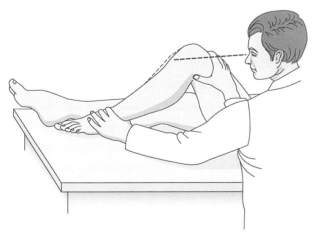

Figure 7–6: Quadriceps active test.
The quadriceps active test is used to test the integrity of the posterior cruciate ligament. If it is torn, the tibia will start subluxated posteriorly on the femur. (Redrawn from Daniel DM, Stone ML, Barnett P, Sachs R [1988]. Use of the quadriceps active test to diagnose posterior cruciate-ligament disruption and measure posterior laxity of the knee. *J Bone Joint Surg Am* 70:386-391.)

problems, but they should be obtained in patients taking anticoagulants. A history of bleeding tendencies and physical examination are more valuable in assessing hemostasis.

- Urinalysis is not helpful in identifying patients at risk for infectious conditions.
  - Asymptomatic bacteriuria can be found in 25% to 50% of elderly patients, and treatment does not guarantee eradication of the bacteria.
  - It is advisable to treat asymptomatic bacteriuria preoperatively, especially given that patients may undergo urologic catheterization in the perioperative period.
  - Patients with symptomatic cystitis should be treated preoperatively and should not undergo surgery until symptoms resolve.

- The history of obstructive or irritative symptoms along with bacterial counts found in culture can help to guide preoperative decision making (Fig. 7–8).
- Chest radiograph abnormalities are common in patients who are older than 60 years and have little influence in identifying abnormalities that affect the outcome of surgery. Patients with chronic obstructive lung disease and heart failure should undergo careful scrutiny, but even in these patients, the history and physical examination are more important in assessing pulmonary or cardiac risk (Callaghan et al. 1998).
- The preoperative electrocardiogram is a valuable test, given that up to 53% of orthopedic patients may have an abnormality on routine electrocardiography (Goldman 1983).

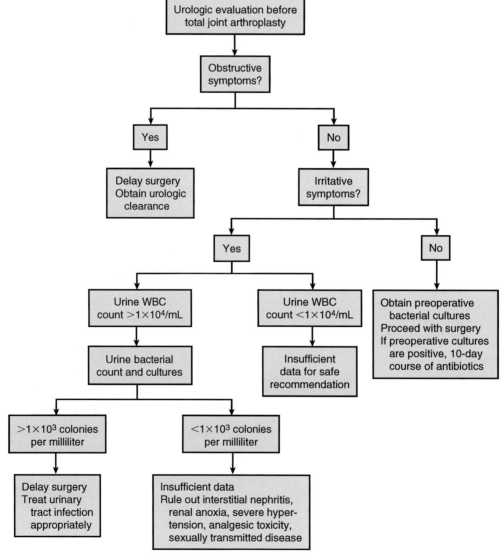

Figure 7–8: Algorithm for urologic evaluation of patients before total joint arthroplasty. WBC, white blood cell. (From David TS, Vrahas MS [2000]. Perioperative lower urinary tract infections and deep sepsis in patients undergoing total joint arthroplasty. *J Am Acad Orthop Surg* 8:66-74.)

Factors Associated With Surgical Risk

- American Society of Anesthesiology (ASA) classification system is used to stratify patients according to surgical risk. There is some predictive value in determining anesthetic complications and postoperative deaths. Patients with certain categories of risk should receive special attention.

Cardiovascular Disorders (Goldman 1983)

- It is difficult to assess the cardiovascular fitness of the elderly and arthritic patient because of functional limitations.
- Although stable angina and recent coronary artery bypass grafting do not appear to increase perioperative risk, unstable angina or angina at low levels of activity are considered high-risk factors, and patients should be evaluated preoperatively.
- Noninvasive pharmacologic studies such as dipyridamole, adenosine thallium, and dobutamine hydrochloride echocardiography are effective in determining the extent of coronary disease.
- Patients with global ischemia or two or more significant areas of myocardium at risk should be studied with coronary arteriography before surgery.
- Patients with a recent myocardial infarction should wait 6 months to have their elective arthroplasty procedure.
- Patients with preexisting congestive heart failure should have their condition optimized before surgery. The presence of an S_3 gallop, jugular venous distention, or rales indicates a high perioperative risk, and consideration should be given to using a Swan-Ganz catheter and arterial line monitoring.
- Patients with aortic stenosis or mitral stenosis are intolerant of significant shifts in fluid balance; therefore perioperative fluid balance should be monitored closely.
- In patients with atrial fibrillation who are taking warfarin sodium to prevent stroke, most physicians stop the warfarin 3 to 5 days preoperatively and then resume the medication the night of surgery.
- In high-risk patients undergoing surgery, the use of perioperative β-blockers has been shown to be effective in reducing perioperative ischemia (Mangano et al. 1996).

Pulmonary Disorders

- The patient's functional capacity is best assessed through a history and physical examination because no pulmonary risk stratification indices exist (Gass and Olsen 1986).
- If patients have no limitation of function and no pulmonary disease, no further evaluation is necessary.
- Patients with chronic obstructive airway disease, asthma, morbid obesity, and neuromuscular disorders should be considered for the following before surgery:
  - Smoking cessation
  - Spinal or epidural anesthesia
  - Aggressive management with inhalers and oral steroids
  - Antibiotics specific to the bacterial infection of the airway
- All patients undergoing joint replacement should have the following preoperative and postoperative interventions to decrease perioperative complications:
  - Instruction in use of incentive spirometry
  - Coughing
  - Deep breathing exercises
  - Early ambulation after surgery

Hypertension

- Patients with systolic blood pressure greater than 200 mm Hg or diastolic pressure greater than 110 mm Hg should have surgery postponed until blood pressure is adequately controlled.
- Patients should be given their antihypertensive medications preoperatively, and these medications should be resumed postoperatively.
- Consideration should be given to discontinuing diuretics 2 to 3 days preoperatively and correcting any hypokalemia.

Diabetes Mellitus

- All patients with diabetes should be evaluated for renal, peripheral vascular, and neuropathic conditions. An electrocardiogram should be obtained in all patients because the incidence of coexisting cardiovascular disease and silent ischemia is higher in the diabetic population.
- Good control of blood glucose levels should be attained for at least 7 days preoperatively.
- Glucose management on the day of surgery:
  - Patients with brittle diabetes should have their surgery earlier in the day to avoid prolonged periods without eating. Management with an insulin drip should be considered for patients with severe brittle diabetes.
  - A half dose of insulin on the morning of surgery should be given with blood glucose testing every 4 hours to follow with a sliding scale.
  - Oral hypoglycemic agents should be held on the day of surgery.
  - 5% Dextrose fluids should be administered to avoid starvation ketosis.
  - Patients with autonomic neuropathy have a higher incidence of postoperative nausea and gastroparesis, and an agent that improves gastric emptying should be given (e.g., metoclopramide).

Cerebrovascular Disease

- Patients with asymptomatic carotid stenosis have a 1% to 2% risk of stroke after anesthesia.

- Patients with carotid stenosis greater than 75% should be evaluated for carotid endarterectomy.
- Patients with recent transient ischemic attack (≤6 weeks) should be thoroughly evaluated, and carotid endarterectomy should be performed if the stenosis is greater than 75%.

Rheumatoid Arthritis

- Of patients with rheumatoid arthritis, 30% to 40% have atlantoaxial subluxation. Preoperative history, physical examination, and flexion-extension radiographs can help to identify this problem.
- It is important to identify these patients because endotracheal intubation can cause subluxation of diseased atlantoaxial joint during endotracheal intubation and may compromise the respiratory center of the medulla.
- Other conditions found in the this population include the following:
  - Restrictive lung disease
  - Heart disease (pericarditis, myocarditis, conduction defects)
  - Anemia of chronic disease

Long-Term Glucocorticoid Use

- For patients who have taken the equivalent of 7.5 mg of prednisone daily for more than 7 days, stress-dose steroids should be given.
- 100 mg of hydrocortisone should be given intravenously 30 minutes preoperatively, then each 8 hours postoperatively for 24 to 48 hours (Callaghan et al. 1998).

Obesity

- During the history and physical examination, special attention should be given to respiratory symptoms, functional abilities in day-to-day life, and sleep disturbance.
- Perioperative risks result from the association of obesity with other medical conditions such as hypertension, hyperlipidemia, atherosclerotic vascular disease, left ventricular hypertrophy, changes in pulmonary function, diabetes mellitus, cholelithiasis, and gout.
- Morbidly obese patients are at higher risk for complications such as wound complications. These issues should be discussed with the patient during the preoperative consultation.
- Pulmonary complications pose the greatest risk in the postoperative period. Because of the decreased compliance of the chest wall and redundant tissue surrounding the upper airway, common findings seen include increased minute ventilation, shallow breathing, and an increase in the energy expenditure of breathing, all to maintain a normal partial pressure of oxygen and to reduce the partial pressure of carbon dioxide.
- Anesthesiologists should pay special attention to airway management in these patients to avoid the need for emergency intubation in these difficult airways.

Imaging

- Imaging of the hip and knee is a critical component in the patient evaluation. It is also instrumental in preoperative planning and allows the surgeon accurately to predict the type, size, and position of components placed at surgery.
- Safety issues are important to recognize. Although ionizing radiation is minimal, it poses a real somatic and genetic risk. Appropriate steps should be taken to reduce exposure, including prescreening women of childbearing age for the possibility of pregnancy, shielding of genitals, and accurate examination procedures.
- Hallmark findings of osteoarthritis include the following:
  - *Joint space:* The loss of joint space indicates loss of cartilage
  - *Osteophytes:* The formation of marginal osteophytes is an early sign of osteoarthritis.
  - *Subchondral sclerosis:* Increased radiodensity in the subchondral zone represents increased bone deposition in response to the loss of overlying cartilage.
  - Other findings that should be sought on each film include subchondral cysts, loose bodies, subtle fractures, and bony lesions indicating underlying neoplastic processes.

Hip

Plain Radiography

- Plain radiographs are used in the initial study of the hip joint. Several common radiographic views are utilized:
  - Anteroposterior (AP) view (Fig. 7–9)
    - For the AP view, internally rotating the hip accommodates femoral anteversion and brings the femoral neck into a plane perpendicular to the x-ray beam.
    - Bony landmarks should be used to determine the adequacy of radiographs. On AP radiographs, the greater and lesser tuberosity should not significantly overlap the femoral neck. The calcar femoris should be clearly visible, and there should be very little elliptic overlap between the anterior and posterior margins of the femoral head-neck junction.
    - The most common error is allowing the hip to rotate externally. This results in overlap of the greater trochanter with the femoral neck and medially profiles the lesser tuberosity. Also, femoral offset is usually underestimated in this situation, and this can lead to inaccuracies in preoperative templating. In patients with an external rotation contracture who are unable to rotate their hips internally, a posteroanterior view of the hip should be obtained (Fig. 7–10).
    - Acetabular landmarks include the iliopubic (or iliopectineal) line marking the anterior column, the ilioischial line marking the posterior column, the teardrop outline at the inferior margin of the medial

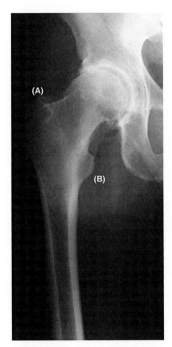

Figure 7–9: Anteroposterior view of the hip in external rotation.
Note the overlap of the greater trochanter on the femoral neck *(A)* and the relative prominence of the lesser trochanter *(B)*. Offset is underestimated in this example.

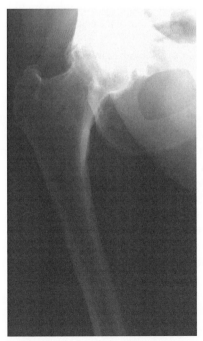

Figure 7–10: Posteroanterior view of the hip.
The patient is positioned prone and is tilted until the hip is in the plane of the film. Note how the lesser trochanter is less noticeable on this view, and the greater trochanter does not overlap with the femoral neck. This view more accurately displays femoral offset.

acetabular border, and the anterior and posterior acetabular rims (Fig. 7–11).

- Frog-leg lateral view
  - For a frog-leg lateral view, the patient's hip is flexed and externally rotated so the leg is flat on the x-ray table, and the x-ray beam is directed anteroposteriorly (Fig. 7–12).
  - The greater trochanter overlaps the femoral neck, and the lesser trochanter can be seen in profile posteriorly.
  - Because this is only a lateral view of the femur, acetabular anatomy is unchanged in the frog-leg lateral view.
- An AP view of the pelvis is taken to examine the contralateral hip, leg-length discrepancy, sacrum, and sacroiliac joints (Fig. 7–13).
  - Preoperative leg-length discrepancy can be estimated by drawing a horizontal line between the corresponding teardrops, obturator foramina, or ischial tuberosities. By comparing the point at which this line intersects with a fixed landmark on each hip (e.g., lesser tuberosity) and measuring the difference with a radiographic ruler, leg-length discrepancy can by obtained. The physical examination described earlier is of greater importance in deciding the amount of length to restore intraoperatively (see Fig. 7–13).
- Special views of the pelvis: Inlet and outlet views
  - The *inlet view* is used to visualize the ring of the pelvis, mainly in traumatic injuries to evaluate for fractures.

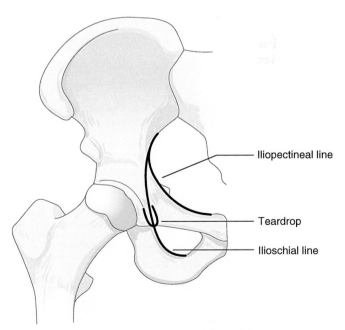

Figure 7–11: Anteroposterior view of the pelvis.
This view includes the iliopectineal line, the ilioischial line, and the teardrop. (Redrawn from Hak DJ, Gautsch TL [1995]. A review of radiographic lines and angles used in orthopedics. *Am J Orthop* 24:597.)

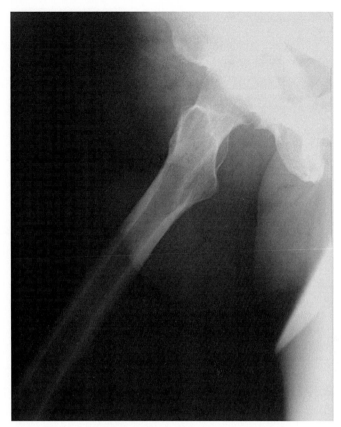

Figure 7–12: Frog-leg lateral view.
The hip is flexed and externally rotated with the x-ray beam directed anteroposteriorly.

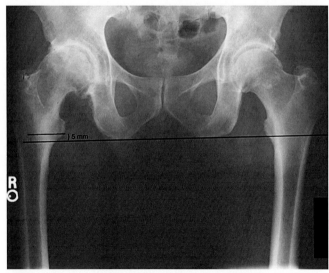

Figure 7–13: Bilateral anteroposterior view of the pelvis. A transverse line is drawn on the radiograph, in this example connecting the ischial tuberosities. By comparing the point that this line intersects with the femur on each hip, an estimation of leg-length discrepancy can be made.

- The film is taken in the AP projection with the beam angled caudally 40 degrees.
  - The *outlet view* can delineate vertical translation or malalignment of pelvis, as well as fractures or lesions of the sacrum. This view is obtained by taking an AP projection angled cranially 40 degrees.
- Anterior and posterior oblique views of the acetabulum: Judet's views
  - When better visualization is needed of acetabular anatomy, these views are a valuable component in the evaluation.
  - For an iliac or posterior oblique view, rotate the patient 45 degrees from supine position with the involved side down, and direct the beam anteroposteriorly. The posterior (ilioischial) column and the anterior rim are seen with this view.
  - To obtain an obturator or anterior oblique view, the pelvis is rotated 45 degrees with the involved side up, and the beam is directed anteroposteriorly. The anterior (iliopubic) column and posterior rim are best delineated in this view.
- Other views available for evaluation of the acetabulum can be obtained, such as the false profile view, sitting AP, sitting lateral, and Chassard-Lapiné semiaxial views, but computed tomography is more readily utilized, given the superior and reliable visualization obtained.
- Standard radiographic measurements include femoral neck-shaft angle, femoral neck version, acetabular protrusio, acetabular index, Shenton's line, and center edge angle of Wiberg (Table 7–3).

Computed Tomography

- The most common use of CT is to evaluate traumatic injuries such as pelvic and acetabular fractures and dislocations.
- When a neoplasm is suspected, CT helps to characterize the lesion with better clarity than plain films.
- For the evaluation of a prosthetic hip, CT can be valuable as well. Although significant scatter artifact can result from the metallic components, the position of the components, periacetabular bone loss, and the presence of prosthetic loosening can be evaluated. Clinical situations in which this can be valuable include a patient with recurrent dislocations to evaluate component position, a patient with a painful hip with normal radiographs, and the preoperative evaluation of a patient with a failed total hip arthroplasty and significant acetabular bone loss (Fig. 7–14).

Magnetic Resonance Imaging

- Advances in the field of MRI have made this test more readily available, cost-effective, sensitive, and specific for the diagnosis of numerous conditions. Although plain films

Table 7–3   Standard Radiographic Measurements

RADIOGRAPHIC LANDMARK	DESCRIPTION	NORMAL FINDING
Femoral neck-shaft angle	Measured between the central axes of the femoral neck and shaft	125 (range, 120–140) degrees
Femoral neck version	Comparison of femoral neck center line with the epicondylar axis of the distal femur	14 degrees anteversion
Acetabular protrusio	Construction of a line (of Köhler) from the medial border of the body of the ischium to the tangent of the medial border of the ilium	Protrusion exists if the acetabulum passes medial to that line
Acetabular index	The angle between a line drawn between the triradiate cartilage of the acetabulum (Hilgenreiner's line) and a second line drawn from the triradiate cartilage to the lateral border of the acetabulum	<25 degrees
Shenton's line	The confluent arch made by the inferior border of the superior pubic ramus and the medial border of the femoral neck	Smooth connection between these two arches
Center edge angle of Wiberg	Measured between a line from the center of the femoral head to the lateral edge of the acetabulum and a line drawn directly cephalocaudad from the center of the femoral head	20–40 degrees

show the diagnosis in a majority of patients, MRI can be useful in the following situations:

- *Occult hip fracture:* MRI has been shown to be superior to bone scintigraphy because of its superior accuracy as well as to its ability to diagnose a fracture shortly after the fall, whereas a bone scan is negative for the first 48 to 72 hours after injury.
- *Stress fractures:* Both compressive and tensile stress fractures can be diagnosed early with MRI scanning, best seen as increased bone marrow edema on T2-weighted sequences (Beltran et al. 1988).
- *Avascular necrosis* (AVN): Early detection and staging of AVN is done with MRI scanning. In patients with a painful hip and normal radiographs, especially those with risk factors for AVN, an MRI scan should

be obtained. Early diagnosis and treatment in earlier stages of this disease are associated with higher success rates.

- *Labral tears:* In patients with a history and physical examination consistent with a labral tear, an MRI arthrogram can help to visualize these tears. Early diagnosis and intervention with hip arthroscopy may help to prevent degenerative arthritis.

Knee

Plain Radiography

- Standing AP and lateral views of the knee are the routine views obtained in the knee series. Obtaining a weight-bearing AP film is critical, and this should be confirmed when reviewing films taken at outside facilities.
- On the AP film, the following should be studied (Fig. 7–15):
  - *Alignment:* The anatomic tibiofemoral axis should be in 5 to 7 degrees of valgus. This can be measured be drawing a line from the center of the femoral shaft proximally to the center of femoral sulcus, and a second line from the center of the tibial shaft distally to the center of the tibial plateau proximally. The angle between these two lines makes the anatomic *tibiofemoral angle.*
- The *lateral view* is usually non–weight bearing and can be taken in 30 or 90 degrees of flexion (Fig. 7–16). Examine the film for the following findings:
  - The position of the patella in relation to the knee joint can be measured (Fig. 7–17).
  - In the 90-degree flexed view, the amount of femoral rollback on the tibia can indicate PCL integrity. If the femur is rolled back excessively on the tibia, this indicates a PCL contracture; if the femur articulates anteriorly on the tibia (tibial sag), this indicates PCL incompetence.
  - In an acute trauma setting, a "fat-fluid" level in the suprapatellar bursa may be seen, indicating the presence of an intra-articular fracture.

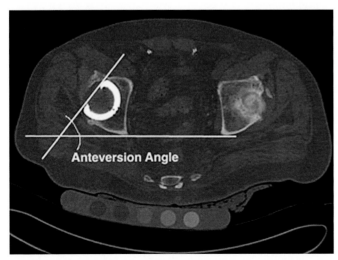

Figure 7–14: Computed tomography (CT).
CT can be valuable in assessing component positioning, peri-acetabular bone loss, and the presence of prosthetic loosening. Clinical situations in which CT can be valuable include dislocations and preoperative evaluations of failed total hip arthroplasties.

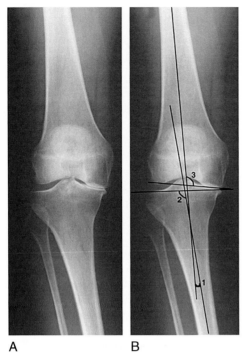

A   B

Figure 7–15: Angles of the knee.
A, Standing anteroposterior view of the knee. **B,** The
shown angles should be measured preoperatively:
(1) tibiofemoral angle (average range, 5 to 7 degrees valgus);
(2) proximal tibial angle (average 93 degrees, referred to as
3 degrees varus); and *(3)* distal femoral angle (average
99 degrees, referred to as 9 degrees valgus).

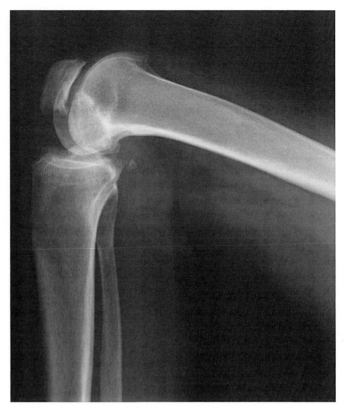

Figure 7–16: Flexion lateral view of the knee.
Examine the film for the position of the patella in relation to
the knee joint. In addition, the amount of femoral rollback on
the tibia can indicate the integrity of the posterior cruciate
ligament.

- The *patellofemoral joint* can be visualized by taking a film
  with the patient's knee flexed 45 degrees and the beam
  directed tangentially through the patellofemoral joint at a
  60-degree angle. The space between the patella and
  femoral trochlea can be evaluated for arthrosis, along with
  patellar tilt and malalignment (Fulkerson and Shea 1990)
  (Fig. 7–18).
- *Posteroanterior weight-bearing views* of the knee are taken
  while the patient is standing with the knee flexed
  45 degrees and the beam directed 10 degrees caudad. This
  specifically evaluates the posterior aspect of the femoral
  condyles to demonstrate focal cartilage loss over the
  posterior femorotibial joint compartment.
- The *tunnel view* (intercondylar notch) is taken when
  clinical signs of decreased range of motion or locking are
  seen. This is useful in diagnosing a fracture of the tibial
  spines, loose bodies in the intercondylar notch, and
  osteochondral lesions involving the inner margin of the
  femoral condyles (Messieh et al. 1990).
- In the presence of any extra-articular malalignment such as
  congenital deformities, prior surgery, or malunion from a
  previous fracture, a standing *long alignment film* from hip to
  ankle should be taken to assist in preoperative planning.

- The *mechanical axis* of the lower extremity is drawn by
  connecting the center of the femoral head to the center of
  the ankle. This line should pass through the center of the
  knee; when it passes medially, this represents a varus knee,
  and when it passes laterally, it represents a valgus knee.

Computed Tomography

- With the increased availability and decreased cost of MRI,
  CT plays less of a role in the preoperative evaluation.
  CT can be useful for assessing the following:
  - Fractures can be visualized.
  - Patellofemoral tilt can be measured with dynamic
    CT scanning with the knee in 15, 30, and 45 degrees of
    flexion. Patellar maltracking and malalignment
    may be seen.
  - Femoral anteversion can be measured. The difference
    between the femoral neck angle and the transcondylar
    axis represents the amount of femoral anteversion or
    retroversion.
  - Tibial torsion can also be determined. The difference
    between the proximal tibial angle and the transmalleolar
    angle represents the amount of internal or external
    rotation.

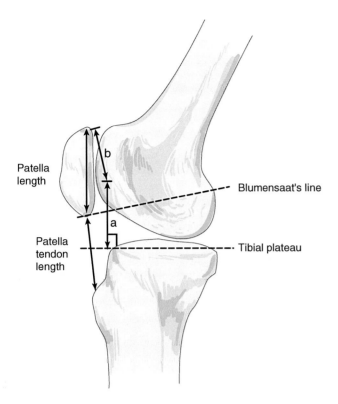

Figure 7–17: Three ways to measure for patella alta or patella baja.
First, the lower border of the patella should lie on Blumensaat's line. Second, the Insall-Salvati index is the ratio of patella length to patella tendon length (should be 1.0). Third, the Blackburne-Peel index is the ratio between *(a)* the distance from the tibial plateau to the inferior articular surface of the patella and *(b)* the length of the patella articular surface (should be 0.8). (Redrawn from Weissman B, Sledge C [1985]. *Orthopedic Radiology.* Philadelphia: WB Saunders, p 498.)

Magnetic Resonance Imaging

- The superior soft tissue clarity and multiplanar imaging capability of MRI has made this technique valuable in the evaluation of knee pain. In the routine evaluation of a patient undergoing arthroplasty when plain radiographs indicate advanced arthritic changes, MRI is rarely indicated (Boden et al. 1992). However, MRI provides excellent visualization of the structures of the knee that can assist in surgical decision making.
- Meniscal disease
  - Intrasubstance increased signal intensity generally indicates degenerative meniscal tears. These tears typically originate at the inferior articular surface of the posterior horn of the medial meniscus. Signal changes that communicate with the surface of the meniscus are more likely true meniscus tears (Stoller et al. 1987) (Fig. 7–19).
  - Increasing medial compartment pressures resulting from degenerative arthrosis cause the anterior margin of the posterior horn to appear blunted on the sagittal images.
  - Remodeling of the condyle and increasing contact pressures of the knee leading to meniscal extrusion beyond the tibia on coronal images can be indicative of radial displacement of the medial meniscus.
  - Sensitivity of MRI in detecting lateral meniscal tears has been reported to be less than that detecting medial meniscus tears, particularly in the setting of an ACL tear.

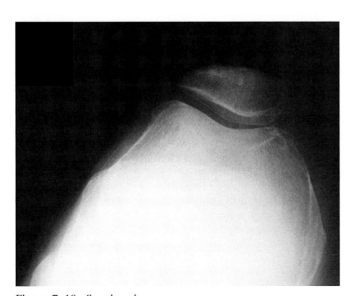

Figure 7–18: Sunrise view.
Examine for asymmetry of patella in groove, joint space narrowing, and osteophytes.

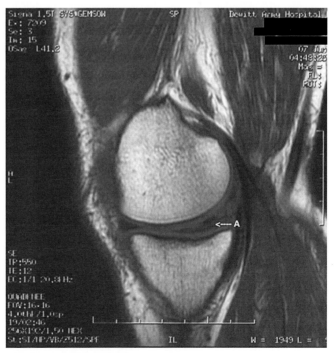

Figure 7–19: Posterior horn tear.
Note the intrasubstance signal change in the meniscus (*A*) consistent with a meniscal tear.

- Articular cartilage
  - MRI is more sensitive than plain radiographs in detecting focal chondral lesions that may exist before joint space narrowing, as well as depicting subchondral bony abnormalities before development of subchondral sclerosis on conventional radiographs (Boegard et al. 1998, Potter et al. 1998).
  - Early degeneration of articular cartilage is manifested at arthroscopy as areas of softening as well as a disruption of collagen network and decreased proteoglycans, which, in turn increase their hydrophilic characteristics.
  - Later stages of chondromalacia include surface fibrillation and erosion, which would correspond to fissures and fibrillation on MRI.
  - In stage IV chondromalacia, MRI shows complete loss of articular cartilage signal.
  - After acute traumatic chondral injury without preexisting osteoarthrosis, however, a bone marrow edema pattern may be helpful in localizing the site of chondral injury.
  - Cartilage imaging in the clinical setting lies in its ability to disclose full-thickness cartilage defects in patients with normal plain radiographs and to discriminate meniscal from chondral pathologic features, as in a displaced chondral flap, which may simulate a displaced meniscal tear, causing locking symptoms.

References

Beltran J, Herman LJ, Burk JM, et al. (1988). Femoral head avascular necrosis: MR imaging with clinical-pathologic and radionuclide correlation. *Radiology* 166:215-220.

A retrospective evaluation of MRI for the detection of AVN of the femoral head was performed in 49 patients (85 hips) with clinical suspicion of AVN. A comparison between MRI scans and bone scans showed MRI to be superior, with a sensitivity of 88.8% (versus 77.5%) and a specificity of 100% (versus 75%). Bone morphogenetic protein was the most sensitive (92%) but least specific test (57%).

Boden SD, Davis DO, Dina TS, et al. (1992). A prospective and blinded investigation of magnetic resonance imaging of the knee: Abnormal findings in asymptomatic subjects. *Clin Orthop Relat Res* 282:177-185.

The purpose of this study was to evaluate MRI scans of meniscal, ligamentous, and bony abnormalities in patients without clinical symptoms. It was concluded that the high incidence of abnormal MRI findings in asymptomatic subjects underscores the danger of relying on a diagnostic test without careful correlation with clinical signs and symptoms. These findings also emphasize the importance of access to relevant clinical data when interpreting MRI scans of the knee.

Boegard T, Rudling O, Petersson IF, et al. (1998). Correlation between radiographically diagnosed osteophytes and magnetic resonance detected cartilage defects in the tibiofemoral joint. *Ann Rheum Dis* 57:401-407.

The purpose of this study was to assess the correlation between the presence of radiographically diagnosed osteophytes in the tibiofemoral joint and (1) MRI-detected cartilage defects and meniscal lesions in the same joint and (2) knee pain. A correlation ($P < .05$) between osteophytes at the medial tibial condyle and knee pain was found. With the presence of marginal osteophytes in the tibiofemoral joint, there is a high prevalence of MRI-detected cartilage defects in the same joint whether joint space narrowing (<3 mm) is present or not.

Butler DL, Noyes FR, Grood ES (1980). Ligamentous restraints to anterior-posterior drawer in the human knee. *J Bone Joint Surg Am* 62:259-270.

This study utilized a testing method to rank the importance of each ligament based on the force provided by each ligament in resisting the drawer tests. The following conclusions were drawn: (1) proposed surgical procedures for knee stability must be analyzed in terms of all ligament restraints; (2) secondary restraints may block clinical laxity tests, but they often stretch out and do not provide knee stability under higher functional forces of activity; (3) the ACL and PCL provide the overwhelming resistance to these respective tibial displacements.

Callaghan JJ, Rosenberg AG, Rubash EH, eds. (1998). *The Adult Hip.* Philadelphia: Lippincott-Raven, pp 315-393.

This two-volume reference provides comprehensive coverage of the evaluation and surgical management of problems of the hip, including the anatomy and biomechanics of the hip, the biomaterials used in hip reconstruction, the biology of bone autografts and allografts, pathology of the hip, osteonecrosis of the hip and related disorders, perioperative considerations, surgical anatomy, and surgical approaches to the hip.

Daniel DM, Stone ML, Barnet P, et al. (1988). Use of the quadriceps active test to diagnose posterior cruciate ligament disruption and measure posterior laxity of the knee. *J Bone Joint Surg Am* 70: 386-391.

In this study, orthopedic surgeons evaluated the integrity of the ligaments of the knee using a quadriceps active test in which the muscle contractures of the subject served as the displacing force. With the knee joint in 90 degrees of flexion, contraction of the quadriceps resulted in anterior translation of the tibia in 41 of 42 knees that had a documented disruption of the PCL. This anterior translation did not occur in the contralateral normal knee of the same subjects, in the knees of the 25 normal subjects, or in 25 knees that had a known unilateral ACL disruption.

Fulkerson JP, Shea KP (1990). Disorders of patellofemoral alignment. *J Bone Joint Surg Am* 72:1424-1429.

This report presented the many ailments associated with patellofemoral alignment as well as the etiology of these disorders. The specific pattern of patellar alignment or malalignment can help localize the resulting articular and retinacular lesions and therefore help one to understand more clearly the cause of pain in the anterior aspect of the knee. Possible treatments discussed included nonoperative rehabilitation, débridement operation, patellar subluxation and dislocation, and combined patellar tilt and subluxation.

Gass GD, Olsen GN (1986). Preoperative pulmonary function testing to predict postoperative morbidity and mortality. *Chest* 89:127-135.

This review attempted to assess critically the numerous pulmonary function techniques available for predicting postoperative pulmonary complications and to suggest which tests may be outmoded. The investigators concluded two observations. First, patients whose history and physical examination suggest underlying pulmonary dysfunction are at increased risk if they demonstrate abnormal pulmonary function tests (spirometry). Second, it is not clear exactly which test should then be performed in the patient with abnormal spirometry who faces pulmonary resectional surgery.

Goldman L (1983). Cardiac risks and complications of noncardiac surgery. *Ann Intern Med* 98:504-513.

This article addresses the care needed for patients who have recently undergone noncardiac surgery. Preoperative exercise testing and cardiac catheterization to assess risk are not routinely indicated, but perioperative hemodynamic monitoring to improve management is recommended in patients at high risk. Postoperative hypertension, arrhythmias, and heart failure commonly occur in the first 2 days after surgery, but the risk of myocardial infarction persists for at least 5 or 6 days postoperatively. Effective perioperative consultation must include careful postoperative observation to detect cardiac complications at an early stage and to assist in their management.

Ireland J, Kessel L (1980). Hip adduction/abduction deformity and apparent leg-length inequality. *Clin Orthop Rel Res* 153:156-157.

The amount of apparent leg-length inequality attributable to given angles of hip adduction/abduction has been expressed quantitatively. The inequality is related to the sine of the angle of adduction/abduction and the distance between the centers of the femoral heads. In a study of 50 adults, the mean figure for this distance in men and women was 18.6 cm. As a rough guide, each 10 degrees of deformity up to 40 degrees produce approximately 3 cm of inequality.

Mangano DT, Layug EL, Wallace A, et al. (1996). Effect of atenolol on mortality and cardiovascular morbidity after noncardiac surgery. *N Engl J Med* 335:1713-1720.

This study performed a randomized, double-blind, placebo-controlled trial to compare the effect of atenolol with that of a placebo on overall survival and cardiovascular morbidity in patients with or at risk for coronary artery disease who were undergoing noncardiac surgery. The study concluded that in patients who have or are at risk for coronary artery disease who must undergo noncardiac surgery, treatment with atenolol during hospitalization can reduce mortality and the incidence of cardiovascular complications for as long as 2 years after surgery.

Messieh SS, Fowler PJ, Munro T (1990). Anteroposterior radiographs of the osteoarthritic knee. *J Bone Joint Surg Br* 72:639-640.

This study observed the accuracy in using radiographs to diagnose osteoarthritis in the knee. Arthroscopy confirmed that cartilage loss occurs in a more posterior portion of the femoral condyles than revealed by radiographs taken in full extension. The radiographs of 64 patients were used to compare the conventional with the standing tunnel view. In 10 knees in which the conventional view suggested normal cartilage, the standing tunnel view revealed severe degeneration.

Murray MP, Gore DR, Clarkson BH, et al. (1971). Walking patterns of patients with unilateral hip pain due to osteoarthritis and avascular necrosis. *J Bone Joint Surg Am* 53:259-274.

This historic study used interrupted-light photography to study multiple simultaneous displacement patterns of walking patients whose primary complaint was unilateral hip pain. This report describes the common features of coxalgic gait as well as the variations found in different patients. The goal of the study was to understand the role hip pain played in gait impairment.

Outerbridge RE (1961). The etiology of chondromalacia patellae. *J Bone Joint Surg Br* 43:752-757.

This classic article explains the key characteristics of patellae chondromalacia. First, chondromalacia of the patella starts most frequently on the medial facet. Second, the anatomy of the medial femoral condyle is described, including the rim at its superior border and the different arrangement at the upper border of the lateral femoral condyle. Finally, rubbing of the medial patellar facet on the rim at the upper border of the medial femoral condyle can partly explain the etiology of chondromalacia.

Potter HG, Linklater JA, Allen AA, et al. (1998). MR imaging of articular cartilage in the knee: A prospective evaluation utilizing fast spin echo imaging. *J Bone Joint Surg Am* 80:1276-1284.

The purpose of this study was to demonstrate that specialized MRI provides an accurate assessment of lesions of the articular cartilage of the knee. Arthroscopy was used as the comparative standard. With use of this readily available modified MRI sequence, it is possible to assess all articular surfaces of the knee accurately and thereby identify lesions that are amenable to arthroscopic treatment.

Stoller DW, Martin C, Crues JV III, et al. (1987). Meniscal tears: Pathologic correlation with MR imaging. *Radiology* 163:731-735.

Menisci from 12 autopsies and above-knee amputations were imaged with MRI at 1.5 T and then were sectioned for gross and histologic examination. A histologic staging system was developed and showed a one-to-one correlation with corresponding grades of MRI signal intensities. Histologic stages 1 and 2 represented a continuum of degeneration culminating in stage 3 fibrocartilaginous tears, seen most frequently in posterior horn segments of the medial meniscus. Correlation of histologic stages with MRI signal intensity allows for an improved diagnostic reading of MRI findings.

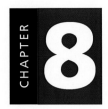

Total Hip Arthroplasty

Sharat K. Kusuma* and Jonathan P. Garino[†]

*MD, MBA, Resident and Clinical Instructor, Department of Orthopaedic Surgery,
University of Pennsylvania School of Medicine, Philadelphia, PA
[†]MD, Director, The Joint Reconstruction Center at Penn-Presbyterian Medical Center;
Director, the Adult Reconstruction Fellowship and Associate Professor, Department of
Orthopaedic Surgery, University of Pennsylvania School of Medicine, Philadelphia, PA

Introduction

- Total hip arthroplasty (THA) is one of the most successful and efficacious procedures performed by orthopaedic surgeons. Annually, hundreds of thousands of patients gain functional improvements and pain relief after undergoing THA (Berry 2001).
- Currently, the most common methods of performing THA utilize combinations of cemented or noncemented acetabular and femoral components. Many historical studies demonstrate excellent long-term longevity of THA. This chapter reviews basic concepts of degenerative hip disease and THA.

Indications and Contraindications

- Despite the fantastic success of THA since the mid-1970s, the procedure does have specific indications and contraindications. Patients who have significant hip pain, ambulatory dysfunction, and radiographic evidence of hip joint arthrosis and in whom attempts at conservative management have failed are generally excellent candidates for hip replacement.
- Examples of conservative treatments for hip joint disease include weight loss, nonsteroidal anti-inflammatory drugs, activity modification, intra-articular injections, and ambulation assistive devices. However, patients with significant dysfunction who do not meet all the preceding criteria may also receive strong consideration for THA; however, in such patients, the physician must more carefully determine with the patient whether the risks of the procedure warrant the potential improvement in the patient's function and quality of life that can result from THA.

- The pathologic processes that can lead to hip dysfunction are many and include osteoarthritis (the most common diagnosis), rheumatoid arthritis, other inflammatory arthritides (systemic lupus erythematosus, psoriatic arthritis), post-traumatic arthrosis, avascular necrosis (AVN), developmental dysplasia of the hip (DDH), and neoplasia with joint involvement.
- Contraindications to THA are generally few but must be carefully sought out in patients who are otherwise excellent candidates for the procedure. Patients who are of advanced age and who have medical comorbidities may be contraindicated to undergo THA. Such patients are medically unfit to tolerate the physiologic stresses of THA and are therefore not candidates.
- However, advanced age in an otherwise medically stable patient is in no way a contraindication to THA. Conversely, very young patients with significant hip disease are also suboptimal candidates because their higher activity levels accelerate the wear rate of the prostheses; such patients often require repeated revision surgery for failure of the prostheses. Such patients should be temporized with nonarthroplastic methods of alleviating their hip dysfunction until they are older (Berger et al. 1997, Callaghan et al. 1998).
- Other contraindications include patients with active bacterial infection either locally near the hip or at distant locations, such as the oral cavity. Patients who are in such a debilitated state that THA is unlikely to provide any functional gains are also suboptimal candidates for THA. Additionally, patients with pain near the hip joint that is unassociated with radiographic or other objective evidence of hip disease are poor candidates. Finally, patients with

psychiatric, cognitive, or behavioral dysfunctions that place them at high risk for postoperative complications (e.g., dislocation) are not ideal candidates (Berry 2001).

Specific Disorders Requiring Total Hip Arthroplasty

- Certain disorders that result in hip joint arthrosis deserve special attention and preoperative consideration.

Avascular Necrosis

- AVN of the hip is one such condition (Fig. 8–1). Traumatic causes of AVN include hip dislocation and femoral neck fracture. Nontraumatic causes of AVN include high doses of steroids, which are often used to treat underlying diseases such as systemic lupus erythematosus and rheumatoid arthritis (Koval 2002b, Lieberman et al. 2002, Mont et al. 2000). AVN is also associated with high levels of alcohol intake. Other disorders associated with AVN include sickle cell disease, Gaucher's disease, caisson disease, human immunodeficiency virus, pancreatitis, and liver and kidney disease.
- It is important to differentiate AVN from a similarly presenting disorder known as transient osteoporosis of the hip. Transient osteoporosis is most commonly seen in middle-aged men and pregnant women in the third trimester of pregnancy and is differentiated on magnetic resonance imaging (MRI) by increased signal throughout the femoral head

and neck (Fig. 8–2). This finding is in contrast to AVN, which appears as a discrete lesion in the femoral head on an MRI scan (Guerra and Steinberg 1995, Urbanski et al. 1991). Transient osteoporosis is self-limiting and is treated conservatively, whereas AVN often requires surgical treatment. This important distinction also highlights that MRI is the most sensitive and specific study for the diagnosis of AVN (Glickstein et al. 1998, Harkess 2003, Steinberg 1994).

Acetabular Fracture

- Fractures of the acetabulum that meet criteria for operative intervention are most often best treated acutely with open reduction and internal fixation (Harkess 2003). Only in rare, isolated situations would THA be considered appropriate initial treatment for such fractures. However, despite anatomic reduction of such fractures, patients can often develop post-traumatic arthritis in the hip joint. Additionally, patients who are treated nonoperatively may have residual joint incongruities and possible malunion that will render subsequent THA more technically challenging.
- *Overall, the results of THA after initial acetabular fracture are inferior to those of routine primary THA. The most often reported mode of THA failure after acetabular fracture is aseptic loosening of the acetabular component.* Several reasons are proposed for this association, including diminished acetabular bone quality and blood supply (Jimenez et al. 1997, Mears and Velyvis 2001, Romness and Lewallen 1990). Additionally, the

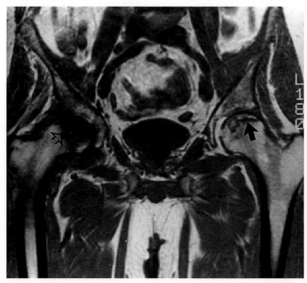 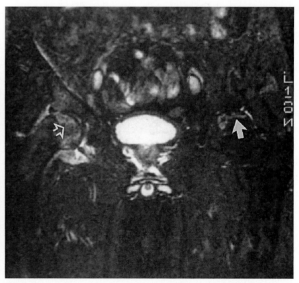

A   B

Figure 8–1: Corticosteroid-induced bilateral avascular necrosis of the femoral head. **A and B,** Coronal T1-weighted and inversion recovery images through both hips reveals a geographic focus of bone marrow replacement in the weight-bearing aspect of the left femoral head that indicates avascular necrosis *(solid arrows).* More advanced disease is seen in the right femoral head with collapse of the articular surface, adjacent marrow edema *(open arrows),* and effusion. (From Canale ST, ed. [2002]. *Campbell's Operative Orthopaedics,* 10th ed. Philadelphia: Mosby.)

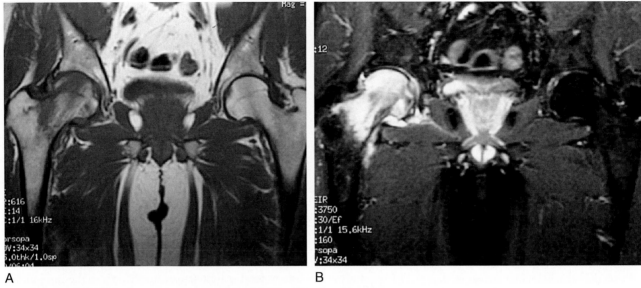

A   B

Figure 8–2: Transient osteoporosis of the hip in a 30-year-old man.
A, Coronal T1-weighted image reveals diminished signal intensity within the right femoral head and neck.
B, Coronal inversion recovery sequence demonstrated hyperintense bone marrow edema in a more diffuse pattern than seen in osteonecrosis. (From Canale ST, ed. [2002]. *Campbell's Operative Orthopaedics*, 10th ed. Philadelphia: Mosby.)

presence of increased scar tissue, possible prior nerve palsy, prior hardware placement, and heterotopic bone can compromise the results of THA following acetabular fracture (Mears and Velyvis 2001).

Developmental Dysplasia of the Hip

- *Patients with DDH also pose treatment challenges.* In general, patients with DDH have acetabular malorientation with bony deficits in the anterolateral aspect of acetabulum.
- A useful radiographic parameter that can be used to determine the degree of acetabular insufficiency is the center edge angle of Wiberg, which is determined on an anteroposterior radiograph of the pelvis (Fig. 8–3). Current published data indicate that for a patient with an angle of 15 degrees or less, a periacetabular osteotomy can be performed. The false profile or faux provil radiograph is also an important component of the preoperative evaluation of a patient with DDH, and it demonstrates sagittal plane acetabular deficits (Ganz et al. 1988, Klaue et al. 1988).

Chronic Hip Dislocation

- THA in the patient with congenital dislocation is technically more difficult than the same procedure in an unaffected individual. The classification systems that are most commonly used include those of Hartofilakidis and associates and the Crowe classification system (Hartofilakidis et al. 1996, Jaroszynski et al. 2001, Numair et al. 1997).
- Hips with low and high dislocations present the surgeon with the most technically demanding problems, particularly

with the issue of limb-length discrepancy. In general, a limb cannot be lengthened more than 4 cm without putting the sciatic nerve at great risk (Jaroszynski et al. 2001). In patients with Crowe type IV hips, which are high dislocated hips that correspond to Hartofilakidis type III hips, the best results have been achieved with femoral shortening osteotomy combined with cementless, modular implants, which provide great flexibility in component size during the reconstruction.

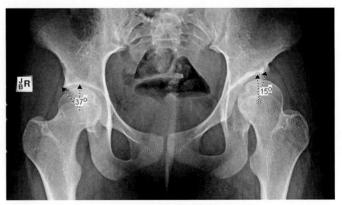

Figure 8–3: Radiograph demonstrating the technique for measuring the center edge angle.
The center edge angle of the right hip is 37 degrees and is within normal limits, whereas that of the left hip is only 15 degrees and therefore could warrant treatment.

- Despite these modifications however, patients with dislocated hips demonstrate a much higher rate of revision surgery than patients with preoperatively unaffected or even subluxated hips. Additionally, the incidence of postoperative nerve injury is increased in dislocated hips because of the femoral lengthening discussed earlier (Schmalzried and Callaghan 1999).

Methods of Treating Hip Disease Other than Arthroplasty

- As discussed earlier, good candidates for THA are those with severely debilitating hip pain that interferes with normal ambulation who also have radiographic evidence of hip joint arthrosis. However, contraindications such as medical illness, young age, and infection may preclude patients from undergoing THA. In such patients, one must consider nonarthroplastic methods of treating hip arthrosis. This section covers such nonarthroplastic treatments, ranging from simple functional and activity modifications to more aggressive surgical treatments.

Conservative Management

- Treatments generally classified as conservative include such modalities as nonsteroidal anti-inflammatory medications, weight loss, activity modification, and the use of an assistive device such as a cane or walker.
- *When patients are using a cane, they should be instructed to place the device in the hand that is contralateral to the affected hip.*
- *In terms of activity modifications, patients should be instructed that if they are required to carry objects in their hands, they can reduce the forces across the diseased hip if they carry such objects using the upper extremity on the same side as their affected hip.* Although this may seem counterintuitive, studies have demonstrated that hip joint forces are smaller when patients carry loads using the upper extremity that is on the same side as the affected hip (Tan et al. 1998).

Osteotomies About the Hip

- Relatively young patients with a history of DDH who have mild to moderate joint arthrosis and severe hip pain can benefit from pelvic osteotomies. *Ideally, pelvic osteotomies are done before the occurrence of severe joint degenerative changes.* The best predictor of success of such procedures is still a simple functional radiograph, such as an abduction hip radiograph or a fluoroscopic study, which demonstrates an improved cartilage space interval with hip abduction maneuvers (Murphy and Deshmukh 2002, Sanchez-Sotelo et al. 2002).
- The most common redirectional osteotomies include the Ganz periacetabular, Salter (single innominate), Sutherland (double innominate), and Steel (triple innominate) (Sanchez-Sotelo et al. 2002).

- Patients with DDH who have a painful but concentric, reduced hip joint are good candidates for a *Ganz osteotomy* (Fig. 8–4). This procedure has several advantages, including the requirement of only one incision and its allowance for large amounts of rotational correction of the acetabulum. The Ganz procedure allows for early patient mobilization because of the limited need for internal fixation. Finally, this procedure maintains the vascular supply of the acetabulum through the inferior gluteal artery (Millis et al. 1996, Sanchez-Sotelo et al. 2002).
  - Potential drawbacks of the Ganz procedure include its technical difficulty and the possibility of anterior displacement of the hip joint, which may ultimately result in limited hip flexion (Hussell 1999, MacDonald et al. 1999, Trousdale et al. 1995).
- Although a *Salter (single innominate) osteotomy* may also be a reasonable option, this procedure offers only a limited amount of correction and lateralizes the hip joint, thereby increasing the joint reactive force (Millis et al. 1996).
- Other osteotomies that may be performed in younger patients include the *Dial (spherical) osteotomy*, which is an intra-articular redirectional osteotomy that does not alter the position of the teardrop (Fig. 8–5).
- The *Chiari osteotomy* is a salvage procedure that does not redirect the acetabulum and does not alter the position of the teardrop (Lack et al. 1991, Ninomiya and Tagawa 1984). It is best utilized in patients with incongruent, subluxated hips (Pellicci et al. 2000, Pemberton 1965, Trousdale and Ganz 1998).

Intertrochanteric Osteotomies in Younger Patients

- Another group of patients who are suboptimal candidates for THA include younger individuals with a history of femoral developmental anomalies such as coxa valga, coxa vara, Perthes disease, or slipped capital femoral epiphysis (Harkess 2003, Pellicci et al. 2000). Patients may also have traumatic proximal femoral deformities such as malunited intertrochanteric fractures or malunited femoral neck fractures with an intact femoral head.
- In such patients, the primary hip joint abnormality occurs in the proximal femur rather than in the acetabulum; therefore, this group of patients can benefit from proximal femoral osteotomies that redirect the femoral head. However, *in such patients, the major abnormality must be present in the proximal femur; if significant acetabular changes are present, then a femoral osteotomy alone is unlikely to address the hip disease fully.* Additionally, similar to pelvic osteotomy, the procedure should be performed before the development of advanced degenerative changes in the hip joint.
- *Varus intertrochanteric osteotomy* can be used in patients with coxa valga; however, patients must have at least 15 degrees

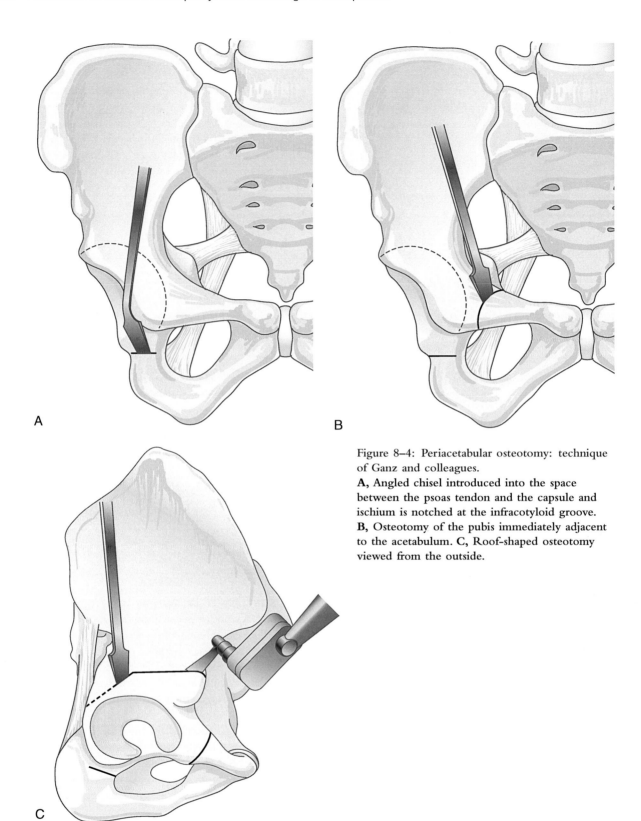

A

B

C

Figure 8–4: Periacetabular osteotomy: technique of Ganz and colleagues.
A, Angled chisel introduced into the space between the psoas tendon and the capsule and ischium is notched at the infracotyloid groove.
B, Osteotomy of the pubis immediately adjacent to the acetabulum. **C,** Roof-shaped osteotomy viewed from the outside.

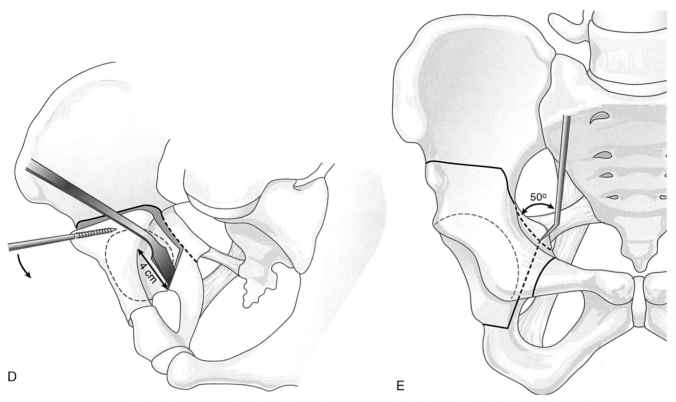

D

E

Figure 8–4, cont'd: **D,** Shanz screw introduced into the supra-acetabular bone, tilting the fragment laterally.
E, Using a distance of 4 cm from the pelvic brim, a 50-degree angle between the blade of the chisel and the
quadrilateral surface results in osteotomy posterior to the acetabulum. (**A,** From Canale ST, ed. [2002].
Campbell's Operative Orthopaedics, 10th ed. Philadelphia: Mosby. B to E, From Ganz R, Klaue K, Vinh TS,
Mast JW [1988]. A new periacetabular osteotomy for the treatment of hip dysplasias: Technique and preliminary
results. *Clin Orthop Relat Res* 232:26.)

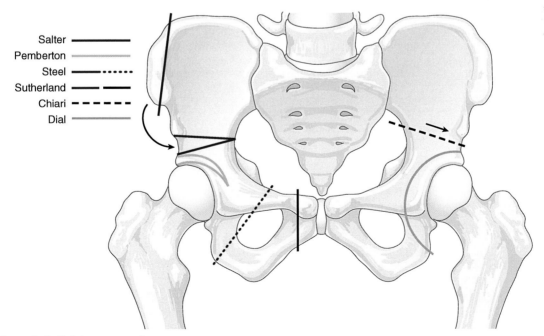

Salter
Pemberton
Steel
Sutherland
Chiari
Dial

Figure 8–5: Pelvic osteotomies.
Common pelvic osteotomies for treatment of developmental dysplasia of the hip. (From Miller MD, ed. [2004].
Review of Orthopaedics, 4th ed. Philadelphia: WB Saunders.)

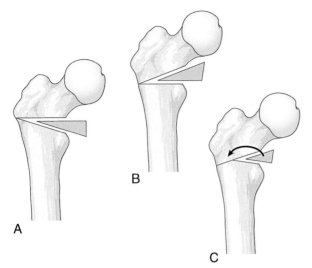

Figure 8–6: Three types of wedges cut for varus osteotomy. **A,** Original technique of Pauwels with a proximal osteotomy made transversely at the distal end of the greater trochanter. This type of osteotomy makes it more difficult to correct rotation and to use a right-angled blade plate. **B,** Original Müller technique of excision of a wide wedge based medially with the distal osteotomy cut transversely across the shaft at just above the level of the lesser trochanter. **C,** Later technique of Müller using a small half-wedge cut medially and transposed laterally.

of passive hip abduction preoperatively to be considered for the procedure (Santore and Kantor 2004) (Fig. 8–6). The procedure is effective because it gives the hip more femoral offset, which increases the tension of the abductor muscles and thereby reduces hip joint reactive forces. This osteotomy does not affect the center edge angle. Complications of the procedure include abductor lag, abductor lurch, and leg-length discrepancy, which results from shortening of the osteotomized extremity (Millis et al. 1996).

- *Valgus intertrochanteric osteotomy* is most commonly performed for nonunion of a Pauwel class II or III femoral neck fracture (Fig. 8–7). It can also be effectively used to treat early-stage osteoarthritis of the hip (Santore and Kantor 2004).
- *Hip arthrodesis:* The most common indications for hip fusion are severe, unilateral hip pain and decreased range of motion in a young patient. Hip arthrodesis is often thought to be a better option than proximal femoral osteotomy in patients who are heavy laborers (Callaghan et al. 1985a).
  - *The optimal position for fusion* is as follows: 30 degrees of flexion, which allows the hip to swing efficiently during gait; 5 degrees of adduction; and 5 degrees of external rotation; this positioning maximizes gait efficiency while allowing the patient to stand appropriately during stance phases of gait (Callaghan et al. 1985a, Koval 2002b). A hip fusion on one side is likely to increase the rate of

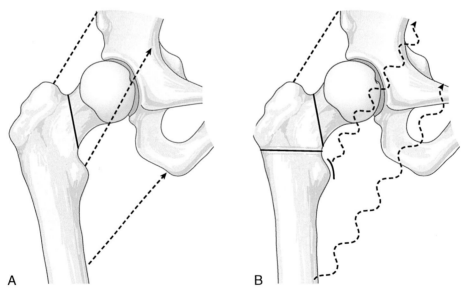

Figure 8–7: Valgus osteotomy.
As demonstrated in this figure, valgus intertrochanteric osteotomy increases the vertical orientation of the femoral neck. Such an osteotomy therefore can convert the vertical orientation (**A**) of a Pauwel II or III femoral neck fracture to an orientation that is more horizontal (**B**). This change in orientation converts shear forces (in vertical orientation) to compressive forces (horizontal orientation). The compressive forces can significantly augment the healing of a femoral neck nonunion.

failure of a contralateral THA by up to 40% (Gore et al. 1975, Romness and Morrey 1992, Waddell 2001). The reason is that the hip fusion requires increased range of motion of the contralateral hip, thus increasing stress and wear.

- *Complications of hip arthrodesis* are many and include lower back pain, lumbar degenerative disease, accelerated degenerative disease of the contralateral hip, and ligamentous laxity with joint degeneration of the ipsilateral knee. Therefore, patients who have lumbar, ipsilateral knee, or contralateral hip degeneration preoperatively are not good candidates for arthrodesis.
- Technical considerations in hip arthrodesis include the fact that the surgeon must avoid damage to the abductor musculature during the procedure; extensive damage to the abductor complex may prohibit the patient from undergoing conversion of the fusion to a THA in the future.
- Sexual function in both sexes and birthing in female patients are not reported to be adversely affected by fusion (Sponseller et al. 1984).
- The most common indication for conversion of a fused hip to THA is debilitating lower back pain. The back pain can often be significantly alleviated through conversion. However, pain and degeneration in the ipsilateral knee or contralateral knee often do not resolve as a result of conversion to THA (Callaghan et al. 1985a, Santore 1995). Overall, the failure rate of fused hips converted to THA is higher than that of primary THA in previously unfused hips.

Preoperative Evaluation

- Preoperative evaluation has several critical components, including a thorough history and physical examination, preoperative radiographs, and medical evaluation; other planning includes templating of the preoperative radiographs and choosing a surgical approach and technique.
- The history and physical examination should help to determine whether the patient's pain is actually emanating from the hip joint, whether the patient's hip pain is sufficiently hampering lifestyle to consider THA, and whether the patient is a good surgical candidate. Patients with hip joint degeneration generally complain of pain anterior and lateral to the hip, with pain in the groin area that can radiate into the anterior thigh. Less commonly, patients also complain of buttock and knee pain.
  - Generally, patients with pain of spinal origin complain of pain in the buttocks and posterior thigh.
  - Two physical examination findings that are indicative of hip disease include Duchenne's sign and a positive Stinchfield test. Duchenne's sign is present when the patient increases the normal lateral displacement of the hip during the stance phase of gait, thus leading to an antalgic gait. Such accentuation of lateral displacement

toward the affected hip reduces the joint reactive force during gait and thereby reduces hip pain.
  - A Stinchfield test is performed by positioning the patient supine, followed by the patient's performing a resisted straight leg raise (Berry 2001). Reproduction of pain in the groin and hip region in this position is indicative of hip joint disease.
- Preoperative radiographs are a critical component of the preoperative workup. Such radiographs can define the extent of joint arthrosis and can also help to identify certain pathologic conditions that warrant special preoperative consideration.
  - Examples of such conditions include rheumatoid arthritis, in which radiographs demonstrate certain distinctive characteristics (Fig. 8–8). These include a more symmetric pattern of medial and lateral joint space destruction, osteopenia, and in late stages, protrusion of the femoral head. In patients with rheumatoid arthritis who have protrusio acetabuli, the center of rotation of the femur is moved to a more medial and posterior position. In these patients, the acetabular component is best placed in an anterior and inferior anatomic position (Crowninshield et al. 1983, Lachiswicz 1997, Ranawat et al. 1980).
  - This finding is in contrast to osteoarthritis, in which images demonstrate more irregular patterns of joint space narrowing.
  - Ankylosing spondylitis also manifests itself in hip radiographs as sacroiliac ankylosis, which is seen on the anteroposterior pelvis view.
  - Standard preoperative radiographs include an anteroposterior view of the pelvis. This radiograph should image as far cephalad as the iliac crest, including the caudal portion of the spine. Additionally, anteroposterior views of the proximal femur are helpful in determining the size of the femoral canal for preoperative implant sizing. Frog-leg lateral views also assist in sizing the proximal femur, whereas true cross-table lateral views are best for viewing the acetabulum. One other special view that is helpful in characterizing dysplastic hips is the false profile view, as discussed earlier. This view demonstrates the extent of anterior coverage of the femoral head in patients with DDH and can be a useful adjunct (Ganz et al. 1988, Klaue et al. 1988).

Special Preoperative Considerations
Specific Disorders

- As discussed earlier, an important component of the preoperative evaluation is to discover certain concurrent medical and musculoskeletal conditions that can adversely affect the outcome of THA. Examples of such conditions include the following:

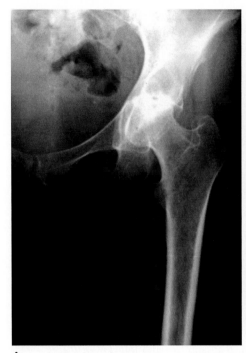
A

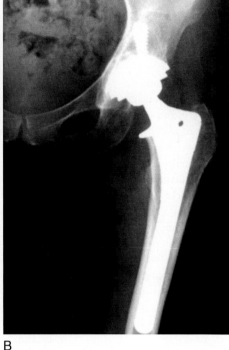
B

Figure 8–8: Total hip arthroplasty for rheumatoid arthritis. **A,** Advanced disease with articular cartilage destruction. **B,** After total hip arthroplasty. (From Canale ST, ed. [2002]. *Campbell's Operative Orthopaedics*, 10th ed. Philadelphia: Mosby.)

- *Ankylosing spondylitis:* Although patients with ankylosing spondylitis can be expected to have a greater than 95% rate of pain relief, studies show that just 65% of patients have good or excellent results. These diminished functional scores are usually the consequence of concurrent medical illnesses or preexistent spinal abnormality. Additionally, patients with ankylosing spondylitis demonstrate a higher rate of postoperative infection and heterotopic ossification (HO) (Joshi et al. 2002).
- *Hypertrophic arthritis:* Patients with hypertrophic arthritis deserve special preoperative management because they are at increased risk for HO; therefore, they should be given perioperative prophylaxis for the development of postoperative ossification (Goel and Sharp 1991, Nollen and van Douveren 1993).
- *DDH:* Patients with DDH also require special preoperative consideration in that they may require smaller acetabular components with smaller femoral head implants. Such smaller implants will allow for improved coverage of the acetabular component, whereas the small femoral head implants will allow for polyethylene of sufficient thickness.
  - Currently, the best positioning of cementless acetabular components in such patients is considered to be anatomic, with supplementary medialization of the component to improve coverage. The femoral component can be implanted with or without cement, based on the clinical situation. Overall, cemented THAs in patients with DDH have demonstrated reduced survivorship in comparison with the general population (Dorr et al. 1999, Jasty et al. 1991, Sanchez-Sotelo et al. 2002).
- *Immunosuppression:* One final group of patients requiring special preoperative planning comprises those who have undergone organ transplantation and who are receiving immunosuppressive medications. Studies demonstrate that such patients have a higher risk of postoperative infection than unaffected patients. This increased infection rate may imply that organ transplant recipients should undergo special perioperative treatments with broad-spectrum antibiotics and possibly antibiotic-impregnated bone cement in the cases of cemented THA (Tannenbaum and Matthews 1997).

Preoperative Planning

- Other important aspects of preoperative planning include the operative approach, patient positioning, cemented versus noncemented technique, use of femoral offset, and avoidance of limb-length discrepancy.
- The most commonly used surgical approaches for THA are the *posterior approach and the anterolateral approaches*. Each approach has advantages and disadvantages.
  - The posterior approach does not involve a true internervous plane; rather, it involves the splitting of the

muscle fibers of the gluteus maximus to gain deeper exposure (Fig. 8–9). The patient is positioned in the lateral decubitus position. This approach has the advantage of providing good access to the femur, and it also does not require violation of the abductor musculature, thus minimizing the incidence of postoperative limp. It also demonstrates a lower HO rate than the direct lateral approach (Pellicci et al. 2000).

- The main disadvantage of the posterior approach is a higher dislocation rate (Masonis and Bourne 2002, Woo and Morrey 1982). For these reasons, many surgeons increase the anteversion of the acetabular component when posterior approaches are used, to decrease the incidence of posterior dislocation.
- The anterolaterally directed techniques generally allow for patient positioning in the supine or lateral decubitus position.
- The *Smith-Petersen approach utilizes the internervous plane between the sartorius/rectus femoris muscles (femoral nerve)*

and tensor fasciae latae/gluteus medius-minimus muscles (superior gluteal nerve) (Fig. 8–10).

- The *Watson-Jones approach uses the plane between the tensor fasciae latae and the gluteus medius muscles* (Fig. 8–11).
- Both these approaches have the advantages of decreased dislocation rate and excellent acetabular exposure.
- The main disadvantage is the incidence of postoperative limp and abductor dysfunction. In such approaches, less anteversion of acetabular components may be used because there is less risk of posterior dislocation. The *Hardinge approach requires the patient to be in the lateral position* and also involves violation of the hip abductors complex.
- The advantages of these approaches include a lower rate of sciatic nerve palsy and postoperative dislocation (Mulliken et al. 1998). Disadvantages of this approach also include postoperative limp and increased risk of HO.

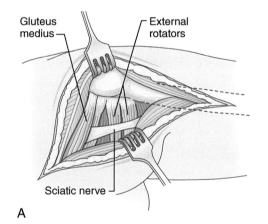

A

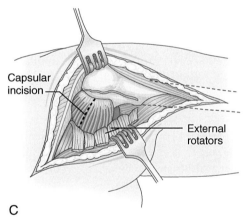

C

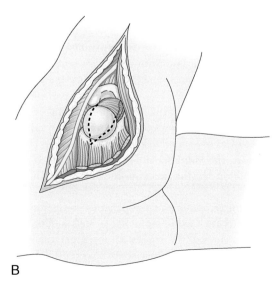

B

Figure 8–9: The Moore approach to hip arthroplasty.
A, The iliotibial band is split proximally and posteriorly. The gluteus maximus is split bluntly in line with its fibers. The sciatic nerve is identified and protected. The short external rotators are identified and transected at their insertion. **B,** The external rotators are retracted posteriorly and provide additional protection for the sciatic nerve. The capsular incision runs obliquely from the acetabular rim to the level of the lesser trochanter. **C,** The hip is dislocated posteriorly by adduction and internal rotation. (From Morrey BF, ed. *Joint Replacement Arthroplasty,* 3rd ed. New York: Churchill Livingstone.)

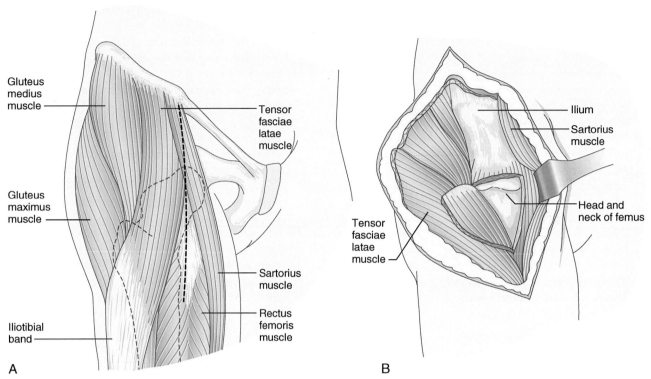

Figure 8–10: The Smith–Petersen anterior iliofemoral approach to the hip.
A, Line of skin incision. **B,** Exposure of the joint after reflection of the tensor fasciae latae and gluteal muscles from the lateral surface of the ilium and the division of the capsule. (From Canale ST, ed. [2002]. *Campbell's Operative Orthopaedics,* 10th ed. Philadelphia: Mosby.)

- One issue that should not go unconsidered preoperatively is that of patient positioning during surgery. For the surgical approaches described earlier, patients are usually positioned supine or laterally. Each of these positions has merit.
  - When the patient is positioned laterally, care must be taken to ensure that the pelvis is maintained in a true lateral position because any rotation of the pelvis intraoperatively makes appropriate version of the acetabular component more difficult.
  - Additionally, with the lateral position, comparison of leg lengths is more difficult than it is with supine positioning. One major advantage of lateral positioning is that it allows for either anterior or posterior approaches to be performed, whereas supine positioning accommodates only anterior approaches.

How to Avoid Limb-Length Discrepancy

- Another important preoperative issue to consider is the avoidance of postoperative limb-length discrepancy. Certain preoperative preventative measures can be used to reduce the chances of postoperative leg-length discrepancy.

- First and foremost, the components must be positioned to confer maximum stability. Such positioning obviates the need to lengthen the leg to achieve acceptable stability. Although increasing neck length may confer stability to the prosthesis, excessive use of neck length can result in a clinically perceivable limb-length discrepancy by the patient.
- In this situation, the concept of femoral offset is important. Technically defined, *femoral offset* is the distance measured by a horizontal line that is perpendicular to two lines, namely, the vertical line through the center of the femoral head and the vertical line through the center of the femoral shaft (Fig. 8–12). Hip prosthesis systems offer offset options of varying lengths. Increasing femoral offset allows reestablishment of appropriate abductor tension, and thereby confers hip stability without increases in leg length. Therefore, the judicious use of femoral offset is an important adjunct in the prevention of limb-length discrepancy.
- Finally, careful measurements of the patient's preoperative limb-length discrepancy radiographically as well as clinically give the surgeon clues to the leg length intraoperatively. Overall, patients with preoperative limb-length discrepancy are at increased risk for postoperative limb-length discrepancy (Ranawat and Rodriguez 1997).

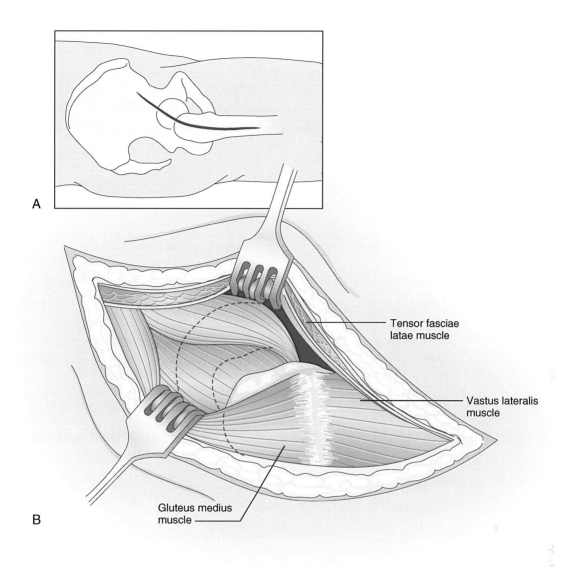

Figure 8–11: The Watson-Jones lateral approach to the hip joint.
A, Skin incision. **B,** Approach has been completed except for incision of the joint capsule. (From Canale ST, ed. [2002]. *Campbell's Operative Orthopaedics*, 10th ed. Philadelphia: Mosby.)

Fixation Methods for Primary Total Hip Arthroplasty

- Each method of THA fixation has advantages and disadvantages, and certain methods are more appropriate in particular patients.

Cement Fixation

- Cement fixation of femoral and acetabular implants is based not on the concept that the cement functions as an adhesive, but rather on the principle that the cement interdigitates within the bone. The cement itself is composed of polymethylmethacrylate (PMMA), which is stronger in compression than in tension (Maloney 1998).

- One conceptual disadvantage of cement is that its use creates two separate interfaces that may fail, namely, the cement–host bone interface and the cement-implant interface. The cement-implant and cement-bone interfaces are static, with no remodeling potential; thus, any areas of failure of the cement mantle do not have the ability to remodel. Nonetheless, numerous studies have shown that cement can provide stable, long-term fixation (Berry 2001).

- However, to be successful over the long term, the cement must be prepared and implanted carefully at the time of surgery. The size of the cement mantle of the femoral component is thought to be best maintained at 2 mm or greater, particularly in the proximal medial aspect of the femur. Studies have shown that a mantle smaller than 2 mm

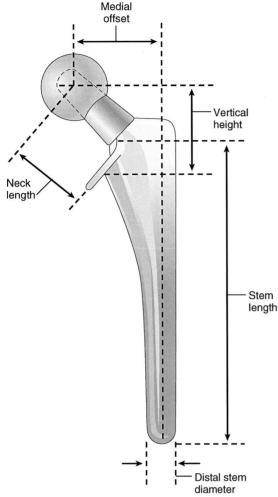

Figure 8–12: Features of the femoral component. Neck length is measured from the center of the head to the base of the collar; head-stem offset, from the center of the head to a line through the axis of the distal part of the stem; stem length, from the medial base of the collar to the tip of the stem; and angle of neck, by the intersection of a line through the center of the head and neck with another along the lateral border of the distal half of the stem. The platform is the medial extension of the collar. (From Canale ST, ed. [2002]. *Campbell's Operative Orthopaedics*, 10th ed. Philadelphia: Mosby.)

demonstrates increased cracking and breakdown (Ebramzadeh et al. 1994, Jasty et al. 1991, Maloney 1995).

- Other technical nuances that increase the success of cemented THA include avoidance of varus stem positioning of the femoral stem and avoidance of gaps in the cement mantle. Varus positioning of cemented femoral stems is detrimental because it results in a thin cement mantle in the proximal medial and distal lateral femur (Callaghan et al. 1998, Maloney 1995). These are two of the areas where the cement mantle experiences the highest stress levels. Thus, varus positioning can contribute to early cracking

and failure of the cement mantle in these areas (Crowninshield et al. 1980, Noble et al. 1998).
  - Gaps in the cement mantle result in areas of prosthesis-bone direct contact, stress concentration, and early failure (Crowninshield et al. 1980, Noble et al. 1998).

Generations of Cement Technique and Characteristics

- Cementing technique has undergone continuous evolution that has been consolidated in the literature into three "generations" of cement technique (Table 8–1). Each "generation" is characterized by certain key technical practices.
  - First-generation technique involved very elementary methods of cement preparation including manual finger packing of cement into the femoral canal without the use of cement gun, cement plug, or cement pressurization, absence of formal femoral canal preparation, and cast metal stems with sharp borders and thin medial borders.
  - Second-generation technique introduced some major improvements, including femoral canal preparation with pulsatile washing and brushing, use of a cement gun with cement restrictors, and alloy femoral components with rounded, broad medial edges and collars. Femoral canal preparation is important because it greatly improves the initial quality of the cement bone interdigitation. Use of femoral stems with rounded medial borders is also a significant improvement because it reduces stress concentration at the medial cement mantle, where failure can occur (Mulray and Harris 1990).
  - Third-generation technique, which best represents present-day practices, includes such advances as vacuum preparation of cement to reduce porosity, pressurization of cement, and use of stem centralizers. Porosity reduction and vacuum preparation of cement are important

Table 8–1	Characteristics of Generations of Cement Technique
GENERATION	**KEY CHARACTERISTICS**
First generation	Finger packing
	Unplugged femoral canal
	Femoral components: sharp corners, narrow medial borders, stainless steel
Second generation	Plugging of medullary canal
	Pulse lavage cleaning of canal
	Cement gun
	"Superalloy" components
	Removal of sharp corners
	Broad medial border
Third generation	Vacuum preparation of cement (porosity reduction)
	Surface modifications of implants
	Polymethylmethacrylate application
	Stem centralization proximally and distally

because these practices increase the ultimate strength of the cement.

Cemented Femoral Components

- Overall, cemented femoral components have demonstrated excellent long-term survivorship and several series have shown revision rates of 0% to 5% at 10-year follow-up (Barrack et al. 1992, Smith et al. 1998).
- The *Dorr classification* of the femur can be helpful in determining which technique of femoral fixation to use. This system radiographically characterizes the morphology of the proximal femur based on the size and shape of the femoral canal and the thickness of the cortices.
  - *Dorr Type A femora*, which have small medullary canals, may be better suited for uncemented implants because of the difficulty in establishing a sufficient cement mantle.
  - *Dorr Type B femora* are equally treated with cemented or uncemented components.
  - Alternatively, *Dorr C femora* may be better suited for cemented femoral components. Additionally, patients with poor bone quality that will not support uncemented implants may be better treated with cemented femoral components.
- Factors associated with early failure of cemented femoral components include varus stem positioning, obesity, and cement mantle defects (Callaghan et al. 1985b, Robinson et al. 1989).
- With regard to precoating of femoral stems, studies do demonstrate that implants precoated with PMMA improve the interface between the stem and the cement mantle. However, this mechanical improvement has not resulted clinically in lower rates of loosening, infection, or wear in such precoated stems compared with stems that are not precoated (Schulte et al. 1993, Sporer et al. 1999).

Cemented Acetabular Components

- On the acetabular side, cemented components have become less popular than cementless components. Studies have shown higher rates of loosening for cemented components in younger patients and in patients with rheumatoid arthritis, acetabular protrusio, hip dysplasia, and bleeding diatheses (Ranawat and Peters 1997).
- However, in patients without such comorbidities, several series demonstrated failure rates of such components at 17 to 20 years of 10% to 23% (Callaghan et al. 1998, Schulte et al. 1993, Smith et al. 1998). Overall, cemented acetabula perform better in older, lower-demand patients. However, regardless of patient age or comorbidity, loosening depends on the quality of the bone-cement interface achieved intraoperatively.

Uncemented Components: General Principles

- Uncemented implants can have either a porous-coated or a grit-blasted surface. Uncemented fixation, unlike

cemented fixation, is a truly biologic method of implantation in that the coated surface of the metal implant is conducive to ingrowth or ongrowth of bone. The cortical bone actually grows into the porous channels within the metal implant to create a rigid interface. Of course, this implies that for uncemented technique to be successful, the implants must be seated against cortical bone and not against cancellous bone (Mont and Hungerford 1997).
- Unlike the cement-bone interface, the metal-bone interface has remodeling potential; if there is disruption of the bony intercalation into the implant, the bone can remodel and reestablish the rigid interface. Therefore, it is theoretically conceivable that uncemented implants may maintain rigid fixation longer than is possible with cemented implants.
- In recent years, as more THAs have been performed in younger patients who place higher demands on their prostheses, there has been an increase in the use of noncemented hips because of the potential lifelong bond between the implant and the host bone. Many studies have demonstrated that cemented components have increased failure rates in younger patients, whereas other complementary studies have shown in the short to medium term that uncemented components demonstrate improved performance and decreased loosening in young patients (Berger et al. 1997). Additionally, cementless implants may be ideal when patients have thick cortices, narrow femoral canals, and good bone quality.
- Uncemented implants can have a surface that is porous coated or grit blasted. The term *porous coated* describes a metallic surface that has been treated to have many microscopic pores of varying depths into which bone may grow. The term *grit blasted* describes a slightly different uncemented metal surface; these implants have been bombarded with microscopic particles that create innumerable indentations on the metal surface onto which bone can grow. These indentations are analogous to jagged peaks and valleys on the metal surface. Technically speaking, porous-coated implants allow for bony ingrowth into the pores, whereas grit-blasted implants allow for bony ongrowth on the peaks and valleys.
- With porous-coated implants, particular size distributions of the pores optimize bony ingrowth (Table 8–2). Studies have demonstrated that the optimum pore size is from 100 to 400 μm (Berry et al. 1995, Cook et al. 1988, Spector 1987). The optimum porosity or pore density on the metal surface is on the order of 40% to 50% (Berry 2001).

Table 8–2	Optimal Characteristics of Cementless Implants
Optimum pore size	100–400 μm
Optimum porosity	40%–50%
Limits of micromotion	150 μm
Bone-implant distance	50 μm

When the surface porosity exceeds 50%, the porous coating can actually be sheared off the metal surface of the implant.

- Other conditions that are required for optimal porous ingrowth include a rigid, motion-free interface between the implant and the host bone. Micromotion between the implant and bone should be reduced to a maximum of 150 μm. If motion between the bone and implant exceeds this value, weak fibrous tissue will grow into the pores. If micromotion is maintained at less than this amount, a rigid bony interface will develop (Callaghan 1993).

- Another equally important parameter is the actual physical distance between the metal surface and the cortical bone. This distance should be kept at a maximum of 50 μm because osteogenic cells and factors are unable to bridge a distance greater than this to create a rigid bony interface.

- With cementless implants, there are two techniques of achieving rigid fixation, namely, line-to-line and press-fit techniques.
  - *Line-to-line technique* is performed by reaming the acetabulum or femur to the same size as the component that is to be placed. With line-to-line acetabular technique, the use of supplemental fixation such as bone screws may be required to maintain a rigid, motionless interface between the host cortical bone and the component.
    - The literature demonstrates disadvantages to the use of acetabular screws. Studies have shown up to 99.1% 12-year survivorship of acetabular shells without screw fixation. Additionally, data show that the bone tracts created for the screws result in decreased acetabular surface area for bony ingrowth; these tracts also provide a conduit for wear debris that can increase the extent of osteolysis. Finally, the screws are subject to backing out, which places them in direct contact with the nonarticular surface of the polyethylene and can contribute to abrasive backside wear (Udomkiat and Dorr 2002).
    - With *press-fit technique*, the femur or acetabulum is reamed to a size that is 1 to 2 mm smaller than the component to be implanted. Press-fit technique does not often require supplemental fixation and relies on hoop stresses to maintain rigid fixation.
  - *Grit-blasted implants* also have certain physical characteristics that increase the rigidity of the bone-implant interface. The key characteristic of grit-blasted implants is the surface roughness; the roughness describes the average of the distance between all the peaks and valleys on the metal implant surface. Bone grows onto the peaks and valleys. Implants with a higher surface roughness concurrently exhibit a more rigid bone-metal interface.
    - One theoretical disadvantage of grit-blasted components is that they require a larger proportion of their surface

to be covered with a blasted surface; additionally, such components with large surface roughness values could abrade the cortical bone surface and produce metal debris (Harkess 2003).

- The manner by which uncemented components have most frequently malfunctioned is through polyethylene failure and osteolysis (Berry et al. 1994).
  - The mechanisms by which the polyethylene fails have included cracking or breaking of the polyethylene, excessive wear, and disengagement of the polyethylene from the metal shell as a result of inadequate locking mechanisms.
  - However, many recent technologic advances in implant design have largely curtailed the occurrence of such failures. Improvements in shell-liner engagement mechanisms have reduced the occurrence of dissociation between these two components. However, osteolysis continues to be one of the more elusive problems in joint replacement surgery; this topic is covered in a subsequent section.

Uncemented Acetabular Components

- Uncemented acetabular components have an excellent track record. As mentioned earlier, medium-term data demonstrate that cementless acetabular components perform as well or even better than cemented components, particularly in patients who place high mechanical demands on their prostheses. Survival rates as high as 98.8% at 10-year follow-up have been reported (Berger et al. 1997).
- Overall, among uncemented acetabular metal shells, the best-performing designs have been of the porous-coated variety. Shells with smooth metal backs have not performed as well (Smith and Harris 1997).

Uncemented Femoral Components

- Despite initial difficulties with thigh pain and loosening, cementless femoral implants now enjoy a success rate very similar to that of the best cemented implants. Annual loosening rates of less than 0.5% have been demonstrated repeatedly in the literature (Pellicci et al. 2000).
- As discussed earlier, with cementless femoral implants, the surgeon must achieve rigid, motionless fixation between the host bone and the implant. The micromotion between the bone and implant should be maintained at a maximum of 150 μm to reduce the probability of fibrous ingrowth into the porous-coated femoral component.
- Various types of surface coating materials have been used on porous-coated femoral components with the goal of improving the quality of the bony ingrowth interface. Among these various coating materials, hydroxyapatite may have a theoretical advantage in achieving bony ingrowth because it is an osteoconductive substance.

Extent of Porous Coating and Stress Shielding

- Another design characteristic that has been heavily analyzed in recent years is the effect of the longitudinal extent of porous coating of the femoral implant on the femoral bone stock.
- Femoral implants can have a porous coating that covers only the proximal portion or the entire length of the prosthesis. The critical conceptual issues that relates to fully versus partially coated implants are *stress shielding and osteolysis.*
- *Fully coated implants generally achieve rigid fixation throughout the length of the implant*, with a large component of the fixation occurring in the more distal aspects of the femur. This distal fixation is evidenced radiographically as spot welds in the femoral diaphysis. *Spot welds* are areas of dense bony ingrowth between the cortex and femur seen on plain radiographs that indicate distal fixation. When such distal fixation occurs, the force loads are transmitted to the more distal aspects of the femur. This results in stress shielding in the proximal aspect of the femur, which leads to bone loss and osteopenia in this area (Fig. 8–13).
- However, fully coated stems do have the advantage of providing a very large surface area for rigid fixation to occur. *Femoral stems that are porous coated only proximally achieve rigid fixation only in these proximal regions of the femur.* Therefore, force loads are transmitted in a more physiologic fashion, through the proximal femur, resulting in less stress shielding and proximal bone loss.

- The circumferential extent of porous coating around the implant is also important in the clinical outcome of cementless femoral implants. Various designs of cementless femoral implants have utilized partial versus full proximal circumferential coating of the stem. These two design principles are important as they relate to the effective joint space and osteolysis.
  - Implants that have only partially circumferentially coated designs have demonstrated failure to establish bony ingrowth around the entire perimeter of the proximal femur. Thus, such designs have left a conduit in the proximal femur where polyethylene wear debris can access the femoral diaphysis, thereby increasing the effective joint space. This wear debris has clinically resulted in greater osteolysis in the femoral diaphysis when such noncircumferentially coated designs have been used (Emerson et al. 1999, Urban et al. 1996).
  - This is in contrast to femoral stems that are fully coated proximally. Such stems allow for full bony ingrowth around the entire perimeter of the proximal femur, thus effectively sealing off the femoral diaphyseal cavity from the effective joint space. Such circumferentially proximally porous-coated stems have performed better than noncircumferentially coated stems with regard to loosening, thigh pain, and osteolysis (Emerson et al. 1999, Urban et al. 1996).
- Stress shielding is also highly influenced by the stiffness of the femoral stem. Generally, stems that have increased mechanical stiffness are able to absorb more of the loads transmitted during weight bearing.

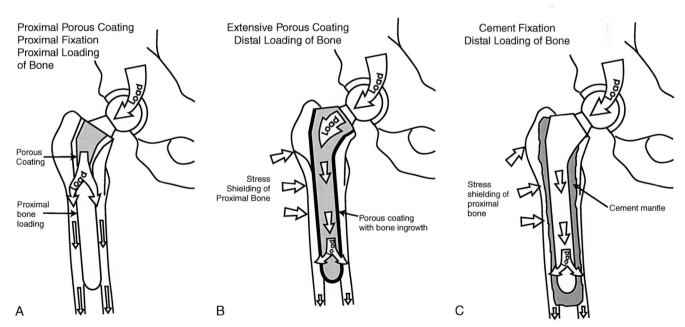

Figure 8–13: Diagram of bone loading in relation to femoral stem fixation.
A, Proximal porous coating, no cement. **B**, Extensive porous coating, no cement. **C**, Cement fixation.
(From Miller MD, ed. [2004]. *Review of Orthopaedics*, 4th ed. Philadelphia: WB Saunders.)

- Therefore, *stiffer stems result in more stress shielding.* Factors that influence the stiffness of stems include the radius of the stem, the geometry of the stem, and the intrinsic stiffness of the metal used for the stem.
- The radius of the stem is of critical importance because the stiffness is proportional to the fourth power of the radius. Therefore, small increases in stem radius lead to large increases in stiffness. The geometry of the stem also determines stiffness because stems that have flutes or that have been hollowed out have decreased stiffness.
- Finally, certain metals are intrinsically stiffer than others; concurrently, stems fashioned from cobalt chrome are stiffer than those fashioned from titanium because cobalt chrome itself is stiffer than titanium.

Complications

- Although THA has been an extremely successful procedure, it is not without complications.
- Complications of THA can be divided into several categories based on the timing of their occurrence.

Perioperative Complications

- The first group of complications occurs perioperatively.
- The major intraoperative complications include fracture of the femur or acetabulum, nerve injury, and vascular injury.

Fractures

- *Intraoperative fractures are more common in the femur than in the acetabulum, and they are more common during the implantation of uncemented components* (Berry 1999a). The insertion of such components requires large amounts of force with the use of impacting devices to achieve the initial rigid fixation required for bony ingrowth.
- In the *acetabulum,* fractures occur when there is a large difference between the size of the last reamer used and the actual implant that is impacted. Fortunately, most intraoperative acetabular fractures involve only partial cortical disruption of the posterior wall, and therefore they can be treated conservatively. Studies have suggested that the intraoperative detection of such a fracture is a good indication for the use of acetabular screws (Sharkey et al. 1999). The combination of the metal acetabular shell with the screw fixation actually allows the shell to function as an internal fixation device for the acetabular fracture. More extensive acetabular fractures may require formal open reduction and internal fixation with plating.
- *On the femoral side, intraoperative fractures occur during broaching and implantation of the final component.* As with the acetabulum, femur fractures happen when inappropriately large broaches and or final implants are impacted with great force.

- Additionally, fractures may also occur in patients who have exceptionally poor bone quality or who have irregularly shaped metaphyseal and diaphyseal regions of the femur.
- Preoperative templating of femoral components with careful attention to the morphology of the femur can prevent intraoperative femoral fracture. The literature suggests that fractures of the metaphyseal region of the femur occur when proximally porous-coated implants are used, whereas fully porous-coated implants are more often associated with diaphyseal fractures (Beals and Tower 1996, Schwartz et al. 1989).
- Most intraoperative femur fractures are partial cortical disruptions that can be treated with cerclage wiring. More extensive fractures that are full cortical disruptions with distal propagation may require the use of longer stem femoral implants with supplemental cerclage wiring.

Nerve Injury

- Another observed intraoperative complication is *nerve injury.* Perioperative nerve injury can be caused by compression, traction, or ischemia (Lewallen 1997) (Box 8–1).
- Nerve injury can be caused by *errant retractor placement or by excessively forceful retraction* for prolonged periods of time.
- Nerve injury can also be observed in the postoperative period when a large hematoma forms and compresses an adjacent peripheral nerve. In this situation, in which hematoma compression is thought to be the cause of the injury, surgical exploration and hematoma evacuation are indicated.
- Nerve injury has been observed and documented in the literature in the sciatic, femoral, obturator, superior gluteal, and lateral femoral cutaneous nerves (Lewallen 1997). *The most commonly observed injury is to the peroneal branch of the sciatic nerve followed by the femoral nerve.*
- The obturator nerve can be injured during cemented THAs when cement escapes the confines of the pelvis. The lateral femoral cutaneous nerve can be injured secondary to positioning or pressure from pelvic positioners.
- The patients who are most vulnerable to intraoperative nerve injury are women, patients with DDH, patients of small stature, patients with lumbar disk disease, patients with peripheral neuropathy, and patients who are having

Box 8–1	Risk Factors for Intraoperative Nerve Injury

1. Female sex
2. Developmental dysplasia of the hip
3. Small stature
4. Associated lumbar disease
5. Peripheral neuropathy
6. Leg lengthening during total hip arthroplasty

significant amounts of leg lengthening performed at the time of THA. In general, neurapraxia associated with leg lengthening can be avoided if a nerve is not stretched by more than 6% of its preoperative length. Studies have also shown that lengthening of greater than 4 cm is associated with much greater risk of postoperative neurapraxia (Edwards et al. 1987, Johanson et al. 1983, Lewallen 1997, Schmalzried et al. 1997, Solheim and Hagen 1980).

Vascular Injury

- Vascular injury, although rare, also represents an observed and reported intraoperative complication of THA.
- The most commonly damaged structures are the *common femoral artery and the external iliac artery* (Shoenfeld et al. 1990). Injury can be caused by careless placement of sharp retractors, by direct insult to a vascular structure with a knife or electrocautery, and by careless placement of acetabular screws that perforate a pelvic vessel.
- Errant placement of acetabular screws can be avoided by the surgeon's recognition of the *acetabular quadrant system* (Wasielewski and Cooperstein 1990). This system divides the acetabulum into four equal quadrants: the anterior inferior and superior quadrants and the posterior superior and inferior quadrants (Fig. 8–14). The compartments are delineated by two lines, the first of which starts at the anterior superior iliac spine and bisects the acetabulum and the second of which is perpendicular to the first and also bisects the acetabulum. The safest area for screw placement is the posterior superior compartment, followed by the posterior inferior quadrant. The anterior inferior and anterior superior quadrants are both generally unsafe for screw placement (Keating et al. 1990).

Early Postoperative Complications

- The second category of THA complications can be considered as those that occur in the early postoperative period.
- Such complications include infection, thromboembolic disease, and dislocation. The topics of infection and thromboembolic disease are covered here, but the subject of dislocation, because of its complexity, is covered in its own subsequent section.
- Although it is quite uncommon, infection after THA represents a potentially devastating complication that can necessitate numerous repeat surgical procedures and long-term antibiotic treatments. The literature is clear that the most important factor for the prevention of infection is the administration of antibiotics approximately 1 hour before the surgical incision is made (Espehaug et al. 1997).
  - Other perioperative measures that have been shown to reduce infection include laminar flow operating rooms and full-body operative suits (Garvin and Hanssen 1993).

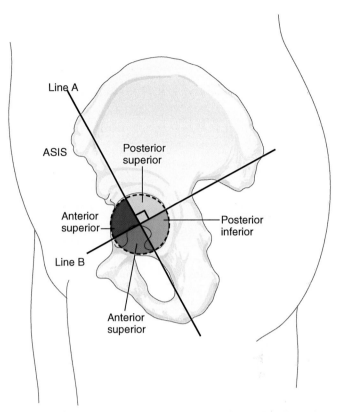

Figure 8–14: Acetabular quadrant system of Wasielewski and colleagues.
Acetabular quadrant system described by Wasielewski et al. for determining safe screw placement (see text). Quadrants are formed by the intersections of lines *A* and *B*. Line *A* extends from the anterior superior iliac spine *(ASIS)* through the center of the acetabulum to the posterior aspect of the fovea, dividing the acetabulum in half. Line *B* is drawn perpendicular to line *A* at the midpoint of the acetabulum, dividing it into quadrants: anterosuperior, anteroinferior, posterosuperior, and posteroinferior. (Redrawn from Wasielewski RC, et al. [1990]. Acetabular anatomy and the transacetabular fixation of screws in total hip arthroplasty. *J Bone Joint Surg Am* 72:501.

- Patients who have hip pain in the first 3 months after surgery with no radiographic evidence of dislocation or periprosthetic fracture must be evaluated for infection. For such patients, aspiration of the hip joint is the most specific and sensitive method by which to diagnose such early infection (Drancourt et al. 1993, Duncan and Beauchamp 1993, Oyen et al. 1990). Other useful tests for the diagnosis of infection include C-reactive protein and erythrocyte sedimentation rate. The sensitivity of these tests has been reported from 61% to 96%, whereas their specificity has ranged between 85% and 100%.
- Studies such as technetium-99m bone scans are not helpful in the early postoperative stages for diagnosis of infection because such studies universally show increased uptake in the setting of recent THA.

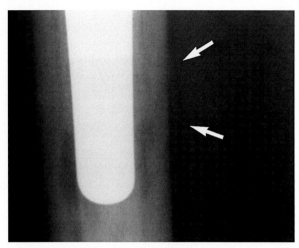

Figure 8–15: Periosteal new bone.
Periosteal new bone in infection 18 months after surgery in a 74-year-old woman with persistent pain. Note the focal osteolysis at the tip of the stem and faint periosteal elevation *(arrows)*. *Staphylococcus aureus* was isolated from hip aspirate. (From Canale ST, ed. [2002]. *Campbell's Operative Orthopaedics*, 10th ed. Philadelphia: Mosby.)

- Additionally, patients with infected THA may not demonstrate systemic symptoms such as fever and chills, and they do not often have an elevated white blood cell count.
- Plain radiographs of recent THAs that demonstrate periosteal reaction are suggestive of infection (Simon 1994) (Fig. 8–15).
- *Overall, the expeditious diagnosis of infection in recent THA may be critical because it may allow for early aggressive surgical irrigation and débridement with avoidance of removal of the components.*
- Another issue related to early postoperative infection is that of antibiotic prophylaxis for surgical procedures that may result in the temporary seeding of the blood with bacteria. Such procedures include dental, urologic, and gastrointestinal procedures. *Current American Academy of Orthopaedic Surgeons guidelines recommend antibiotic prophylaxis for 2 years following THA for such transient bacteremia-inducing procedures.* Oral amoxicillin, at a dose of 2 g, is the most commonly recommended agent for penicillin-tolerant patients; alternatively recommended agents include cephalexin, clindamycin, and ciprofloxacin. Patients with special immunodeficiencies usually are advised to employ lifetime antibiotic prophylaxis for dental, urologic, and gastrointestinal procedures after THA.
- Thromboembolic disease includes the occurrence of such complications as intraoperative and perioperative fat or bone marrow emboli and postoperative deep venous thrombosis (DVT) that can result in pulmonary embolus.

- *Thromboembolic disease is the most common complication following THA; however, most of these occurrences are of subclinical significance and do not adversely affect the outcome.*
- It is currently thought that most thromboembolic phenomena originate during the actual surgical procedures, particularly during reaming and broaching of the femoral canal, insertion of the femoral stem, and relocation of the dislocated hip (Pitto et al. 2002, Sharrock et al. 1995). During insertion of femoral components, studies demonstrate that thrombogenic factors such as tissue thromboplastin are extruded into the femoral veins. Increased intramedullary pressure during insertion of the femoral component has been demonstrated to be a critical event in the deposition of fat, bone marrow, and other thrombotic factors into the circulation (Breed 1974, Kallos et al. 1974, Pitto et al. 2002).
- The occurrence of intraoperative thrombotic events is much more common with cemented femoral implants than with uncemented implants (Pitto et al. 2002). The twisting of the femoral vessels that occurs during dislocation and relocation of the hip causes temporary venous stasis with subsequent release of thrombogenic substances into the circulation (Binns and Pho 1990, Sharrock et al. 1995).

Late Complications

- The final category of complications following THA includes those that occur in a delayed fashion, usually more than 3 months after performance of the procedure.
- Delayed or chronic infections can occur many months or years after THA and are included in this category; periprosthetic fractures and HO are also seen many months after the index procedure.

Delayed or Chronic Infections

- Late infection after THA can occur at any point, several months or years after the primary THA, and therefore this complication can be considered both an early and a late complication.
- The main difference between early and late infection is that early postoperative infection is more often the result of direct inoculation of the operative site during the primary THA, whereas late infection usually occurs through hematogenous seeding of the prosthetic joint. The infection originates at a distant body site and is hematogenously spread to the prosthetic joint.
- Late infections can be characterized as late acute or late chronic infections. Late acute infections are those that are discovered within approximately 3 weeks of the origination of infection in the prosthetic joint. Such infections can usually be treated with aggressive irrigation and débridement of the prosthesis with component retention and extended intravenous antibiotic treatment.
- Late chronic infections are those that have been present for more than 4 weeks.

- On the microscopic level, chronic infections are differentiated from acute infections by the presence of *biofilm*, which is a biologic polysaccharide deposited by infecting bacteria onto the prosthetic implants. The formation of such a layer necessitates the removal of all the components because irrigation and débridement of such chronic infections will not likely eradicate the bacteria.
- As with early postoperative infections, the diagnostic tests that are most helpful include hip aspiration, C-reactive protein, and erythrocyte sedimentation rate.
- The one disadvantage of hip aspiration is the false-positive rate of 15%, but in combination with the erythrocyte sedimentation rate and C-reactive protein, aspiration is still extremely valuable (Barrack and Harris 1993, White 1998). Bone scans are useful tests in differentiating septic and aseptic loosening if they are performed after a hip aspiration sample tests negative for infection.

Periprosthetic Hip Fracture

- *Periprosthetic hip fracture* is most often a delayed complication that occurs several months or years after the index procedure.
- In general, cementless femoral stems fracture earlier than cemented stems because the aggressive broaching and reaming required for the placement of uncemented stems can create minute stress risers and cortical cracks that can propagate. This finding is in contrast to cemented femoral components, which are more often associated with fractures distal to the stem tip.
- Periprosthetic fractures are considered most simply by analyzing two main factors: (1) the level of the fracture about the femur, and (2) the quality of the fixation of the femoral stem at the time of the fracture. A careful assessment of these two factors can often guide management of periprosthetic fractures.
- The *Vancouver classification* is one of the more widely used systems to grade periprosthetic fractures (Duncan and Masri 1995, Lewallen and Berry 1997) (Table 8–3). Vancouver type A fractures are peritrochanteric fractures, whereas type B includes those around the stem or distal to the stem tip; type C fractures are those well distal to the stem tip.

- *Type B fractures* are subclassified as follows: B1, or those surrounding a rigidly fixed stem; B2, or those surrounding a loose stem; and B3, or those surrounding a stem with extensive osteolysis and bony destruction.
- Generally, *type A fractures* can be treated nonoperatively, unless there is extensive osteolysis in the peritrochanteric region, in which case the debris-generating polyethylene component should be replaced along with débridement of sites of osteolysis.
- *Type B1 fractures* (Fig. 8–16) are treated with open reduction and internal fixation with the prosthesis left intact, with a combination of plating, cerclage wires, and screws.
- The preferred treatment for *type B2 fractures* (Fig. 8–17) is revision of the femoral stem with a longer stem femoral component with supplemental cerclage wires or strut grafts.
- *Type B3 fractures* exhibit extensive proximal femoral bone loss and generally require reconstruction of the proximal femur with an allograft or tumor-type prosthesis.
- *Type C fractures,* which are well distal to the femoral component, are best treated with open reduction and internal fixation (Harkess 2003).

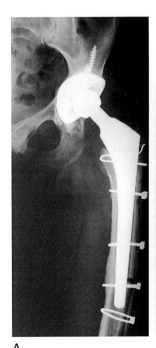
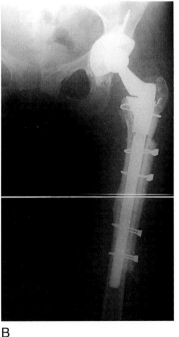

A   B

Figure 8–16: Type B1 femoral fracture with plate fixation. **A,** Total hip replacement in a 68-year-old woman 6 months after surgery with a good result. A fall down steps resulted in spiral femoral fracture below the tip of the stem. The stem remains well fixed. Note the nondisplaced distal fracture extension. **B,** After fixation with a cable plate and bone grafting. The fracture was united at 3 months with good function. (From Canale ST, ed. [2002]. *Campbell's Operative Orthopaedics,* 10th ed. Philadelphia: Mosby.)

Table 8–3	Vancouver Classification of Periprosthetic Hip Fractures	
TYPE	**LOCATION**	**SUBTYPE**
A	Peritrochanteric	A$_G$: greater trochanter A$_L$: lesser trochanter
B	Around or just distal to stem	B1 : prosthesis stable B2 : prosthesis unstable B3 : prosthesis unstable with extensive osteolysis
C	Well below stem	

From Duncan C, Masri BA (1995). Fracture of the femur after hip replacement. *Instr Course Lect* 44:293-304.

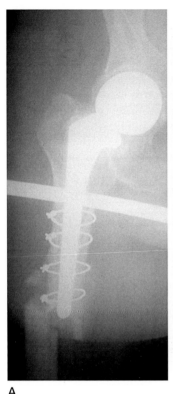
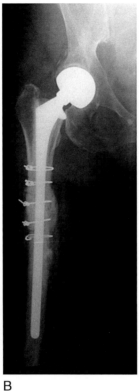
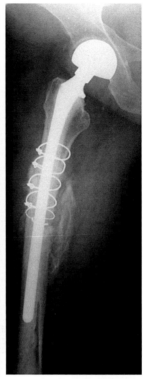

Figure 8–17: Type B2 femoral fracture. **A,** Elderly, debilitated woman referred for femoral fracture. The proximal femur apparently had been fractured during initial arthroplasty. The distal cement mantle is disrupted, and the stem is loose. Reduction in traction is unsatisfactory. Malunion would greatly complicate subsequent revision. **B and C,** Six months after revision of the femoral component to the long stem with additional cerclage wires and extensive bone grafting. (From Canale ST, ed. [2002]. *Campbell's Operative Orthopaedics*, 10th ed. Philadelphia: Mosby.)

A   B   C

Heterotopic Ossification

- The formation of heterotopic bone after THA is quite common, but fortunately it is not often painful or clinically significant. The incidence in the literature is reported to be anywhere from 0.6% to 84% (Pellegrini and Gregoritch 1996). HO is more common in male patients and also in patients with hypertrophic arthritis, ankylosing spondylitis, diffuse idiopathic skeletal hyperostosis, those who have post-traumatic arthritis, and patients with hip fusion that is converted to THA. HO is more commonly associated with anterior and lateral approaches to the hip, and it is related to the length of the surgical procedure and the extent of soft tissue disruption inflicted during surgery (Healy et al. 1995, Iorio and Healy 2002).
- HO is often classified using the *Brooker system* (Box 8–2; Fig. 8–18). Patients with grade III or IV disease that

Box 8–2	Brooker Classification of Heterotopic Ossification
I:	Islands of bone within the soft tissues
II:	Bone off the pelvis or the proximal end of the femur with at least a 1-cm gap
III:	Bone off the pelvis or the proximal end of the femur with a less than 1-cm gap
IV:	Bone connecting the pelvis and femur (ankylosis of the hip)

restricts motion are generally good candidates for surgical removal (Iorio and Healy 2002). Generally, HO need not be excised unless it causes significant restriction of motion or impingement of the hip. Surgical excision of HO is normally performed approximately 1 year after index THA. Additionally, postexcision prophylaxis in the form of radiation or pharmacotherapy should be utilized.
- Prophylactic measures for prevention of HO include radiation and pharmacotherapies; such treatments must generally be initiated within the first 72 hours after surgery to achieve maximal efficacy. The usual radiation protocol for prevention is to deliver 700 rad in one single dose within 24 hours after surgery (Healy et al. 1995, Pellegrini and Gregoritch 1996, Pellegrini et al. 1992). If radiation therapy is to be used, then cementless components should be protected because excessive radiation to such components can retard rigid bony ingrowth into the prostheses.
- Pharmacotherapies that are efficacious include indomethacin (75 mg/day for 6 to 8 weeks postoperatively), ibuprofen, and high-dose aspirin (Pellicci et al. 2000).

Miscellaneous Complications

- Hypersensitivity to the metals used in THA has also been reported in the literature. Although rare, it is thought that nickel in cobalt-chromium components is the substance that most often induces hypersensitivity reactions.

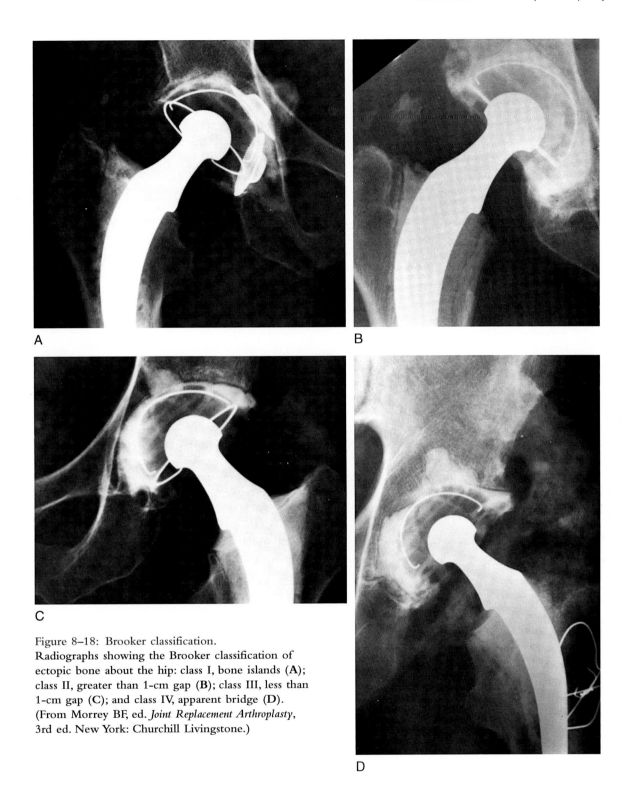

A

B

C

Figure 8–18: Brooker classification.
Radiographs showing the Brooker classification of
ectopic bone about the hip: class I, bone islands (**A**);
class II, greater than 1-cm gap (**B**); class III, less than
1-cm gap (**C**); and class IV, apparent bridge (**D**).
(From Morrey BF, ed. *Joint Replacement Arthroplasty*,
3rd ed. New York: Churchill Livingstone.)

D

Postoperative Management

- Two areas of THA postoperative protocol that deserve special focus include management of blood loss and transfusions and anticoagulation.

Transfusions

- Because of the elective nature of THA, patients have the option to autodonate blood before the surgical procedure or to undergo preoperative treatment with bone marrow stimulating agents to increase preoperative hemoglobin levels.
- However, studies have shown that patients with normal preoperative hemoglobin levels (>15 g/dl) rarely require transfusions postoperatively. Additionally, the preoperative autologous donation of blood in such patients increases the probability that such patients will require postoperative transfusions (Billote et al. 2002). Thus, the more recent literature has called into question the cost-effectiveness of preoperative donation of blood in patients with normal preoperative hemoglobin levels (Bierbaum et al. 1999, Pellicci et al. 2000).
- The preoperative use of marrow stimulating agents such as erythropoietin has been shown to reduce postoperative transfusion requirements in prospective, randomized, controlled trials (Feagan et al. 2000, Waddell 2001). Such agents can be particularly useful in patients whose preoperative hemoglobin levels are too low to tolerate autodonation. Erythropoietin use does entail small risks of increased thrombotic events and hypersensitivity. For these reasons, its use is not currently indicated in patients who have a preoperative hemoglobin level of more than 13 g/dl or in those who have recent history of DVT, myocardial infarction, or stroke.

Anticoagulation

- The postoperative management of DVT is also a controversial topic in total joint replacement. Currently popular agents for DVT prophylaxis include warfarin, low-molecular-weight heparin (LMWH), aspirin, unfractionated heparin, dextran, and mechanical devices such as sequential compression devices. Each of these agents has advantages and disadvantages.
- Unfractionated heparin, despite its high efficacy in preventing thrombotic events, is associated with at least a 2.6% risk of major bleeding events, compared with only a 0.4% risk with aspirin, a 1.3% risk with warfarin, and a 1.8% risk with LMWH (Colwell et al. 1994, Salvati et al. 2000). Unfractionated heparin also results in a higher rate of thrombocytopenia. Unfractionated heparin exerts its effects by binding with antithrombin III to inactivate thrombin and factor Xa (Colwell et al. 1999).
- LMWH imparts its effects by facilitating binding to antithrombin, which subsequently inactivates antithrombin III (Hirsh et al. 1998). LMWH offers the further advantage over unfractionated heparin in that it demonstrates

improved bioavailability, with a longer half-life and a more consistent dose-response curve (Bara 1985, Colwell et al. 1994, Paiement 1998). Both these heparin–related agents have the disadvantage that they cannot be used in patients with indwelling epidural anesthetic catheters.
- Warfarin functions by preventing the production of vitamin K–dependent clotting factors by the liver. These factors include II, VII, IX, and X. Warfarin has the disadvantage of requiring frequent international normalized ratio monitoring along with its very slow onset of action.
- Dextran functions through its dilutional effects on the blood.
- Sequential compression devices improve venous return to the heart while they stimulate endothelium to release fibrinolytic factors.
- Aspirin functions by retarding thromboxane A_2 synthesis and inhibiting platelet aggregation.

Hip Stability

- The topic of hip stability is critical in the discussion of primary THA because dislocation is a relatively common, preventable, and distressing complication whose incidence is most likely underreported in the literature.
- Dislocation rates of primary THAs are reported anywhere from 1% to 9% in the literature, with the true incidence most likely falling in the 2% to 3% range. The most common direction of dislocation is posteriorly; approximately three fourths of dislocations occur in this direction (Pellicci et al. 2000).
- The highest dislocation rate and risk occur within the first 3 months after surgery. Early hip dislocations are considered to be those that occur roughly within 1 year after the index procedure, whereas late dislocations are categorized as those that occur many years after the primary THA.
- Particular groups of patients at increased risk for postoperative dislocation include women, who have twice the risk of men, older patients, and, as discussed earlier, patients who have had posterolateral approaches to the hip (Berry 1999b).
- Additionally, patients who have THA after acute femoral neck fracture also have increased dislocation rates.
- Finally, the literature has shown association between psychiatric problems, such as dementia, depression, and alcohol abuse, and increased dislocation (Pellicci et al. 2000).

Assessment

- Several key aspects of the primary THA greatly influence its subsequent stability. These factors include the component configuration, the positioning of the components, and the abductor musculature.

Component Configuration

- Several aspects of the component configuration affect the ultimate stability of the prosthetic hip. The parameters of the ball head and acetabular articulation are one of the

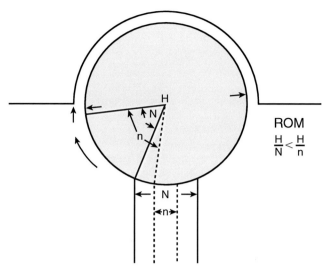

Figure 8–19: Head-to-neck ratio influencing motions before impingement.

The motion "N" of the head-to-neck ratio (H/N) is less than that "n" of the more narrow neck (H/n). *ROM*, range of motion. (From Morrey BF, ed. *Joint Replacement Arthroplasty*, 3rd ed. New York: Churchill Livingstone.)

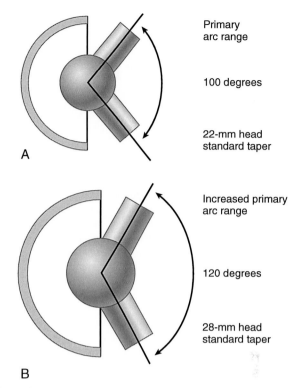

Figure 8–20: Comparison of the primary arc range between 22- and 28-mm heads.

A, Primary arc range with a 22-mm head. **B,** Primary arc range with a 28-mm head. The only change in this illustration is head size. This increases the head-to-neck ratio, which in turn allows for an increased arc range. (From Miller MD, ed. [2004]. *Review of Orthopaedics*, 4th ed. Philadelphia: WB Saunders.)

most critical factors. Maximizing the femoral head-to-neck ratio through the use of larger ball heads and smaller diameter femoral necks can improve this ratio by improving the primary arc range and the excursion distance of the hip (Fig. 8–19).

- The *primary arc range* (Fig. 8–20) is defined as the full range of motion that the prosthetic articulation can tolerate before the femoral neck contacts the acetabular implant at the extremes of motion (Scifert et al. 1998). At the limits of the primary arc range, the femoral neck will impinge on the acetabulum. Therefore, it is clear that a larger head coupled with a thin femoral neck will allow for the largest primary arc range.

- Once the primary arc range has been reached, the implant still tolerates further motion before dislocation. The distance of this limit of motion after the primary arc range has been reached is defined as the *excursion distance*. This distance is normally half the diameter of the ball head.

- In relation to the head-to-neck ratio, studies have shown that the use of a larger femoral head while preserving the same head-neck ratio can result in improved stability without compromising the range of motion (Cobb et al. 1996, Urquhart et al. 1998). However, larger femoral heads do have the disadvantage of increased volumetric wear of the polyethylene liner.

- Other component design factors that influence range of motion and stability include the use of elevated liners. Surgeons may choose to use posteriorly elevated acetabular liners to increase the posterior stability of the hip. Although such liners are effective in improving posterior

stability, they also result in increased impingement and decreased primary arc range when the hip is extended. Therefore, the increased posterior stability afforded by posteriorly elevated liners comes at a cost.

- Finally, hip components that utilize constrained liners, in which the acetabular component nearly completely envelopes the femoral head, provide excellent stability, but at the expense of a severely reduced primary arc range (Fig. 8–21).

- Additionally, such constrained components result in transmittal of a large amount of force to the interface between the acetabular shell and the acetabular bone. This can result in accelerated mechanical loosening of the acetabular component.

Component Alignment

- The orientation of the hip components within the patient's femur and acetabulum also critically influences hip stability.

- On the acetabular side, generally, implants that are placed in inadequate anteversion have increased risk of posterior

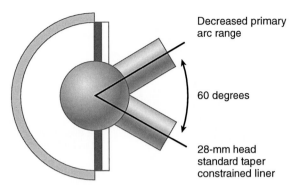

Figure 8–21: Diagram of a constrained acetabular liner. A constrained liner covers the femoral head past its equator. This keeps the ball from coming out of the socket and has the adverse effect of severely restricting the primary arc range. (From Miller MD, ed. [2004]. *Review of Orthopaedics*, 4th ed. Philadelphia: WB Saunders.)

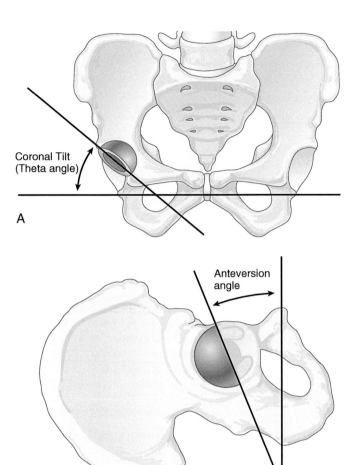

Figure 8–22: Diagram showing the acetabular cup position in the coronal and sagittal planes.
A, Coronal tilt (also known as theta angle) should be 35 to 45 degrees. **B,** In the sagittal plane, cup anteversion should be 15 to 30 degrees. (From Miller MD, ed. [2004]. *Review of Orthopaedics*, 4th ed. Philadelphia: WB Saunders.)

dislocations, whereas those placed in excessive anteversion increase the risk of anterior dislocation (Paterno et al. 1997).

- However, the surgical approach also affects the degree of desired version. When posterior approaches are used, acetabula are better placed in slightly higher ranges of anteversion to reduce the probability of posterior dislocation. Studies have demonstrated that for posteriorly implanted hips, a range between 15 and 20 degrees of anteversion results in excellent stability (Morrey 1997, Pellicci and Bostrom 1998). This concept also extends to hips implanted through anterior approaches, which do not require the same increased anteversion that benefits the stability of posteriorly approached hips.

- The vertical orientation of the acetabular component also affects the stability because implants that are inserted with an extreme vertical orientation, or that have a large theta angle, have a higher risk of superior dislocation. The *theta angle* describes the degree of abduction or vertical alignment of the acetabular component (Fig. 8–22).

- In summary, although the optimal position of the acetabular component is a controversial issue, studies have demonstrated that the abduction should be between 30 and 50 degrees, whereas the anteversion should fall between 0 and 30 degrees, depending on the surgical approach used. On the femoral side, studies have shown that the stem should be positioned between 0 and 15 degrees of anteversion (Barrack 2003, Barrack et al. 2001).

- One final important concept is that the position of the hip components does not affect the absolute value of the primary arc range of the prosthesis; as discussed earlier, this primary arc range is a mechanical phenomenon that is a function of the primary femoral head–acetabular articulation. Changing component position results in a change in the position of this primary arc range within space. *The goal of primary THA is to position the primary arc range of the prosthetic hip in the center of the functional range of motion required by the patient. Such alignment will result in overall decreased dislocation and maximal range of motion.*

Tightness of the Abductor Complex

- Another key factor affecting the stability of the implant is the tension conferred to the patient's hip abductor muscles by the prosthesis; this tension plays a critical role in generating sufficient force to maintain the prosthetic head within the acetabulum.

- The hip abductor muscles, consisting primarily of the gluteus medius and minimus, must be appropriately tensioned by the placement of the hip prosthesis. The maintenance of correct postoperative tension in these muscles requires that the femoral component have sufficient length and lateral

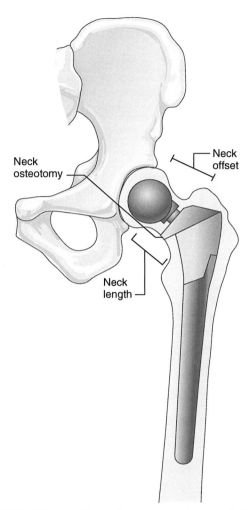

Figure 8–23: Diagram illustrating preoperative templating for proper femoral stem positioning.
The prosthetic stem should be positioned such that femoral stem offset (center of the head to the greater trochanter) matches the native hip. In addition, femoral neck length must be restored. Restoring head offset and neck length optimizes abductor tension and provides stability. (From Miller MD, ed. [2004]. *Review of Orthopaedics*, 4th ed. Philadelphia: WB Saunders.)

offset to produce sufficient resting tension within these muscles to maintain a reduced prosthetic hip (Fig. 8–23).
- If the implant has a femoral neck that is too short in the cranial-caudal dimension, this will result in lax abductor muscles and compromised stability. The lateral offset of the implant is defined as the horizontal distance between the center of the femoral head and the center of the femoral shaft. An insufficient lateral offset will also result in lax abductor muscles and compromised stability (Berry 2001).
- Therefore, placement of femoral components that maintain tension in abductors both in the craniocaudal direction and medial-lateral direction is critical to achieving a stable THA.

- In general, increasing the femoral offset has the advantage of improving abductor tension and decreasing joint reactive force, but it has the disadvantage of increasing torsional loads on the femoral component, which could lead to earlier loosening. Finally, increased femoral offset is associated with trochanteric bursitis.

Soft Tissue Function

- The final critical component of THA stability relates to the actual preoperative status and functioning of the patient's abductor muscle complex. If the patient has very weak or damaged abductor muscles, even the perfect combination of lateral offset and neck length in the prosthesis will not result in a stable hip.
- Patients with deficient abductor function include those with central nervous system damage from cerebrovascular accidents, cerebral palsy, multiple sclerosis, Parkinson's disease, and cervical myelopathy.
- Peripheral nervous system dysfunction that results in weakened abductor muscles includes damage to the superior gluteal nerve, lumbar stenosis, and myelopathy. In such patients with abductor dysfunction, restoration of maximal abductor tension is even more critical than in unaffected patients.
- In extreme situations in which the abductor complex is completely nonfunctional, the use of a constrained acetabular liner at the time of primary THA may be warranted.

Management of Dislocations

- Most first and even second dislocations can be treated with closed reduction, abduction bracing, and patient education. The duration of bracing is usually on the order of 3 months, to allow adequate scar tissue to form around the hip joint to augment stability. Approximately 66% of patients with dislocations will successfully maintain long-term stability with this protocol (Pellicci et al. 2000).
- The occurrence of a third dislocation is associated with an unfavorable prognosis, with a slim likelihood that nonoperative management will result in long-term stability. In such situations with repeated dislocations, the causes are many and include component malposition, component impingement, and abductor complex dysfunction.
- Surgical techniques that can be used to correct such issues include repositioning of malaligned components and increasing the femoral head-to-neck ratio; surgical techniques that may improve the tensioning of the abductor complex and thereby stability include increasing the femoral offset or neck length and possible advancement of the greater trochanter (Goetz et al. 1998, Woo and Morrey 1982).
- As described earlier, when the abductors are severely dysfunctional, a constrained liner, in which the femoral head locks into the acetabular liner, may be utilized. Constrained liners increase stability but severely decrease primary arc range; they also transmit larger mechanical

forces to the acetabulum, which can result in accelerated component failure. They generally do not result in any increased polyethylene wear (Anderson et al. 1994, Lachiewicz and Kelley 2002).

Hip Loosening

- Aseptic loosening of either the femoral or acetabular implant continues to be the most common indication for reoperation on a primary THA.
- *Generally, with cemented THAs, the acetabulum is the first component to fail from loosening, whereas with cementless hips, the femoral component loosens more often as a result of osteolysis.*
- Patients with loose implants generally complain of pain in three stages; the first stage occurs at startup, when weight bearing is initially commenced. In the second stage, after a short ambulation distance, the pain subsides somewhat, only to increase again after the patient ambulates further. Loose acetabular components generally cause buttock and groin pain, whereas loose femoral implants cause thigh pain.
- The diagnosis of loosening is best made by serial plain radiographs, which demonstrate progressive radiolucencies around the components in consecutive images (Miniaci et al. 1990).
- Radiolucencies that involve the entire perimeter of a given component and develop during a very brief time are more suggestive of a septic process (Barrack 2003, Garvin and Hanssen 1993).
- Authors have systematically described the radiographic patterns of loosening. Femoral component loosening is characterized by the *Gruen system*, which divides the femur as visualized on an anteroposterior radiograph into seven zones. Radiolucent lines documented in all seven

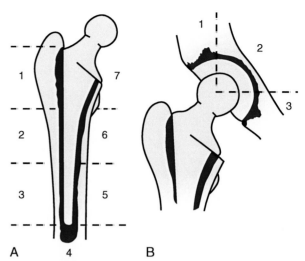

Figure 8–24: Zones about the cement mass.
Zones about the cement mass in the femur (**A**), as described by Gruen, and in the pelvis (**B**), as described by DeLee and Charnley. (**A**, From Canale ST, ed. [2002]. *Campbell's Operative Orthopaedics*, 10th ed. Philadelphia: Mosby. **B**, Redrawn from Amstutz HC, Smith RK [1979]. Total hip replacement following failed femoral hemiarthroplasty. *J Bone Joint Surg Am* 61:1161.)

zones are highly indicative of a loose component (Fig. 8–24).

- The Gruen system also incorporates a description of four modes of cemented femoral component failure (Fig. 8–25). The four mechanisms are as follows: (1) pistoning behavior, in which the stem and cement subside into the femur; (2) medial stem pivoting, in

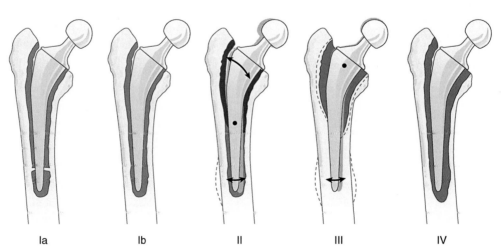

Figure 8–25: Stem loosening.
Mechanisms or modes of stem loosening according to Gruen and associates: mode *Ia*, subsidence of the stem in the cement mantle; *Ib*, subsidence of the cement mantle and stem; *II*, medial stem pivot with the center of axis of rotation of the stem illustrated by a *dot* on the stem; *III*, calcar pivot with the axis of rotation of the stem in the proximal area illustrated by a *dot* on the stem; and *IV*, cantilever bending. (From Canale ST, ed. [2002]. *Campbell's Operative Orthopaedics*, 10th ed. Philadelphia: Mosby.)

which a varus positioned stem fails at the proximal medial and distal lateral areas; (3) calcar pivoting, in which the distal aspect of the stem can shift within the distal cement mantle; and (4) cantilever bending, in which actual stem fracture may occur because of loss of the cement mantle proximally, resulting in proximal stem bending and eventual breakage. With cantilever bending, the stem undergoes fatigue failure proximally because of repetitive loading at a compromised proximal cement-implant interface (Gruen et al. 1979).

- Radiolucencies on the femoral side can also be the result of *bone remodeling.*

Osteolysis and Wear Debris

- It is currently thought that wear particles generated from the acetabular polyethylene are the main inducers of the macrophage and histiocytic response that leads to osteolysis.
- However, other wear sources are present within the total hip construct, including the PMMA cement, the hydroxyapatite coating of the implants, and the metals of the implants such as cobalt, chromium, and titanium. Nonetheless, polyethylene is considered the major wear component that triggers the pathway for osteolysis (Harkess 2003).
- Wear particles are thought to be engulfed by macrophages, which excrete several osteolytic cytokines and trigger the pathway of bony destruction and resorption.

Mechanisms of Wear

- The two main mechanisms by which wear particles are produced in the hip are abrasive wear and adhesive wear.
  - *Abrasive wear* occurs when a rough surface contacts another surface and results in removal of particles from the less abrasive substance with less surface hardness. The mechanism is similar to the effect of sandpaper on wood. Abrasive wear can also be caused by third-body particles, which become entrapped between two closely contacting surfaces. Such third-body particles include cement, metal, or bone particles.
  - The second major wear mechanism is that of *adhesive wear.* This type of wear takes place at the femoral head-polyethylene articulation, when submicron polyethylene particles are sheared off and are deposited within the joint space. These particles are then engulfed by macrophages and trigger the histiocytic osteolysis reaction. The size of the wear particles that induce the osteolytic response is on the order of 0.2 to 7 μm (Campbell et al. 1995, Maloney et al. 1995, Shanbhag 1994).

Reduction of Wear at the Head-Liner Interface

- Reduction of adhesive wear at the head-liner interface has been addressed in several ways, one of which is by improving the wear properties of the polyethylene.

- Since the late 1980s, it has been recognized that the process utilized for polyethylene sterilization and shelf packaging significantly affects the wear rate of the acetabular liner. For many years, acetabular polyethylene had been sterilized with γ-irradiation in oxygen-rich environments. Such caustic environments compromised the wear profile of the polyethylene and led to faster in vivo wear rates and ultimately to greater osteolysis (Archibeck et al. 2001, Bartel et al. 1986, Fisher et al. 1995).
- Oxygen-rich environments result in the formation of free radicals that damage polyethylene. When polyethylene is irradiated, the end result on its wear and material properties depends on the environment.
- When irradiation occurs in an oxygen-rich environment, oxidation occurs, which produces delamination under the polyethylene surface, with cracking on the surface. In an inert milieu such as gas plasma/ethylene oxide, cross-linking of the polyethylene occurs and thus makes the substance less susceptible to abrasive and adhesive wear.
- However, this improved wear profile comes at the cost of increased brittleness and diminished mechanical properties. The sterilization of polyethylene in environments that do not cause high levels of oxidation, such as gas plasma and ethylene oxide, has significantly reduced the problem of oxidative degradation of polyethylene (Simon 1994, Wright 1991).
- The shelf storage environment of the polyethylene after sterilization has also been recognized to affect the in vivo wear profile of the acetabular liner. When such components are packaged and stored in oxygen-containing environments, the oxygen can further degrade the polyethylene. Thus improvements in the intrapackage environment of the polyethylene components have further improved their wear properties.
- Other factors recognized over the years to increase the rate of polyethylene wear included the use of larger femoral heads. Such larger heads increased the volumetric wear at the ball head-liner interface and ultimately led to increased wear debris and osteolysis. Although such larger heads reduced the linear wear that is more characteristic of smaller, 22-mm femoral heads, the increased volumetric wear resulted in an overall higher production of wear debris.
- In more recent years, the use of polyethylene with improved wear properties has allowed the use of 32-mm femoral heads without the production of prohibitive amounts of wear debris. Finally, attempts to reduce the effective joint space in the total hip construct through elimination of holes in the metal shell have yielded mixed results.

Effective Joint Space

- The *effective joint space* is a concept that describes the entire volumetric area within a hip joint construct that can be infiltrated by polyethylene wear particles and

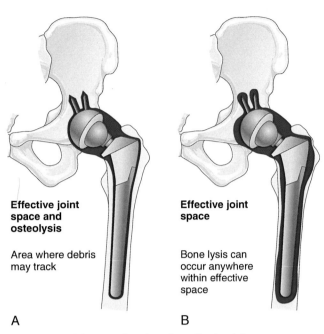

Effective joint space and osteolysis

Area where debris may track

Effective joint space

Bone lysis can occur anywhere within effective space

A   B

Figure 8–26: Diagram showing the effective joint space. **A,** Area of the effective joint space, which includes any area around the prosthetic construct, including screws. **B,** Osteolysis can occur in any region of the effective joint space. Particles are pumped via the path of least resistance. (From Miller MD, ed. [2004]. *Review of Orthopaedics,* 4th ed. Philadelphia: WB Saunders.)

macrophages (Fig. 8–26). Bone breakdown can occur anywhere within the effective joint space.

- The theory implies that reductions in the effective joint space may reduce the amount of osteolysis that can occur. The use of bone screws for the fixation of metal shells is thought to create new voids in the acetabular bone that increase the effective joint space. Therefore, the elimination of bone screws for acetabular components could decrease the effective joint space and therefore decrease the osteolysis rate.
- Finally, the use of circumferential proximal porous coating for the femoral stem effectively seals off the diaphyseal component of the femoral canal from the effective joint space and therefore has been recognized to reduce osteolysis in the proximal femur (Archibeck et al. 2001, Bartel et al. 1986, Fisher et al. 1995).

Wear at the Shell–Liner Interface

- It has been recognized in recent years that polyethylene wear debris can also be produced at the interface between the metal acetabular shell and the polyethylene liner.
- The mechanism by which this occurs is through motion between the shell and liner, which can result in the production of wear particles. This phenomenon is implant specific and should become less problematic with newer,

better-designed locking mechanisms. This phenomenon is more prevalent when modular acetabular components are used because these components may have suboptimal locking mechanisms between the shell and liner that allows relatively increased motion and consequent wear debris at this interface (Archibeck et al. 2001, Bartel et al. 1986, Fisher et al. 1995).

Treatment of Osteolysis

- The treatment for osteolysis is variable, depending on the extent of bony destruction in both the acetabulum and the femur. However, it is possible for significant pelvic osteolysis to occur without loosening the acetabular shell. In such cases, when pelvic osteolysis occurs with a well-fixed acetabular shell, treatment includes retention of the metal shell, bone grafting of the osteolytic defects, and exchange of the worn polyethylene liner (Pellicci et al. 2000).
- For more significant osteolysis with loosening of the acetabular and femoral components, more extensive revision surgery is required, with replacement of loose components and grafting of bony defects.

Prosthetic Articular Bearing

- The topic of articular bearings and the search for more durable bearing surfaces have been the subjects of significant debate and research in recent years.
- Traditional surface couplings have included polyethylene acetabular liners with combinations of metal heads. These bearing surfaces are referred to as *hard-on-soft combinations* (Schmalzried and Callaghan 1999).
  - Of these metals, the results have been least favorable for titanium heads because this metal is associated with higher rates of volumetric wear and the production of third-body wear particles (Harkess 2003). The problem with titanium is that its surface hardness is inferior to that of other alloys; therefore, it scratches more easily than other metals and is vulnerable to third-body abrasive wear (Agins et al. 1988).
  - However, the traditional combination of cobalt and chromium on polyethylene has produced a record of predictable, long-term success. Despite this success, the search for improvements in the wear rate of hard-on-soft coupling continues.
  - As discussed earlier, great enhancements have been made in the surface hardness of the polyethylene component. Ultrahigh-molecular-weight polyethylene (UHMWPE), which has excellent wear properties, is now frequently used for acetabular liners. This polyethylene has increased surface hardness and wear properties in comparison with older generations of polyethylene.
  - Recent advances in UHMWPE have included processes to achieve cross-linking of the polyethylene molecules to produce new, highly cross-linked UHMWPEs. This newer

generation of UHMWPEs is produced when the polyethylene is γ-irradiated in an inert environment. Such highly cross-linked UHMWPEs have even better surface hardness and improved resistance to adhesive and abrasive wear. However, these improved wear properties come at the expense of decreased material properties such as Young's modulus of elasticity and yield strength; these new components are more susceptible to fracture.

- Attempts to improve the femoral head component of the coupling have utilized new materials such as alumina, ceramic, or zirconium. Alumina components have the advantage of better scratch resistance than traditional cobalt-chromium heads and therefore demonstrate lower rates of third-body abrasive wear. The wear rates of ceramic-polyethylene couplings have been reported anywhere between 0 and 150 μm/year. This represents a 10% to 50% decrease in the wear rates reported for traditional metal-polyethylene couplings (75 to 250 μm/year) (Jazrawi et al. 1998, McKellop et al. 1996, Schmalzried and Callaghan 1999).
- However, ceramic components do have the disadvantage of increased susceptibility to fracture. Rates of fracture have been reported in the literature to be on the order of 0.004% (Heisel et al. 2003).
- In recent years, interest has increased in *hard-on-hard bearings*, in which the "soft" polyethylene component of the coupling is replaced with a "hard" bearing such as ceramic or metal.
  - The most common combinations of hard-on-hard bearings have been ceramic-ceramic and metal-metal bearings. Both these combinations have demonstrated significantly lower wear rates than those of hard-on-soft bearings. Additionally, these hard-on-hard bearings are advantageous because the wear particles that are produced are on the order of 0.015 to 0.12 μm. These particles are significantly smaller than those produced by hard-on-soft combinations and are so small that they are believed to be immunologically inert, failing to activate the osteolytic pathway in the manner of larger polyethylene wear particles.
  - Ceramic-ceramic combinations have the best wear profile of currently available bearings, with annual wear rates of 0.5 to 2.5 μm/year.
  - Metal-metal couplings also have extremely low wear rates on the order of 2.5 to 5.0 μm/year (Jazrawi et al. 1998, McKellop et al. 1996, Schmalzried and Callaghan 1999).
  - However, these new hard-on-hard bearings are not without their disadvantages. As a material, ceramic is extremely brittle and therefore is more susceptible to fracture than is metal or polyethylene. Therefore, concerns persist that catastrophic failure of ceramic-ceramic couplings can occur with component fractures. For metal-metal couplings, the potential

carcinogenic effects of metal particles is a concern. Although no reports have directly correlated metal-metal bearings with neoplasia, investigators have demonstrated increased concentrations of metal ions in the urine and blood of patients with metal-metal THAs (Jazrawi et al. 1998).

Conclusions

- In summary, THA is one of the most successful and efficacious procedures performed in the modern medical era.
- Significant improvements in design of the prosthetic components combined with advanced, more durable materials and refined surgical techniques have improved the results of THA since the mid-1970s. However, efforts to improve the results of THA continue.

References

Agins HJ, Alcock NW, Bansal M, et al. (1988). Metallic wear in failed titanium-alloy total hip replacements: A histologic and quantitative analysis. *J Bone Joint Surg Am* 70:347-356.

> The authors conducted histologic examination of the tissues that were adjacent to the prosthesis in nine hips with a failed total arthroplasty. These investigators found that femoral components made of titanium alloy can undergo severe wear of the surface and on the stem, where it is loose, with liberation of potentially toxic local concentrations of metal debris into the surrounding tissues.

Anderson MJ, Murray WR, Skinner HB, et al. (1994). Constrained acetabular components. *J Arthroplasty* 9:17-23.

> The authors evaluated 21 constrained acetabular components that were placed for unstable hips; at average 31 months follow-up, these investigators found a 30% dislocation rate but no component loosening or osteolysis.

Archibeck MJ, Jacobs JJ, Roebuck KA, Glant TT (2001). The basic science of periprosthetic osteolysis. *Instr Course Lect* 50:185-195.

> This article reviews the immunology and basic science of the osteolytic process in total joint arthroplasty.

Bara L, Billaud E, Kher A, Samama M (1985). Increased anti-Xa bioavailability for a low-molecular weight heparin (PK 10169) compared with unfractionated heparin. *Semin Thromb Hemost* 11:316-317.

> The authors discuss the pharmacokinetics of LWMH and unfractionated heparin and demonstrate increased bioavailability and half-life of LWMH.

Barrack RL (2003). Dislocation after total hip arthroplasty: implant design and orientation. *J Am Acad Orthop Surg* 11:89-99.

> This review discusses the causes of unstable THA, ideal component positioning, and the treatment of persistently dislocating THAs.

Barrack RL, Harris WH (1993). The value of aspiration of the hip joint before revision total hip arthroplasty. *J Bone Joint Surg Am* 75:66-76.

> The authors reviewed 270 THAs in which aspiration was performed before revision. They concluded that aspiration should be performed before THA revision only if the clinical history and radiographs strongly suggest infection.

Barrack RL, Lavernia C, Ries M, et al. (2001). Virtual reality computer animation of the effect of component position and design on stability after total hip arthroplasty. *Orthop Clin North Am* 32:569-77.

The authors used virtual reality technology to determine the effects of component design and orientation on the range of motion before dislocation in THA. Computer animations were used to determine the propensity for dislocation with the components in various positions.

Barrack RL, Mulroy RD, Harris WH (1992). Improved cementing techniques and femoral component loosening in young patients with hip arthroplasty: A 12 year radiographic review. *J Bone Joint Surg Br* 74:385-389.

The authors reviewed 50 THAs performed using "second-generation" cement technique at an average follow-up of 12 years and found a very low rate of femoral component loosening and a high rate of acetabular component loosening.

Bartel DL, Bicknell VL, Wright TM (1986). The effect of conformity, thickness, and material on stresses in ultra-high molecular weight components for total joint replacement. *J Bone Joint Surg Am* 68:1041-1051.

Finite-element analysis and elasticity data were utilized to determine the fatigue stresses imparted on polyethylene from contact with metal femoral heads and metal total knee arthroplasty (TKA) femoral components. The authors determined that tibial TKA components are more likely to suffer surface damage from fatigue than are acetabular components of THAs.

Beals RK, Tower SS (1996). Periprosthetic fractures of the femur: An analysis of 93 fractures. *Clin Orthop Relat Res* 327:238-246.

The authors reviewed 93 periprosthetic femur fractures and demonstrated that the type of prosthesis utilized and preexisting stress rises may help to predict where such fractures will occur.

Berger RA, Jacobs JJ, Quigley LR, et al. (1997). Primary cementless acetabular reconstruction in patients younger than 50 years old: 7-to 11-year results. *Clin Orthop Relat Res* 344:216.

The authors reviewed 79 consecutive primary THAs in patients less than 50 years old at an average follow-up of 106 months. Cementless acetabular components were used in all cases. The authors demonstrated a survival rate of 98.8% and concluded that osteolysis was the most common problem.

Berry DJ (2001). Primary total hip arthroplasty. In: Chapman MW, ed. *Chapman's Orthopaedic Surgery*. Philadelphia: Lippincott Williams & Wilkins, pp 2769-2790.

This review chapter describes all aspects of primary THA including indications, anatomy, and complications.

Berry DJ (1999a). Epidemiology: Hip and knee. Periprosthetic fractures after major joint replacement. *Orthop Clin North Am* 333:183-190.

This review article discusses the epidemiology of periprosthetic fractures associated with THA and TKA. Causes of intraoperative and postoperative fractures are described.

Berry DJ. Dislocation (1999b). In: Steinberg ME, ed. *Revision Total Hip Arthroplasty*. Philadelphia: Lippincott Williams & Wilkins, pp 463-482.

This textbook review chapter describes the etiology and treatment of unstable THA.

Berry DJ, Barnes CL, Scott RD, et al. (1994). Catastrophic failure of the polyethylene liner of uncemented acetabular components. *J Bone Joint Surg Br* 76:575-578.

Ten cases of catastrophic failure of the polyethylene component of THA were reviewed. The authors demonstrated that polyethylene with thickness of less than 5 mm is associated with a much higher risk of catastrophic failure.

Berry DJ, Harmsen WS, Ilstrup D, et al. (1995). Survivorship of uncemented proximally porous-coated femoral components. *Clin Orthop Relat Res* 319:168-177.

The authors reviewed 375 consecutive THAs with 6 different proximally porous-coated designs. The average postoperative follow-up was 4.7 years. A survivorship of 58% free from revision for aseptic failure was demonstrated.

Bierbaum BE, Callaghan JJ, Galante JO, et al. (1999). An analysis of blood management in patients having a total hip or knee arthroplasty. *J Bone Joint Surg Am* 81:2-10.

The authors prospectively reviewed 9482 hip and knee replacement procedures with respect to requirements for postoperative blood transfusions. These authors demonstrated that revision THA, bilateral primary TKA, and patients with preoperative hemoglobin values less than 13.0 were associated with the highest transfusion requirements.

Billote D, Glisson SN, Green D, et al. (2002). A prospective, randomized study of preoperative autologous donation for hip replacement surgery. *J Bone Joint Surg Am* 84:1299-1304.

In this report, 96 patients were divided into two groups, one of which preoperatively donated autologous blood and one that did not. This prospective randomized trial demonstrated that preoperative autologous donation of blood is not cost-effective in patients who have a normal hemoglobin value preoperatively.

Binns M, Pho R (1990). Femoral vein occlusion during hip arthroplasty. *Clin Orthop Relat Res* 255:168-172.

The authors studied the mechanism of femoral vein occlusion during the THA procedure in fresh-frozen cadaveric specimens. The authors demonstrated that the dislocation maneuver is associated with femoral vein occlusion, which may lead to thrombotic activity.

Breed AL (1974). Experimental production of vascular hypotension, and bone marrow and fat embolism with methylmethacrylate cement: Traumatic hypertension of bone. *Clin Orthop Relat Res* 102:227-244.

The author utilized an in vivo model to demonstrate that methylmethacrylate causes adverse physiologic effects when it is introduced into the vascular space.

Callaghan JJ (1993). The clinical results and basic science of total hip arthroplasty with porous-coated prostheses. *J Bone Joint Surg Am* 75:299-310.

This review article discusses the results of cementless THA. The basic science underlying the principles of biologic bony ingrowth of cementless prosthesis is also discussed.

Callaghan JJ, Brand RA, Pedersen DR (1985a). Hip arthrodesis: A long-term follow-up. *J Bone Joint Surg Am* 67:1328-1335.

The authors retrospectively reviewed 28 hip fusions at an average of 35 years postoperatively. The most common complications included ipsilateral knee pain, back pain, and contralateral hip pain.

Callaghan JJ, Forest EE, Olejniczak JP, et al. (1998). Charnley total hip arthroplasty in patients less than fifty years old: A twenty to twenty-five year follow-up note. *J Bone Joint Surg Am* 80:705.

In this article, 93 consecutive cemented Charnley THAs performed by a single surgeon with a minimum of 20-year follow-up were reviewed; 29% of these THAs required revision surgery of some type.

Callaghan JJ, Salvati EA, Pellicci PM, et al. (1985b). Results of revision for mechanical failure after cemented total hip replacement, 1979 to 1982: A two to five-year follow-up. *J Bone Joint Surg Am* 67:1074-1085.

The results of 146 aseptic revision cemented THAs were reviewed retrospectively. At the time of latest follow-up (2 to 5 years), 15.8% of the revision THAs exhibited failure.

Campbell P, Ma S, Yeom B, et al. (1995). Isolation of predominantly submicron-sized UHMWPE wear particles from periprosthetic tissues. *J Biomed Mater Res* 29:127-131.

A novel method of retrieval and characterization of submicron-sized UHMWPE particles from in vivo samples is described.

Cobb TK, Morrey BF, Ilstrup DM (1996). The elevated rim acetabular liner in total hip arthroplasty: Relationship to postoperative dislocation. *J Bone Joint Surg Am* 78:80-86.

The results of 2469 acetabular components with an elevated-rim liner were compared with 2698 acetabular components with a standard liner. These authors demonstrated that elevated liners are associated with a lower rate of dislocation than are standard liners.

Colwell CW Jr, Collis DK, Paulson R, et al. (1999). Comparison of enoxaparin and warfarin for the prevention of venous thromboembolic disease after total hip arthroplasty: Evaluation during hospitalization and three months after discharge. *J Bone Joint Surg Am* 81:932-940.

The authors reviewed 3011 patients in a multicenter study to compare the efficacy and complications of enoxaparin and warfarin. These authors demonstrated that during hospitalization, patients given enoxaparin had a lower rate of venous thromboembolic disease. However, at 3 months postoperatively, the two groups had converged with regard to rates of venous thromboembolic disease.

Colwell CW, Spiro TE, Trowbridge AA, et al. (1994). Use of enoxaparin, a low-molecular weight heparin, and unfractionated heparin for the prevention of deep venous thrombosis after elective hip replacement: A clinical trial comparing efficacy and safety. *J Bone Joint Surg Am* 76:3-14.

A randomized trial of 601 patients was conducted to compare the safety and efficacy and enoxaparin and unfractionated heparin after elective THA. Patients who received enoxaparin had a lower DVT rate than those who received heparin.

Cook SD, Thomas KA, Haddad RJ Jr (1988). Histologic analysis of retrieved human porous-coated total joint components. *Clin Orthop Relat Res* 234:90-101.

The authors histologically and microradiographically analyzed 90 retrieved human uncemented, porous-coated implants; 62 TKA components and 28 THA components were reviewed. These authors found that none of the components had greater than 10% of surface involvement with bony ingrowth.

Crowninshield RD, Brand RA, Johnston RC, et al. (1980). The effect of femoral stem cross-sectional geometry on cement stresses in total hip reconstruction. *Clin Orthop Relat Res* 146:71-77.

The authors described the findings of a three-dimensional numeric stress analysis model of a prosthesis-cement proximal femur. They demonstrated that stresses to the model were distributed best when the prostheses had broad medial and lateral surfaces.

Crowninshield RD, Brand RA, Pedersen DR (1983). A stress analysis of acetabular reconstruction in protrusio acetabuli. *J Bone Joint Surg Am* 65:495-499.

A finite-element model was used to examine the stresses of acetabular components in the reconstructions of protrusio acetabuli. The authors demonstrated that during such reconstructions, the acetabular component should be placed in a normal and not a protruded position. Metal-backed components reduce stress levels of the medial pelvic bone in such patients.

Dorr LD, Tawakkol S, Moorthy M, et al. (1999). Medial protrusio technique for placement of a porous-coated, hemispherical acetabular component without cement in total hip arthroplasty in patients who have acetabular dysplasia. *J Bone Joint Surg Am* 81:83-92.

The authors reviewed 24 THAs in patients with varying types of Crowe developmentally dislocated hips. These authors described the technique of placing the acetabular cups in an exaggerated medial position. They concluded that the technique is advantageous because it allows the use of uncemented implants in such patients, and it permits earlier weight bearing.

Drancourt M, Stein A, Argenson JN, et al. (1993). Oral rifampin plus ofloxacin for treatment of staphylococcus-infected orthopedic implants. *Antimicrob Agents Chemother* 37:1214-1218.

A prospective cohort study was conducted in which 51 patients from whom *Staphylococcus* organisms susceptible to rifampin and ofloxacin were treated with oral formulation of these drugs for infected total joint prostheses. These authors concluded that this oral regimen is a viable alternative to conventional intravenous therapy.

Duncan CP, Beauchamp C (1993). A temporary antibiotic-loaded joint replacement system for the management of complex infections involving the hip. *Orthop Clin North Am* 24:751-759.

The authors described a novel method for constructing an antibiotic spacer device that can be utilized during two-stage revision for infected THA. They concluded that such devices are valuable adjuncts to treatment in such situations.

Duncan C, Masri BA (1995). Fracture of the femur after hip replacement. *Instr Course Lect* 44:293-304.

This review article describes the etiology, classification, and treatment of periprosthetic femur fractures after THA.

Ebramzadeh E, Sarmiento A, McKellop HA, et al. (1994). The cement mantle in total hip arthroplasty: Analysis of long-term radiographic results. *J Bone Joint Surg Am* 76:77-87.

The authors examined the relationship among the size of the thickness of the cement mantle, the medullary canal fill, and the positioning of the stem on the long-term radiographically evident loosening of 836 cemented femoral components. These authors demonstrated that a cement mantle of 2 to 5 mm is associated with the best results.

Edwards BN, Tullos HS, Noble PC (1987). Contributory factors and etiology of sciatic nerve palsy in total hip arthroplasty. *Clin Orthop Relat Res* 218:136-141.

The authors reviewed 23 peroneal and sciatic nerve palsies after primary THA. They demonstrated that risk factors include revision surgery, female sex, and limb lengthening.

Emerson RH Jr, Sanders SB, Head WC, Higgins L (1999). Effect of circumferential plasma-spray porous coating on the rate of femoral osteolysis after total hip arthroplasty. *J Bone Joint Surg Am* 81: 1291-1298.

The authors compared two study groups, one of which had a circumferentially porous-coated femoral stem implanted (90 patients), and the other of which had a noncircumferentially porous-coated femoral stem implanted (126 patients). These authors demonstrated that the osteolysis was greater in the group with noncircumferentially porous-coated implants.

Espehaug B, Engesaeter LB, Vollset SE, et al. (1997). Antibiotic prophylaxis in total hip arthroplasty: Review of 10,905 primary cemented total hip replacements reported to the Norwegian arthroplasty register, 1987 to 1995. *J Bone Joint Surg Br* 79:590-595.

This review of a nearly 11,000 primary THAs from the Norwegian arthroplasty register demonstrated that for cemented THA, the lowest revision rate for septic failure was achieved in patients who received perioperative systemic antibiotics in addition to antibiotic-impregnated bone cement.

Feagan BG, Wong CJ, Kirkley A, et al. (2000). Erythropoietin with iron supplementation to prevent allogeneic blood transfusion in total hip joint arthroplasty: A randomized, controlled trial. *Ann Intern Med* 133:845-854.

A randomized, double-blind, multicenter trial was conducted to compare two different regimens of erythropoietin with regard to their efficacy in preventing allogeneic blood transfusions after THA. The authors concluded that both regimens of erythropoietin were effective in reducing transfusions after THA.

Fisher J, Hailey JL (1995). The effect of aging following irradiation on the wear of UHMWPE. *Trans Orthop Res Soc* 20:12.

The authors performed wear studies on three groups: UHMWPE, unirradiated polyethylene; irradiated polyethylene aged for 2 months; and irradiated polyethylene aged 5 years. These authors found that irradiation and aging increased the wear experienced by the polyethylene.

Ganz R, Klaue K, Vinh TS, Mast JW (1988). A new periacetabular osteotomy for the treatment of hip dysplasias: Technique and preliminary results. *Clin Orthop Relat Res* 232:26-36.

The authors described a technique for periacetabular osteotomy that is performed through an anterior Smith-Petersen approach. This new osteotomy allows for early weight bearing and requires minimal hardware fixation.

Garvin KL, Hanssen AD (1993). Infection after total hip arthroplasty: Past, present, and future. *J Bone Joint Surg Am* 75:66-76.

In this review of the history of infected THA, current treatment algorithms and results are also discussed.

Garvin KL, Pellicci PM, Windsor RE, et al. (1989). Contralateral total hip arthroplasty or ipsilateral total hip arthroplasty in patients who have long-standing fusion of the hip. *J Bone Joint Surg Am* 71:1355-1362.

These authors reviewed 22 patients with previous hip fusion who underwent subsequent ipsilateral TKA (8 patients) or contralateral THA (13 patients). The authors noted loosening as a common complication in THA. Patients with TKAs after hip fusion demonstrated a frequent need for manipulation.

Glickstein MF, Burk DL Jr, Schiebler ML, et al. (1998). Avascular necrosis versus other diseases of the hip: Sensitivity of MR imaging. *Radiology* 169:213-215.

The authors had blinded radiologists review the MRI scans of 22 cases of non-AVN hip disease and 23 cases of biopsy-proven cases of AVN. They found that MRI was 85% sensitive in differentiating AVN from other causes of hip disease.

Goel A, Sharp DJ (1991). Heterotopic bone formation after hip replacement: The influence of the type of osteoarthritis. *J Bone Joint Surg Br* 73:255-257.

Forty-three THAs were examined to determine whether the type of arthritis encountered preoperatively influenced the incidence of postoperative heterotopic bone formed. Hypertrophic arthritis was associated with the highest incidence of heterotopic bone.

Goetz DD, Capello WN, Callaghan JJ, et al. (1998). Salvage of a recurrently dislocating total hip prosthesis with use of a constrained acetabular component: A retrospective analysis of fifty-six cases. *J Bone Joint Surg Am* 80:502-509.

Fifty-six recurrently dislocating hips that were treated with constrained acetabular liners were reviewed. A 4% postrevision dislocation rate was observed.

Gore DR, Murray MP, Sepic SB, Gardner GM (1975). Walking patterns of men with unilateral surgical hip fusion. *J Bone Joint Surg Am* 57:759-765.

The authors described the ambulation characteristics of men with hip fusion, including increased transverse and sagittal pelvic rotation, increased motion in the unfused hip, and increased knee flexion during the gait cycle.

Gruen TA, McNiece GM, Amstutz HC (1979). "Modes of failure" of cemented stem–type femoral components: A radiologic analysis of loosening. *Clin Orthop Relat Res* 141:17-27.

The authors described the findings of radiographic review of 389 THAs and identified several modes of failure of the femoral stem, including stem pistoning, stem-cement pistoning, medial stem pivoting, calcar pivoting and bending, and cantilever bending.

Guerra JJ, Steinberg ME (1995). Distinguishing transient osteoporosis from avascular necrosis of the hip. *J Bone Joint Surg Am* 77:616-624.

The authors reviewed MRI findings of transient osteoporosis in comparison with MRI appearance of AVN of the hip.

Harkess JW (2003). Arthroplasty of hip. In: Canale ST, ed. *Campbell's Operative Orthopaedics,* 10th ed. Philadelphia: Mosby, pp 315-471.

This review chapter covers all aspects of THA including biomechanics, implant design, indications, and complications.

Hartofilakidis G, Stamos K, Karachalios T, et al. (1996). Congenital hip disease in adults: Classification of acetabular deficiencies and operative treatment with acetabuloplasty combined with total hip arthroplasty. *J Bone Joint Surg Am* 78:683-692.

Three distinct types of congenital hip dysplasia in adults were described. The authors also described the procedure and results of acetabuloplasty for adults with this disorder who undergo THA.

Healy WL, Lo TC, DeSimone AA, et al. (1995). Single-dose irradiation for the prevention of heterotopic ossification after total hip arthroplasty: A comparison of doses of five-hundred and fifty and seven hundred centigray. *J Bone Joint Surg Am* 77:590-595.

One hundred seven hips that were identified as high-risk for postoperative HO after THA were divided into two groups, one of which received a single 550-centigray dose of postoperative radiation, and the other of which received 700 centigray. These authors concluded that a dose of 700 centigray is effective for HO prophylaxis.

Heisel C, Silva M, Schmalzried TP (2004). Bearing surface options for total hip replacement in young patients. *Instr Course Lect* 53:49-65.

This comprehensive review article discusses the basic science of tribology and various bearing surfaces including UHMWPE, ceramics, and metals.

Hirsh J, Dalen JE, Anderson DR, et al. (1998). Oral anticoagulants: Mechanism of action, clinical effectiveness, and optimal therapeutic range. *Chest* 114:445S-469S.

This comprehensive review article discusses various types of oral anticoagulants.

Hussell JG, Rodriguez JA, Ganz R (1999). Technical complications of the Bernese periacetabular osteotomy. *Clin Orthop Relat Res* 363:81-92.

The authors retrospectively reviewed 500 cases of periacetabular osteotomy to determine the most common complications.

Iorio R, Healy WL (2002). Heterotopic ossification after total hip and total knee arthroplasty: Risk factors, prevention, and treatment. *J Am Acad Orthop Surg* 10:409-416.

This review article discusses all aspects of HO after THA and TKA procedures.

Jaroszynski G, Woodgate IG, Saleh KJ, Gross AE (2001). Total hip replacement for the dislocated hip. *Instr Course Lect* 50:307-316.

This review article discusses all aspects of the etiology and management of THA for hips with DDH.

Jasty M, Maloney WJ, Bragdon CR, et al. (1991). The initiation of failure in cemented femoral components of hip arthroplasty. *J Bone Joint Surg Br* 73:551-558.

Sixteen femora that were from cadaveric specimens that had previously undergone cemented THA were examined for evidence of loosening. The authors concluded that the loosening process in cemented implants begins at the cement-prosthesis interface and progresses further into the cement mantle.

Jazrawi LM, Kummer FJ, DiCesare PE (1998). Alternative bearing surfaces for total joint arthroplasty. *J Am Acad Orthop Surg* 6:198-203.

This review article discusses polyethylene wear-induced osteolysis and alternative bearing surfaces with more favorable wear characteristics such as ceramic and metal.

Jimenez ML, Tile M, Schenk RS (1997). Total hip replacement after acetabular fracture. *Orthop Clin North Am* 28:435-446.

This review article discusses preoperative, intraoperative, and postoperative management of THA in the setting of acetabular fractures.

Johanson NA, Pellicci PM, Tsairis P, Salvati EA (1983). Nerve injury in total hip arthroplasty. *Clin Orthop Relat Res* 179:214-222.

This is a retrospective review of 34 patients who suffered nerve injury after THA was performed. Risk factors for nerve injury are discussed. The authors demonstrated that 79% of patients had persistent neurologic dysfunction at an average of 3.7 years after the index THA.

Joshi A, Markovic L, Hardinge K, Murphy JC (2002). Total hip arthroplasty in ankylosing spondylitis: An analysis of 181 hips. *J Arthroplasty* 17:427-433.

The authors reviewed 181 patients who underwent THA with a concurrent diagnosis of ankylosing spondylitis at an average of 10.3 years postoperative follow-up. At latest follow-up, 96% of hips had excellent pain scores, and 29.2% of hips had nearly normal function.

Kallos T, Enis JE, Gollan F, Davis JH (1974). Intramedullary pressure and pulmonary embolism of femoral medullary contents in dogs during insertion of bone cement and a prosthesis. *J Bone Joint Surg Am* 56:1363-1367.

This seminal study, performed in an in vivo canine model, demonstrated the deleterious physiologic effects that resulted from the release of bone cement and marrow contents into the intravascular space.

Keating EM, Ritter MA, Faris PM (1990). Structures at risk from medially placed acetabular screws. *J Bone Joint Surg Am* 72:509-511.

The authors performed anatomic analysis of 10 cadaveric acetabula and 4 acetabula in vivo during gynecologic operations. These studies were used to construct models that demonstrate dangerous areas for the placement of acetabular screws.

Klaue K, Wallin A, Ganz R (1988). CT evaluation of coverage and congruency of the hip prior to osteotomy. *Clin Orthop Relat Res* 232:15-25.

A computer model that could better characterize the areas of deficiency of femoral head coverage and acetabular dysplasia in patients with DDH was described.

Koval KJ, ed (2002a). *Orthopaedic Knowledge Update* 7. Rosemont, IL, American Academy of Orthopaedic Surgeons, pp 47-53.

This review chapter discusses biomaterials and bearing surfaces in total joint arthroplasty.

Koval KJ, ed (2002b). *Orthopaedic Knowledge Update* 7. Rosemont, IL, American Academy of Orthopaedic Surgeons, pp 417-451.

This review chapter discusses hip and pelvis reconstruction.

Lachiewicz PF (1997). Rheumatoid arthritis of the hip. *J Am Acad Orthop Surg* 5:332-338.

This review article discusses the radiographic findings seen in patients with rheumatoid arthritis. The results of cemented and uncemented THA in rheumatoid patients are also discussed.

Lachiewicz PF, Kelley SS (2002). Constrained components in total hip arthroplasty. *J Am Acad Orthop Surg* 10:233-238.

This review article discusses the use of highly constrained THA devices in patients with recurrently unstable THAs. Various device designs are described.

Lack W, Windhager R, Kutschera HP, Engel A (1991). Chiari pelvic osteotomy for osteoarthritis secondary to hip dysplasia: Indications and long-term results. *J Bone Joint Surg Br* 73:229-234.

The authors reviewed 18 patients who underwent Chiari pelvic osteotomy for osteoarthritis and hip dysplasia at an average postoperative follow-up of 15.5 years. These authors concluded that patients who were more than 44 years old at the time of osteotomy had worse results and also that Chiari osteotomy has advantages over intertrochanteric osteotomy.

Lewallen DG (1997). Instructional Course Lectures, The American Academy of Orthopaedic Surgeons: Neurovascular injury associated with hip arthroplasty. *J Bone Joint Surg Am* 79:1870-1880.

> This comprehensive review article describes neurologic complications after THA. Central and peripheral nervous system complications and anatomic considerations in neurovascular injury are discussed.

Lewallen DG, Berry DJ (1997). Instructional Course Lectures, The American Academy of Orthopaedic Surgeons: Periprosthetic fracture of the femur after total hip arthroplasty. Treatment and results to date. *J Bone Joint Surg Am* 79:1881-1890.

> This comprehensive review article covers the history, prevalence, etiology, treatment, and results of periprosthetic femur fractures after THA.

Lieberman JR, et al. (2002). Osteonecrosis of the hip: Management in the twenty-first century. *J Bone Joint Surg Am* 84:834-853.

> This comprehensive review article discusses the etiology, pathophysiology, treatment options, and results of treatment of avascular necrosis of the hip.

MacDonald SJ, Hersche O, Ganz R (1999). Periacetabular osteotomy in the treatment of neurogenic acetabular dysplasia. *J Bone Joint Surg Br* 81:975-978.

> The authors reviewed Bernese periacetabular osteotomy performed in 13 dysplastic hips in patients with a concurrent neurologic disorder. Patients were on average 23 years of age at the time of the procedure and had 6.4 years of postoperative follow-up. These authors concluded that Bernese periacetabular osteotomy can be used successfully to treat dysplastic hips with a neurogenic etiology.

Maloney WJ III (1998). The cemented femoral component. In: Callaghan JJ, Rubash HE, Rosenberg AG, eds. *The Adult Hip.* Philadelphia: Lippincott-Raven, pp 959-979.

> This review chapter discusses all aspects of cemented femoral components in THA. Surgical technique, complications, and results are described.

Maloney WJ III (1995). Primary cemented total hip arthroplasty. In: Callaghan JJ, Dennis, DA, Paprosky WG, Rosenberg AG, eds. *Orthopaedic Knowledge Update: Hip and Knee Reconstruction.* Rosemont, IL: American Academy of Orthopaedic Surgeons, pp 179-189.

> This review chapter discusses many aspects of cemented THA.

Maloney WJ, Smith RL, Schmalzried TP, et al. (1995). Isolation and characterization of wear particles generated in patients who have had failure of a hip arthroplasty without cement. *J Bone Joint Surg Am* 77:1301-1310.

> The authors characterized wear particles that were isolated from tissue membranes obtained from 35 hips undergoing revision surgery. These authors determined that debris surrounding failed THA components are less than 1 μm in size and are found in a density of greater than 1 billion particles/g of tissue.

Masonis JL, Bourne RB (2002). Surgical approach, abductor function, and total hip arthroplasty dislocation. *Clin Orthop Relat Res* 405:46-53.

> This is a systematic literature review of articles pertaining to surgical approach and dislocation after THA was performed. The authors concluded that the current literature is insufficient to determine definitively whether certain surgical approaches are associated with higher dislocation rates.

McKellop H, Park SH, Chiesa R, et al. (1996). In vivo wear rates of three types of metal on metal hip prostheses during two decades of use. *Clin Orthop Relat Res* 329:S128-S140.

> The authors studied the wear patterns of 21 metal-metal THAs that were retrieved from patients after varying time periods of implantation. Light and scanning electron microscopy was performed. The patterns and volume of wear observed were described in detail.

Mears DC, Velyvis JH (2001). Primary total hip arthroplasty after acetabular fracture. *Instr Course Lect* 50:335-354.

> This comprehensive review article discusses in detail the complications encountered when performing THA in hips that previously suffered acetabular fractures.

Millis MB, Murphy SB, Poss R (1996). Osteotomies about the hip for the prevention and treatment of osteoarthritis. *Instr Course Lect* 45:209-226.

> This review article discusses in detail the various types of osteotomies available for treatment of osteoarthritis of the hip resulting from various causes including DDH and prior trauma.

Miniaci A, Bailey WH, Bourne RB, et al. (1990). Analysis of radionuclide arthrograms, radiographic arthrograms, and sequential plain radiographs in the assessment of painful hip arthroplasty. *J Arthroplasty* 5:143-149.

> The authors utilized and compared the efficacy of three radiographic modalities in the diagnosis of loose THA components; 65 painful THAs were evaluated over a 2-year period. The authors concluded that sequential plain radiographs were the most useful studies.

Mont MA, Hungerford DS (1997). Proximally coated ingrowth prostheses: A review. *Clin Orthop Relat Res* 344:139-149.

> This review article discusses the history of proximally porous-coated devices and the evolution of their design.

Mont MA, Jones LC, Sotereanos DG, et al. (2000). Understanding and treating osteonecrosis of the femoral head. *Instr Course Lect* 29:169-185.

> This comprehensive review article discusses the pathophysiology, etiology, treatment, and results of femoral head avascular necrosis.

Morrey BF (1997). Difficult complications after hip joint replacement: Dislocation. *Clin Orthop Relat Res* 344:179-187.

> The incidence and risk factors for persistent instability after THA are discussed. The results of various treatment options including acetabular reorientation, abductor advancement, and constrained liner implantation are also described.

Mulliken BD, Rorabeck CH, Bourne RB, Nayak N (1998). A modified direct lateral approach in total hip arthroplasty: A comprehensive review. *J Arthroplasty* 13:737-747.

> The authors reviewed 770 consecutive primary THAs performed utilizing a modified lateral approach to the hip joint that incises the anterior third of the abductor complex. The authors concluded that this approach significantly reduces the postoperative complications of instability and results in an acceptable level and severity of postoperative limp.

Mulroy RD Jr, Harris WH (1990). The effect of improved cementing techniques on component loosening in total hip replacement: An 11-year radiographic review. *J Bone Joint Surg Br* 72:757-760.

The authors reviewed 105 cemented THAs in which techniques that improved on first-generation cementing were utilized. They concluded that the use of devices such as cement guns and medullary plugs with advanced cement technique resulted in a significant decline in femoral component loosening.

Murphy S, Deshmukh R (2002). Periacetabular osteotomy: Preoperative radiographic predictors of outcome. *Clin Orthop Relat Res* 405:168-174.

The authors prospectively reviewed 95 consecutive hips that underwent periacetabular osteotomy for a minimum of 2 years after surgery. The authors concluded that periacetabular osteotomy is effective for improving coverage of hips with even grade 3 arthrosis and that preoperative functional radiographs are useful in predicting outcome.

Ninomiya S, Tagawa H (1984). Rotational acetabular osteotomy for the dysplastic hip. *J Bone Joint Surg Am* 66:430-436.

The authors reviewed 45 hips that underwent a rotational acetabular osteotomy at an average postoperative follow-up of 4.5 years. They concluded that the procedure was effective in reducing pain and limp and in improving range of motion.

Noble PC, Collier MB, Maltry JA, et al. (1998). Pressurization and centralization enhance the quality and reproducibility of cement mantles. *Clin Orthop Relat Res* 355:77-89.

The authors performed two laboratory studies in cadaveric and acrylic model femora to assess the effects of cement technique on the longevity of the cement mantle. They concluded that optimizations in the design of cement plugs and stem centralizers are important factors that can improve the longevity and quality of the cement mantle.

Nollen JG, van Douveren FQ (1993). Ectopic ossification in hip arthroplasty: A retrospective study of predisposing factors in 637 cases. *Acta Orthop Scand* 64:185-187.

These authors reviewed 673 hip arthroplasties to determine risk factors for the development of HO. The major risk factors identified for HO include male sex and cemented arthroplasty.

Numair J, Joshi AB, Murphy JC, et al. (1997). Total hip arthroplasty for congenital dysplasia or dislocation of the hip: Survivorship analysis and long-term results. *J Bone Joint Surg Am* 79:1352-1360.

The authors reviewed 141 THAs that were performed on patients with congenital acetabular dysplasia or hip dislocation. These authors demonstrated a 10% failure rate of the acetabular component and 3% for the femoral stem at 10-year follow-up.

Oyen WJ, Claessens RA, van Horn JR, et al. (1990). Scintigraphic detection of bone and joint infections with indium-111–labeled nonspecific human immunoglobulin G. *J Nucl Med* 31:403-412.

The authors evaluated the diagnostic sensitivity of indium-111 immunoglobulin G nuclear scans to detect infection in 32 patients with culture-verified infections of bone at the time of surgery. These authors determined that the technique is highly sensitive for diagnosing infection.

Paiement GD (1998). Prevention and treatment of venous thromboembolic disease complications in primary hip arthroplasty patients. In: Cannon WD Jr, ed. *Instructional Course Lectures 47*. Rosemont, IL: American Academy of Orthopaedic Surgeons, pp 331-335.

This brief review article discusses the efficacy of enoxaparin and warfarin in reducing post–total joint arthroplasty DVT and fatal pulmonary embolus.

Paterno SA, Lachiewicz PF, Kelley SS (1997). The influence of patient-related factors and the position of the acetabular component on the rate of dislocation after total hip replacement. *J Bone Joint Surg Am* 79:1202-1210.

This retrospective review discussed 446 patients who underwent either primary THA or revision THA performed to determine the predisposing factors for dislocation. These authors concluded that excessive alcohol intake may predispose patients to dislocation, whereas revision surgery was associated with increased dislocation. No association was noted between version or abduction of the acetabular component and dislocation.

Pellegrini VD Jr, Gregoritch SJ (1996). Preoperative irradiation for the prevention of heterotopic ossification following total hip arthroplasty. *J Bone Joint Surg Am* 78:870-881.

A prospective randomized trial comparing preoperative versus postoperative radiation dose of 800 centigray was conducted using 85 patients who were determined to have risk factors for HO after THA. The investigators concluded that preoperative radiation is effective for the prevention of HO after THA.

Pellegrini VD Jr, Konski AA, Gastel JA, et al. (1992). Prevention of heterotopic ossification with irradiation after total hip arthroplasty: Radiation therapy with a single dose of eight hundred centigray administered to a limited field. *J Bone Joint Surg Am* 74:186-200.

In this study, 62 hips considered at high risk for HO were given either 800 or 1000 centigray of radiation. The authors concluded that single-dose limited-field radiation is effective for preventing postoperative HO without affecting the fixation of uncemented implants.

Pellicci PM, Bostrom M (1998). Posterior approach to total hip replacement using enhanced posterior soft tissue repair. *Clin Orthop Relat Res* 355:224-228.

The authors demonstrated a significant reduction in postoperative dislocation of THA when an enhanced posterior soft tissue repair was used at the time of initial THA.

Pellicci PM, Tria AJ, Garvin KL (2000). *Orthopaedic Knowledge Update: Hip and Knee Reconstruction 2*. Rosemont, IL: American Academy of Orthopaedic Surgeons, pp 3-217.

A comprehensive review section covers the basic science of total joint arthroplasty, bearing surfaces, and outcomes. The section also covers several aspects of THA including biomechanics, cemented and uncemented THA, osteolysis, and revision THA.

Pemberton PA (1965). Pericapsular osteotomy of the ilium for the treatment of congenital subluxation and dislocation of the hip. *J Bone Joint Surg Am* 47:65-86.

This is the original article in which the surgical technique of Pemberton osteotomy is described.

Pitto RP, Hamer H, Fabiani R, et al. (2002). Prophylaxis against fat and bone-marrow embolism during total hip arthroplasty reduces the incidence of postoperative deep-vein thrombosis: A controlled, randomized clinical trial. *J Bone Joint Surg Am* 84:39-48.

The authors conducted a prospective, randomized study on 130 consecutive patients who had THA to determine whether reduction of fat and marrow content embolization during the insertion of cemented femoral components during THA could reduce postoperative DVT and pulmonary embolus. They utilized a bone vacuum device to reduce embolic events during THA and also to reduce postoperative DVT.

Ranawat CS, Dorr LD, Inglis AE (1980). Total hip arthroplasty in protrusion acetabuli of rheumatoid arthritis. *J Bone Joint Surg Am* 62:1059-1065.

The authors reviewed 35 THAs performed in patients with rheumatoid arthritis and protrusion acetabuli with an average follow-up of 4.3 years; 66% of patients had good or excellent results. The authors concluded that improved fixation can be achieved by use of bone graft, mesh, or an acetabular shell.

Ranawat CS, Peters LE (1997). Fixation of the acetabular component: The case for cement. *Clin Orthop Relat Res* 344:207-215.

The authors discussed the benefits of using cemented THA in patients older than 60 years of age.

Ranawat CS, Rodriguez JA (1997). Functional leg-length inequality following total hip arthroplasty. *J Arthroplasty* 12:359-364.

The authors reviewed a consecutive series of 100 patients who underwent primary THA to assess the prevalence of functional leg-length inequality; 14% of patients were found to have functional leg-length inequality 1 month after surgery, but symptoms had resolved in all patients after 6 months.

Robinson RP, Lovell TP, Green TM, Bailey GA (1989). Early femoral component loosening in DF-80 total hip arthroplasty. *J Arthoplasty* 4:55-64.

The authors reviewed 47 DF-80 THAs and demonstrated that early failure and loosening of femoral components may be related to weakening of the proximal cement-bone interface combined with a proximally loading stem design.

Romness DW, Lewallen DG (1990). Total hip arthroplasty after fracture of the acetabulum: Long-term results. *J Bone Joint Surg Br* 72:761-764.

The authors retrospectively reviewed 55 THAs that were performed after previous acetabular fracture and demonstrated increased rates of loosening and revision of both the femoral and acetabular components compared with THAs that did not have a history of previous acetabular fracture.

Romness DW, Morrey BF (1992). Total knee arthroplasty in patients with prior ipsilateral hip fusion. *J Arthroplasty* 7:63-70.

The authors reviewed 16 TKAs in patients with prior ipsilateral hip fusion and concluded that conversion of hip fusion to THA before ipsilateral TKA can improve the outcome in these patients.

Salvati EA, Pellegrini VD Jr, Sharrock NE, et al. (2000). Recent advances in venous thromboembolic prophylaxis during and after total hip replacement. *J Bone Joint Surg Am* 82:252-270.

This comprehensive review article discussed the entire spectrum of currently available agents for prophylaxis against DVT after THA.

Sanchez-Sotelo J, Berry DJ, Trousdale RT, Cabanela ME (2002). Surgical treatment of developmental dysplasia of the hip in adults II: Arthroplasty options. *J Am Acad Orthop Surg* 10:334-344.

This review article discusses the surgical difficulties encountered in implanting THAs in patients with DDH.

Santore RF (1995). Hip reconstruction: Nonarthroplasty. In: Callaghan JJ, Dennis DA, Paprosky WG, Rosenberg AG, eds. *Orthopaedic Knowledge Update: Hip and Knee Reconstruction.* Rosemont, IL: American Academy of Orthopaedic Surgeons, pp 109-115.

This review chapter discusses hip and femoral osteotomies for the treatment of hip arthritis.

Santore RF, Kantor SR (2004). Intertrochanteric femoral osteotomies for developmental and posttraumatic conditions. *J Bone Joint Surg Am* 86:2542-2553.

The advantages of using intertrochanteric femoral osteotomy over THA for the treatment of post-traumatic arthritis are discussed in detail.

Schmalzried TP, Callaghan JJ (1999). Wear in total hip and knee replacements. *J Bone Joint Surg Am* 81:115-136.

This comprehensive review article describes the basic and clinical science of polyethylene-induced wear in total joint arthroplasty.

Schmalzried TP, Noordin S, Amstutz HC (1997). Update on nerve palsy associated with total hip replacement. *Clin Orthop Relat Res* 344:188-206.

This review article discusses the incidence, etiology, prognosis, and treatment of nerve palsy after THA.

Schulte KR, Callaghan JJ, Kelley SS, Johnston RC (1993). The outcome of Charnley total hip arthroplasty with cement after a minimum twenty-year follow-up: The results of one surgeon. *J Bone Joint Surg Am* 75:961-975.

The authors reviewed 330 Charnley THAs at an average 20-year postoperative follow-up. A 10% revision rate was demonstrated, with 2% revised for infection, 7% for aseptic loosening, and 1% for dislocation.

Schwartz JT, Mayer JG, Engh CA (1989). Femoral fracture during noncemented total hip arthroplasty. *J Bone Joint Surg Am* 71:1135-1142.

The authors reviewed 1318 consecutive uncemented THAs and found an intraoperative fracture rate of 3%, of which only 50% were diagnosed intraoperatively. These authors concluded that such fractures did not adversely affect the long-term outcome.

Scifert CF, Brown TD, Pedersen DR, Callaghan JJ (1998). A finite element analysis of factors influencing total hip dislocation. *Clin Orthop Relat Res* 355:152-162.

A validated three-dimensional finite element model was used to determine that increasing the femoral head size significantly improved stability, as did increased component anteversion. However, increased anteversion did increase the probability of anterior dislocation.

Shanbhag AS, Jacobs JJ, Glant TT, et al. (1994). Composition and morphology of wear debris in failed uncemented total hip replacement. *J Bone Joint Surg Br* 76:60-67.

The membranes found at the bone-prosthesis interface at time of revision in 11 failed cementless THAs were analyzed for wear particles. Polyethylene particles, titanium particles, bone, stainless steel, and silicate particles were all found in these membranes.

Sharkey PF, Hozack WJ, Callaghan JJ, et al. (1999). Acetabular fracture associated with cementless acetabular component insertion: A report of thirteen cases. *J Arthroplasty* 14:426-341.

A retrospective review of 13 cases of intraoperative acetabular fracture during insertion of cementless acetabula during primary THA demonstrated that oversized components and osteoporotic bone may indicate the use of line-to-line technique and even cemented acetabula to prevent this complication.

Sharrock NE, Go G, Harpel PC, et al. (1995). The John Charnley Award. Thrombogenesis during total hip arthroplasty. *Clin Orthop Relat Res* 319:16-27.

The authors discussed the findings that increased thrombogenic activity occurs during placement of the femoral component during THA and that measures to prevent DVT may be taken intraoperatively to reduce the risk of this complication postoperatively.

Shoenfeld NA, Stuchin SA, Pearl R, Haveson S (1990). The management of vascular injuries associated with total hip arthroplasty. *J Vasc Surg* 11:549-555.

The authors reviewed a total of 68 cases of intraoperative vascular injury during THA to demonstrate that increased risk for this complication exists during revision procedures, left-sided procedures, and when there is protrusion of the acetabular component into the pelvis.

Simon SS, ed (1994). Orthopaedic Basic Science. Rosemont, IL: American Academy of Orthopaedic Surgeons, pp 449-496.

Smith SE, Harris WH (1997). Total hip arthroplasty performed with insertion of the femoral component with cement and the acetabular component without cement: Ten to thirteen-year study. *J Bone Joint Surg Am* 79:1827-1833.

The authors retrospectively reviewed 52 consecutive hybrid THAs (uncemented acetabulum with screws and cemented femoral component with second generation technique). The authors demonstrated that such prostheses performed well at the 10- to 13-year follow-up interval, but with a relatively high dislocation rate.

Smith SW, Estok DM 2nd, Harris WH (1998). Total hip arthroplasty with use of second-generation cementing techniques: An eighteen-year-average follow-up study. *J Bone Joint Surg Am* 80:1632-1640.

The authors reviewed 140 patients who underwent cemented THA with a "second-generation" cementing technique. They demonstrated that femoral components implanted with these techniques performed better than acetabular components implanted with the same technique.

Solheim LF, Hagen R (1980). Femoral and sciatic neuropathies after total hip arthroplasty. *Acta Orthop Scand* 51:531-534.

The authors reviewed six patients who had sciatic, femoral, or combined neuropathies after THA. The incidence of such nerve injury was 0.7%.

Spector M (1987). Historical review of porous-coated implants. *J Arthoplasty* 2:163-177.

This review article described the origins, evolution, and results of cementless THA.

Sponseller PD, McBeath AA, Perich M (1984). Hip arthrodesis in young patients: A long-term follow-up study. *J Bone Joint Surg Am* 66:853-859.

The authors reviewed 53 hip arthrodeses at an average postoperative follow-up of 38 years; 78% of patients had reported satisfaction with their functional status at latest follow-up.

Sporer SM, Callaghan JJ, Olejniczak JP, et al. (1999). The effects of surface roughness and polymethylmethacrylate precoating on the radiographic and clinical results of the Iowa hip prosthesis: A study of patients less than fifty years old. *J Bone Joint Surg Am* 81:481-492.

The authors compared the results of two different types of THAs with different surface finishes (grit-blasted versus bead-blasted). They concluded that femoral components with a polished surface fixed with cement performed better than the grit-blasted components.

Steinberg ME (1994). Early diagnosis, evaluation, and staging of osteonecrosis. *Instr Course Lect* 43:513-518.

This comprehensive review article discusses the diagnosis, imaging, radiographic staging, prognosis, and treatment of femoral head avascular necrosis.

Tan V, Klotz MJ, Greenwald AS, Steinberg ME (1998). Carry it on the bad side! *Am J Orthop* 27:673-677.

The authors used free-body diagram analysis to determine that carrying heavy objects on the side of the body most affected by pain and arthritis will result in decreased load and pain to that joint.

Tannenbaum DA, Matthews LS (1997). Infection around joint replacements in patients who have a renal or liver transplantation. *J Bone Joint Surg Am* 79:36-43.

The authors reviewed 35 joint replacements in patients who had previously undergone organ transplantation. They demonstrated an infection risk of 19% after joint arthroplasty in such patients.

Trousdale RT, Ekkernkamp A, Ganz R, Wallrichs SL (1995). Periacetabular and intertrochanteric osteotomy for the treatment of osteoarthrosis in dysplastic hips. *J Bone Joint Surg Am* 77:73-85.

This report described 42 patients who underwent periacetabular osteotomy with and without intertrochanteric femoral osteotomy. These patients were followed for an average of 4 years. The investigators demonstrated an average improvement in Harris hip score of 24 points for these patients.

Trousdale RT, Ganz R (1998). Periacetabular osteotomy. In: Callaghan JJ, Rosenberg AG, Rubash HE, eds. *The Adult Hip*. Philadelphia: Lippincott-Raven, pp 789-802.

This review chapter discusses in detail the various types of periacetabular osteotomies, including indications and technique.

Udomkiat P, Dorr LD (2002). Cementless hemispheric porous-coated sockets implanted with press-fit technique without screws: Average ten-year follow-up. *J Bone Joint Surg Am* 84:1195-1200.

In this article, 132 primary THAs performed with cementless acetabular components without screws were reviewed. The investigators found a 12-year revision-free survival rate of 95.3%.

Urban RM, Jacobs JJ, Sumner DR, et al. (1996). The bone-implant interface of femoral stems with non-circumferential porous coating. *J Bone Joint Surg Am* 78:1068-1081.

Ten cadaveric specimens that had previously been implanted with noncircumferentially porous-coated femoral stems underwent histologic analysis. The analysis demonstrated that uncoated areas had less bony ingrowth than did coated areas.

Urbanski SR, de Lange EE, Eschenroeder HC Jr (1991). Magnetic resonance imaging of transient osteoporosis of the hip: A case report. *J Bone Joint Surg Am* 73:451-455.

This report described the MRI diagnosis of transient osteoporosis of the hip. The MRI findings of this condition were compared with those of osteonecrosis of the hip.

Urquhart AG, D'Lima DD, Venn-Watson E, et al. (1998). Polyethylene wear after total hip arthroplasty: The effect of a modular femoral head with and extended flange-reinforced neck. *J Bone Joint Surg Am* 80:1641-1647.

The authors reviewed 100 primary THAs to determine the effects of modular femoral heads with extended flanges on polyethylene wear. They determined that this design feature does increase polyethylene wear.

Waddell JP (2001). Evidence-based orthopedics. *J Bone Joint Surg Am* 83:788.

The article showed the findings of a randomized, double-blinded, placebo-controlled trial to determine the efficacy of preoperative erythropoietin in reducing the need for blood transfusion after total joint arthroplasty. The authors demonstrated the erythropoietin does reduce the need for allogeneic blood transfusion after arthroplasty.

Wasielewski RC, Cooperstein L (1990). Acetabular anatomy and the transacetabular fixation of screws in total hip arthroplasty. *J Bone Joint Surg Am* 72:501-508.

The authors performed anatomic dissection and analysis of cadaveric pelvic specimens to determine the safe zones for placement of acetabular screws during THA.

White RE (1998). Evaluation of the painful total hip arthroplasty. In: Callaghan JJ, Rosenberg AG, Rubash HE, eds. *The Adult Hip*. Philadelphia: Lippincott-Raven, vol 2, pp 1377-1385.

This review chapter discusses all aspects of the diagnostic workup and treatment of painful THA.

Woo RY, Morrey BF (1982). Dislocations after total hip arthroplasty. *J Bone Joint Surg Am* 64:1295-1306.

The authors retrospectively reviewed 10,500 THAs. They determined that prior hip surgery was the strongest predictor of dislocation after primary THA. Trochanteric osteotomy nonunion was also a significant risk factor.

Wright TM (1991). Ultra-high molecular weight polyethylene. In: Morrey BF, ed. *Joint Replacement Arthroplasty*. New York: Churchill Livingstone, pp 37-46.

This comprehensive review chapter covers all aspects of polyethylene in total joint arthroplasty.

Total Knee Arthroplasty

Javad Parvizi,* Peter Sharkey,† and James A. Sanfilippo‡

*MD, FRCS, Associate Professor, Jefferson Medical College, Rothman Institute, Thomas Jefferson University, Philadelphia, PA
†MD, Professor of Orthopaedic Surgery, Jefferson Medical College, Rothman Institute, Thomas Jefferson University, Philadelphia, PA
‡MD, MHS, Resident, Department of Orthopaedic Surgery, Thomas Jefferson University Hospital, Philadelphia, PA

Introduction

- Primary total knee arthroplasty (TKA) continues to be a highly successful procedure, resulting in good pain relief and functional improvement.
- Patient selection remains the key to surgical success. The population that demonstrates the best functional results is the older, less active group of patients in whom conservative medical management has failed. Overall, patient selection criteria for primary TKA should include pain, severe arthritis on radiographs, and the inability to perform the activities of daily living.
- Contraindications include nonfunctional extensor mechanism, neuromuscular disease, vascular disease of the affected extremity, and active infection (Box 9–1). Age and body habitus continue to be challenges. Younger, more active patients may place higher demands on implants, leading to earlier wear and the need for revision. Obese patients are technically more challenging, and they place higher stress on implants that leads to early wear and revision (Bugbee et al. 1998).

Nonsurgical Options

- These options are listed in Box 9–2.

Nonpharmacologic Treatment

- Weight loss, muscle strengthening and stretching, and low-impact aerobic exercise play crucial roles in physical therapy for knee osteoarthritis (van Baar et al. 1998).
- Other nonpharmacologic therapies include lateral shoe wedges and unloader braces. Lateral shoe wedges decrease the varus moment of the leg and lead to reduction of the medial compartment load. This approach tends to be more effective in the early stages of disease. Varus or valgus unloader braces work in similar fashion by "unloading" either the medial or lateral compartment by exerting a varus or valgus force on the knee. These braces are useful in compliant patients with severe disease in only one of the compartments and with a correctable deformity (Kirkley et al. 1999, Lindenfeld et al. 1997).

Pharmacologic Treatment

- The first line in this treatment continues to be the nonsteroidal anti-inflammatory drugs (NSAIDs). These are directed at inhibiting the synthesis of the cyclooxygenase (COX) family of enzymes. Traditional NSAIDs inhibit both COX-1 and COX-2. These agents have potentially serious side effects including peptic ulcer disease, impaired renal functioning, liver toxicity, bleeding, and death (Laine et al. 1999).
- Within the past decade or so, selective COX-2 inhibitors were introduced. They provided the same anti-inflammatory effects without these side effects. More recently, however, these drugs have come under scrutiny for potentially increased risks of myocardial infarction, stroke, and sudden cardiac death.

Box 9–1	Contraindications to Total Knee Arthroplasty

- Nonfunctional extensor mechanism
- Neuromuscular disease
- Vascular disease of the affected extremity
- Active infection

Box 9–2	Nonsurgical Options in Total Knee Arthroplasty

- Anti-inflammatory medications: Nonsteroidal anti-inflammatory drugs, cyclooxygenase-2 inhibitors
- Physical therapy
- Weight loss
- Intra-articular injection: Narcotics and steroids versus hyaluronic acid

- Another treatment option, aimed at the inflammatory process, is an intra-articular injection of steroid and local anesthetic. These treatments tend to be less predictable and are often only transiently effective.
- Intra-articular injections of hyaluronic acid, (viscosupplementation), may restore some viscous and elastic properties of the synovial fluid and may result in decreased pain and improved functioning. Clinical studies are not conclusive in their results of knee functional improvement with viscosupplementation. However, this approach has been shown to be at least as equally efficacious as NSAIDs in all areas except activity restriction. One complication of viscosupplementation is a localized, potentially serious, local inflammatory response. This response seems to be additive and can mimic septic arthritis in the severity of the knee effusion after the third injection (Adams et al. 1995, Rosier and O'Keefe 2000).

Implant Selection

- Posterior cruciate ligament (PCL)–sparing, PCL-sacrificing, and mobile bearing/rotating platform knee implants have been used and studied for years (Buechel and Pappas 1990).
- PCL-sparing knees were originally designed to maintain stability and proprioception of the knee. Multiple studies have demonstrated that overall survivorship of cemented PCL-sparing knees is at least 90% at 10 years. However, clinical studies suggest that the PCL does not function properly following arthroplasty, and preoperative, intraoperative, and postoperative damage may even lead to increased knee instability following implantation of a PCL-sparing implant (Ritter et al. 1994).
- Most studies have shown that the use of a PCL-substituting/sacrificing knee implant leads to no increase in instability or range of motion. In addition, clinical evaluation has demonstrated no difference in proprioception between PCL-sparing and PCL-sacrificing knees after TKA. Posterior femoral rollback is reproducible in the clinical studies using these implants (Ranawat et al. 1993).
- The rotating platform, or mobile bearing knee, was designed to try to limit polyethylene wear by reducing metal-polyethylene contact stress, thus leading to increased survivorship of the knee. One study demonstrated excellent results at 10 to 13 years, with no evidence of osteolysis, no bearing dislocations, and no revisions performed for mechanical failure of the implant (Callaghan et al. 2000).

Fixation

- Cementing in the prosthesis has been proven to have the best overall short-term fixation. However, the use of cement has been linked to increased osteolysis from third-body wear, and thus early failure.
- Uncemented implants were designed to limit this third-body wear. One study demonstrated good fixation results at 12 years with uncemented components. This study showed decreased radiolucent lines, evidence of osteolysis (Bassett 1998).

Surgical Approaches

Operating Room Setup

- The patient should be placed supine on the operating table in the middle of the laminar flow area of the room.
- The use of laminar flow rooms has been shown to decrease the overall infection rate during TKA (Ayers et al. 1997).
- A tourniquet may be used during the procedure to limit bleeding into the surgical field. If it is to be employed, it should be placed on the operative leg as proximally on the thigh as possible. The tourniquet should be set for between 250 and 300 psi, depending on the size of the patient, with larger patients requiring increased pressure because of increased soft tissue mass. Tourniquet use has been linked to postoperative nerve palsies and vascular injuries.
- A bump should be placed distally. It should be placed at the level of the foot when the hip is flexed to 45 degrees and the knee flexed to 90 degrees. This bump acts as a foot rest and allows the maintenance of knee flexion at 90 degrees during the procedure. It also precludes the need for an additional assistant to hold the patient's foot to maintain flexion.
- The surgical site should be prepared in the usual sterile fashion and should be draped widely, both proximally to distally and medially to laterally.
- Before the incision is made, the proposed skin incision site should be marked, and the tourniquet should then be inflated.

Approach

- Exposure is essential in performing TKA. When possible, a midline skin incision should be used to ensure good visualization of both the medial and lateral compartments.
- If a prior surgical skin incision exists, it should be used as long as proper exposure can be obtained. If proper exposure cannot be obtained through the prior incision, this former incision site should be ignored, and a midline incision used, with care taken not to compromise skin integrity further.
- Through a midline skin incision, the choice of arthrotomy incisions includes medial and lateral parapatellar, subvastus, and midvastus approaches.

- With the more popular *medial parapatellar approach*, the quadriceps tendon is incised longitudinally, leaving a small medial cuff to help aid in closure. The entire extensor mechanism is then retracted laterally to provide exposure to the joint. The incision into the quadriceps tendon may lead to extensor mechanism weakening.
- The *subvastus approach* was designed to avoid incising the quadriceps tendon and thus protect the integrity of the extensor mechanism. However, with this approach, the potential exists to injure the femoral artery, and exposure to the lateral compartment is limited (Matsueda and Gustilo 2000).
- With the *midvastus, or vastus splitting approach*, danger to the femoral artery is limited. This approach avoids incising the quadriceps tendon, while still proving adequate exposure to the knee joint (Engh and Parks 1998).

Surgical Techniques

- Overall alignment and ligament balancing are vital to proper functioning and survivorship of the TKA. The goal is to provide a slight valgus aligned knee with the tibial component perpendicular to the tibial shaft, full range of motion from at least 0 to 125 degrees, and midline tracking patella throughout that range. In addition, the knee should have good ligament balance at 0, 30, 60, and 90 degrees of flexion.
- The tibial side should be cut perpendicular to the tibial axis. Both intramedullary and extramedullary cutting guides can be employed with equal efficacy.
- On the femoral side, intramedullary guides have been shown to be more accurate than extramedullary guides that rely on often obscured landmarks. The femoral cut should be made with 4 to 6 degrees of valgus.
- If the tibial component is perpendicular to the tibial shaft and the femoral component is in 4 to 6 degrees of valgus, the knee should be in 4 to 6 degrees of valgus, which is ideal.

Ligament Balancing

- Varus deformity, or medial side tightness, is corrected by a stepwise release of the medial soft tissue structures, the capsule, the pes anserine tendons, and the medial collateral ligament.
- In correcting valgus deformity, there is no stepwise sequence. However, preserving the integrity of the iliotibial band and protecting the lateral collateral ligament are thought to prevent overcorrection.
- Flexion contractures can be corrected with a posterior capsule release or by examining the flexion-extension gap and correcting bony cuts or changing implant size.
- The *flexion-extension gap* refers to the knee tightness at 90 degrees of flexion and at full extension (Box 9–3). It is affected by the tibial cut and polyethylene size in both flexion and extension, the distal femoral cut in extension

Box 9–3	Summary of Flexion-Extension Gap Correction in Total Knee Arthroplasty

Knee Balance	Options
Tight in flexion and extension	Remove more tibial bone and/or use smaller polyethylene
Tight in flexion only	Remove more posterior femoral bone and/or use smaller femoral component
Tight in extension only	Remove more distal femoral bone
Loose in flexion and extension	Use larger polyethylene
Loose in flexion only	Use larger femoral component and/or use posterior femoral augments
Loose in extension only	Use distal femoral augments

only, and the posterior femoral cut and femoral component size in flexion only.

- If a knee is tight in both flexion and extension, more bone may be taken from the tibial side or a smaller polyethylene insert may be used.
- If a knee is tight in extension but satisfactory in flexion, more distal femoral bone may be taken.
- If a knee is satisfactory in extension but tight in flexion, more posterior femoral bone may be taken. The size of the femoral component refers to the medial to lateral size as well as to the anterior to posterior size. Thus, by downsizing the femoral component, there is a decreased anteroposterior diameter, which helps restore the flexion gap in a knee tight in flexion only.
- Conversely, if a knee is loose in both flexion and extension, a larger polyethylene insert may be used to restore the gap. For a knee that is loose in extension only, distal femoral augments may be employed. If a knee is loose in flexion only, upsizing the femoral component or using posterior femoral augments may help.

Patellar Tracking

- Rotational positioning of the femoral and tibial components is key to proper tracking. Slight external rotation of both the femoral and tibial components, essentially medializing the patella, has been shown to provide good patellar tracking and to limit patellar dislocation following TKA (Lewonowski et al. 1997, Olcott and Scott 1999).
- Patellar resurfacing has been shown to reduce anterior knee pain, and by resurfacing at the time of the initial surgical procedure, the need for revision surgery for recalcitrant knee pain is reduced. However, patellar resurfacing remains controversial. The advantages of not resurfacing include shorter operative and tourniquet times, maintenance of the bone stack, and a decreased risk of patellar fracture.

Postoperative Management
Postoperative Pain Management

- Common methods of pain control include epidural anesthesia, patient-controlled analgesia, and parenteral narcotics.
- The increased use of epidural anesthesia during TKA has led to an increased use of epidural analgesia postoperatively. The epidural catheter is left in place for 1 to 3 days, and narcotics or anesthetics can be injected. With this technique, a high degree of pain control can be achieved. Studies have demonstrated that patients with epidural analgesia have shorter hospital stays and an increase in early knee range of motion. Potential side effects with epidural analgesia are nausea, hypotension, and respiratory depression. Another concern is the need for patient-controlled analgesia or parenteral narcotics following catheter removal. In addition, nerve palsies, particularly peroneal nerve palsy, may go undiagnosed for a longer period of time because of a high level of anesthesia control (Horlocker et al. 1994, Ilahi et al. 1994).
- Parenteral narcotic injections have been used for years following TKA. With this approach comes a familiarity with their use and with proper dosing. These injections are normally administered on an as-needed basis. Limitations with this type of pain control include administration in elderly patients, who may be more sensitive, the inability to "stay out in front" of the pain, especially after sleep, and the strict nature of the timed dosing of these agents.
- Patient-controlled analgesia was designed to allow patients to have control over their own analgesia. Narcotics are administered in set doses and/or at a set rate that the patient can receive with a push of a button. Careful monitoring of the patient-controlled analgesia machine setup is required to ensure that the correct dose and the correct rate are set.

Physical Therapy and Range-of-Motion Exercises

- Many patients begin ambulating as early as the first day postoperatively. The use of a walker, cane, or crutches is dependent on the patient and the institution.
- Early range-of-motion goals include flexion and full extension. The use of continuous passive motion (CPM) machines is controversial. Proponents of CPM machines show that the patients achieve greater flexion arcs sooner than without the use of this device. In addition, there are reports of decreased analgesia, deep vein thrombosis, and manipulations with the use of the CPM machine. Opponents show that flexion is unchanged at 1 year postoperatively and there is no increase in the rate of manipulation. In addition, CPM machines may lead to wound healing complications and larger postoperative blood loss (Kumar et al. 1996, McInnes et al. 1992, Ververeli et al. 1995).

Results

- The cemented PCL-retaining knee has been used since the early 1980s. Most recent studies show a 10-year survivorship between 92% and 97%. The reasons for revision include aseptic loosening, extensor mechanism rupture or malfunction, polyethylene wear, and patella failures. The Knee Society scores have shown good to excellent results ranging between 88% and 94% (Ritter et al. 1994).
- The PCL-sacrificing, posteriorly stabilized TKA has been looked at since the mid-1990s. Most studies report a Knee Society score with good to excellent results ranging between 90% and 98%. Furthermore, 7- to 10-year survivorship ranges between 88% and 97% in the studies with the longest follow-up. Failures are attributed to aseptic loosening, patellar tracking problems, fracture, and flexion instability (Colizza et al. 1995).
- The mobile bearing knee has been used since 1977. Multiple designs, including bicruciate sparing, PCL sparing, and rotating platform, have all been employed. Published results seem to be very similar to those with the PCL-retaining knee. Although no large studies exist, Knee Society scores average near 93% at 10 to 15 years. In addition, 10- to 18-year survivorship ranges between 88% and 94% (Buechel 1998).
- Uncemented TKA is newer than cemented TKA and has had 33% to 94% good and excellent results at 5 to 10 years of follow-up. There is also a higher revision rate, with some studies quoting between 10% and 21% at 10 years. One study showed a 90% rate of osteolysis at 7 years and a 50% rate of patellar loosening. Once again, polyethylene wear was also noted in all these studies (Bassett 1998).
- Successful results have been obtained in young patients, those less than 50 years old, with inflammatory arthritis. Three studies investigated results in this population and showed marked improvement in pain and range of motion. Survivorship at 7 to 10 years ranges between 95% and 98%. In all patients with rheumatoid arthritis, successful improvement in pain and range of motion is also seen. Knee Society scores are less reliable secondary to the differing functioning levels preoperatively, but survivorship at 10 years seems to be between 88% and 93% (Dalury et al. 1995, Gill et al. 1997).

Complications

- Complications include infection, patellar difficulties, fracture, wound healing, and neurovascular problems.
- These complications not only lead to revision surgery and increased recovery times, but also place an enormous load on the economy. With an estimated 300,000 TKAs performed per year, the estimated cost to treat the infections alone is more than $250 million annually.

Infection

- The current overall infection rate is approximately 1% to 2%. The overall infection rate in revision TKA is 5% to 7%. The infection rates following primary TKA are higher in patients with rheumatoid arthritis (4% to 10% in the literature) and in diabetic patients (3% to 7%). Both these subsets of patients tend to have higher rates of malnutrition, skin breakdown, and wound healing complications, thus predisposing them to deeper infections. Other factors associated with increased infection rates include obesity, malignancy, concurrent other site infection, and oral steroid use (Ayers et al. 1997).
- Prevention of infection relies strongly on prophylactic perioperative antibiotics. The first dose should be given 5 to 30 minutes preoperatively and then for 24 hours postoperatively. Cefazolin, vancomycin, and clindamycin continue to be the drugs of choice in TKA (Friedman et al. 1990).
- Other important methods in infection prevention include the use of sterile surgical technique, ultraviolet light, closed-air exhaust suits, laminar flow operating room systems, antibiotic irrigation, and antibiotic-impregnated cement.
- Infections can be classified in multiple ways. *Superficial infection* refers to any infection of the skin or subcutaneous tissues. It does not cross the fascial layer and enter the joint space. It has a very good prognosis with early antibiotic and surgical treatment. *Deep infection* refers to subfascial infection, meaning it is deep to the fascial layer and in the joint space (Mont et al. 1997).
  - Identifying the infection as superficial or deep may be challenging, but with a good history and physical, laboratory analysis, and joint aspiration, an accurate diagnosis can be made (Duff et al. 1996).
  - Another way to classify infection is based on the length or duration of the infection. Most authors use 2 weeks as the line between acute and chronic infections. The studies show that when treatment is based on duration of symptoms, results can be predictable and successful.
- Diagnosing the infection is the first step to successful treatment (Box 9–4).
  - The history should include any fevers or chills, any recent infections, any drainage, and increased pain with ambulation, weight bearing, or range of motion.
  - Physical examination should note the presence of edema, erythema, increased warmth of the knee, or any drainage or skin sloughing.
  - Laboratory analysis is helpful in making this diagnosis. The overall white blood cell count may or may not be elevated in an acute infection. The erythrocyte sedimentation rate is elevated, but although it is very sensitive, it is not very specific. C-reactive protein levels are also elevated, and this value is more specific than the

Box 9–4	**Diagnosing Infections After Total Knee Arthroplasty**

- History and physical examination: Fever and chills, recent infections, increased pain with range of motion and ambulation, swelling, redness, increased warmth, drainage
- Laboratory analysis: White blood cell count, C-reactive protein, erythrocyte sedimentation rate very sensitive but not very specific (especially within the first 3 weeks following total knee arthroplasty)
- Joint aspiration: Note the quality and quantity of fluid, white blood cell count (>2500 consistent with infection), Gram stain, culture

erythrocyte sedimentation rate. However, in the 2 to 3 weeks immediately postoperatively, these values are less specific in diagnosing infection because they are elevated from the inflammation of surgery.
- The standard in diagnosing postoperative infection remains *joint aspiration.* Aspirate can be sent for Gram stain and culture to identify the bacteria, as well as a cell count in which a white blood cell count greater than 2500 in a prosthetic joint is consistent with infection (Duff et al. 1996).
- Several treatment options exist, but aggressive treatment of the infection is essential to its eradication and prevention of deep sepsis.
- Nonsurgical options, such as long-term intravenous antibiotics, have an eradication rate between 10% and 15%. This is because the antibiotics cannot penetrate the bacterial glycocalyx that forms. In addition, bacteria may be present between the bone and components, thus making antibiotic penetration impossible. For this reason, most authors recommend intravenous antibiotics only for patients in whom the infection was diagnosed within 48 hours, an infection with penicillin-sensitive streptococcus, and those that cannot tolerate more aggressive surgical débridement.
- Open irrigation and débridement with retention of the components potentially offer more thorough débridement, possibility for polyethylene exchange, and a lower morbidity than a more aggressive surgery. However, eradication rates for open incision and drainage are reported between 25% and 75% (Mont et al. 1997).
- One-stage prosthesis exchange allows for removal of infected components and cement with extensive débridement. The reported eradication rates for the one-stage revision range from 30% to 80%.
- The standard for treatment of deep infection remains a two-stage revision, with removal of infected components, implantation of antibiotic-impregnated spacer, a course of intravenous antibiotics, and reimplantation at a later surgery. Success rates for this procedure are between 77% and 90% survivorship at 10 years (Ayers et al. 1997, Backe et al. 1996).

Patellofemoral Complications

- These complications range from 2% to 10%, and many patients with these complications require revision surgery.
- *Patellar clunk* is one of these complications. A soft tissue nodule forms on the undersurface of the quadriceps tendon and during active extension rides over the femoral component and makes a painful clunking sensation. More recent femoral component designs and the use of smaller patellar components have led to a reduction in patellar clunk (Berger et al. 1998, Hozack et al. 1989).
- *Patellar component failure* is another type of patellofemoral complication. The result is poor polyethylene wear, peg failure, and component fracture. It is usually associated with large polyethylene size, oversizing of the femoral component, obesity, increased patient activity, and the use of metal-backed patellar components.
- *Patellar fractures* are uncommon, although one study reported an incidence of 21%. Improper patellar resection, cementing of the patellar component, maltracking, avascularity, obesity, and increased patient activity have all been implicated (Akagi et al. 1999).

Nerve Injury

- The most common neuronal injury following TKA is to the peroneal nerve. *Peroneal nerve palsy* has a reported incidence between 0.3% and 4%. It is usually associated with correction of a severe valgus or severe flexion deformity. This is the result of traction on the nerve during the limb correction. Risk factors include valgus and flexion deformities, epidural anesthesia, previous lumbar laminectomy, and previous proximal tibial valgus osteotomy (Horlocker et al. 1994, Idusuyi and Morrey 1996).
- Treatment should include dressing removal and flexion of the knee.
- Recovery is variable following peroneal nerve injury.

Revision Total Knee Arthroplasty

- The need for TKA revision continues to increase because of the aging population and the increasing numbers of primary TKAs performed.
- The same basic principles used in primary TKAs are also used in revisions. The need for surgical exposure is still vital because the surgeon must be able to visualize the component and cement being removed. Incision should be made through the previous incision whenever possible. Soft tissue balancing remains a must, and the joint line must be restored to ensure proper function (Partington et al. 1999).
- Bone defects are a major problem in performing a revision TKA.
- The *Anderson Orthopaedic Research Institute* classification is used to guide the use of metal augments and bone grafts. It is based on the severity of bone loss. Type 1 defects have healthy metaphyseal bone, good cancellous structure, and a

relatively normal joint line. Type 2 defects have bone loss that includes cancellous structures that need repair to restore the joint line. Type 2A defects have this lesion on only one condyle, whereas type 2B lesions have these lesions on both condyles. Type 3 defects have large osteolytic lesions and represent severe tibial bone loss. With type 1 defects, a component similar to the primary component may be used. Type 2 defects usually require either modular or stemmed components. Type 3 defects are managed with hinged or custom-designed components, or the defect is bone grafted, and a long-stemmed prosthesis is used (Engh 1997).

Surgical Alternatives
Arthroscopic Débridement

- *Arthroscopic débridement* of an arthritic knee has had variable results. Proper patient selection is essential to its success. A patient with symptoms for less than 6 months, with mild or moderate unicompartmental disease, and with normal limb alignment may be considered for arthroscopy if nonsurgical management is unsuccessful. Indications include a discrete chief complaint such as joint line pain, catching or locking, and mild to moderate degenerative changes (Rand 1991).
- *Synovectomy*, or the removal of the hypertrophied, inflamed synovium, has been recommended for the relief of pain and chronic effusions in rheumatoid arthritis, pigmented villonodular synovitis, synovial chondromatosis, and other inflammatory arthritis. Good to excellent results with arthroscopic synovectomy have been reported to be between 80% and 96% in patients with rheumatoid arthritis at 2 years (Ishikawa et al. 1986).

Tibial Osteotomy

- *Tibial osteotomy* attempts to restore the proper mechanical axis of the knee. The ideal patient for osteotomy has single-compartment disease and ligamentous stability and is young and physically active.
- The goal of realignment osteotomy is to redistribute the forces through the knee from the diseased compartment to the compartment with better articular cartilage. Good to excellent results with tibial osteotomy are reported to range from 73% to 95% at 5 years. Ten-year results are less impressive, with a range from 45% to 80% (Billings et al. 2000, Coventry et al. 1993).
- Absolute contraindications include inflammatory arthritis, tricompartmental disease, flexion arc less than 90 degrees, tibiofemoral subluxation, and previous meniscectomy in the contralateral compartment.
- Relative contraindications include age older than 60 years, patellofemoral disease, ligamentous instability, lateral tibial subluxation, or a varus deformity greater than 10 degrees.
- Varus deformities are corrected with a lateral closing wedge. For large varus deformities, a tibiofemoral angle

greater than 12 degrees, a dome osteotomy may be more appropriate.

- A medial closing wedge may be used to correct a mild valgus deformity, an angle less than 12 degrees.
- Larger valgus deformities may require a distal femoral osteotomy to maintain the joint line and to prevent tibial subluxation. Internal fixation allows for early range of motion and weight bearing (Healy et al. 1998).
- Complications associated with tibial osteotomy include infection (higher rates when external fixators are used), peroneal nerve palsy, undercorrection, nonunion, overcorrection, and compartment syndrome postoperatively.
- It is very important to perform the osteotomy at least 2 cm below the joint line to prevent fracture through the proximal fragment and extension into the joint space. TKA following tibial osteotomy can be difficult. The lateral plateau may be deficient and may require an augment. If a stemmed tibial component is to be used, an offset stem may be required to ensure passage down the canal (Meding et al. 2000, Naudie et al. 1999).

Distal Femoral Osteotomy

- Distal femoral osteotomy is commonly used to correct a valgus deformity. Ninety percent of 5-year results are good to excellent (Healy et al. 1998).
- A medial closing wedge with internal fixation is the usual method of choice.
- Contraindications are similar to those to tibial osteotomy and also include significant joint medial thrust with ambulation.
- TKA following femoral osteotomy may be difficult. The femoral shaft is displaced in relation to the joint line. A component with an offset stem may be required. In addition, the knee following femoral osteotomy has a varus alignment in extension and a valgus alignment in flexion that make soft tissue balancing difficult.
- Constrained components may be necessary to achieve proper soft tissue balance.

Unicompartmental Knee Replacement

- A unicompartmental knee replacement may be employed in the presence of isolated unicompartmental disease. Medial replacement is more common than lateral. Success rates have been lower than with TKA. Survivorship has ranged from 87% to 98% at 10 years. Failures have been associated with excessive polyethylene wear and progression of disease of the contralateral compartment. Contraindications include inflammatory arthritis, a flexion contracture of 15 degrees or more, angular deformity, patellofemoral disease, and ligamentous instability (Cartier et al. 1996, Squire et al. 1999).
- Conversion to a TKA following unicompartmental knee replacement is technically more demanding and may require bone graft or augments (Chakrabarty et al. 1998).

References

Adams ME, Atkinson MH, Lussier AJ, et al. (1995). The role of viscosupplementation with hylan G-F 20 (Synvisc) in the treatment of osteoarthritis of the knee: A Canadian multicenter trial comparing hylan G-F 20 alone, hylan G-F 20 with non-steroidal anti-inflammatory drugs (NSAIDs) and NSAIDs alone. *Osteoarthritis Cartilage* 3:213-225.

This randomized, controlled, multicenter clinical trial was conducted in patients with osteoarthritis of the knee. At 26 weeks, groups receiving hylan G-F 20 were significantly better than the group receiving NSAIDs alone. Hylan G-F 20 is a safe and effective treatment for osteoarthritis of the knee and can be used either as a replacement for or an adjunct to NSAID therapy.

Akagi M, Matsusue Y, Mata T, et al. (1999). Effect of rotational alignment on patellar tracking in total knee arthroplasty. *Clin Orthop Relat Res* 366:155-163.

Patients who underwent identical condylar-type TKA were evaluated retrospectively. Postoperative measurements performed using computed tomography scans showed the mean angle between the prosthetic posterior condylar axis and the transepicondylar axis. The external rotation setting of the femoral component diminished the need for lateral retinacular release and may decrease the rate of patellofemoral complications that occur after TKA.

Ayers DC, Dennis DA, Johanson NA, et al. (1997). Common complications of total knee arthroplasty. *J Bone Joint Surg Am* 79:278-311.

This study focused on the common complications following TKA, including infection, and it also described the prevention and treatment of knee infection.

Backe HA, Wolff DA, Windsor RE (1996). Total knee replacement infection after 2-stage reimplantation: Results of subsequent 2-stage reimplantation. *Clin Orthop Relat Res* 331:125-131.

This study reviewed patients who underwent salvage of an infected TKA with removal, débridement, 6 weeks of parenteral antibiotics, and reimplantation and who subsequently acquired another infection in the same knee. These patients were again treated with the same protocol, followed by reimplantation or arthrodesis, and were observed for an average of 31 months.

Bassett RW (1998). Results of 1,000 Performance knees: Cementless versus cemented fixation. *J Arthroplasty* 13:409-413.

Patients with Performance total knee prostheses were retrospectively studied. The mean follow-up was 5.2 years. The average subjective and functional Knee Society scores were higher with cementless knees than with cemented replacements. An absence of osteolysis around screw fixation was noted, and at 5 years, there was 99% implant survival.

Berger RA, Crossett LS, Jacobs JJ, et al. (1998). Malrotation causing patellofemoral complications after total knee arthroplasty. *Clin Orthop Relat Res* 356:144-153.

Patients with isolated patellofemoral complications after TKA were compared with patients with well-functioning TKAs without patellofemoral complications. The group with patellofemoral complications had excessive internal component rotation. This finding suggests that internal component rotation may be a cause of patellofemoral complications.

Billings A, Scott DF, Camargo MP, et al. (2000). High tibial osteotomy with calibrated guide, rigid internal fixation, and early motion: Long-term follow-up. *J Bone Joint Surg Am* 82:70-79.

This study reviewed patients who underwent high tibial osteotomy with a calibrated osteotomy cutting guide and rigid internal fixation. This series showed good early motion and a low rate of complications; approximately two thirds of the knees had a good or excellent clinical result at an average of 8.5 years. Conversion to a TKA was accomplished without difficulty in the patients who had this procedure.

Buechel FF (1998). Mobile-bearing joint replacement options in post-traumatic arthritis of the knee. *Orthopedics* 21:1027-1031.

Buechel FF, Pappas MJ (1990). Long-term survivorship analysis of cruciate-sparing versus cruciate-sacrificing knee prosthesis using meniscal bearings. *Clin Orthop Relat Res* 260:162-169.

This study examined cumulative survivorship analysis using an end point of implant revision or a poor knee score. It revealed a small early failure rate of each implant in the first 3 years. This study indicated a predictable long-term survival of both cruciate-retaining and cruciate-sacrificing mobile bearing knee prostheses as well as rotating bearing patellar prostheses in primary knee arthroplasty.

Bugbee WD, Ammeen DJ, Parks NL, et al. (1998). 4 to 10-year results with the anatomic modular total knee. *Clin Orthop Relat Res* 348:158-165.

This minimally constrained PCL-retaining modular design performed well at intermediate follow-up. The absence of patellofemoral complications and of aseptic loosening was notable. Wear-related phenomena were the most common indications for reoperation, and these occurred in younger, active individuals with relatively thin polyethylene bearings.

Callaghan JJ, Squire MW, Goetz DD, et al. (2000). Cemented rotating-platform total knee replacement: A nine to twelve-year follow-up study. *J Bone Joint Surg Am* 82:705-711.

This study reviewed patients after 9 to 12 years of follow-up. The cemented LCS rotating-platform knee replacement was found to be performing well, with durable clinical and radiographic results.

Cartier P, Sanouiller JL, Grelsamer RP (1996). Unicompartmental knee arthroplasty surgery: 10-year minimum follow-up period. *J Arthroplasty* 11:782-788.

Patients in this study were followed a minimum of 10 years after unicompartmental knee arthroplasty surgery. The 10- to 12-year survivorship for the entire cohort was 93%. Slight undercorrection of varus alignment and adequate polyethylene thickness of the tibial component appeared to be important contributors to a successful outcome.

Chakrabarty G, Newman JH, Ackroyd CE (1998). Revision of unicompartmental arthroplasty of the knee: Clinical and technical considerations. *J Arthroplasty* 13:191-196.

This study reviewed patients with failed unicompartmental arthroplasties. In 73 unicompartmental arthroplasties of the knee that were revised, the major causes of failure were progression of arthritis and implant failure. Seventy-nine percent of these knees had excellent or good function at an average follow-up period of 56 months.

Colizza WA, Insall JN, Scuderi GR (1995). The posterior stabilized total knee prosthesis: Assessment of polyethylene damage and osteolysis after a ten year minimum follow-up. *J Bone Joint Surg Am* 77:1713-1720.

The long-term results of use of the posterior stabilized total knee prosthesis were evaluated with regard to clinical performance, survival of the implant, polyethylene wear, osteolysis, and loosening.

Coventry MB, Ilstrup DM, Wallrichs SL (1993). Proximal tibial osteotomy: A critical long-term study of eighty-seven cases. *J Bone Joint Surg Am* 75:196-201.

This study looked at the predisposing factors to failure of high tibial osteotomies. There is a considerable risk of failure of a proximal tibial osteotomy if the alignment is not overcorrected to at least 8 degrees of valgus angulation and if the patient is substantially overweight.

Dalury DF, Ewald FC, Christie MJ, et al. (1995). Total knee arthroplasty in a group of patients less than 45 years of age. *J Arthroplasty* 10:598-602.

The long-term follow-up evaluation of TKA in patients younger than 45 years old was reviewed. The results demonstrated that the success of TKA in this patient population is comparable to that for TKA in elderly patients.

Duff GP, Lachiewicz PF, Kelley SS (1996). Aspiration of the knee joint before revision arthroplasty. *Clin Orthop Relat Res* 331:132-139.

The erythrocyte sedimentation rate, peripheral leukocyte count, radiographs, and presenting symptoms correlate poorly with infection. Preoperative aspiration of the knee is the most helpful study for the diagnosis or exclusion of infection in a prosthetic knee joint.

Engh GA (1997). Bone defect classification. In: Engh GA, Rorabeck CH, eds. *Revision Total Knee Arthroplasty*. Baltimore: Williams & Wilkins, pp 63-120.

This chapter is a review of the Anderson Orthopaedic Research Institution Bone Defect Classification System.

Engh GA, Parks NL (1998). Surgical technique of the midvastus arthrotomy. *Clin Orthop Relat Res* 352:270-274.

The midvastus muscle splitting approach achieves surgical exposure equivalent to that of the standard medial parapatellar approach. The limited disruption of the extensor mechanism improves the rapid restoration of quadriceps muscle control.

Friedman RJ, Friedrich LV, White RL, et al. (1990). Antibiotic prophylaxis and tourniquet inflation in total knee arthroplasty. *Clin Orthop Relat Res* 260:17-23.

The standard 1 g of cefazolin with a 5-minute interval between administration and tourniquet inflation resulted in adequate mean soft tissue and bone concentrations for prophylaxis during TKA with a tourniquet time less than 2 hours. Additional doses are not warranted after tourniquet release.

Gill GS, Chan KC, Mills DM (1997). 5 to 18-year follow-up study of cemented total knee arthroplasty for patients 55 years old or younger. *J Arthroplasty* 12:49-54.

This study demonstrated that cemented TKA in younger patients with osteoarthritis and rheumatoid arthritis can attain results comparable to the excellent results obtained in older age groups.

Healy WL, Anglen JO, Wasilewski SA, et al. (1998). Distal femoral varus osteotomy. *J Bone Joint Surg Am* 70:102-109.

A varus osteotomy of the distal part of the femur is a reliable and effective surgical procedure for the treatment of gonarthrosis associated with valgus deformity resulting from osteoarthritis or trauma. It is not recommend for use in patients who have rheumatoid arthritis or in those who have inadequate motion of the knee before the operation.

Horlocker TT, Cabanela ME, Wedel DJ (1994). Does postoperative epidural analgesia increase the risk of peroneal nerve palsy after total knee arthroplasty? *Anesth Analg* 79:495-500.

Postoperative epidural analgesia was used in 108 cases and was not a significant risk factor for the development of peroneal palsy. Because the diagnosis of peroneal nerve palsy may be delayed in patients with postoperative epidural analgesia, these patients must be monitored closely.

Hozack WJ, Rothman RR, Booth RE, et al. (1989). The patellar clunk syndrome: A complication of posterior stabilized total knee arthroplasty. *Clin Orthop Relat Res* 241:203-208.

This retrospective review described patients with a painful, audible, "clunk" following TKA with a posterior stabilized prosthesis. Impingement of the suprapatellar fat pad on the femoral component when extending the knee led to this phenomenon.

Idusuyi OB, Morrey BF (1996). Peroneal nerve palsy after total knee arthroplasty: Assessment of predisposing and prognostic factors. *J Bone Joint Surg Am* 78:177-184.

A retrospective chart review of postoperative patients with peroneal nerve palsies was performed. Comparison of this group with a control group showed that epidural anesthesia for postoperative control of pain, previous laminectomy, and preoperative valgus deformity were all significantly associated with peroneal nerve palsy.

Ilahi OA, Davidson JP, Tullos HS (1994). Continuous epidural analgesia using fentanyl and bupivacaine after total knee arthroplasty. *Clin Orthop Relat Res* 299:44-52.

When compared with previous experiences using morphine (Duramorph) and bupivacaine for the first 3 days after TKA, the group using fentanyl and bupivacaine had shorter average hospitalization and earlier return of flexion. Confusion and pruritus were significantly less common with fentanyl, but the incidence of hypotension was increased. Nausea, hypoventilation, and respiratory depression were equally problematic in both groups.

Ishikawa H, Ohno O, Hirohata K (1986). Long-term results of synovectomy in rheumatoid patients. *J Bone Joint Surg Am* 68:198-205.

This study showed that synovectomy of the knee is a good treatment alternative for selected patients with early stage I rheumatoid arthritis that has proved resistant to standard medical therapy.

Kirkley A, Webster-Bogaert S, Litchfield R, et al. (1999). The effect of bracing on varus gonarthrosis. *J Bone Joint Surg Am* 81:539-548.

This study indicated that patients with varus gonarthrosis may benefit significantly from the use of a knee brace in addition to standard medical treatment. The unloader brace was, on average, more effective than the Neoprene sleeve.

Kumar PJ, McPherson EJ, Dorr LD, et al. (1996). Rehabilitation after total knee arthroplasty: A comparison of 2 rehabilitation techniques. *Clin Orthop Relat Res* 331:93-101.

This randomized prospective study compared patients who used a CPM machine with patients who were rehabilitated with early passive flexion of the knee (the drop and dangle protocol). Range of motion and hospital discharge can be achieved in a similar time interval with the drop and dangle technique as with using a CPM

device, and such a device is not required for postoperative knee rehabilitation.

Laine L, Harper S, Simon T, et al. (1999). A randomized trial comparing the effects of rofecoxib, a cyclooxygenase-2 specific inhibitor, with that of ibuprofen on gastroduodenal mucosa of patients with osteoarthritis. *Gastroenterology* 117:776-783.

Rofecoxib, at doses two to four times those demonstrated to relieve symptoms of osteoarthritis, caused significantly less gastroduodenal ulceration than ibuprofen, and ulcer rates were comparable to those with placebo.

Lewonowski K, Dorr LD, McPherson EJ, et al. (1997). Medialization of the patella in total knee arthroplasty. *J Arthroplasty* 12:161-167.

This study concluded that, for proper patellar tracking, it is recommended that the patellar component be placed on the medial two thirds of the patella. This additionally helps to reduce the occurrence of lateral release.

Lindenfeld TN, Hewett TE, Andriacchi TP (1997). Joint loading with valgus bracing in patients with varus gonarthrosis. *Clin Orthop Relat Res* 344:290-297.

This study showed that pain, function, and biomechanical knee loading can be altered by a brace designed to unload the medial compartment of the knee.

Matsueda M, Gustilo RB (2000). Subvastus and medial parapatellar approaches in total knee arthroplasty. *Clin Orthop Relat Res* 371:161-168.

This retrospective study compared the outcome of two consecutive groups of patients having primary TKA. The subvastus approach led to improved patellar tracking and stability.

McInnes J, Larson MG, Daltroy LH, et al. (1992). A controlled evaluation of continuous passive motion in patients undergoing total knee arthroplasty. *JAMA* 268:1423-1428.

The use of CPM increased active flexion and decreased swelling and the need for manipulations but did not significantly affect pain, active and passive extension, quadriceps strength, or length of hospital stay. At 6 weeks, no differences were noted between the two groups in either range of motion or function. In this series, the use of CPM resulted in a net savings of $6764 over conventional rehabilitation in achieving these results.

Meding JB, Keating EM, Ritter MA, et al. (2000). Total knee arthroplasty after high tibial osteotomy: A comparison study in patients who had bilateral total knee replacement. *J Bone Joint Surg Am* 82:1252-1259.

This study suggested that the clinical and radiographic results of primary TKA in knees with and without a previous high tibial osteotomy are not substantially different.

Mont MA, Waldman B, Banerjee C, et al. (1997). Multiple irrigation, debridement, and retention of components in infected total knee arthroplasty. *J Arthroplasty* 12:426-433.

This study showed that in selected circumstances, irrigation, débridement, and retention of the components can result in low morbidity with high success rates.

Naudie D, Bourne RB, Rorabeck CH, et al. (1999). Survivorship of the high tibial valgus osteotomy: A 10 to 22 year follow-up study. *Clin Orthop Relat Res* 367:18-27.

The results of 106 high tibial valgus osteotomies in 85 patients were evaluated after a minimum 10-year follow-up to determine survivorship, complications, and risk factors associated with failure. A body mass index of greater than 25, the presence of a lateral tibial thrust, and the development of delayed union or nonunion were significantly associated with probability of early failure. These results suggested that survival of high tibial osteotomy can be improved through careful patient selection and surgical technique.

Olcott CW, Scott RD (1999). Femoral component rotation during total knee arthroplasty. *Clin Orthop Relat Res* 367:39-42.

This study showed that the transepicondylar axis most consistently recreated a balanced flexion space, whereas the finding of 3 degrees of external rotation off the posterior condyles was least consistent, especially in knees in valgus.

Partington PF, Sawhney J, Rorabeck C, et al. (1999). Joint line restoration after revision total knee arthroplasty. *Clin Orthop Relat Res* 367:165-171.

This study concluded that joint line elevation after revision TKA is a problem. Excessive elevation may result in worse clinical outcomes. Distal femoral augments should be used more often and with greater thicknesses. Standard implants used for revision surgery should have increased distal dimensions.

Ranawat CS, Flynn WF, Saddler S, et al. (1993). Long-term results of total condylar knee arthroplasty: A 15-year survivorship study. *Clin Orthop Relat Res* 286:94-102.

This study showed that the total condylar knee arthroplasty had a 94.6% clinical survival at 15 years, with predictably good clinical results.

Rand JA (1991). Role of arthroscopy in osteoarthritis of the knee. *Arthroscopy* 7:358-363.

This study compared arthroscopic partial meniscectomy with limited débridement versus arthroscopic abrasion arthroplasty in patients with osteoarthritis. Abrasion arthroplasty appeared to offer little benefit over partial meniscectomy and débridement in the degenerative knee.

Ritter MA, Herbst SA, Keating EM, et al. (1994). Long-term survival analysis of a posterior cruciate–retaining total condylar total knee arthroplasty. *Clin Orthop Relat Res* 309:136-145.

This study reviewed patients with PCL-retaining total condylar knee arthroplasties. These patients were observed for 1 to 18 years, and the crude survival estimate at 12 years was 98.1%.

Rosier RN, O'Keefe RJ (2000). Hyaluronic acid therapy. *Instruct Course Lect* 49:495-502.

This article reviewed the evidence suggesting a beneficial effect of intra-articular hyaluronate preparations in treating the symptoms of osteoarthritis.

Squire MW, Callaghan JJ, Goetz DD, et al. (1999). Unicompartmental knee replacement: A minimum 15 year follow-up study. *Clin Orthop Relat Res* 367:61-72.

This study concluded that disease progression and tibial component subsidence with wear were the major long-term problems in this group of patients.

van Baar ME, Dekker J, Oostendorp RA, et al. (1998). The effectiveness of exercise therapy in patients with osteoarthritis of the hip or knee: A randomized clinical trial. *J Rheumatol* 25:2432-2439.

This randomized, prospective study showed that after 12 weeks, exercise therapy is effective in reducing pain and disability in patients with osteoarthritis of the knee.

Ververeli PA, Hozack WJ, Rothman RR (1995). Continuous passive motion after total knee arthroplasty: Analysis of cost and benefits. *Clin Orthop Relat Res* 321:208-215.

This study concluded that CPM is efficacious in increasing short-term flexion and decreasing the need for knee manipulation without raising costs.

CHAPTER 10

Ankle Arthroplasty

Sudheer Reddy,★ David I. Pedowitz,† and Enyi Okereke‡

★MD, Instructor, Department of Orthopaedic Surgery, University of Pennsylvania School of
Medicine, Philadelphia, PA
†MD, Chief Resident, Department of Orthopaedic Surgery, Hospital of the University of
Pennsylvania, Philadelphia, PA
‡MD, PharmD, Associate Professor and Chief, Orthopaedic Foot and Ankle Services,
University of Pennsylvania School of Medicine, Philadelphia, PA

Introduction

- Although primary degenerative ankle arthritis is not seen with nearly the frequency as in the hip or knee, degenerative disease in the ankle is a significant orthopaedic problem.
- Despite having an estimated prevalence of degenerative disease nine times lower than in the hip or knee, the ankle joint is subjected to more injuries and more force per square centimeter during weight bearing than any other joint in the body (Cushnaghan and Dieppe 1991; Huch et al. 1997).
- Patients with ankle arthritis have difficulty using the affected limb predominantly because of pain and stiffness with any weight-bearing activities.
- Arthrodesis has historically remained the "gold standard" for the treatment of end-stage arthritides of the ankle despite its notable shortcomings.
- Although total ankle arthroplasty (TAA) has not been met with the same success seen in primary hip and knee reconstruction, numerous advances in the design, operative techniques, and instrumentation of TAAs have occurred in the past decade.
- As results improve with these advances in technology and technique, one can anticipate an expansion of indications for TAA and greater use of these devices among recon-structive surgeons (Soohoo and Kominski 2004).
- This chapter is an overview of the predominant causes of ankle arthritis and reviews the current reconstructive tools available to diagnose and manage these patients effectively.

Patient Selection

Etiology of the Arthritic Ankle and Patient Demographics (Coughlin 1999, Walling 2004)

- Arthritis of the ankle falls into one of three main categories: primary osteoarthritis (OA), inflammatory arthritis, and post-traumatic degenerative arthritis.

Primary Osteoarthritis

- Primary OA of the ankle is uncommon. Although it does occur, practically speaking, it is even rare in elderly patients.
- The primary pathologic process of ankle OA involves distortion of the articular surface. Increased water content and proteoglycan breakdown at the level of the articular cartilage lead to a biochemically altered surface that, because of its decreased compliance, ultimately transmits greater forces to the subchondral bone. Repetitive injury in this setting leads to classic joint space narrowing, subchondral sclerosis, and osteophyte formation (Fig. 10–1).
- Osteoarthritic patients often lose ankle motion, and most patients complain of pain at the extremes of motion.

Inflammatory Arthritis

- Although seronegative and crystalline arthropathies are not uncommon in the foot, they infrequently lead to disabling ankle arthritis. The most common inflammatory arthritis of the ankle is rheumatoid arthritis (RA).

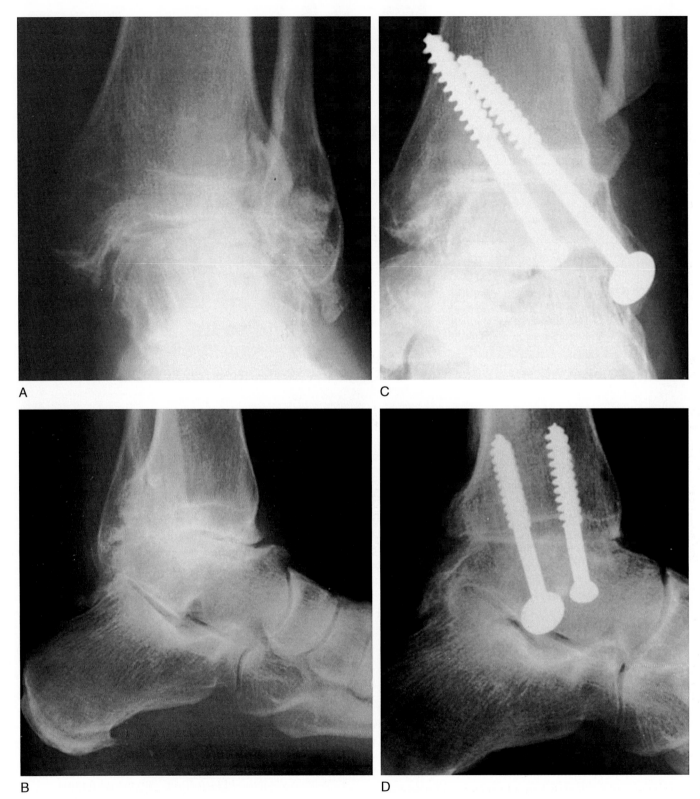

A

B

C

D

Figure 10–1: Degenerative arthritis of the ankle.
Anteroposterior (**A**) and lateral (**B**) preoperative radiographs demonstrate degenerative arthritis of the ankle joint. Anteroposterior (**C**) and lateral (**D**) radiographs demonstrate arthrodesis of the ankle joint. (From Coughlin MJ [1999]. Arthritides. In: Coughlin MJ, Mann RA, eds. *Surgery of the Foot and Ankle*, 7th ed. St. Louis: Mosby.)

- RA manifests early in the disease process mainly as a synovitis without a significant painful articular deformity.
- Foot deformity in RA is very common. The feet are generally involved slightly more often than the hands in RA (15.7% versus 14.7%). The ankle specifically, however, is typically involved less frequently and is seen in only 4% to 16% of patients.
- RA affects approximately 1% to 2% of the population, with a peak incidence in the third to fifth decades. Patients are predominantly white women and often have a lower functional demand of their ankles relative to patients with OA or post-traumatic arthritis.
- The underlying course of RA is that of pain and synovitis leading to progressive disability.
- Most patients with RA of the ankle have pain as a result of significant soft tissue inflammation that is often mistaken for ankle joint pain of bony origin.

- Arthritic joint changes with symmetric joint narrowing and pannus formation are eventually seen in long-standing cases, and patients may present with concomitant distal tibia stress fractures (Fig. 10–2).
- With disease progression, ligamentous destruction can also occur, leading to instability with resultant fibular impingement.

Post-traumatic Arthritis

- With the high incidence of ankle trauma, it is no surprise that post-traumatic arthritis of the ankle is the most common cause of degenerative changes in the ankle joint.
- Although reported prevalences of post-traumatic arthritis of the ankle have varied considerably, this condition has been estimated to occur in 13% of ankle fractures following open reduction and internal fixation and in 47% to 97% of talus fractures.

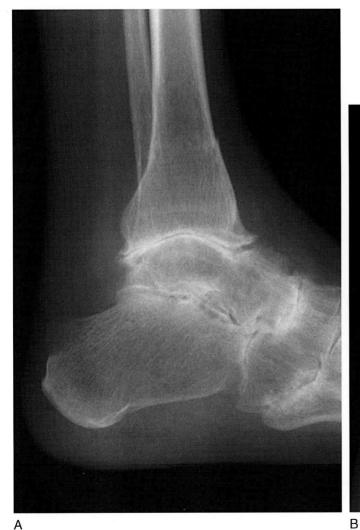
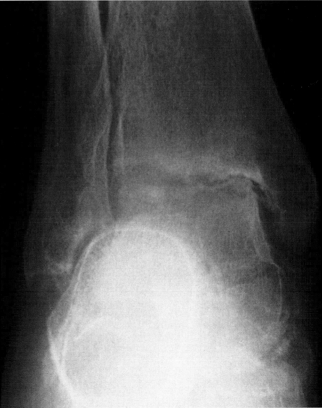

A   B

Figure 10–2: Rheumatoid arthritis.
A and B, Degenerative changes associated with rheumatoid arthritis. Although no significant deformity occurs, severe chondrolysis is associated with pain and difficult ambulation. (From Coughlin MJ [1999]. Arthritides. In: Coughlin MJ, Mann RA, eds. *Surgery of the Foot and Ankle,* 7th ed. St. Louis: Mosby.)

- Unlike RA or primary OA, post-traumatic arthritis of the ankle can affect patients of any age or sex. It is most commonly seen following intra-articular comminuted fractures of the ankle that heal with residual incongruity of the articular surface. Despite meticulous open reduction and internal fixation of intra-articular and periarticular fractures, the resulting injury to the articular cartilage from the initial trauma predisposes these patients to post-traumatic arthritis.
- Medial or lateral ligamentous insufficiency may also lead to articular wear and progressive arthritis in the post-traumatic ankle.
- Pain is often the main complaint in patients with post-traumatic arthritis of the ankle.
- Although treatment for OA and RA is more standardized, treatment in this case is individualized depending on the functional demands, age, occupation, and degree of injury of the patient.

Evaluation of the Patient With Ankle Arthritis

History and Physical Examination

- As with any condition affecting the musculoskeletal system, a detailed history and physical examination are important.
- The history is guided, to look for symptoms of pain, instability, increasing stiffness, or mechanical symptoms (catching, clicking, or locking) that could be suggestive of loose bodies or osteochondral lesions.
- Additionally, any neurologic symptoms should be discerned.
- Previous trauma and surgery of the ankle should also be discussed.
- Physical examination of the ankle should follow a structured, anatomic approach that adheres to a rigorous routine.
- Additionally, one must avoid the tendency to focus in on the ankle itself while disregarding pathologic features elsewhere in the distal lower extremity.
- Gait is examined over an appreciable distance to observe overall limb alignment, the degree of dynamic deformity, and the position of the foot and ankle in all stages of locomotion, as well as to note any compensatory motions or tendencies.
- Gait should be visualized with and without shoe wear.
- Shoe wear and any orthotic should also be inspected for appropriateness and specifically for areas of excessive wear or of prominence.
- Inspection of the ankle allows for visualization of the orientation of the resting extremity (aids in identifying malunion or nonunion), examines for swelling (inflammation), and reveals skin changes and previous surgical scars.
- Passive range of motion (ROM) is assessed with the knee in flexion and in full extension because knee flexion relaxes the gastrocnemius muscle, which originates on the femur.
- Of particular importance is testing for ankle ROM with the midfoot inverted.

- Midfoot inversion locks the transverse tarsal joint (as occurs during the push-off phase of gait) and allows one to evaluate specifically for ankle ROM. Foot eversion unlocks the transverse tarsal joint (seen when the foot encounters the floor) and allows significant motion (including dorsiflexion) to occur through the midfoot.
- Examining the ankle with the foot everted may erroneously yield an overestimation of ankle dorsiflexion.
- Active ROM should similarly be evaluated.
- Although the ankle is essentially a hinge, the axis is skewed in the transverse and coronal planes to allow for approximately 6 degrees of rotation of the talus relative to the tibia.
- For purposes of the physical examination, the ankle goes through a range of plantar flexion and dorsiflexion (extension) and consists of motion occurring at the tibiotalar articulation.
- Because the ankle is the gateway into the terminal weight-bearing portion of the lower extremity, special attention should be given to examination of the entire foot as well as to the ankle.
- Failure to appreciate coexisting deformity or neurologic deficit distal to the ankle makes appropriate decision making regarding the treatment of ankle disease impossible.
- Normal ankle ROM varies but should be symmetric and should come into some dorsiflexion. Various normal ROM measurements have been reported. Dorsiflexion ranges from 10 to 23 degrees, whereas plantar flexion ranges from 23 to 48 degrees.
- Dorsiflexion of 5 degrees and plantar flexion of 20 degrees are generally required for adequate gait.
- Walking upstairs, however, requires 36 degrees of total motion, whereas descending stairs requires 56 degrees.
- Palpation of the ankle can identify tenderness or swelling and should follow anatomic structures:
  - Medial malleolus, deltoid ligament, posterior tibial tendon, posterior tibial artery, posteromedial ankle joint, Achilles tendon complex, posterolateral ankle joint, peroneal tendons, lateral malleolus, lateral ligamentous complex, anterolateral ankle joint, tibialis anterior tendon, dorsalis pedis artery, long extensor tendons, anterior ankle joint, talar neck and head, and anteromedial ankle joint
- Prominent osteophytes can often be palpated at the anterior lip of the tibial plafond. Concomitant lesions on the talar neck are common.
- Provocative examination of the ankle includes assessment of stability and muscle function.
- Laxity of the deltoid ligament may be primary or secondary and is seen with valgus instability or deformity.
- Similarly, on the lateral side, attenuation of the lateral ligamentous complex (anterior and posterior talofibular ligaments [ATFL and PTFL] and calcaneofibular ligaments [CFL]) contributes to resultant varus instability and a deformity pattern.

- The anterior drawer test done in plantar flexion evaluates the integrity of the ATFL, whereas dorsiflexion determines CFL incompetence.
- Syndesmotic injury must also be assessed and can manifest as a global instability pattern because the talus is poorly constrained within the bony mortise.
- Plantar flexion strength is manually tested with the patient in a sitting position, which assesses the gastrocnemius-soleus complex. The ability to perform single limb heel-rises reflects more accurately the strength of plantar flexion but may be painful or significantly limited in the significantly arthritic tibiotalar joint.

Radiographic Examination

- Standard anteroposterior, lateral, and mortise views are the mainstay of radiographic evaluation of the arthritic ankle. The anteroposterior and lateral radiographs must be weight-bearing films to appreciate the degree of arthritic change fully.
  - Oblique views of the ankle provide additional information about the ankle mortise, talar dome, and malleoli.
  - The surgeon must scrutinize all radiographs for degenerative changes, which may be present at adjacent joints because such patients may require additional procedures at the time of primary arthroplasty. For this reason, weight-bearing views of the foot are also mandatory in the preoperative evaluation for TAA.
  - Radiographs can identify osteophytes, loose bodies, abnormal osseous anatomy, and loss of articular cartilage.
  - These radiographs also assist in determining available bone stock for future arthroplasty.
  - Lateral views help to reveal osteophytes on the plafond and talar neck as well as the degree of articular collapse and subluxation.
  - The anteroposterior view can reveal osteophytes, cysts, joint space narrowing, and proliferative changes in the medial or lateral gutters.
  - The ankle mortise is composed of the medial malleolus, lateral malleolus, and tibial plafond surrounding the talar dome. This view, an anteroposterior view in 15 to 20 degrees of internal rotation, demonstrates syndesmotic widening and talar tilt or shift within the aforementioned bony constraints.
  - Stress radiographs are used to evaluate for instability as needed, and the following are considered abnormal when affected/stressed sides are compared to the unaffected/unstressed sides:
    - More than 3 mm of medial or lateral widening of the mortise
    - More than 4 mm of anterior displacement on the anterior drawer test compared with unstressed findings or more than 2 mm compared with the unaffected side
    - 10 degrees of difference in talar tilt

- Computed tomography scans may be helpful to evaluate more complex situations with bone loss, malunion, or ankylosis of the ankle but are not used routinely.
- Magnetic resonance imaging is infrequently used in the evaluation of the patient with ankle arthritis, but it may help to visualize ligamentous anatomy or evaluate the integrity of the posterior tibial tendon.
- The typical radiographic findings for each cause of ankle arthritis follow:
  - OA
    - Radiographic features of the ankle with OA correlate strongly with the clinical features.
    - Primary OA of the ankle is quite rare but manifests radiographically as it does in other large joints with the characteristic appearance of osteophytes, asymmetric joint space narrowing, subchondral sclerosis, and subchondral cysts (see Fig. 10–1).
  - RA
    - Radiographic signs of RA are also characteristic (see Fig. 10–2).
    - Periarticular osteopenia, juxta-articular erosions with symmetric joint space narrowing in the absence of deformity, and proliferative changes are seen.
  - Post-traumatic arthritis
    - Radiographic changes of post-traumatic arthritis typically reflect the underlying trauma to the joint.
    - Evidence of malunion or articular incongruity can be observed on plain radiographs. Computed tomography may be helpful in these patients.

Nonoperative Treatment (Thomas and Daniels 2003)

- Nonoperative management of ankle arthritis centers on preserving ROM and on alleviating stiffness and inflammation.
- As for all patients with disease of the foot and ankle, proper footwear is paramount when considering a treatment strategy.
- Several available modalities are aimed at managing the pain and stiff ankle, including medications, bracing, and injections.
- Because the ankle is the recipient of tremendous compressive and shear stresses, physical therapy tends to aggravate the condition and is therefore not traditionally used in conservative management.

Bracing

- This is a popular method of treating ankle pain.
- The rationale behind this treatment is that limiting ROM can increase ambulatory capacity and decrease pain.
- Braces consisting of a molded leather ankle brace, a polypropylene ankle-foot orthosis, or a rocker-bottom shoe can be successful.

Oral Medications

- Common to any arthritic condition, aspirin and other nonsteroidal anti-inflammatory drugs are commonly used to control pain.
- Long-term use of these agents may increase the risk of gastrointestinal complications.
- More potent agents such as antimalarial drugs, gold salts, and immunosuppressives such as corticosteroids can be beneficial, especially in the treatment of RA.
  - Newer antirheumatic agents have been recently found to be very effective in controlling painful synovitis in these patients.
  - Administration of these medications should be reserved for the rheumatologist.

Injections

- Corticosteroid injections can prove useful in alleviating symptoms of acute flare-up of arthritis or synovitis.
- These often temporary interventions may be repeated every few months (no more than three times/year).
- Viscosupplementation has only recently been used in the ankle.
- When available, published outcomes data must be scrutinized before widespread use of this modality can be endorsed.
- This approach is unlikely to be deleterious to the ankle, however, and, as it has in the knee, it may represent an additional form of treatment for relief of arthritic symptoms.

Implant Selection

Anatomy and Biomechanics of the Ankle

- Familiarity and recognition of normal and pathologic anatomy of the arthritic ankle are critical to successful management of ankle arthritis.
- Additionally, anatomic and biomechanical considerations dictate to some degree ankle arthroplasty design.

Osteology

- The *ankle*, also known as the *talocrural joint*, is composed of the distal tibia (plafond), including the medial and lateral malleoli, and the talus.
- The medial malleolus has two prominences distally known as the anterior and posterior colliculi.
- The talus has a head, neck, and body, which participate in different articulations.
  - The talar head articulates distally with the navicular at the talonavicular joint.
  - The talar dome articulates with the distal tibia at the ankle joint.
  - The talar body articulates inferiorly with the calcaneus in the subtalar joint.

- For the purposes of arthroplasty, the tibiotalar joint is the articulation that is replaced.
- In the coronal plane, the talar dome has a saddle-shaped trochlear surface dorsally, which articulates with the tibial plafond above it.
- In the axial plane, the dome is larger anteriorly than posteriorly by an average of 4.2 mm.
- The distal tibia is similarly narrowed posteriorly and is wider anteriorly.
  - This feature may have the effect of some instability in maximum plantar flexion when the narrowest diameter of the talus is residing in the mortise, which essentially remains unchanged in size.
- In the coronal plane medially and laterally, the talus has slightly concave surfaces to accommodate the medial and lateral malleoli.

Capsuloligamentous Anatomy

- The ankle joint is encased within the capsule, and the ligaments ensure the integrity of the precise articular surface alignment required for normal gait.
- On the medial and lateral sides of the joint, thickenings of the capsule comprise the ligamentous complexes.
- Between the distal tibia and fibula is the syndesmotic complex.

Medial Collateral Ligament Complex/Deltoid Ligament

- The deltoid ligament is subdivided into the superficial and deep ligaments (Fig. 10–3).
- The superficial deltoid originates from the anterior colliculus of the medial malleolus and has no discrete bands of tissue.
  - This broad fan of medial tissue has three insertions separately named the tibionavicular, tibiocalcaneal, and posterior tibiotalar ligaments.
  - The superficial deltoid resists hindfoot eversion.
- The deep deltoid originates from the intercollicular groove and the posterior colliculus of the medial malleolus.
  - It is confluent with the medial capsule of the ankle joint and is usually thought of as having two parts: the anterior and posterior tibiotalar ligaments.
  - The deep deltoid is a stronger structure than the superficial component and is largely responsible for resisting medial opening (valgus), lateral translation, and external rotation of the talus.

Lateral Collateral Ligament Complex

- The lateral collateral ligament complex is composed of three distinct components: (1) the ATFL, (2) the PTFL, and (3) the CFL (Fig. 10–4).
- The ATFL originates on the distal anterior fibula and inserts on the body of the talus slightly anterior to the tibiotalar articular surface proximal to the talar neck.

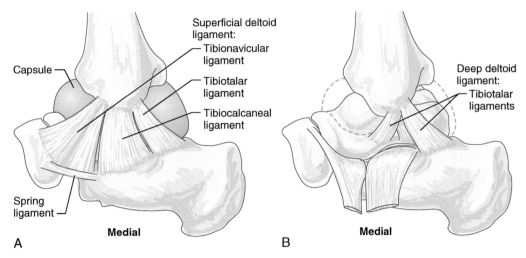

Figure 10–3: Deltoid ligament.
A, Diagrammatic view of the superficial deltoid ligament. **B,** Deep deltoid ligament. (From Morrey BF [2003]. *Joint Replacement Arthroplasty*, 3rd ed. New York: Churchill Livingstone.)

- It forms an angle of approximately 104 degrees with the CFL.
- It is the most frequently torn ligament in ankle sprains.
- The PTFL courses from the medial surface of the lateral malleolus to the posterior aspect of the talus.
- The CFL originates anteriorly on the distal lateral malleolus (slightly distal to the ATFL origin) and inserts on a

small tubercle posterior and superior to the peroneal tubercle of the calcaneus.

Syndesmotic Complex

- This complex has four components: the anterior inferior tibiofibular ligament, the posterior inferior tibiofibular ligament, the interosseous ligament, and the interosseous membrane (which runs the entire length of the tibia and fibula) (Fig. 10–5).

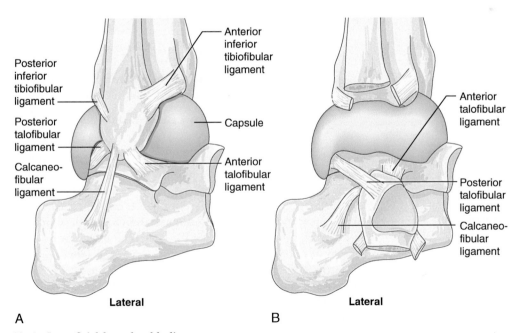

Figure 10–4: Superficial lateral ankle ligaments.
A, Diagrammatic view of the superficial lateral ankle ligaments. **B,** Deeper view with the fibula transected and reflected inferiorly. (From Morrey BF [2003]. *Joint Replacement Arthroplasty*, 3rd ed. New York: Churchill Livingstone.)

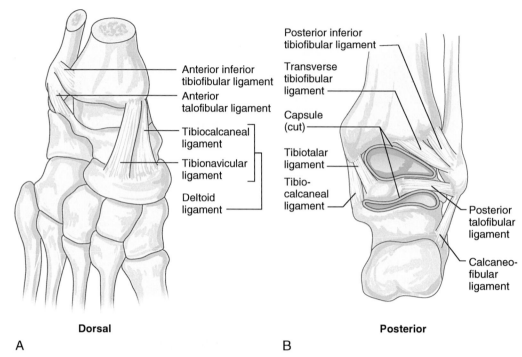

Dorsal

A

Posterior

B

Figure 10–5: Anterior and posterior tibiofibular ligaments.
A, Diagrammatic view of the anterior tibiofibular ligament. The anterior deltoid and lateral ligaments are also seen. **B,** The posterior tibiofibular ligament and other posterior stabilizers are also seen. (From Morrey BF [2003]. *Joint Replacement Arthroplasty*, 3rd ed. New York: Churchill Livingstone.)

- These fascial condensations stabilize the distal tibiofibular joint.

Muscular Anatomy

- Numerous muscles cross the ankle joint and have a role in dorsiflexion (extension) and plantar flexion.
- Although these muscles tend to move the ankle through its flexion and extension ROM, they also facilitate different movements at joints distal to the ankle.
- This section briefly mentions the major muscles involved in motion of the ankle.
- Muscles about the ankle can broadly be described by the compartment within the leg in which they reside (anterior, posterior, or lateral).
- From medial to lateral, the anterior compartment muscles consist of the tibialis anterior, extensor hallucis longus, and extensor digitorum longus.
  - All anterior compartment muscles facilitate dorsiflexion of the ankle
  - All also run beneath the superior extensor retinaculum just proximal to the joint to prevent bowstringing
- The posterior compartment has both deep and superficial portions.
  - The superficial posterior compartment contains the gastrocnemius and soleus muscles, which plantar flex the ankle.

- The deep posterior musculature consists of the flexor hallucis longus, the tibialis posterior, and the flexor digitorum longus.
  - All posterior compartments plantar flex the ankle
- Although they are extremely important for overall foot function, the two muscles in the lateral compartment, the peroneus longus and brevis muscles, contribute little to overall tibiotalar joint movement.

Neurovascular Anatomy

- The ankle has complex neurovascular anatomy, which necessitates a thorough understanding of the anatomic relationships and of three-dimensional anatomy.
- Both motor and sensory nerves cross the ankle joint.
- Three sensory nerves cross the ankle, all supplying cutaneous innervation to the dorsum of the foot.
- Medially, the saphenous nerve courses along with its vein, anterior to the medial malleolus.
  - It supplies the medial side of the foot and hindfoot.
- The superficial peroneal nerve is a terminal branch of the common peroneal nerve and is purely sensory (Fig. 10–6).
  - It crosses the ankle roughly just lateral to the midline as it travels along the path of the extensor digitorum longus.
  - It provides innervation to the majority of the dorsum of the foot.

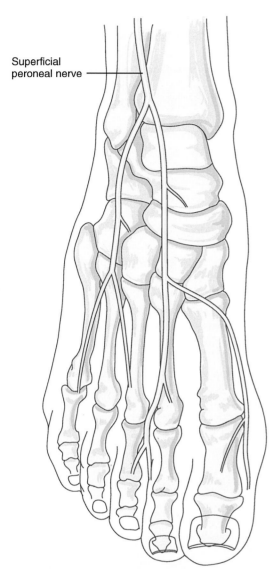

Superficial
peroneal nerve

Figure 10–6: Superficial peroneal nerve.
Dorsal diagrammatic representation of the superficial peroneal
nerve distribution. (From Morrey BF [2003]. *Joint Replacement
Arthroplasty*, 3rd ed. New York: Churchill Livingstone.)

- The sural nerve is a terminal branch of the tibial nerve
  and runs laterally posterior to the distal fibula but anterior
  to the Achilles tendon.
  - The sural nerve supplies the skin on the lateral border
    of the foot.
- The tibial nerve innervates all posterior compartment
  musculature and is the medial division of the sciatic nerve.
  - It travels just posterior to the flexor digitorum longus
    tendon behind the medial malleolus.
  - When the nerve enters the foot, it forms the calcaneal,
    medial, and lateral plantar nerves.
- The deep peroneal nerve is a terminal branch of the
  common peroneal nerve. It travels with the anterior tibial
  artery just medial to it.

- Supplying the extensor digitorum and extensor hallucis
  brevis muscles, the nerve also provides cutaneous
  sensation in the first dorsal webspace.
- Proximal to the ankle joint, the nerve and the artery are
  located between the tibialis anterior and the extensor
  hallucis tendons.
- At the level of the ankle and distally, the nerve and
  artery lie lateral to the extensor hallucis longus tendon.
- The anterior tibial artery becomes the dorsalis pedis
  artery distal to the ankle.
- The posterior tibial artery is a branch of the popliteal
  artery, which runs posterior to the medial malleolus
  with the tibial nerve and the deep posterior tendons as
  they cross the ankle.

Biomechanics

- The ankle joint is not a true hinge. With weight bearing,
  tibiotalar motion is closely linked with subtalar motion.
- It is important to recognize the contributions the subtalar
  joint makes to overall ankle motion when tibiotalar
  arthroplasty is considered.
- The ankle allows approximately 60 to 70 degrees of
  motion with as much as 7.5 degrees of axial rotation of
  the talus relative to the tibia.
- During the gait cycle, rotation at the ankle joint occurs
  with inversion/eversion at the subtalar joint.
- During the first contact phase of gait, the subtalar joint everts
  and then undergoes progressive inversion until toe-off.
- If the subtalar joint is degenerative, these linked motions will
  transmit significantly increased stress to the tibiotalar joint.
- The axis of rotation of the trochlea of the talus within the
  mortise is not fixed.
  - The axis rotates in dorsiflexion/plantar flexion,
    inversion/eversion, and internal/external rotation.
- The ankle is externally rotated approximately 23 degrees.

Joint Forces

- The ankle can experience substantial joint contact and
  reaction force with normal daily activities.
- During normal gait, approximately 5.2 times body weight
  is distributed to the ankle in vertical load.
- Shear in the lateral plane and shear in the anteroposterior
  plane are estimated to be one and two times body weight,
  respectively.
- It is critical that the surgeon considers the strength of the
  underlying cancellous bone of the tibia and talus when
  performing arthroplasty. If this is not done, failure of the
  cancellous bone at the bone-implant interface may result.

Types of Implants

- This section is an overview of current design differences of
  available TAAs (Alvine 2000).
- Although more than 20 TAAs have been developed since
  the first use of a total ankle prosthesis by Lord and
  Marrotte in 1970, only one prosthesis was approved by the

Food and Drug Administration (FDA) for use in the United States until recently. One other implant is widely used in Europe and is just completing clinical trials in this country.

- Several other total ankle replacement devices have recently received FDA approval, including the following:
  - Topez Total Ankle System (Topez Orthopaedics, Boulder, CO)
  - Salto Talaris Anatomic Ankle (Tornier, Stafford, TX)
  - Eclipse Total Ankle (Kinetikos Medical Inc., Carlsbad, CA)
- We anticipate myriad new designs to enter the market in the near future. However, because these two implant designs are unique and represent the two current design philosophies in TAA development, the discussion is limited to these two implants.
- Historically, ankle prosthetic designs have been classified based on their resistance to the forces to which they are subjected.
  - This presented three categories: constrained, semiconstrained, and unconstrained.
- For simplicity, current implants are now generally categorized based on the number of components in the arthroplasty system.

Two-Component Design

- The prototypical two-component design is the Agility ankle arthroplasty (DePuy Johnson and Johnson, Warsaw, IN) (Fig. 10–7) (Alvine 2000).
- The Agility ankle is a semiconstrained implant with a titanium tibial component and a cobalt-chromium talar component (see Fig. 10–7).
- A modular polyethylene component is secured within the tibial component.
- There is some freedom for axial rotation as well as some medial-lateral translation of the talar component within the polyethylene component.

- The implant allows for a flexion-extension arc of 60 degrees.
- FDA approval is for implantation with the use of bone cement; however, the trend is toward a press-fit implantation of these implants, with encouraging results.
- Implantation of the Agility device requires arthrodesis of the tibiofibular syndesmosis to allow transfer of weight to the fibula.
- The tibial component is obliquely rectangular and is positioned so its articulating surface is in 20 degrees of external rotation.
- The tibial component has a porous coating on its entire superior surface as well as along the medial and lateral sides that are in contact with the medial and lateral malleoli.
- The talar component has a porous coating on the inferior surface that is exposed to the talar bone.
- Like the native talus, the talar component is slightly wider anteriorly than posteriorly.
- Like the tibial side, the talar component is placed in 20 degrees of external rotation. The implant is semiconstrained, allowing rotation and medial and lateral shift.
- The body of the talus is tapered posteriorly to facilitate insertion.
- Depending on the size of implant that is used, the minimum thickness of the polyethylene liner varies from 3.73 to 4.70 mm.

Three-Component Design

- The prototypical three-component design is the Scandinavian total ankle replacement (STAR; Waldemar Link, Hamburg, Germany) (Fig. 10–8) (Kofoed 2004).

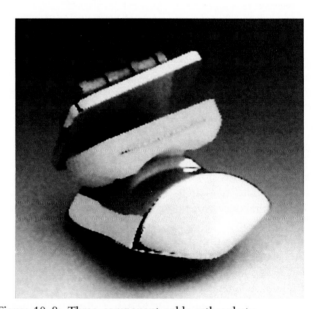

Figure 10–8: Three-component ankle arthroplasty. Scandinavian total ankle replacement (STAR) three-component ankle arthroplasty. (From Morrey BF [2003]. *Joint Replacement Arthroplasty*, 3rd ed. New York: Churchill Livingstone.)

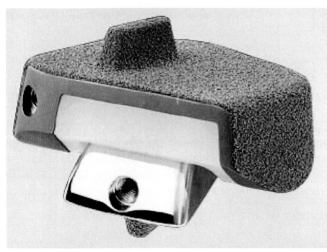

Figure 10–7: Two-component ankle replacement. Two-component Agility ankle replacement. (From Morrey BF [2003]. *Joint Replacement Arthroplasty*, 3rd ed. New York: Churchill Livingstone.)

- The STAR device was designed in 1978 and is currently a three-component anatomic unconstrained prosthesis.
- The tibial component is a cobalt-chrome alloy implant with a highly polished flat articular surface and two cylindrical fixation bars positioned on the tibial surface for anchoring into subchondral bone. The more recent versions of this component have a plasma-sprayed hydroxyapatite layer that is 100-μm thick and is applied to the two fixation bars.
- The talar component is also cobalt-chrome alloy with a ridge in the middle from anterior to posterior that matches a groove in the mobile polyethylene insert. The undersurface of the implant is similarly coated with hydroxyapatite.
- The talar components come in right-sided and left-sided implants.
- The meniscal component is a sliding mobile bearing made of ultrahigh-molecular-weight polyethylene (UHMWPE).
- It ranges in thickness from 6 to 10 mm and is sterilized by γ-irradiation in air.
- The UHMWPE sliding core has a smooth plane surface, which articulates with the tibial component, and a concave undersurface that matches the convex surface of the talar component.
- As stated earlier, a ridge in the talar component matches a groove in the polyethylene component. This fit ensures stability of the mobile bearing in the coronal plane.
- The design rationale for a UHMWPE meniscus between the metal parts is to allow only compressive forces to be translated to the talar and tibial components and to avoid rotational stresses at the bone-prosthesis interface.
- Implantation of the STAR prosthesis does not rely on syndesmotic fixation.

Surgical Techniques for Total Ankle Arthroplasty

- Because of the difficulties related to implant insertion, myriad exposures have been developed to aid in the implantation of specific ankle prosthetics.
- As a result of the tenuous soft tissue envelope around the ankle, many of these exposures have been abandoned because of less than favorable wound healing.
- Additionally, alternative exposures developed for specific implants have fallen out of favor as have their respective implants because of poor outcomes.
- Most arthroplasty procedures require wide exposure of the articular surface of the ankle but necessarily cross internervous planes.

Anteromedial Exposure

- Most TAAs implanted with modern designs utilize an anteromedial exposure.

- Some implant designs, such as the Agility, also require fusion of the syndesmosis.
  - This requires a second incision, which is usually a direct lateral exposure, as would be used in fixation of distal fibular fractures.
- The anterior tibiofibular ligament is reflected, the tibiofibular syndesmosis is distracted, and its soft tissues are removed.
- Because of the ease of view, surgeon familiarity, good healing rates, and accessibility to all areas of the tibiotalar joint, this exposure is preferred under most circumstances.
- Because of the bony and soft tissue constraints on the ankle joint, arthroplasty must be accomplished while the tibiotalar joint is distracted.
  - This is facilitated by the temporary use of a medially based distraction/compression device before the ankle joint is exposed (Fig. 10–9A).
  - Half-pins are placed in the talar head-neck junction, the posterior calcaneus, and the tibia.
  - The talar pin is placed first, with attention directed at positioning it in the talus in line with the deformity, if one exists.
  - By doing so, the varus/valgus deformity can be corrected before pins are placed in the tibia and calcaneus.
  - The external fixator is removed following fixation of the implants.
- Once the distractor has been assembled and the leg exsanguinated, a thigh tourniquet is inflated.
- A 15-cm anterior midline incision is then made centered over the ankle between the extensor hallucis longus and the tibialis anterior tendons.
- The superficial peroneal nerve lies directly beneath this incision and must be protected throughout the operation.
- The nerve is retracted laterally with the lateral skin flap.
- Dissection is carried out, splitting the extensor retinaculum and entering the tendon sheath of the extensor hallucis longus tendon to enter the ankle joint.
- An attempt is made to avoid violating the tendon sheath of the tibialis anterior.
- The deep peroneal nerve and anterior tibial artery are found beneath the extensor hallucis longus tendon and are retracted laterally as a unit with the tendon.
- Once this dissection has been completed, the entire distal tibia and ankle joint are visible in the surgical exposure (see Fig. 10–9C).
- The joint capsule is incised longitudinally, and subperiosteal dissection of the distal tibia is then continued medially and laterally to expose the joint from the medial malleolus to the fibula.
- Osteophytes should be excised at this time to restore as much normal anatomy as is possible.
- Further exposure of the ankle joint and of the fibula/syndesmosis is then dictated by the instrumentation

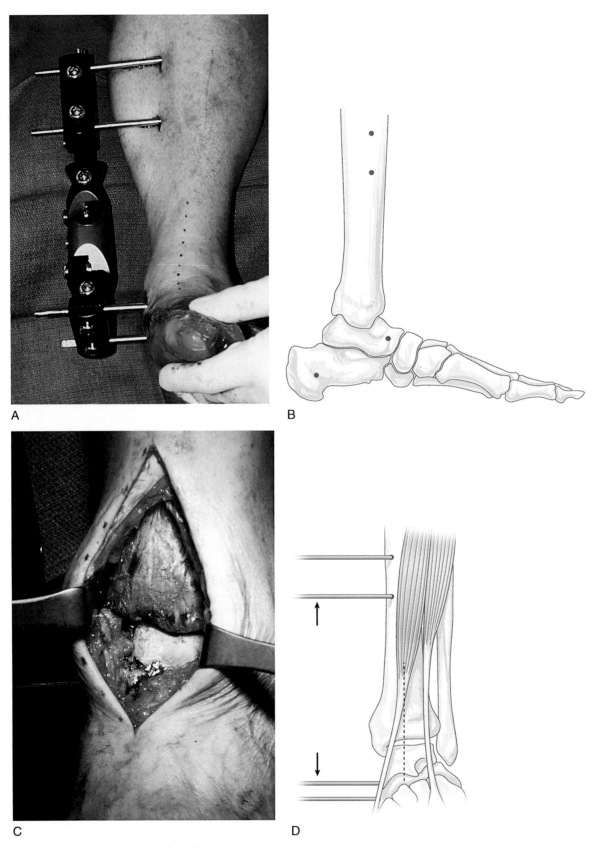

Figure 10–9: Agility total ankle replacement.
A, A medial external fixator is applied. Correction of any fixed equinus deformity is required before this step.
B, Diagram showing pin placement. **C,** The anterior ankle exposure is completed. **D,** Traction is applied at this time to correct any deformity and to restore ligamentous balance.

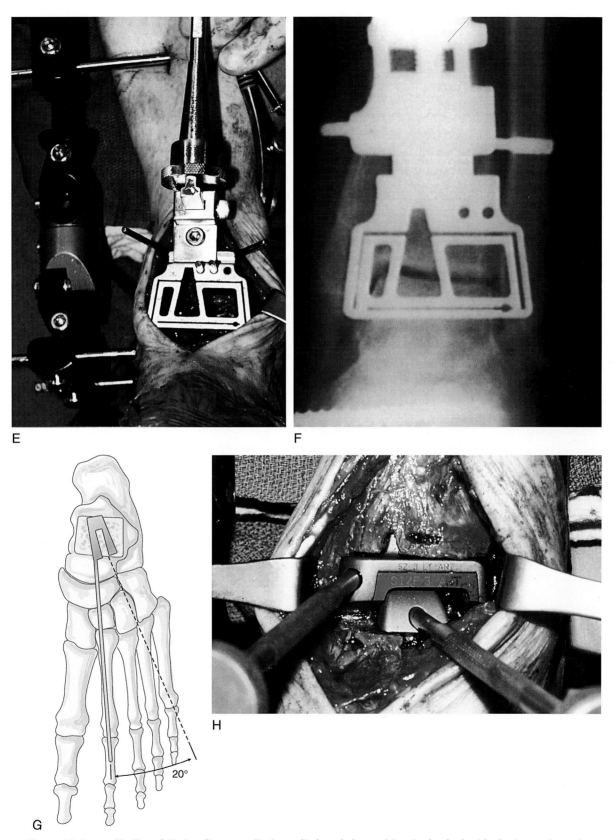

E

F

G

H

Figure 10–9, cont'd: **E** and **F**, An alignment jig is applied, and the position is checked with the image intensifier. **G**, The keel for the talar component is cut in 20 degrees of external rotation. H, The position of the trial components is checked, followed by insertion of the final components. (From Morrey BF [2003]. *Joint Replacement Arthroplasty*, 3rd ed. New York: Churchill Livingstone.)

and cutting jigs specific for the chosen implant (see Fig. 10–9E).

- The alignment jig is secured to the tibia with a unicortical half-pin, and the ankle is slightly distracted in the neutral position. The correct size of tibial jig is chosen to remove as little bone as possible while ensuring removal of all cartilaginous surfaces, including the cartilage from the lateral malleolus.
- Approximately 5 mm of bone are removed from the distal aspect of the tibia, and an additional 5 to 6 mm are removed from the talar dome.
- Using the provided instrumentation, trials are placed, and the final implants are seated in appropriate position.
- Once the components are in place, graft consisting of bone obtained from the resected articular surfaces is placed at the site of the syndesmosis, after which the syndesmosis is stabilized with lag screws.
- The fixator is then removed, and the skin is closed. After dressings are applied, a well-padded posterior splint is placed with the foot in neutral position. (Fig. 10–10).

Postoperative Management

- Although postoperative regimens remain controversial and are largely determined by surgeon preference, general trends are for the patient to remain non–weight bearing for 6 weeks postoperatively in a well-padded splint.
- During this 6-week period, the patient is encouraged to remove the splint and to move the ankle several times a day to prevent contracture and stiffness.
- Lengthy non–weight bearing prevents subsidence of the implants and impaction and weakening of the underlying cancellous bone.
- It is recommended that during the first postoperative 6 weeks, the patient wear the splint, on average, for more than 23 hours each day.
- Gradual progression to weight bearing as tolerated is then achieved over the next 6 weeks in a cam walker boot.
- Routine radiographs are obtained at 4 weeks, 8 weeks, 3 months, 6 months, and yearly thereafter.

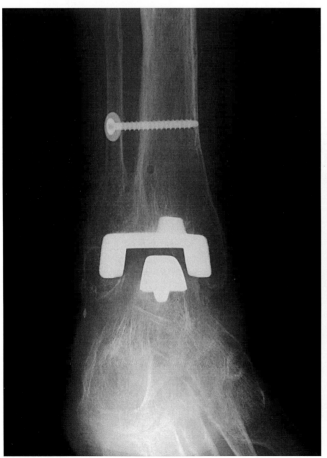

A

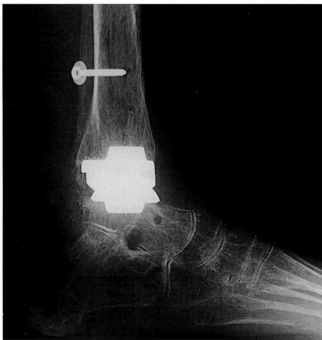

B

Figure 10–10: Agility total ankle replacement.
Mortise (**A**) and lateral (**B**) views of Agility total ankle replacement with a good alignment and ingrowth at 2 years. (From Morrey BF [2003]. *Joint Replacement Arthroplasty*, 3rd ed. New York: Churchill Livingstone.)

Surgical Alternatives to Arthroplasty

Distraction Arthroplasty

- *Distraction arthroplasty* is a relatively new method of treating OA and is based on the premise that patients with OA have some reparative ability. It is thought that mechanical unloading via joint distraction helps to relieve the osteoarthritic cartilage of additional mechanical stress. Joint distraction is maintained via an external fixator that eliminates contact between the arthritic surfaces (Fig. 10–11). Furthermore, patients are allowed to ambulate within a few days of the placement of the external fixator, which allows cyclic loading and unloading of the distracted joint.

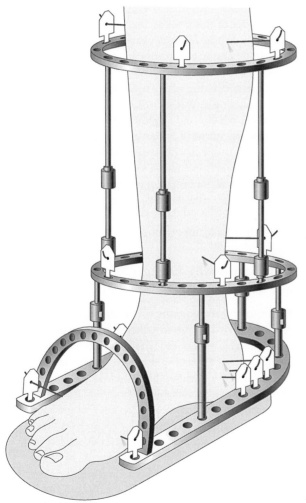

Figure 10–11: Ilizarov external ring fixator. Demonstration of the application of the Ilizarov external ring fixator for distraction of the ankle joint in the treatment of severe ankle osteoarthritis. (From Marijnissen ACA, van Roermund PM, van Melkebeek J, et al. [2002]. Clinical benefit of joint distraction in the treatment of severe osteoarthritis of the ankle. *Arthritis Rheum* 46:2893-2902.)

This, in turn, allows intermittent changes within the synovial fluid pressure, which is important for lubrication of the joint and cartilage nutrition.

- In a prospective study, Marijnissen and associates analyzed the clinical outcome of 57 patients with severe OA of the ankle who were treated with joint distraction via an Ilizarov external ring fixator (Marijnissen et al. 2002). Once the external fixator was placed, the joint was distracted by 0.5 mm each day until a total distraction of 5 mm was reached. Full weight bearing was allowed within 1 week after placement of the fixator, and ankle distraction was maintained at 5 mm for a period of 3 months.
    - With a mean follow-up of 2.8 years, there was a significant clinical improvement in terms of reduced pain, increased joint mobility, and improved function. Furthermore, there was also radiographic improvement of the distracted joint, in which joint space width had increased by 17% at 1 year following surgery. The joint space width had increased by an additional 10% for those patients who were followed for at least 3 years postoperatively.
    - Of note, 35 of the 57 patients underwent arthroscopic débridement so the foot could be placed in a plantigrade position that is requisite for distraction arthroplasty. However, the authors also compared the effects of joint distraction with arthroscopic débridement alone in a group of 17 patients (9 patients in the distraction group and 8 in the débridement group) and found significant improvements with regard to pain and function in the distraction group relative to the débridement group. Furthermore, within this group, three patients in the débridement group continued to have persistent severe pain, underwent distraction arthroplasty, and then experienced improvements in pain and function.
- Although studies on distraction arthroplasty have limited follow-up, this approach presents a potentially viable option for treating severe ankle arthritis. It could potentially delay the need for arthrodesis (thus potentially sparing adjacent joints from increased stress) or ankle arthroplasty, especially if the patient is young. With regard to this study in particular, approximately 25% of these patients did not experience an improvement with distraction arthroplasty, a finding indicating that patient variability has a definite role in affecting the clinical outcome of this procedure.

Open and Arthroscopic Débridement

- Débridement can be performed either arthroscopically or through an open approach, although arthroscopy is generally preferred.
- This method is best used when the degree of arthritis is mild to moderate, but it is not favored for severe end-stage arthritis, deformity, or arthrofibrosis. It can be used to remove impinging osteophytes and loose bodies and to address focal chondral defects.

Arthrodesis

- Arthrodesis is considered the gold standard treatment of severe arthritis of the ankle. It can reliably provide a stable, painless, plantigrade foot. Rates of successful fusion of 80% to 100% have been reported in various studies. It can be used to address arthritis of the ankle of all causes, including post-traumatic arthritis, OA, RA, or even failed TAAs.

- Although a detailed description of ankle arthrodesis is beyond the scope of this chapter, methods of stabilization of an arthrodesis include either internal fixation or external fixation. Internal fixation is generally preferred because it results in a higher fusion rate and provides a stronger biomechanical construct without the added burden of having an external fixator. However, external fixation has a role in the treatment of the infected ankle or in cases with a compromised soft tissue envelope.

- The optimal position of an ankle arthrodesis is in neutral dorsiflexion, 5 degrees of hindfoot valgus, and external rotation of the foot, similar to the contralateral extremity. The talus should also be shifted posteriorly relative to the tibia when fused. Fusion of the foot in neutral dorsiflexion also maximizes the amount of plantar flexion occurring through the midfoot (approximately 10 degrees) that aids in recreating a more efficient gait pattern.

- However, although arthrodesis remains the best current standard, it is not without complications. The most common are infection, nonunion, or malunion, but other complications such as neurovascular injury, tibial stress fracture, and adjacent joint arthritis can also occur.

- Coester and associates analyzed the long-term (mean follow-up, 22 years) results of ankle arthrodesis for post-traumatic arthritis in a series of 23 patients (Coester et al. 2001). These investigators found that the prevalence of OA in the ipsilateral subtalar, talonavicular, calcaneocuboid, naviculocuneiform, tarsometatarsal, and first metatarsophalangeal joints was increased (Fig. 10–12). The limb with the ankle arthrodesis was also more symptomatic relative to the contralateral extremity. Although ankle arthrodesis can reduce pain and can provide a stable foot for ambulation, it can result in long-term adjacent joint degeneration associated with significant dysfunction.

Results

First-Generation Implants

- Initial TAA implants had largely disappointing clinical results attributed to overall design flaws in the components.

- Design flaws seen in the first-generation implants included poor instrumentation, inaccurate positioning of implants, poor implant design (lack of metal-backed components on the tibial side), and excessive bone resection in preparation for implantation.

- Additional flaws with the first-generation ankle arthroplasties included failure to produce normal ankle kinematics, failure to correct angular deformities at the ankle, and inadequate recognition of the need for proper soft tissue balancing.

- Clinical problems frequently encountered included lateral ankle pain, antalgic and abnormal gait, and stiffness.

- In analyzing a series of 204 primary TAAs performed with the Mayo TAA system, 36% of arthroplasties were considered to be a failure (removal of the implant). The investigators recommended that this implant not be used to treat end-stage arthritis of the ankle.

- Other poor clinical results with similar types of implants led to the discontinuation of first-generation ankle arthroplasty systems.

Second-Generation Implants

- Because of the lack of clinical success with first-generation implants and as a result of the success observed with arthroplasties of other joints (e.g., the knee and hip), second-generation implants were developed to provide a favorable treatment for terminal ankle arthritis.

- Second-generation implants were designed with the aim of more closely reproducing normal ankle anatomy, ankle kinematics (including sliding and rotational motions of the ankle), ligamentous stability, and alignment. Reproduction of normal ankle anatomy included replacement of all three articulations of the ankle (talofibular, tibiotalar, and medial malleolar–talar). Additional features included a porous metal backing for each component to allow for biologic fixation to reduce the amount of bone needed to be resected for implantation.

- Second-generation implants that have been utilized include the two-component design with syndesmosis fusion and the three-component design.

Two-Component Design With Syndesmosis Fusion

- The prototypical two-component design is the Agility TAA. The early and intermediate-term results of the Agility prosthesis were evaluated by Pyevitch and associates (Pyevich et al. 1998). One hundred consecutive Agility prostheses were evaluated. Eighty-two patients (85 ankle arthroplasties) were available at a mean follow-up period of 4.8 years (range, 2.8 to 12.3 years). The preoperative diagnoses for the 100 TAAs included post-traumatic OA in 45 ankles, RA in 26 ankles, primary OA in 26, septic arthritis in 2 ankles, and psoriatic arthritis in 1 ankle.
  - Patients were available for both clinical and radiographic evaluation. Five of the 85 ankle arthroplasties had been revised. The reasons for revision included persistent pain (1 patient, converted to an ankle arthrodesis), tibial component fracture (1 patient), talar component loosening (2 patients), and talar component malpositioning (1 patient).
  - Sixty-five patients stated they were extremely satisfied with the procedure, 11 were satisfied, 3 were indifferent, and an additional 3 patients were dissatisfied.

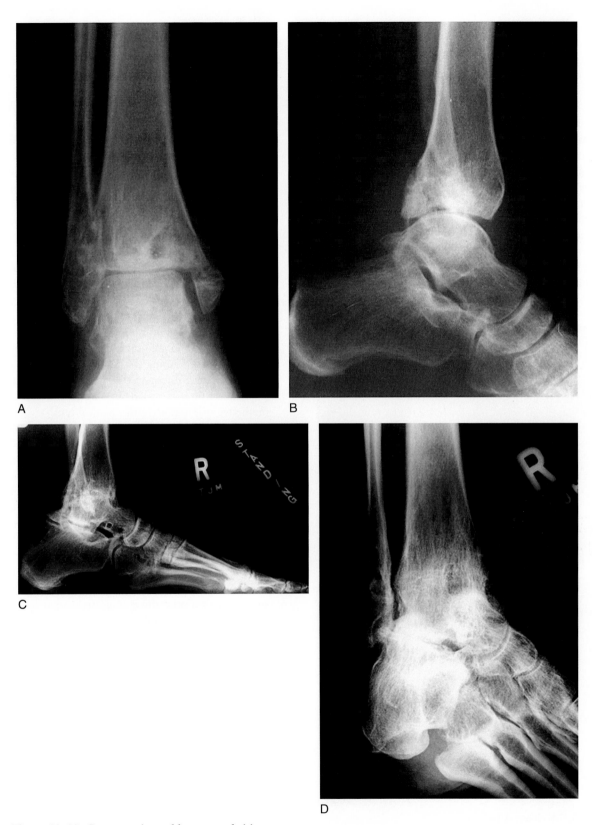

Figure 10–12: Postoperative ankle osteoarthritis.
A and **B,** Ankle osteoarthritis 1 year following an open fracture dislocation of the ankle; the patient had undergone ankle arthrodesis. **C** and **D,** Severe osteoarthritis of the subtalar joint observed 21 years postoperatively. (From Coester LM, Saltzman CL, Leupold J, Pontarelli W [2001]. Long-term results following ankle arthrodesis for post-traumatic arthritis. *J Bone Joint Surg Am* 83:219-228.)

- Patients who had post-traumatic arthritis reported significantly more pain than patients who had either RA or primary OA.
- Critical to the success of the Agility ankle is fusion of the syndesmosis. In this study, of the ankles available for follow-up, 61 ankles had a successful fusion, and 28 ankles had a delayed fusion (requiring >6 months for fusion), whereas 9 had a syndesmotic nonunion. Eight of 12 tibial component migrations were associated with a syndesmotic nonunion, with nonunion significantly increasing the risk of tibial component migration. Mechanical lysis in the presence of either a delayed union or a nonunion of the syndesmosis occurred along the lateral margin of the tibial component, between the fibula and the lateral aspect of the tibial component (Fig. 10–13). These investigators concluded that syndesmotic union is a requisite for stability of the tibial component.

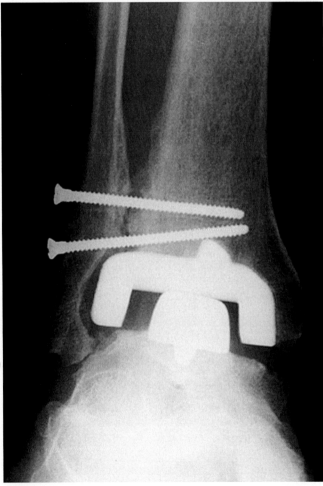

Figure 10–13: Mechanical lysis.
Mechanical lysis present along the lateral aspect of the tibial component observed with nonunion of the tibiofibular syndesmosis. (From Pyevitch MT, Saltzman CL, Callaghan JJ, Alvine FG [1998]. Total ankle arthroplasty: A unique design. *J Bone Joint Surg Am* 80:1420-1420.)

- Knecht and associates reported longer-term results with the Agility prosthesis (Knecht et al. 2004); 132 TAAs were performed in 126 patients. Eighty-one ankles were available at a mean follow-up period of 9 years. Sixty-seven patients (69 ankles) were available for clinical evaluation, and 90% of patients stated that they had reduced pain and were satisfied with the procedure.
- Fourteen major revisions were performed, and *major revisions* were defined as removal or replacement of one or both of the components. Of these patients, 7 underwent conversion to an arthrodesis, whereas the remaining 7 had a revision ankle arthroplasty. The reasons for failure included component subsidence/settling (5 patients), component loosening (4 patients), tibial component fracture (2 patients), talar component malalignment (1 patient), and infection (1 patient). In the entire cohort of patients, 32 nonrevision procedures were performed, with syndesmotic screw removal the most common.
- With regard to adjacent joint arthritis, only 19% had arthritic progress at the subtalar joint, whereas only 15% had progression at the talonavicular joint.
- Mean time to syndesmotic union was 10 months (range, 2 to 60 months). Syndesmotic nonunion was predictive of progressive mechanical lysis.
- Seventy-six percent of ankles demonstrated radiographic signs of lucency, and 42% demonstrated evidence of mechanical lysis. Mechanical lysis present in the lateral aspect of the tibial component was predictive of increased pain, along with syndesmotic nonunion or delayed union.
- With regard to component subsidence, talar subsidence was more common and was more likely to be progressive than tibial subsidence.
- These authors concluded that although problems and complications were related to the Agility ankle, the low incidence of progressive hindfoot arthritis and percentage of revision procedures indicated that it was a viable treatment for severe ankle arthritis.

Three-Component Design

- Three-component designs require less bone resection than two-component designs. Both the tibial and talar components have a porous metal backing and rely on biologic fixation. A polyethylene bearing is placed between the two components. The prototypical three-component design is the STAR device.
- Results of 51 consecutive STAR ankles were reported by Anderson and associates, with an average follow-up of approximately 4 years (range, 3 to 8 years) (Anderson et al. 2003).
  - Twelve ankles had to be revised, 7 revised for component loosening (3 done within the first 6 months following the index procedure); 2 ankles were revised for meniscal fracture, and an additional 3 were revised for unspecified reasons.

- Thirty-nine unrevised ankles were available for follow-up. The average ROM of the ankles was approximately 28 degrees (range, 10 to 55 degrees). The overall 5-year clinical survival rate was 0.70, with revision for any reason as the end point.
- Despite the high incidence of revision in this population, these authors concluded that because of the limited number of alternatives in treating terminal ankle arthritis, the STAR TAA could be a viable option compared with arthrodesis in treating ankle arthritis.

Complications

- Complications following use of the first-generation TAA implants were frequent and often precluded the use of the first-generation implants. As stated previously in a study analyzing the use of the Mayo total ankle replacement system, 36% of patients were considered to have failures, defined as removal of the implant for any reason. Invariably, all these reoperations resulted from persistent ankle pain (Kitaoka and Patzer 1996).
- Given that ankle arthroplasties are technically challenging procedures, it is not unexpected that they would have several types of complications. Complications in TAA can be divided as follows:
  - Wound complications and infection
  - Malalignment
  - Loosening
  - Nerve or tendon damage
  - Fracture

Wound Complications and Infection

- Various studies reported the incidence of minor wound complications such as delayed wound healing, wound edge necrosis, and superficial infection as ranging from 2% to 40%.
- Most wound complications involve wound edge necrosis that can typically be treated with wound care and oral antibiotics. Wound complications are potentially disastrous because skin breakdown can lead to superficial and potentially deep infection that may necessitate removal of the components. Additionally, wound complications can necessitate prolonged immobilization that leads to stiffness and limited ROM.
- Meticulous attention must be paid to the soft tissues and particularly to the extensor retinaculum, to reestablish its role as a protective layer.
- Myerson and Mroczek stated that avoidance of unnecessary and excessive retraction on the wound edges, by retracting only on one side at a time or at different levels of the wound, is critical in avoiding soft tissue complications (Myerson and Mroczek 2003). In their study analyzing the first 50 TAAs performed by a single surgeon, there was a 24% rate of minor wound complications in the first 25 surgical procedures compared with 8% in the next 25

patients who underwent TAA. These investigators concluded that familiarity with the total ankle exposure and with meticulous soft tissue management reduces the incidence of wound complications (Myerson and Mroczek 2003).
- As with other joint replacements, deep infections can also occur. Diagnosis of a deep infection should follow the algorithms of diagnosing infections of other joint prostheses, such as the hip or knee. Infection laboratory values such as a white blood cell count, erythrocyte sedimentation rate, and C-reactive protein should be obtained along with synovial fluid cultures and imaging studies. In a study analyzing complications and failures after TAA, Spirt and associates performed irrigation and débridements with retention of the components for acute deep infections (those infections that occurred ≤3 months following implantation of the prosthesis) (Spirt et al. 2004). Patients with late deep infections (those occurring >3 months following implantation of the prosthesis) were treated with extirpation of the components and implantation of an antibiotic spacer.

Malalignment

- Parameters used to measure component migration and malpositioning were developed by Pyevich and associates, who used both lateral and mortise radiographic views (Fig. 10–14) (Pyevich et al. 1998). These investigators defined *migration* of a component as a shift of at least 5 degrees in the measured angle that indicated the position of the component. A learning curve exists with ankle arthroplasties, and several studies have concluded that greater surgeon expertise with the instrumentation leads to improved positioning.
- As an example, with regard to avoiding valgus tilting of the talus, Myerson and Mroczek concluded that improper tension or distraction by the medially placed external fixator could lead to valgus tilting of the talus (Myerson and Mroczek 2003). In addition, setting the external fixator off the tibia will also help to avoid a plantar flexed tibial cut and thus avoid reduction of the overall motion allowed by the prosthesis.
- Malpositioning of components can lead to worse functional outcome. In particular, Pyevich and associates found that tibial components placed in greater than 4 degrees of valgus were associated with significantly higher rates of pain (Pyevich et al. 1998). Proper alignment with both components inserted to within 4 degrees of varus/valgus alignment is key to having a successful outcome.

Loosening

- In a study by Spirt, Assal, and Hansen analyzing 306 Agility TAAs, the authors found that component migration and subsidence typically involved the talar component (Spirt et al. 2004).
- Pyevitch and associates defined lucency and lysis as related to TAA components strictly (Pyevich et al. 1998).

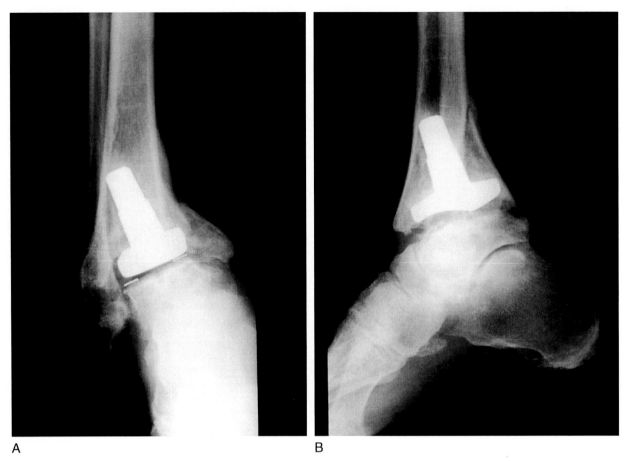

A   B

Figure 10–14: Failed total ankle arthroplasty.
A, Anteroposterior radiograph reveals an acute malleolar fracture and varus deformity. **B,** Lateral view shows malposition of the tibial component. The subtalar joint does not appear to be compromised. (From Morrey BF [2003]. *Joint Replacement Arthroplasty*, 3rd ed. New York: Churchill Livingstone.)

Radiolucent lines smaller than 2 mm were defined as *lucencies,* whereas radiolucent areas larger than 2 mm were defined as *lysis.*

- It is important to serially evaluate components radiographically for evidence of lucency and lysis.
- For the two-component design with syndesmotic fusion, nonunion and delayed union of the syndesmosis were related to increased lysis of the tibial component that was progressive. Pyevich and associates concluded that syndesmotic fusion is vital to a stable tibial component (Pyevich et al. 1998). For those implants that had problems with syndesmotic union, the areas of lysis were typically seen along the lateral margin of the tibial component (an area of high shear stress within the bone-implant interface). However, this progressive lysis ceased once syndesmotic union was achieved.
- Talar component migration and loosening are related to component subsidence as a result of the axial loads placed on it. These complications have not been found to be related to syndesmotic union. Unfortunately, talar component migration is more common and more problematic

with regard to the overall survival of the implant. Talar component migration will likely be encountered more frequently as longer-term results are obtained with TAA.

Nerve or Tendon Damage

- Nerve and tendon lacerations are possible complications of TAA.
- The posteromedial tendons (posterior tibial, flexor hallucis longus, flexor digitorum longus) appear to be the most at risk when one advances the saw blade posteriorly. The posterior extent of the talar and tibial cuts should be performed with caution, especially when cutting the posteromedial aspect of the tibia. This is particularly a problem with posttraumatic arthritic ankles, in which exposure can be difficult.
- Nerve lacerations can occur with extreme medial and lateral extents of the bone cuts, particularly the superficial and deep peroneal nerves. Nerve injuries can also occur through excessive retraction on soft tissue structures. This necessitates surgeon expertise and proper soft tissue technique in performing TAAs.

Fracture

- Intraoperative fracture of either the tibia or the talus can occur during the bone cuts or during insertion of the components.
- Preoperative templates and intraoperative fluoroscopy should be used to determine prosthesis size. Intraoperative fluoroscopy is especially helpful in ensuring proper cutting block placement and to verify the accuracy of the cuts once they are made.
- Other technical tips that should be followed to avoid fracture include the following:
  - The lateral malleolus is located posterior and angled 30 degrees relative to the tibial plafond. Knowledge of its exact anatomic location is imperative to proper bone cuts and implant positioning. Placing a laminar spreader between the tibia and fibula to distract the lateral malleolus away from the saw when performing the tibial and talar cuts will aid in protecting the lateral malleolus. If the surgeon is unsure of the exact position of the lateral malleolus before making the tibial and talar bone cuts, the lateral malleolus can be cut freehand.

- The medial apex of the tibial cut should be conservative and should leave enough medial malleolus to prevent a medial malleolar fracture. The tibial cutting guide can be lateralized to allow for sufficient medial malleolar bone, to ensure safe tibial component insertion.

Revision Surgery

- Salvage of a failed TAA is a difficult challenge. The surgeon faces obstacles involving bone loss, wound complications (possible compromised soft tissue envelope), infection, or even a combination of these problems. As a result, salvage procedures have a high risk of failure and morbidity. If the reason for failure is infection, then the infection must be eradicated before salvage surgery can be considered.
- Three treatment options exist in salvaging failed TAA: (1) revision arthroplasty, (2) arthrodesis, or (3) below-the-knee amputation. Arthrodesis is likely the most favorable option in a revision situation when bone quality is poor or is insufficient to support the implantation of a new prosthesis. An arthrodesis can help either to restore or to maintain limb length or alignment. Fig. 10–15 demonstrates

Figure 10–15: Arthrodesis techniques for failed total ankle arthroplasty.
A, Malleolar resection. **B,** Modified Chuinard arthrodesis. **C,** Modified Campbell arthrodesis. **D,** Posterior tibiotalocalcaneal arthrodesis. (From Morrey BF [2003]. *Joint Replacement Arthroplasty*, 3rd ed. New York: Churchill Livingstone.)

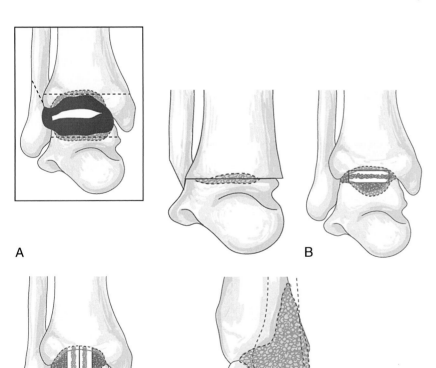

A

B

C

D

various arthrodesis techniques for failed TAA. Revision arthroplasty is a technically difficult procedure with high risk (provided sufficient bone stock remains to support a new prosthesis), and little information, mainly in the form of anecdotal cases, exists on the clinical outcome of these cases.

- Carlsson and associates analyzed a series of 21 patients who underwent ankle arthrodesis following failed TAA (Carlsson et al. 1998). Of the 21 patients, 4 had arthrodesis resulting from infection, 14 had aseptic loosening, and 3 had unexplained pain. The primary diagnoses leading to TAA included RA in 12 patients, psoriatic arthritis in 2 patients, and post-traumatic arthritis in 3. Four of the 21 ankles had a failed arthrodesis, whereas 17 had a successful, functional arthrodesis. Of these 17 patients, 4 required a repeat arthrodesis to gain successful fusion. Those patients who had successful fusion had a satisfactory clinical outcome. Although these authors concluded that arthrodesis can be a successful salvage procedure following failed TAA, operative approaches need to be individualized because of the possibility of compromised soft tissue envelope, bone loss (including the potential that the entire talus may be missing), and infection.

Conclusion

- The management of patients with ankle arthritis has evolved over the past decade as advancements in implant design and surgical technique have coincided with improved understanding of the normal and pathologic anatomy of the ankle.
- Reports of results of surgical management of the arthritic ankle have been encouraging with respect to pain relief and restoration of function.
- We are cautiously optimistic that with modern design and technique, TAA will remain as a sound alternative to fusion for those with debilitating arthritic conditions of the ankle.

References

Anderson T, Montgomery F, Carlsson A (2003). Uncemented STAR total ankle prostheses. *J Bone Joint Surg Am* 85:1321-1329.

The purpose of this article is to present the results of a consecutive series of STAR prostheses; 51 consecutive prostheses were implanted over a 6-year period. Twelve ankles had to be revised, 7 because of loosening. Thirty-nine unrevised ankles were evaluated at an average follow-up of 52 months, and 31 patients were satisfied overall with the procedure and noted an improvement in the mean Kofoed score. The estimated 5-year survival rate was 0.70, with revision for any reason as the end point. Provided the implants are positioned properly, these authors concluded that ankle replacement can be a realistic option.

Alvine F (2000). Total ankle arthroplasty. In: Myerson M, ed. *Foot and Ankle Disorders*. Philadelphia: WB Saunders, pp 1085-1102.

This is a comprehensive review chapter on TAA.

Carlsson AS, Montgomery F, Besjakov J (1998). Arthrodesis of the ankle secondary to replacement. *Foot Ankle Int* 19:240-245.

The investigators of this study analyzed 21 patients who underwent ankle arthrodesis for failed TAA. Reasons for failure of the prosthesis included unexplained pain, aseptic loosening, and infection. Arthrodesis was successful in 17 patients. All patients undergoing arthrodesis related to infection had a successful result. Ankle arthrodesis can be performed successfully after failed arthroplasty.

Coester LM, Saltzman CL, Leupold J, Pontarelli W (2001). Long-term results following ankle arthrodesis for post-traumatic arthritis. *J Bone Joint Surg Am* 83:219-228.

This cardinal article outlines the problem of adjacent joint arthritis following ankle arthrodesis. The clinical and radiographic results of 23 patients who had an ankle arthrodesis for post-traumatic arthritis were followed for a mean of 22 years. The presence of OA in the ipsilateral subtalar, talonavicular, calcaneocuboid, naviculocuneiform, tarsometatarsal, and first metatarsophalangeal joints was significantly increased and also more severe. Patients reported significant pain and disability, with the ipsilateral side routinely more symptomatic.

Coughlin M (1999). Arthritides. In: Coughlin MJ, Mann RA, eds. *Surgery of the Foot and Ankle,* 7th ed. St. Louis: Mosby.

This is a comprehensive review chapter on the etiology, pathophysiology, and treatment of the various types of ankle arthropathies. A thorough description of TAAs, including surgical technique and postoperative care, is also given.

Cushnaghan J, Dieppe P (1991). Study of 500 patients with limb joint osteoarthritis. I. Analysis by age, sex, and distribution of symptomatic joint sites. *Ann Rheum Dis* 50:8-13.

This epidemiologic study focuses on a series of 500 patients with symptomatic limb joint OA. The distribution of affected joints and associated factors were analyzed including that of ankle OA. The number of sites affected, as well as the distribution, was strongly related to age and gender, a finding suggesting that polyarticular OA arises from slow acquisition of new joint sites in a nonrandom distribution. Generalized OA did not emerge as a distinct entity.

Huch K, Keuttner KE, Dieppe P (1997). Osteoarthritis in ankle and knee. *Semin Arthritis Rheum* 26:667-674.

This review article analyzes the epidemiologic factors leading to OA of the ankle and knee. Ankle and knee joints differ in their susceptibility to OA likely because of differences in joint motion, cartilage thickness, congruency, mechanical forces, and even evolutionary changes. Unlike in the knee, ankle cartilage develops fissures that do not appear to progress to later stages of OA. The possible reason may be that ankle and knee chondrocytes respond differently to stimuli.

Kitaoka HB, Patzer GL (1996). Clinical results of the Mayo total ankle arthroplasty. *J Bone Joint Surg Am* 78:1658-1664.

This study presents the radiographic and clinical results of the Mayo Clinic TAA, a first-generation implant; 160 arthroplasties were analyzed in 143 patients with a mean follow-up period of 9 years. Fifty-seven arthroplasties were removed and were thus defined as failures. Radiographic loosening was observed in 8% of tibial components and in 57% of talar components. Although not invariably associated with failure, most ankles with radiographic evidence of loosening likely had an unsuccessful clinical result.

Because of the high rate of failure and the complications encountered, the authors recommended that the Mayo implant not be used to treat patients with RA or OA of the ankle.

Knecht SI, Estin M, Callaghan JJ, et al. (2004). The Agility total ankle arthroplasty. *J Bone Joint Surg Am* 86:1161-1171.

The authors of this study presented the long-term results of the Agility TAA system as a follow-up study to the intermediate-term results of Pyevitch and associates; 132 arthroplasties were performed in 126 patients. After a mean follow-up period of 9 years, 33 patients (36 implants) died, and 14 patients (11%) had an implant revision or an ankle arthrodesis. More than 90% of the patients followed clinically reported a reduction in pain and were satisfied overall with the outcome of the surgery. Radiographically, 19% had progressive subtalar arthritis, and 76% had evidence of periimplant radiolucency. Syndesmotic nonunion led to progressive mechanical lysis around the prosthesis; syndesmotic union was critical to the integrity of the prosthesis. The authors concluded that the relatively low rates of radiographic hindfoot arthritis and the need for revision procedures at a mean follow-up of 9 years were encouraging and that the Agility TAA system is a viable option for the treatment of ankle arthritis in selected patients.

Kofoed H (2004). Scandinavian total ankle replacement (STAR). *Clin Orthop Relat Res* 424:73-79.

This prospective study analyzed the results of a cemented versus uncemented meniscal-bearing prosthesis (STAR). Nine of 33 patients in the cemented group had revision surgery or fusion, whereas only 1 of 25 patients had revision surgery in the uncemented group. Uncemented implants demonstrated superior survivorship (70% survival rate [confidence limit, 60.3 to 78.5] for the cemented group and 95.4% survival rate [confidence limit, 91.0 to 99.9] for the uncemented group) and improved clinical outcome. It is therefore recommended that unconstrained meniscal-bearing ankle prostheses should be uncemented.

Marijnissen ACA, van Roermund PM, van Melkebeek J, et al. (2002). Clinical benefit of joint distraction in the treatment of severe osteoarthritis of the ankle. *Arthritis Rheum* 46:2893-2902.

The authors presented both an open prospective trial and a randomized controlled study analyzing the benefit of joint distraction for the treatment of ankle arthritis; 75% of patients in the open prospective study reported a clinical benefit. Patients undergoing distraction had a superior clinical result relative to débridement in the randomized study. Although the follow-up was short, the results demonstrated that joint distraction could be a potential option in treating severe OA of the ankle.

Myerson MS, Mroczek K (2003). Perioperative complications of total ankle arthroplasty. *Foot Ankle Int* 24:17-21.

Perioperative complications of the first 50 patients undergoing TAA with the Agility prosthesis were analyzed. The initial 25 patients were compared with the subsequent 25. A higher number of complications (minor wound infections, nerve or tendon laceration, and fractures) was noted in the first group relative to the second, a finding indicating that a learning curve exists when performing TAA.

Pyevich MT, Saltzman CL, Callaghan JJ, Alvine FG (1998). Total ankle arthroplasty: A unique design. *J Bone Joint Surg Am* 80:1410-1420.

This study is a precursor to one conducted by Knecht and associates and presents the intermediate-term (mean follow-up, 4.8 years) of the Agility TAA. Eighty-two patients of the initial 100 formed the basis of the study; 93% of patients reported a satisfactory outcome. Importantly, the authors found that nonunion or delayed union of the syndesmosis resulted in progressive mechanical lysis around the tibial component.

SooHoo NF, Kominski G (2004). Cost-effectiveness analysis of total ankle arthroplasty. *J Bone Joint Surg Am* 86:2446-2455.

These authors created a decision model for the treatment of end-stage ankle arthritis. Although the current literature has not yet demonstrated that TAA is a cost-effective procedure, the analysis presented in this study showed that it could be a financially beneficial alternative to ankle arthrodesis.

Spirt AA, Assal M, Hansen ST (2004). Complications and failure after total ankle arthroplasty. *J Bone Joint Surg Am* 86:1172-1178.

This article analyzed factors that influence reoperation and failure in TAA. Age was the only significant factor found to be predictive of reoperation and failure. The 5-year survival rate, with failure as an end point, was 80% overall and 89% for those patients who were older than 54 years. Reoperations most commonly included débridement of heterotopic bone, correction of axial malalignment, and component replacement.

Thomas RH, Daniels TR (2003). Current concepts review: Ankle arthritis. *J Bone Joint Surg Am* 85:923-936.

This review article outlines the pathophysiology and epidemiology of ankle arthritis as well as the operative options available for treatment. Overviews of ankle arthrodesis and TAA are presented.

Walling A (2004). Arthritis of the ankle and hindfoot. In: Richardson GE, ed. *Orthopaedic Knowledge Update: Foot and Ankle,* 3rd ed. Rosemont, IL: American Academy of Orthopaedic Surgeons, pp 155-166.

This chapter provides an evaluation of ankle arthritis as well as a summary discussion of the nonsurgical and surgical treatments available.

CHAPTER 11

Shoulder Arthroplasty

Joseph A. Abboud,* Charles L. Getz,† and Gerald R. Williams, Jr.‡

*MD, Clinical Assistant Professor, Department of Orthopaedics, University of Pennsylvania
School of Medicine, Philadelphia, PA
†MD, Assistant Professor, Department of Orthopaedic Surgery, University of Pennsylvania;
Assistant Professor, Division of Shoulder and Elbow Surgery, Penn-Presbyterian Medical
Center, Philadelphia, PA
‡MD, Attending Surgeon, The Rothman Institute of Orthopaedic Surgery,
Thomas Jefferson University, Philadelphia, PA

Introduction

- The main articulation of the shoulder is the *glenohumeral joint.*
- The glenohumeral joint normally has smooth hyaline cartilage on the surfaces of the proximal humerus and the glenoid.
- The *rotator cuff* consists of the subscapularis, supraspinatus, infraspinatus, and teres minor.
  - The deltoid's direction of pull causes an abnormal superior migration of the humeral head if the rotator cuff is deficient.
  - The rotator cuff's main function is to act as a fulcrum to depress the humeral head while the deltoid lifts the arm.
  - Loss of the rotator cuff's ability to act as a fixed fulcrum leads to a loss of overhead shoulder function.
- Shoulder replacement is performed most commonly to restore a smooth articulation between the proximal humerus and the glenoid. This results in decreased pain.
- The ability of the shoulder to establish a fixed fulcrum determines overhead function in the replaced shoulder.
- Unless otherwise noted, shoulder replacement is done primarily as a pain-relieving operation, with the secondary benefit of increased function.
- Retroversion of the proximal humerus is quite variable and ranges from 25 to 40 degrees when measured from the intercondylar axis of the elbow (Fig. 11–1*A*).
- *Glenoid version* is determined based on a line drawn perpendicular to the plane of the scapula. Normal glenoid version is from 0 to 7 degrees of retroversion (Fig. 11–1*B*).
- The *head-shaft angle,* defined as the angle subtended by the plane of the anatomic neck and the longitudinal axis of the humeral shaft, ranges from 30 to 55 degrees.
- Reestablishing the normal relationships places the rotator cuff at its most efficient resting tension and gives the best results (Fig. 11–2).
- The greater tuberosity is located 5 to 10 mm inferior to the superiormost part of the humeral head; it should not be placed proximal to the head or more than 10 mm inferior to the head. This relationship is one of the most important parameters to reestablish and maintain when proximal humerus reconstruction is performed.
- The center of the humeral head is offset, on average, 6.9 mm medial and 2.6 mm posterior to the center of the humeral canal (Fig. 11–3) (Boileau et al. 2001).

Patient and Implant Selection
Osteoarthritis

- *Osteoarthritis* is a primary disease of articular cartilage.
- Osteoarthritis involves degeneration of articular cartilage, which causes a roughening of the joint surfaces of both the glenoid and the proximal humerus.

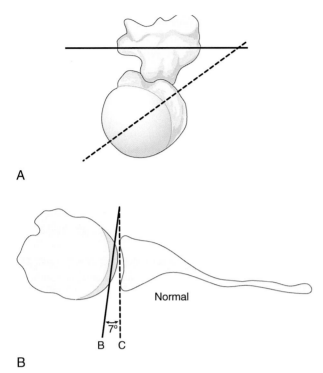

A

B C

Figure 11–1: Glenoid and humeral retroversion.
A and **B,** The range of glenoid and humeral retroversion is quite variable, ranging between 4 and 12 degrees for glenoid and between 25 and 40 degrees for the humerus. (From Rockwood CA Jr, Matsen FA III, Wirth MA, Lippitt SB, eds. [2004]. *The Shoulder*, 3rd ed. Philadelphia: WB Saunders, pp 13, 202.)

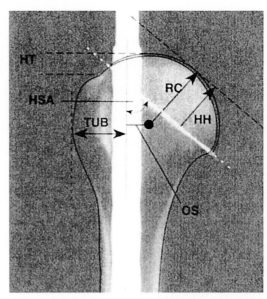

Figure 11–2: Normal anatomic relationships of the proximal humerus.
Plain radiograph marked to demonstrate head height *(HH)*, head to tuberosity height *(HT)*, head-shaft angle *(HSA)*, radius of curvature *(RC)*, and medial offset of the center of rotation to the center of the humeral shaft *(OS)*. TUB, greater tuberosity. (From Pearl ML, Volk AG [1996]. Coronal plane geometry of the proximal humerus relevant to prosthetic arthroplasty. *J Shoulder Elbow Surg* 5:320-326.)

- Patients typically present with pain with or without stiffness, with a progressive onset of the symptoms over many years.
- An inciting event such as minor trauma can make nonpainful arthritis become painful.
- Patients with osteoarthritis of the shoulder tend to be younger than patients with knee or hip arthritis.
- Loss of passive and active range of motion (particularly loss of external rotation with the arm at the side) and pain with range of motion are common physical examination findings.
- The main differential diagnosis for osteoarthritis is adhesive capsulitis.
- Radiographs required to confirm diagnosis should include orthogonal radiographs including anteroposterior, scapular Y, and axillary views.
- Findings on radiographs consistent with osteoarthritis include the presence of an inferior humeral head osteophyte, asymmetric joint space narrowing, subchondral sclerosis, and cyst formation (Fig. 11–4).
- The glenoid is most often worn eccentrically, with asymmetric cartilage and occasional bone loss.

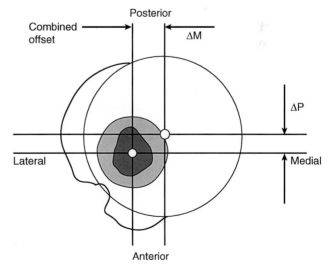

Figure 11–3: Humeral head offset.
The center of the humeral shaft is offset from the center of the humeral head. The center of the shaft is 2 to 4 mm anterior and 7 to 9 mm lateral to the center of the head. ΔM, medial offset; ΔP, posterior offset. (From Boileau P, Walch G [1997]. The three-dimensional geometry of the proximal humerus: Implications, surgical technique and prosthetic design. *J Bone Joint Surg Br* 79:857-865.)

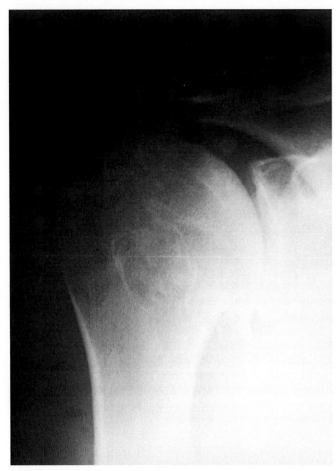

Figure 11–4: Radiographic features of an arthritic shoulder. Plain anteroposterior radiograph of an arthritic shoulder, including asymmetric joint space narrowing, an inferior osteophyte, subchondral cyst formation, and a loose body.

- The best study for evaluating glenoid wear is a computed tomographic (CT) scan (Fig. 11–5).
- An axillary x-ray view and magnetic resonance imaging (MRI) scans can also help to determine glenoid wear, but not as accurately as a CT scan.
- Rotator cuff tears occur in approximately 5% to 10% of shoulders displaying osteoarthritis.
- An MRI scan can show rotator cuff disease in patients with such poor motion that rotator cuff testing cannot be performed.
- Shoulder arthroplasty can relieve the pain associated with osteoarthritis of the shoulder and usually leads to an improvement in shoulder function.

Nonoperative Treatment

- Nonoperative treatment consists of activity modification, medication, physical therapy, and injections.
- Oral medications include nonsteroidal anti-inflammatory drugs and acetaminophen.
- Activity modification includes changing professions (e.g., from manual labor to a desk job), changing hobbies,

(e.g., giving up weight lifting), or modifying activities of daily living (e.g., getting help with household chores).
- Physical therapy consists of gentle range-of-motion exercises with minimal or no strength training.
- Physical therapy is variable in its effect on an arthritic shoulder and in some patients may lead to worsening of the pain.
- Intra-articular corticosteroid injections (e.g., dexamethasone) can provide variable relief from pain.
- Overuse of corticosteroid injections can have deleterious effects such as further degeneration of articular cartilage.
- Injection of viscosupplementary compounds (e.g., hyaluronic acid) is not approved for the treatment of osteoarthritis of the shoulder at this time by the US Food and Drug Administration.
- Surgical intervention is considered for patients with severe symptoms and significant functional disability in whom conservative treatment has failed.

Surgical Options Other Than Arthroplasty

- Shoulder arthritis in the young, active patient (<40 years old) is a difficult problem because of the limited life expectancy of a shoulder replacement.
- In the young, higher-demand patient, traditional arthroplasty (hemiarthroplasty or total shoulder arthroplasty [TSA]) is avoided whenever possible.
- Some patients with early shoulder arthritis on x-ray studies present with loss of motion.
- With minimal bone deformity (humeral osteophytes <1 to 2 cm) on radiography and an examination with loss of motion, arthroscopic débridement and capsular release of the glenohumeral joint can be performed with variable success.
  - Arthroscopic capsular release is believed to allow the joint to wear through a wider area, potentially increasing the contact area of the joint surfaces. This, in turn, leads to a favorable decrease in the contact pressures on the glenoid and proximal humeral surfaces.
  - As a result, the degenerative process may be slowed down and allow for better function, thus delaying or potentially obviating the need for arthroplasty.
- Microfracture arthroplasty (arthroscopic drilling of exposed subchondral bone) may promote the growth of fibrocartilage to fill in the defects on the articular surface and may decrease symptoms.
- In the young, high-demand patient with advanced glenohumeral arthritis, arthroscopic capsular release in combination with débridement or microfracture arthroplasty may not be as successful in diminishing symptoms.
  - In these patients, interpositional arthroplasty without humeral head replacement can be performed, also with variable success.
  - Interposition arthroplasty involves the placement of soft tissue between the humerus and glenoid articular

Figure 11–5: Bilateral arthritis of the shoulder. Computed tomographic image of a patient with bilateral arthritis of the shoulder at the level of the glenohumeral joint. Note the posterior (eccentric) wear of his right glenoid fossa, whereas the left glenoid exhibits central (concentric) wear.

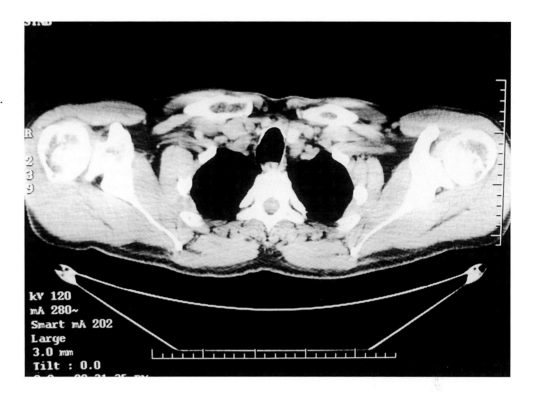

surfaces to improve the bearing characteristics of the joint surfaces.
- The surgical procedure is performed through a standard deltopectoral approach.
- The humeral head is reshaped by removing osteophytes.
- If eccentric glenoid wear is present, the glenoid is reamed to neutral version before the interposition graft is placed.
- The interposition graft can be composed of fascia lata, meniscus allograft, dermis, or anterior joint capsule.
- Releases to improve range of motion are also performed (see the later discussion of technique for TSA).
- Subscapularis advancement or lengthening is also performed in a fashion similar to the method described next for TSA.

Arthroplasty

- The three types of arthroplasty for the patient with an osteoarthritic shoulder are TSA, hemiarthroplasty, and humeral resurfacing arthroplasty (Fig. 11–6).

Total Shoulder Arthroplasty

- TSA is believed to provide the most predictable postoperative pain relief for patients with osteoarthritis of the shoulder.
- TSA consists of a humeral and a glenoid component.
- The humeral component is made of metal, usually a combination of a chrome-cobalt head with a titanium stem; the glenoid component is most commonly made of ultrahigh-molecular-weight polyethylene.

- The glenoid component appears to be the weak link in implant survival because it wears out faster with high activity levels, deficient rotator cuff, and possibly metal backing.
- A deficient rotator cuff allows proximal migration of the humeral component with edge loading of the glenoid that may lead to premature loosening and polyethylene wear.
- Patients with a reparable cuff tear are candidates for TSA. However, when the rotator cuff deficiency is not correctable, hemiarthroplasty or reverse TSA should be considered.
- Metal-backed glenoids have had a higher failure rate than all-polyethylene components.

Hemiarthroplasty

- Hemiarthroplasty for osteoarthritis may result in acceptable pain relief.
- The metal (humeral head) on cartilage (native glenoid) articulation may lead to some residual symptoms of pain, but there is no risk of glenoid component loosening as in TSA.
- Hemiarthroplasty in patients with concentric glenoid wear typically have the best postoperative results.
- Patients with eccentric glenoid wear should have the glenoid wear addressed at the time of implant so the remaining native glenoid surface is concentric with the humeral head.
- As mentioned previously, patients with irreparable rotator cuff tears are not candidates for TSA because proximal migration of the humeral head leads to premature glenoid

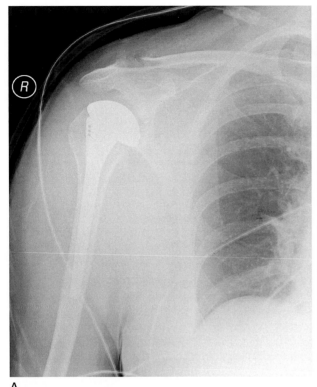

A

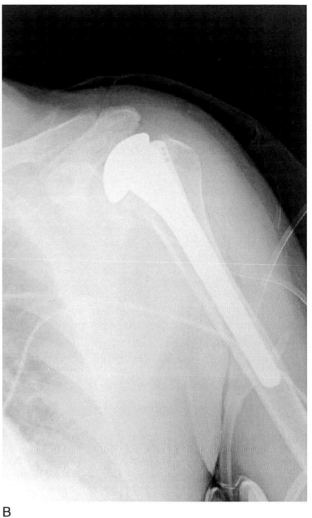

B

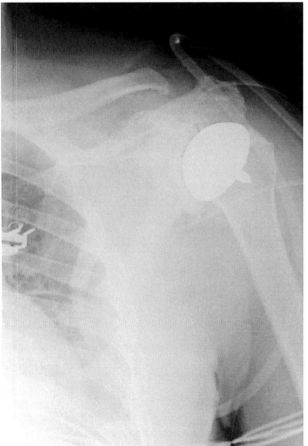

C

Figure 11–6: Humeral resurfacing arthroplasty.
A, Plain anteroposterior radiograph of a total shoulder replacement with restoration of the normal anatomic relationships of the proximal humerus. **B,** Plain anteroposterior radiograph of a patient with a humeral hemiarthroplasty, also with anatomic restoration of the normal relationships of the proximal humerus. **C,** Plain anteroposterior radiograph of a patient with a humeral resurfacing arthroplasty. This procedure may improve results of future revision surgery by preserving humeral metaphyseal and humeral shaft bone stock.

component wear and failure. These patients should be considered for hemiarthroplasty. In these cases, the coracoacromial arch must be preserved at all costs because it is the only remaining restraint to proximal humeral migration.

Humeral Resurfacing Arthroplasty

- Humeral resurfacing arthroplasty is typically indicated in young, high-demand patients with severe shoulder pain resulting from osteoarthritis refractory to nonoperative treatment and who have a concentric glenoid or one that can be made concentric.
- Humeral resurfacing prosthetic components have a peg that enters the metaphysis of the humerus but does not go down the medullary canal of the shaft.
- Humeral resurfacing is thought to preserve humeral bone stock for the future revisions that many young patients will require.
- The exposure of the glenoid may be difficult with a humeral resurfacing prosthesis, so if major deformity of the glenoid exists, removing the humeral head before glenoid preparation will improve glenoid exposure.

Rheumatoid Arthritis and Inflammatory Arthritides

- *Rheumatoid arthritis* is a systemic autoimmune disease in which the patient's synovium incites an inflammatory response.
- Rheumatoid arthritis affects multiple joints and organ systems.
- The inflammatory response destroys soft tissues (e.g., the rotator cuff) and the joint surface (Fig. 11–7).
- Massive glenoid and humeral bone loss can be present.
- Glenoid bone loss usually occurs concentrically.
- As in patients with osteoarthritis, CT scans are the best radiographic modality to assess glenoid bone loss, whereas MRI scans are best to assess rotator cuff integrity.
- Evaluation of the patient with rheumatoid arthritis should assess the extent that the disease is being controlled systemically. In the process of treatment, attempts at medical management to decrease joint pain should be maximized.
- When considering multiple joint reconstructions in the upper extremity, the most proximal joints are typically replaced first.
- When upper and lower extremity joint involvement are equal, the lower extremity joints are addressed first to minimize weight bearing through the replaced upper extremity joint.
- When the ipsilateral shoulder and elbow are to be reconstructed, planning must be made to ensure the stems of both components will fit in the humerus.
- When surgery of any kind is considered on a patient with rheumatoid arthritis, flexion and extension films of the cervical spine are needed to assess cervical spine stability, especially at the C1-C2 level, given the high incidence of atlantoaxial instability in this patient group.

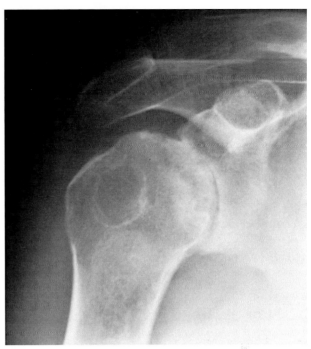

Figure 11–7: Rheumatoid arthritis. Symmetric joint surface destruction, periarticular cyst formation and osteopenia, and central glenoid erosion are characteristic findings on radiographs in rheumatoid arthritis. (From Rockwood CA Jr, Matsen FA III, Wirth MA, Lippitt SB, eds. [2004]. *The Shoulder*, 3rd ed. Philadelphia: WB Saunders, p 903.)

Surgical Treatment Other Than Arthroplasty

- Surgical procedures should be entertained only in patients with severe symptoms and functional disability in whom nonoperative management in the form of medical maximization of systemic treatment of rheumatoid arthritis has failed.

Synovectomy

- Surgical synovectomy (open, arthroscopic) can reduce pain associated with synovitis in arthritic joints.
- Surgical synovectomy is better then medical synovectomy in relieving pain and in improving function.
- The results of synovectomy are temporary because synovitis frequently recurs.
- Synovectomy is mainly used in young patients with minimal joint changes, although results have been encouraging for more patients with advanced rheumatoid arthritis in some series.

Arthroplasty

- In patients with adequate glenoid bone stock and an intact rotator cuff, TSA results in excellent pain relief and modestly improved range of motion and function.
- TSA results in better pain relief and function than hemiarthroplasty (Barrett et al. 1989).

- Hemiarthroplasty is reserved for patients with either massive bone loss or an irreparable rotator cuff.
- A reverse prosthesis can be performed in patients with good glenoid bone stock but an irreparable rotator cuff (Rittmeister and Kerschbaumer 2001).

Other Inflammatory Conditions Associated With Shoulder Arthritis

- Other inflammatory-type arthritides that may affect the shoulder include psoriatic arthritis, arthritis of inflammatory bowel disease, and ankylosing spondylitis.
- Rheumatologic syndromes that are less frequently associated with shoulder involvement include Reiter's syndrome and systemic lupus erythematosus.
- Systemic lupus erythematosus is associated with avascular necrosis (AVN) of the humeral head in approximately 10% of patients with this condition.

Avascular Necrosis of the Humeral Head

- AVN of the humeral head is a disease process that results in bone death of the humeral epiphysis.
- Typically, patients with AVN are younger than patients with osteoarthritis.
- With collapse of supporting bone, the articular surface becomes involved.
- The causes of AVN are varied and include the following:
  - Proximal humerus fractures and dislocations
  - Radiation therapy
  - Sickle cell anemia, Gaucher's disease, and caisson disease
  - Systemic steroid use
  - Alcohol abuse
- AVN is graded according to the system of Ficat and Arlet as follows:
  - Stage I: Pain with a positive MRI but no change in plain radiographs
  - Stage II: Plain radiographic appearance of sclerosis of the subchondral bone with no evidence of joint collapse on plain radiographs
  - Stage III: Plain x-ray presence of the "crescent sign" representing collapse of the subchondral bone with maintenance of the subchondral articular margin (Fig. 11–8)
  - Stage IV: Collapse of the humeral head articular surface (Fig. 11–9)
  - Stage V: Collapse of the humeral head articular surface and degenerative involvement of the glenoid fossa
- Nonoperative treatment for humeral head AVN is similar to the nonoperative treatment of osteoarthritis (see earlier).

Surgery Other Than Arthroplasty

- Pressure studies of femoral head AVN have found increased pressure within the femoral heads affected by AVN.
- Unlike extensive data on the treatment of AVN of the femoral head in the hip, limited studies exist in the shoulder regarding the efficacy of core decompression for AVN of that joint.
- Some evidence suggests success for core decompression treatment in stage I, II, and III humeral AVN.
- Core decompression is most helpful before subchondral collapse and articular incongruity have developed.

Arthroplasty

- Patient's with stage IV or failed core decompression in stages I to III are treated with hemiarthroplasty.
- Patients with stage V AVN are treated with TSA (Parsch et al. 2003).

Rotator Cuff Arthropathy

- Approximately 4% of patients with large irreparable rotator cuff tears go on to develop humeral subchondral collapse, glenohumeral arthritis, and other findings characteristic of rotator cuff tear arthropathy (Fig. 11–10).
- *Milwaukee shoulder* is another term used to describe patients with massive rotator cuff insufficiency, humeral head collapse, and glenohumeral arthritis.
  - Patients with Milwaukee shoulder syndrome have been found to have basic calcium phosphate crystals in their joint fluid.
  - The relationship between basic calcium crystals and cuff arthropathy is unclear.
- Patents with cuff tear arthropathy typically present with complaints of pain, loss of function, or both.
- Some patients with cuff tear arthropathy are able to stabilize the humerus enough to elevate the arm to shoulder height or above. Others, however, have no rotator cuff function and exhibit anterosuperior subluxation or dislocation with attempted humeral elevation.

Nonoperative Treatment

- Options are similar to those used for osteoarthritis (see earlier).
- Rotator cuff, deltoid, and scapular muscle strengthening may result in modest gains in strength and function.

Options Other Than Arthroplasty

- Proximal humerus resection and arthrodesis are options that result in some pain relief but also in major functional deficits, which are not well tolerated in the mostly elderly patient population with this entity.
- Arthroscopic débridement with biceps tenotomy may result in pain relief and maintained function in selected patients with a less aggressive degenerative process.

Arthroplasty

- Unipolar or bipolar hemiarthroplasty, extended-head hemiarthroplasty, and reverse TSA are the primary options for treatment.
- In true cuff tear arthropathy, the rotator cuff is rarely reparable, so unconstrained TSA is not often, if ever, indicated.

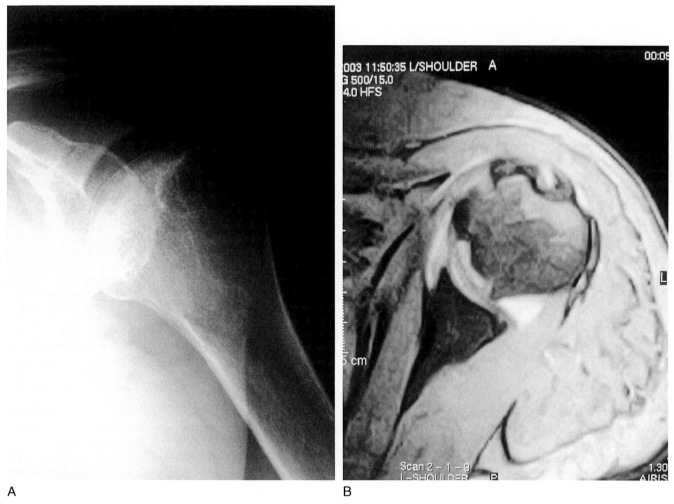

A   B

Figure 11–8: Stage III avascular necrosis.
A, Plain anteroposterior radiograph of the shoulder revealing flattening and sclerosis of the humeral head that
are typical of stage III avascular necrosis with an obvious crescent sign (the presence of a linear radiolucency
below the articular surface of the most proximal aspect of the humeral head). **B,** Magnetic resonance imaging
scan of the same patient revealing greater collapse of the subchondral bone of the humeral head than would be
anticipated by the relatively benign x-ray appearance.

- Unconstrained TSAs often fail rapidly because of superior migration of the humerus and the resulting edge loading and polyethylene wear of the glenoid.
- Hemiarthroplasty has a long track record of pain relief but variable function.
- Function postoperatively is most heavily influenced by function preoperatively.
- Bipolar hemiarthroplasty has shown no increase in function over unipolar hemiarthroplasty and may have more complications.
- Extended-head hemiarthroplasty implants are designed to have a smooth metallic head articulating with the undersurface of the acromion process, but they are otherwise similar to traditional hemiarthroplasties (Fig. 11–11).

- Reverse prosthesis TSA is a constrained prosthesis (Fig. 11–12).
  - The constrained nature of the prosthesis takes the place of the deficient rotator cuff to establish the fixed fulcrum to allow arm elevation.
  - Medium-term follow-up studies reveal better restoration of function than with hemiarthroplasty but a higher complication rate.

Proximal Humerus Fractures

- Fractures of the proximal humerus are most often associated with osteoporosis, parallel the incidence of proximal femoral fractures, and are typically associated with minor trauma such as a fall from a standing height.

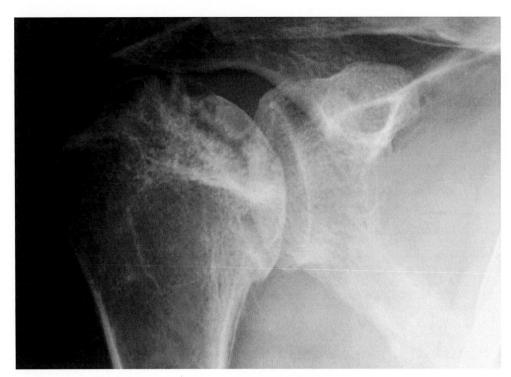

Figure 11–9: Stage IV avascular necrosis.
Plain anteroposterior radiograph of the shoulder reveals progression of avascular necrosis to stage IV, which results in fragmentation and a step-off of the humeral joint surface.

- Plain radiographs are required to determine the presence and type of fracture.
- Proximal humerus fracture lines occur in predictable locations: the surgical neck, the anatomic neck, and near the bicipital groove within the greater tuberosity.

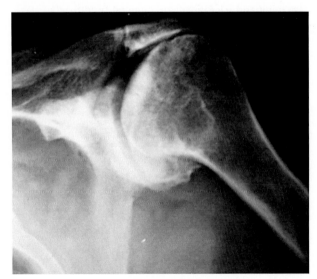

Figure 11–10: Rotator cuff arthropathy.
Plain anteroposterior radiograph of the shoulder revealing superior migration and flattening of the humeral head and joint space narrowing characteristic of rotator cuff arthropathy. (From Rockwood CA Jr, Matsen FA III, Wirth MA, Lippitt SB, eds. [2004]. *The Shoulder*, 3rd ed. Philadelphia: WB Saunders, p 908.)

- The fracture lines separate the proximal humerus into four pieces: the articular surface, the greater tuberosity, the lesser tuberosity, and the humeral shaft.
- The most common classification system for proximal humerus fractures is the Neer classification system.
  - A piece becomes a part by the Neer classification if it is displaced 1 cm or angulated 45 degrees.
  - The Neer classification has been shown to have poor interobserver and intraobserver reliability.
- Nondisplaced fractures are generally treated nonoperatively.
- Of proximal humerus fractures, 80% are nondisplaced and should be treated nonoperatively.

Nonoperative Treatment

- Nonoperative treatment consists of an initial period (7 to 10 days) of immobilization.
- Pendulum exercises can begin as soon as pain allows, usually before 2 weeks. Immobilization lasting longer than 2 weeks has been shown to have a detrimental effect on outcome.
- A repeat examination between 3 and 4 weeks focuses on whether or not the proximal humerus moves as a unit with the shaft. If it does, then passive supine range of motion can begin with limits of 30 degrees of external rotation and 90 degrees of forward flexion. Radiographs at this visit determine whether displacement of the fracture has occurred.
- At 6 to 8 weeks, new radiographs are taken, and the examination focuses on pain with light resistance to the patient's external rotation with the arm at the side. If this

Figure 11–11: Extended-head hemiarthroplasty. Anteroposterior radiograph of a shoulder with extended-head hemiarthroplasty (DePuy Johnson and Johnson, Warsaw, IN). This implant allows articulation of the undersurface of the acromion process and the smooth humeral head prosthetic surface providing for a larger range of motion than a conventional hemiarthroplasty.

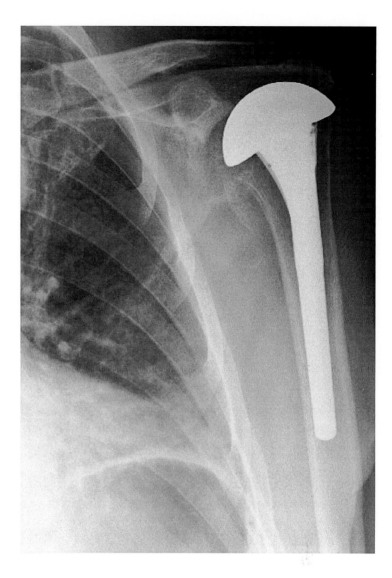

is painless, then full passive supine range of motion is allowed. The sling is discontinued, and the arm can be used for activities of daily living with a 2-lb weight limit restriction. Depending on fracture type, an overhead pulley and light rotator cuff, deltoid, and scapular muscle strengthening may begin.

Operations Other Than Arthroplasty

- Fractures of the proximal humerus consisting of two or three parts are almost always repaired surgically.
- In a physiologically young patient with severe fractures and fracture dislocations, an attempt at repair is undertaken.
- Various repair methods exist for fracture fixation, including closed reduction with percutaneous pinning, open reduction with screws, open reduction with internal fixation of plate and screws, open reduction with internal fixation by a fixed-angle device (blade plate or locked plate), open reduction with interfragmentary suture or wire, and open reduction with internal fixation with intramedullary device.

Arthroplasty

- Patients with four-part fractures, three- and four-part fracture dislocations, three-part fractures with severe comminution and poor bone quality, displaced anatomic neck fractures, and head-splitting fractures are typically treated with prosthetic replacement (Fig. 11–13) (Bosch et al. 1998, Compito et al. 1994).
- Replacement is done in these patients partly because the blood supply to the epiphyseal section of the humeral head becomes disrupted, leading to a high incidence of AVN.
- Hemiarthroplasty is the implant of choice when arthroplasty is performed for fracture.
- Glenoid replacement is only performed acutely when the native glenoid is damaged or arthritic.

Proximal Humeral Malunion and Nonunion

- When a fracture heals in poor position *(malunion)* or fails to heal *(nonunion)*, a patient often experiences pain and significant functional deficit.

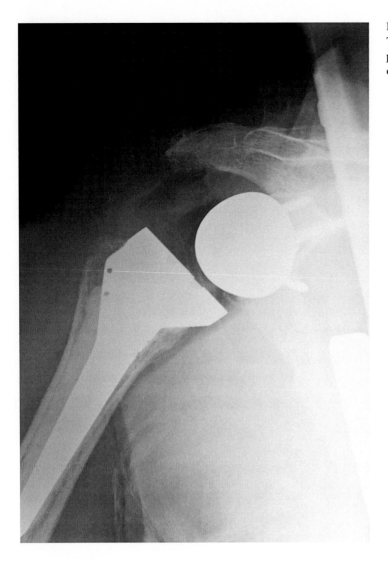

Figure 11–12: Reverse total shoulder prosthesis. The radiographic appearance of a reverse total shoulder prosthesis that is stable because of deltoid tension and component constraint.

- For most nonunions, a diagnosis of infection should be excluded.
- If previous surgery was performed, the location of hardware is assessed by plain radiography and CT scan.
- Physical evidence of neurologic injury should be sought; if there is any concern for any deficit, electrodiagnostic studies should be obtained approximately 4 weeks after the injury or surgical procedure.

Operative Treatment of Nonunions

- Most symptomatic fracture nonunions can be managed with open reduction and internal fixation.
- Open reduction, stable internal fixation (blade plate, locking plate, sutures), and bone grafting are the treatments of choice if the articular surfaces of the humeral head and glenoid fossa remain relatively intact.
- If the patient has joint surface involvement or absence of a large portion of the humeral head, then prosthetic replacement is the treatment of choice (Antuna et al. 2002a,b).

Operative Treatment of Malunions

- Malunions of proximal humerus fractures present several deformities that must be addressed surgically (Fig. 11–14).
- Malunion of the greater tuberosity above the articular surface and a varus neck-shaft angle are two common problems that limit overhead function (Fig. 11–15).
- The greater tuberosity can also heal into an abnormal posterior position limiting external rotation.
- Hardware placed during attempted open reduction and internal fixation may cause pain and limited motion, and its position is therefore assessed with plain radiographs and CT scans.
- Treatment depends on the patient's active motion and extent of pain.
- Treatment options for malunions include acromioplasty, osteotomy with open reduction and internal fixation, osteotomy with arthroplasty, and arthroplasty (Antuna et al. 2002a,b).

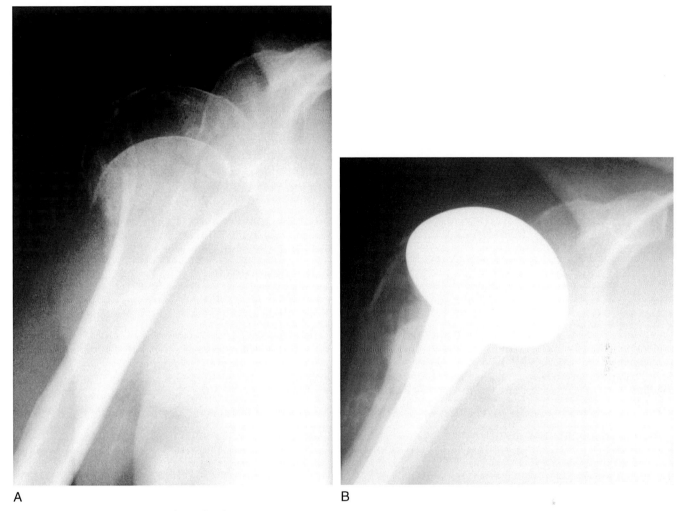

A   B

Figure 11–13: Arthroplasty for fracture.
A, Preoperative radiograph reveals the presence of an anatomic neck fracture that has been impacted to the level of the humeral shaft. **B,** Postoperative radiograph shows restoration of the tuberosity to head height and an anatomic-appearing humeral offset.

Surgical Treatment Other Than Arthroplasty

- Acromioplasty is done for patients with a superiorly migrated malunion of the greater tuberosity who have good overhead function that is painful. Typically, these patients have mild to moderate (1 to 1.5 cm) tuberosity displacement.
- Osteotomy, with reduction and repair, is preferred for patients with greater tuberosity malunions who have decreased range of motion but a normal neck-shaft angle.
- The results following osteotomy depend on the ability to restore the native anatomic relations between the tuberosity and the articular surface.

Arthroplasty for Malunion

- The primary indication for arthroplasty in the presence of a proximal humeral malunion is joint incongruity with subsequent arthritis.

- Replacement is performed for pain relief, and functional improvement is variable.
- A decreased neck-shaft angle can make placement of a prosthesis difficult.
- A superiorly migrated greater tuberosity malunion can also make placing the prosthesis difficult.
- Cementing in a smaller-stemmed prosthesis in varus to reestablish the tuberosity relationship is preferable to tuberosity osteotomy because results deteriorate when tuberosity osteotomy is required.
- Implants that allow for a variable neck-shaft angle can be useful when treating malunions because these devices can be adapted to conform to the altered anatomy.
- Tuberosity osteotomy is avoided if possible when using hemiarthroplasty (Boileau et al. 2001).
- Glenoid resurfacing is performed only if the native glenoid surface is damaged.

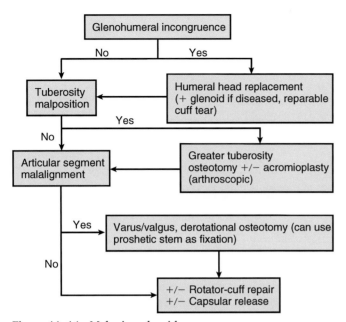

Figure 11–14: Malunion algorithm.
Algorithm for the categorization and operative treatment of malunions of the proximal aspect of the humerus. (Adapted from Beredjiklian PK, Iannotti JP, Norris TR, Williams GR [1998]. Surgical management of proximal humerus fracture malunion. *J Bone Joint Surg Am* 80:1496.)

Chronic Dislocations

- Patients with a large deformity of the humeral head following chronic dislocation may require shoulder replacement if the joint remains unstable following closed reduction (Cheng et al. 1997).
- In general, arthroplasty is considered when dislocations are of more than 6 months' duration or humeral head defects (Hill-Sachs or reverse Hill-Sachs lesions) involve more than 50% of the articular surface of the humeral head (Fig. 11–16).
- Osteoarticular allografts can be considered as an option in young (<40 years of age), active patients with humeral head defects involving approximately 50% of the articular surface of the humeral head and in dislocations of less than 6 months' duration.
- Glenoid bone loss can also contribute to the instability and must be evaluated by CT scan.
- If glenoid bone loss is greater then 25% of the surface of the fossa, autogenous bone grafting from either the iliac crest or the ipsilateral coracoid process may be required to stabilize the joint. Glenoid prosthetic replacement may also be required to achieve stability.

Arthritis of Instability

- Dislocation and chronic recurrent instability of the shoulder lead to an increased incidence of arthritis.
- Several surgical procedures for treatment of recurrent anterior shoulder instability (e.g., Magnuson-Stack

[subscapularis advancement to the greater tuberosity] and Putti-Platt [subscapularis advancement and anterior capsular imbrication] procedures) are now known to increase the risk of arthritis significantly.
- The pattern of glenoid wear resulting from chronic instability is typically posterior (eccentric). A CT scan is needed to evaluate glenoid bone loss.
- The loss of motion, particularly diminished passive external rotation with the arm at the side, can be severe and must be addressed with capsular releases and subscapularis lengthening at the time of prosthetic replacement.
- In patients displaying mild arthritic changes, open or arthroscopic capsular release with manipulation may decrease symptoms, recenter the humeral head on the glenoid fossa, and delay the progression of degenerative changes.

Failed Arthroplasty

- Failed shoulder replacement surgery can result from aseptic loosening, infection, periprosthetic fracture, rotator cuff tear, an overstuffed joint (an overly large humeral head), incorrect version of the humeral component, or incorrect version of the glenoid component.
- Evaluation includes radiographic studies (plain radiographs and CT scan), laboratory studies (sedimentation rate, C-reactive protein, and joint aspiration).

Infection

- Bone scans and white cell–labeled scans (i.e., indium or gallium scans) may aid in the diagnosis of infected arthroplasty.
- Infections are treated with implant removal, irrigation and débridement, placement of antibiotic spacer, and long-term (6 to 8 weeks) intravenous antibiotics.
- Immediate component reimplantation has a higher rate of infection recurrence but may be indicated in very early (2 to 4 weeks) infection, an immune-competent host, and a less virulent organism.
- Most often, reimplantation can be attempted following eradication of the infection as evidenced by normalization of the erythrocyte sedimentation rate and C-reactive protein.
- Choice of implant for revision shoulder replacement (hemiarthroplasty, TSA, or reverse TSA) depends on the glenoid bone stock and the condition of the rotator cuff.

Tumor

- See also Chapter 15.
- Resection of the proximal humerus for tumor can be reconstructed with either standard or custom prosthesis.
- Choice of implant for revision shoulder replacement (hemiarthroplasty, TSA, or reverse TSA) depends on the glenoid bone stock and on the condition of the rotator cuff and deltoid muscle.
- In proximal humerus resections in which excision of the rotator cuff is necessary to eradicate the tumor surgically,

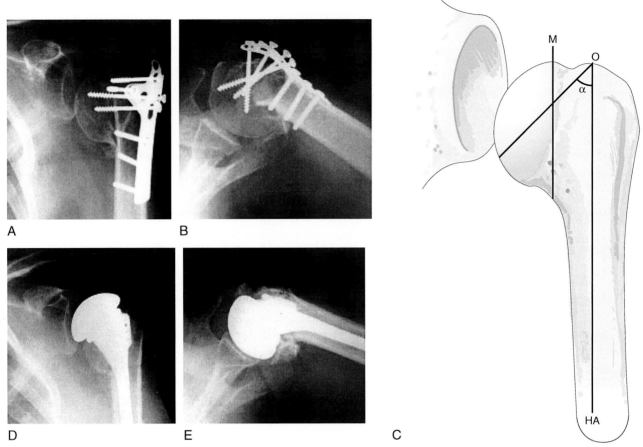

Figure 11–15: Malunion.
A and **B**, Anteroposterior and axillary radiographs, made before operative treatment of the malunion, demonstrating varus malalignment of the articular segment. **C**, Line drawing demonstrating the measurement of varus malalignment of the humeral head segment. α, correct neck-shaft angle of 45 degrees, which represents the correct plane of the osteotomy *(O); HA*, humeral axis; *M*, malalignment of the humeral head, which is parallel to the humeral axis (0 degrees of varus). **D** and **E**, Anteroposterior and axillary radiographs demonstrating correction after hemiarthroplasty. (From Beredjiklian PK, Iannotti JP, Norris TR, Williams GR [1998]. Surgical management of proximal humerus fracture malunion. *J Bone Joint Surg Am* 80:1492.)

a reverse prosthesis may give better function than hemiarthroplasty.

- Allograft arthrodesis is another option if, following resection, there is not enough soft tissue integrity to perform an arthroplasty.

Surgical Approaches
Deltopectoral Approach

- The most common approach used to perform shoulder replacement is the deltopectoral approach. It is used for hemiarthroplasty, TSA, revision shoulder replacement, reverse TSA, and humeral resurfacing.
- The patient is placed in the beach chair position with the back at approximately 40 degrees from the horizontal.
- One uses either a specialized table or lateral braces to secure the patient and allow for full extension and

adduction of the humerus. Complete adduction and extension are required to access the humerus.

- Landmarks for the incision are the tip of the coracoid process and the deltoid tuberosity (Fig. 11–17).
- Loose fascia is divided to expose the anterior fascia of the deltoid and pectoralis major.
- Flaps are raised medially and laterally in the avascular plane just above the deltoid and pectoralis major fascia.
- The cephalic vein is identified within the deltopectoral interval.
- The vein can be retracted laterally, with the deltoid, along with most of its feeding vessels or medially with the pectoralis. Retracting the vein medially places less tension on the vein but sacrifices many of the feeding vessels entering from the deltoid side.
- Self-retaining retractors are placed deep to the deltoid and pectoralis major to expose the clavipectoral

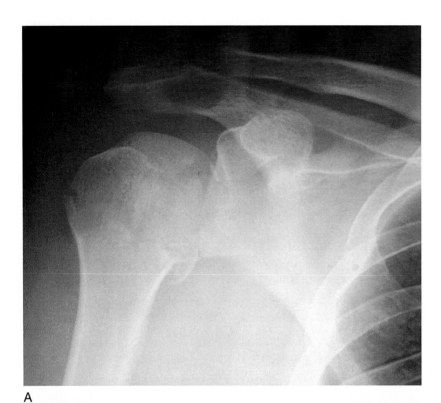

A

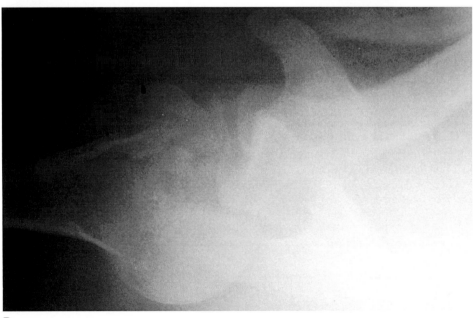

B

Figure 11–16: Chronic dislocation. Plain anteroposterior (A) and axillary (B) radiographs of a chronic locked posterior dislocation. Significant involvement of the humeral head is observed, obviating the possibility of treatment without prosthetic replacement.

fascia and conjoined tendon. Abducting the arm decreases the tension on the deltoid and facilitates placement of the retractors.
• To increase exposure, the proximal portion of the pectoralis major can be divided. This may result in decreased internal rotation strength and therefore is avoided when possible. If partial release of the pectoralis major is required, the amount released should be the minimum required to gain adequate exposure.
• A reliable finding is a small muscle belly on the lateral side of the conjoined tendon. The clavipectoral fascia is incised just lateral to this muscle belly.
• The clavipectoral fascia is opened superiorly to the coracoacromial ligament, but the ligament does not need to be divided.

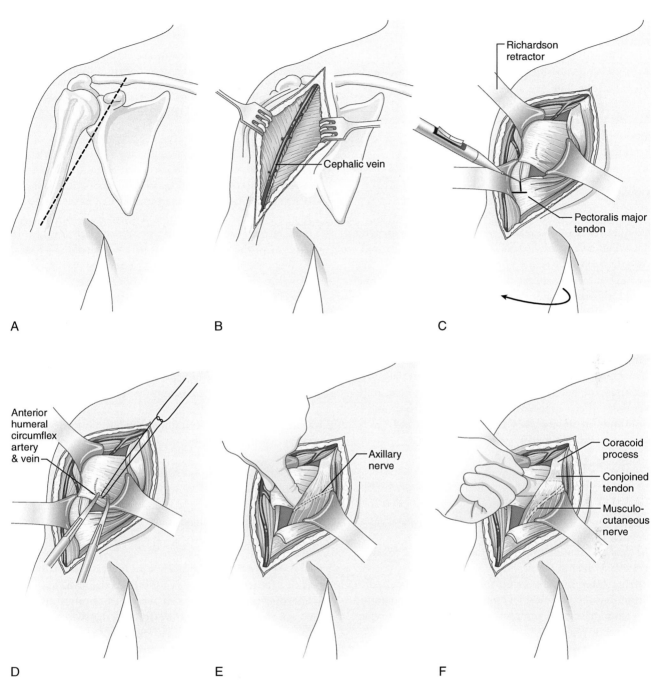

Figure 11–17: Deltopectoral approach.
A, The deltopectoral approach is made through an anterior incision placed from the tip of the coracoid to the humerus at the level of the deltoid insertion. **B,** The cephalic vein is identified in the deltopectoral interval and retracted. **C,** The proximal border of the pectoralis major muscle can be released to improve visualization. **D,** The circumflex vessels are identified and ligated. **E,** Identification of the axillary nerve. **F,** Identification of the musculocutaneous nerve allows for safe completion of the anterior approach. (From Rockwood CA Jr, Matsen FA III, Wirth MA, Lippitt SB, eds. [2004]. *The Shoulder*, 3rd ed. Philadelphia: WB Saunders, pp 964-965.)

- The deep surface of the conjoined tendon is palpated to assess the location of the musculocutaneous nerve. It often enters the deep surface of the conjoined tendon distal to the surgical field but can enter within 1 to 2 cm of the tip of the coracoid.

- A finger can be run along the inferior border of the subscapularis to palpate the axillary nerve.
- If the locations of the nerves allow safe placement of self-retaining retractors deep to the conjoined tendon, the medial blade of the retractor is repositioned to that location.

- The subacromial space deep to the coracoacromial ligament is entered with curved scissors. Into this space, a reverse retractor is placed.
- Any remaining adhesions between the deep surface of the deltoid and the humerus are incised, and a larger reverse deltoid retractor can be placed.
- The arm is externally rotated to put the subscapularis on tension and to identify the anterior circumflex vessels.
- The vessels are dissected out, ligated, and divided.

Superior Approach

- This approach is most commonly used for rotator cuff repairs, but it is also used for reverse TSA in patients with rotator cuff arthropathy because of the excellent glenoid exposure it affords.
- Proximal humerus resurfacing and TSA can be performed through this approach, most commonly by releasing the subscapularis.
- This approach is not extensile and therefore is not frequently used for revision surgery or fracture treatment.
- The patient is positioned into a sitting position with the back approximately 60 degrees from the horizontal.
- One uses either a specialized table or lateral braces to secure the patient and allow for full extension and adduction of the humerus.
- The landmarks for the incision are the anterior and lateral acromion.
- The incision is approximately 4 inches long, with 1 inch proximal to the anterolateral corner of the acromion.
- The direction of the incision is longitudinally parallel to the fibers of the deltoid.
- The skin and loose connective tissue are divided to the level of the deltoid fascia.
- Flaps are raised in the avascular plane just superficial to the deltoid fascia. Frequently, an artery traverses the fascia at the acromioclavicular joint and should be expected when raising the medial flap.
- The raphe between the anterior and lateral heads of the deltoid is a bloodless plane that is divided to gain access to the subacromial space. However, a more posterior deltoid split, in line with the anterior cortical border of the clavicle, can make glenoid exposure easier. The trade-off is more difficulty with humeral exposure.
- Splitting of the deltoid past 5 cm can result in an axillary nerve injury and should be avoided.
- In the cuff-deficient shoulder, the humeral head is exposed after the anterior head of the deltoid is released from the anterior acromion.
- In shoulders with no cuff deficiency, the rotator interval is divided, the subscapularis is tagged and released to expose the proximal humerus.
- The remaining portion of the procedure varies, depending on the operation performed.

Surgical Techniques

- Most prosthetic replacements are performed via the deltopectoral approach and are described as such in this section.

Total Shoulder Arthroplasty for Osteoarthritis

- An examination of the patient's range of motion under anesthesia is assessed, with particular attention to the amount of external rotation with the arm at the side.
- If external rotation is limited to less than neutral, steps must be taken to increase the range of motion, such as medialization or Z-plasty of the subscapularis (Fig. 11–18).
- Z-plasty of the subscapularis is generally avoided because it weakens the muscle. However, if external rotation is less than −20 degrees, Z-plasty should be considered (Fig. 11–19).
- If external rotation is greater than 20 degrees, then the subscapularis can be taken down intratendinously and repaired anatomically. Alternatively, the subscapularis may be released using an osteotomy of the lesser tuberosity.
- Release of the inferior capsule off the humerus, along with a portion of the latissimus dorsi tendon, improves exposure.
- Care must be taken to know the location of the axillary nerve while performing anterior and inferior capsule releases.
- The anterior capsule is excised to increase postoperative external rotation and to improve subscapularis mobility.
- To increase exposure of the proximal humerus, the patient's arm is extended, adducted, and externally rotated. A large Darrach retractor will make this maneuver more effective.
- In patients with osteoporosis, care must be taken, especially with external rotation, not to fracture the arm.
- Osteophytes are removed to allow identification of the native anatomic neck and to decrease the size of the humerus to improve later glenoid exposure.
- Depending on the implant system, intramedullary guides, extramedullary guides, or freehand techniques are used to osteotomize the humerus head.
- The cut should recreate the patient's natural version. This is accomplished by making the osteotomy exit through the anatomic neck, close to the insertion of the rotator cuff superiorly and posteriorly.
- The canal is prepared, and a trial stem is left in place while the glenoid is exposed to prevent fracture.
- The arm is abducted, externally rotated, and extended to allow the posterior capsule to relax and the humerus to be retracted posteriorly.
- Any remaining anterior capsule is released off the anterior glenoid from the top to the bottom of the glenoid.
- A large Darrach retractor is placed onto the anterior glenoid neck. Other retractors may be placed around the

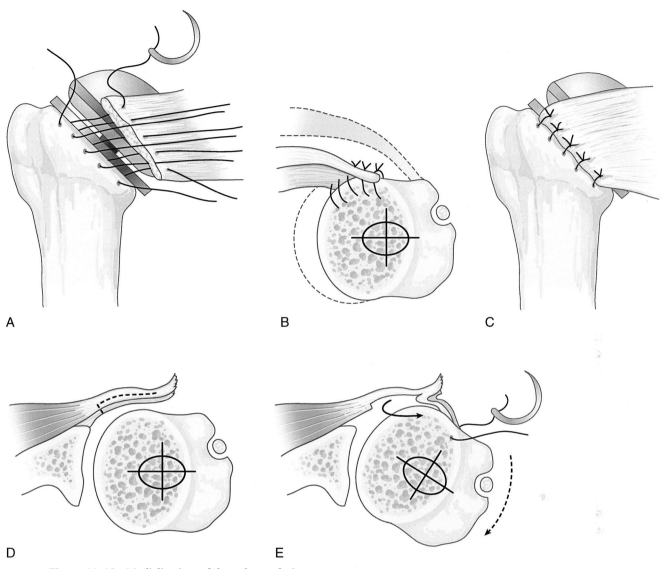

A   B   C

D   E

Figure 11–18: Medialization of the subscapularis.
A to C, Subscapularis tendon repair to drill holes in the anterior humeral neck medial to the lesser tuberosity.
D and E, The inside-out Z-plasty. **D,** Additional length of the subscapularis tendon can be gained by splitting
the capsule from the tendon medially and leaving the connection intact laterally. **E,** The medial end of the split
capsule is reflected and attached to the humeral neck. (From Rockwood CA Jr, Matsen FA III, Wirth MA,
Lippitt SB, eds. [2004]. *The Shoulder*, 3rd ed. Philadelphia: WB Saunders, p 958.)

glenoid to optimize exposure. Such retractors include a
Fukuda ring retractor, a reverse Homan retractor inferiorly,
and a single-prong Bankart retractor superiorly just
posterior to the biceps tendon.
- The labrum is removed, and the long head of the biceps is
  released if it is partially torn or tethered in the bicipital
  groove.
- Reamers are used to prepare the glenoid for implantation
  onto subchondral bone.
- Eccentrically worn glenoids can be reshaped to a neutral
  version by reaming.
- The glenoid is prepared for implantation according to the
  various implants.

- Two major implant designs are currently used:
  pegged and keeled. Most glenoid components are
  cemented.
- Keeled components are easier to implant but are more
  difficult to place so they are uniformly supported by the
  subchondral bone.
- The glenoid must be checked for penetration through the
  deep cortical bone. If the deep cortex is violated, bone
  grafting is performed. Care is also taken not to
  overpressurize to prevent extravasation of the
  cement.
- Once the glenoid placement is complete, the humerus is
  again exposed.

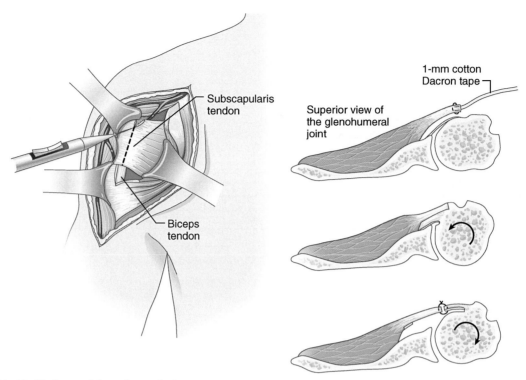

Figure 11–19: Z-plasty of the subscapularis.
A, The subscapularis tendon should be released from its insertion into the lesser tuberosity. **B,** When the patient has −20 degrees or less of external rotation, the subscapularis tendon and capsule should be lengthened with a coronal Z-plasty technique. (From Rockwood CA Jr, Matsen FA III, Wirth MA, Lippitt SB, eds. [2004]. *The Shoulder*, 3rd ed. Philadelphia: WB Saunders, p 966.)

- Any reparable rotator cuff tears should have sutures passed through the tendon and bone but not tied until after the humeral component is placed.
- The optimal humeral head
  - Covers the most cut surface with the least overhang.
  - Provides enough lateral humeral offset to allow at least 50% to 100% displacement posteriorly with spontaneous relocation when the posterior force is removed.
  - Recreates the tuberosity–head height relationship.
- The proper-size component is selected and implanted, by either press-fit or cemented means.
- Patients with poor bone quality and a large diaphysis-to-metaphysis diameter ratio are at increased risk of fracture with press-fit implantation, and consideration should be given to cementing.
- The subscapularis is repaired. Anatomic repair is performed if preoperative external rotation was greater than 20 degrees; medialization is performed if external rotation was between −20 and +20 degrees; Z-plasty is performed if external rotation was less than −20 degrees.
- The maximal external rotation obtained intraoperatively without undue tension on the subscapularis is noted and is used to direct postoperative rehabilitation.

Hemiarthroplasty for Arthritis

- Although the technique is similar to what is used for TSA described earlier, several technical points should be noted.
- The releases of soft tissue performed for total shoulder exposure on both the humerus and glenoid should be performed for hemiarthroplasty even though glenoid exposure is not as critical because it is believed that this intraoperative maneuver improves postoperative motion.
- If the glenoid is eccentrically worn, it should be reamed to a neutral version if remaining bone is adequate. In rare cases, bone grafts may be required to improve glenohumeral concentricity and glenoid version. Occasionally, the glenoid is so deficient that bone grafting is not possible and a less than optimal glenoid position must be accepted (Levine et al. 1997).

Shoulder Replacement in Inflammatory Arthritis

- Several technical considerations should be made when treating patients with inflammatory arthropathy.
- Tissue quality is typically poor, and therefore leaving a portion of the anterior capsule on the subscapularis

tendon may strengthen the tendon repair. However, the retained capsule should still be released from the glenoid.

- Bone quality is often poor, and care must be taken when preparing the humerus and glenoid to prevent fracture, especially with the extension, adduction, and external rotation maneuver to deliver the proximal humerus.
- If adequate glenoid bone and an intact or reparable rotator cuff are present, every effort should be made to resurface the glenoid fossa in addition to the humeral replacement.

Hemiarthroplasty for Rotator Cuff Arthropathy

- The various implants used (extended-head arthroplasty, unipolar hemiarthroplasty, and bipolar arthroplasty) require a review of the manufacturers' recommendations.
- Even when one uses a deltopectoral approach, if the superior defect of the rotator cuff tear is large enough, an implant can be placed through the defect, without detaching any additional subscapularis or posterior rotator cuff tendons. To attempt this, an extramedullary guide can be used to direct the humeral neck cut. Without taking down the subscapularis, postoperative rehabilitation can be accelerated.

Hemiarthroplasty for Fracture

- Exposure of the fracture is via the deltopectoral approach.
- Frequently, the circumflex vessels are disrupted and cannot be found to be ligated. In addition, because the glenoid is exposed by displacing the lesser and greater tuberosity fragments, the anterior circumflex artery can often be preserved.
- The biceps tendon is an important landmark because the anatomic landmarks are often distorted.
- Opening the sheath of the biceps facilitates access to the joint to allow assessment of the fracture.
- Previous fracture lines are used to gain access to joint. Most often, the fracture line separating the lesser and greater tuberosity fragments is 1 to 1.5 cm posterior to the bicipital groove. The result is that the anterior fragment contains both the bicipital groove and the lesser tuberosity.
- The articular fragments are removed, and any portion of articular surface attached to the tuberosities is resected.
- Heavy sutures are placed into the anterior and posterior cuff at the tendon-bone junction.
- The canal is prepared to accept the humeral component.
- Drill holes are placed into the shaft and heavy sutures are passed before cementing.
- The head size is determined by trialing the prosthesis or by sizing the head that was removed.
- The component is cemented into place, with care taken to put in approximately 30 degrees of retroversion. It is also important to reestablish the appropriate greater tuberosity

and humeral head height. This can be done by trial reduction of the fragments and confirmed by intraoperative radiography.

- In the absence of medial comminution, the collar of the prosthesis should be approximately 0.5 to 1.0 cm above the medial neck of the humerus.
- Sutures placed around the prosthesis and brought through the tuberosities (cerclage sutures) provide the greatest resistance to tuberosity pull-off (Fig. 11–20).
- Tuberosity sutures are secured to the prosthesis, with care to restore the proper tuberosity–head height relationship.
- The shaft sutures are sewn to the tuberosities, and the cerclage sutures are fastened, thereby creating both horizontal and vertical fixation.
- External rotation is assessed to help guide postoperative rehabilitation.
- If the biceps tendon is released, soft tissue tenodesis is performed.

Proximal Humerus Resurfacing

- The proximal humerus is exposed through a deltopectoral approach, as described for TSA or hemiarthroplasty.
- The general steps for implantation are as follows:
  - The center of the humeral head is located.
  - A drill hole is made into the center mark of the head at a 135-degree angle for the shaft and perpendicular to the surface.
  - A cup-shaped reamer with a central peg is placed over the proximal humerus, and the head is reshaped to accept the resurfacing component.
  - Areas of bone loss are grafted.
  - The implant is impacted into place.
- The implant relies on bony ingrowth for stability.

Reverse Total Shoulder Prosthesis

- The proximal humerus is exposed as previously described earlier by either a deltopectoral or a superior approach. Typically, a deltopectoral approach is used if a previous implant requires removal, and a superior approach is used if not. The rotator cuff is generally deficient, but any portion that remains can be preserved or repaired.
- The humerus is prepared according to the implant manufacturer and a trial humeral component is implanted.
- The glenoid is exposed and prepared similar to a TSA, with specifics depending on the implant manufacturer.
- Implant selection must be done to put the deltoid under tension.
- If the components are easy to reduce and dislocate, then a spacer or larger components must be selected to increase the deltoid tension (Boulahia et al. 2002).

Revision Surgery

- Revision surgery presents several problems not encountered with primary joint reconstruction, including removal

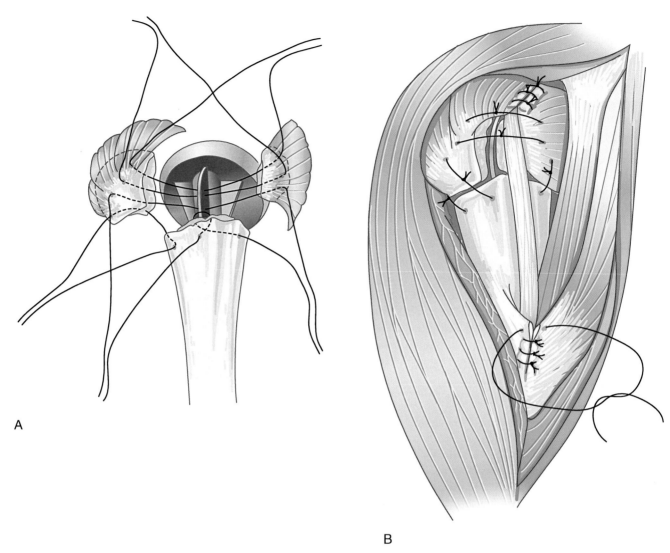

A

B

Figure 11–20: Hemiarthroplasty for fracture.
A, Multiple sutures are used to secure the tuberosities to the implant. This technique involves at least two 1-mm Dacron tapes for the bone-tendon junction of the greater and lesser tuberosities each, two 1-mm Dacron tapes through humeral shaft drill holes, and two 1-mm Dacron tapes placed as cerclage sutures (not shown) around the metaphysis of the implant and passed through the greater and lesser tuberosity. **B,** The reduction of the tuberosities is done under fluoroscopy before the tapes that secure the construct are tied. (From Rockwood CA Jr, Matsen FA III, Wirth MA, Lippitt SB, eds. [2004]. *The Shoulder*, 3rd ed. Philadelphia: WB Saunders, pp 13, 202.)

of hardware, potential rotator cuff deficiency (especially the subscapularis tendon), scarring, and poor bone stock.
- If infection is suspected preoperatively or if there is any appearance of infection intraoperatively, the implants, cement, and all nonabsorbable sutures should be removed, cultures obtained, and an antibiotic cement spacer should be placed. The duration of antibiotic treatment and the timing of reimplantation are determined by culture results.

- Following a standard deltopectoral approach, the subscapularis is incised as indicated earlier in primary shoulder arthroplasty. If external rotation is less than −20 degrees, the thickened periosteum, scar tissue, subscapularis, and biceps can be elevated in a single layer by incising the soft tissue approximately 1 cm lateral to the bicipital groove, thus subperiosteally raising this flap to expose the prosthesis.
  - The lateral edge of this flap can be repaired in a medialized position to improve external rotation on implantation of the prosthesis.

- The biceps tendon should be tenodesed to the humerus when the subscapularis is taken down in this manner.
- Locating the axillary nerve before performing any releases is critical.
- Freeing subdeltoid scar tissue and performing the glenoid and humeral releases (as described for TSA) are essential to improve exposure.
- Deficiencies of the glenoid may require bone grafting or augmentation of the glenoid component. The deficiencies may be anterior, posterior, or central.
- Large central lesions can be bone grafted with cancellous allograft and reamed smooth or impacted with the glenoid impactor. A second surgical procedure to implant a glenoid can be done after the graft has incorporated if pain is present.
- Humeral deficiency usually requires the stem to be cemented. A long-stem prosthesis should be used if there is a cortical deficiency at the tip of a standard stem. The tip of the stem must extend at least two cortical diameters beyond any cortical defect.
- Choice of implant (hemiarthroplasty, TSA, or reverse TSA) depends on the bone stock of the glenoid and the condition of the rotator cuff, as described earlier.

Postoperative Management
Total Shoulder Arthroplasty and Hemiarthroplasty

- The amount of external rotation obtained on the operating table without undue tension on the subscapularis repair should be used as the limit during the early postoperative rehabilitation.
- The first 6 weeks of therapy consist of daily exercises for hand, wrist, and elbow range of motion. Pendulum exercises with passive forward flexion without limitation and passive supine external rotation are recommended (Table 11–1).
- The arm is maintained in a sling full time during the first 2 weeks, except during therapy and hygiene care.
- At 2 weeks, the patient can remove the sling at home and perform unweighted activities of daily living with the arm at the side.
- Three weeks postoperatively, range-of-motion exercises are continued with the addition of stretching of the posterior capsule and light strengthening of the posterior rotator cuff. A 1-lb weight limit is given for activities of daily living.
- Six weeks postoperatively, internal rotation strengthening is initiated, the external rotation strengthening is advanced, and the external rotation limits are lifted.
- Deltoid strengthening can be started when the rotator cuff shows sufficient strength, approximately 3 months from surgery.
- Return to athletic activities such as golf is allowed at 4 months. Heavy weight lifting and vigorous sporting

Table 11–1	Rehabilitation Program Following Total Shoulder Replacement
WEEK	**EXERCISES**
0–3	Use of pendulums, passive forward flexion, passive supine external rotation to safe limit, and elbow and wrist exercises
3–6	Continuation of previous exercises; addition of cross-body adduction stretches, light isometric external rotation strengthening, and scapula stabilizers
6–12	Progressive resistance of external rotation strengthening, initiation of internal rotation strengthening, and lifting of restriction on passive external rotation; may begin deltoid strengthening when cuff strength returns
16–20	Return to sports

activity are discouraged. Maximal recovery takes approximately 1 year.
- Radiographs are taken at yearly intervals to assess for loosening of components.

Inflammatory Arthritis

- Bone and soft tissue quality often require a modification of postoperative rehabilitation.
- In cases with poor bony or soft tissue quality, therapy is limited to pendulum exercises for the first 7 to 10 days. Supine flexion to 90 degrees and external rotation to neutral are then added.
- At 6 weeks, the passive external rotation exercises are restricted to the level observed in the operating room after subscapularis repair, whereas passive forward flexion is limited to 135 degrees. Also at 6 weeks, the patient can begin using the arm for unweighted activities of daily living.
- At 12 weeks postoperatively, restrictions on range of motion are lifted, and rotator cuff and deltoid strengthening is begun. Patients can begin to use the arm for weighted activities with a 2-lb limit.
- Return to all activities except lifting is allowed at 5 months. A plateau in recovery occurs at 1 year.
- Radiographs are taken at yearly intervals to assess for loosening of components.

Hemiarthroplasty for Rotator Cuff Arthropathy When the Subscapularis Muscle Is Spared

- No restrictions are placed on postoperative range of motion when the subscapularis is spared.
- Passive range-of-motion exercises are started immediately, and the arm is allowed to be used for activities of daily living as the pain allows. This is delayed to 6 weeks when the subscapularis has to be detached and repaired during surgery.
- When passive range of motion produces minimal or no pain, cuff and deltoid strengthening exercises are started.

This is delayed to 6 weeks when the subscapularis is taken down and repaired.

Reverse Total Shoulder Prosthesis

- The patient is placed in a sling for 2 weeks with range-of-motion exercises performed for the hand, wrist, and elbow. The sling is removed only for therapy and hygiene.
- After 2 weeks, passive forward flexion and pendulum exercises are initiated. When forward flexion to 90 degrees is achieved passively, deltoid muscle strengthening is started.
- Rotator cuff strengthening exercises are performed only if the posterior cuff remains attached to the humerus.
- Range-of-motion goals include 130 degrees of forward flexion and 30 degrees of external rotation.

Results

Total Shoulder Arthroplasty for Osteoarthritis

- TSA for primary osteoarthritis provides relief of pain, improvement in function, and patient satisfaction.
  - Ninety percent of patients report complete or near complete pain relief.
  - Ninety-five percent of patients demonstrate a good to excellent outcome (pain relief, functional improvement, and satisfaction).
- The degree of postoperative functional improvement is inversely correlated to the preoperative functional level.
- Degree of preoperative stiffness is directly correlated with the postoperative range of motion and function.
- Outcome and patient satisfaction are not significantly different for those patients with reparable rotator cuff tears who received either hemiarthroplasty or TSA, at least in short-term follow-up.
- Large rotator cuff tears and fatty infiltration of the rotator cuff are negative prognostic factors.

Total Shoulder Arthroplasty Versus Hemiarthroplasty for Osteoarthritis

- Hemiarthroplasty and TSA are considered acceptable treatment options for advanced degenerative changes.
- Results of hemiarthroplasty at midterm follow-up have been favorable.
- It is recommended that hemiarthroplasty be reserved for patients with a concentric glenoid.
- No significant functional differences have been found in randomized studies in patients treated for osteoarthritis with either hemiarthroplasty or TSA.
- In spite of the lack of functional differences, patients treated with TSA experienced greater pain relief and had greater internal rotation (Gartsman et al. 2000).
- Persistent pain after hemiarthroplasty is not uncommon when glenoid wear is ignored during the index procedure.

- In these situations, revision from a hemiarthroplasty to a TSA results in symptomatic improvement and increased ROM.

Arthroplasty for Humeral Head Avascular Necrosis

- Results of shoulder arthroplasty for AVN are rarely reported.
- Results are thought to be among the best of any patients undergoing shoulder arthroplasty because of the integrity of rotator cuff in most of these patients.
- The results may not be as good as previously thought, and further investigation is warranted.
- Arthroplasty for patients with steroid-induced osteonecrosis has better results than in patients with other causes of osteonecrosis.
- Glenoid changes are often underestimated at the time of surgery and can be associated with persistent pain and progression of glenoid erosion in patients undergoing hemiarthroplasty.

Reverse Shoulder Arthroplasty for the Arthritic Rotator Cuff–Deficient Shoulder

- Grammont's Delta reverse shoulder prosthesis has been used since 1992.
- Reports have shown excellent results with regard to pain reduction and improvement in active range of motion (Boulahia et al. 2002).
- Patients note significant reduction of pain and significant improvement in forward elevation and function with the use of this prosthesis.
- Reverse shoulder prosthetic replacement has potential benefits with good results shown for the early and midterm follow-up periods, particularly when patients with rotator cuff arthropathy are evaluated separately from those with inflammatory arthritis.
- It is likely that patients undergoing a reverse prosthesis in a revision setting will have a higher complication rate than those treated with standard TSA.

Arthroplasty in Inflammatory Arthritis

- Neer published the first results of shoulder arthroplasty in patients with rheumatoid arthritis (Torchia, et al. 1997).
  - Patients had a longer rehabilitation time when compared with patients with osteoarthritis and achieved less range of motion on average with 57 degrees of forward flexion and 60 degrees of external rotation.
  - Complications noted included continued pain of unclear origin and difficulty in rehabilitation resulting from ongoing problems with the ipsilateral elbow.
- Other authors have reported similar results with standard TSA prostheses (Table 11–2).

AUTHORS	NUMBER OF PATIENTS	OUTCOMES	RADIOGRAPHIC ASSESSMENT

Table 11–2   Results of Arthroplasty in Inflammatory Arthritis

AUTHORS	NUMBER OF PATIENTS	OUTCOMES	RADIOGRAPHIC ASSESSMENT
Barrett et al.*	140	93% of patients with excellent pain relief	Radiographs revealed radiolucent lines on 82% of glenoid components, 10% of which were probably loose, although none had been revised.
Stewart and Kelly†	49	78% of patients reporting complete pain relief	Radiographs also showed loosening around glenoid and humeral components. This raised a concern about uncemented humeral components, and the authors recommended that cemented components do better.
Sneppen et al.‡	51	89% of patients with good pain relief	Of humeral components, 51% showed some proximal migration. Radiographic loosening of the glenoid was noted in 40% of cases. The authors recommended that cemented hemiarthroplasty may be better for end-stage disease.

*Barrett WP, Thornhill TS, Thomas WH, et al. (1989). Nonconstrained total shoulder arthroplasty in patients with polyarticular rheumatoid arthritis. *J Arthroplasty* 4:91-96.
†Stewart MP, Kelly IG (1997). Total shoulder replacement in rheumatoid disease: 7 to 13 year follow-up of 37 joints. *J Bone Joint Surg Br* 76:68-72.
‡Sneppen O, Fruensgaard S, Johannsen HV, et al. (1996). Total shoulder replacement in rheumatoid arthritis: Proximal migration and loosening. *J Shoulder Elbow Surg* 5:47-52.

Resurfacing Arthroplasty

- Results of surface replacement prostheses in rheumatoid arthritis are satisfactory.
- Levy and Copeland and their associates reported their results with the Copeland implant (Levy et al. 2004).
  - Patients achieved an average of 105 degrees of active forward flexion and 45 degrees of external rotation.
  - Overall results were similar to those with stemmed prostheses; complications were less frequent, and revision was easier.

Shoulder Arthroplasty for Chronic Dislocations

- Literature on long-term results after shoulder arthroplasty for chronic dislocation is scarce (Cheng et al. 1997).
- Results from the few studies that analyzed TSA for chronic posterior dislocations are encouraging. However, the results are inferior to those reported for osteoarthritis and AVN.

Arthroplasty for Proximal Humerus Fractures

- Results of hemiarthroplasty for the treatment of severe proximal humerus fractures have been good for pain relief but variable for shoulder function.
- Inconsistent functional outcomes reported by multiple authors are influenced by the following:
  - Variables inherent to the patient's injury
  - Surgical technique
  - Study design
- Neer reported successful treatment of specific proximal humerus fractures with hemiarthroplasty.
  - Of these patients, 39 of 43 of those with displaced proximal humerus fractures who were treated with hemiarthroplasty noted excellent or satisfactory results.
- Over the years, several authors have presented their outcomes (Table 11–3).

- Several studies showed that attention to technical detail can maximize outcome following surgery.
- Appropriate prosthesis position in the presence of successful healing of the tuberosities often results in active elevation motion in the range of 90 to 120 degrees.
- Most patients continue to note weakness of the shoulder and have difficulty working overhead.
- Several other variables have been found to influence the outcome of patients following hemiarthroplasty for proximal humerus fractures.
- Several series containing both acute and chronic proximal humerus fractures showed more predictable improvement in function and superior pain relief in those fractures treated acutely with hemiarthroplasty.
- Decreased function after delayed hemiarthroplasty results from the following:
  - Soft tissue scarring
  - Tuberosity malunion and nonunion
  - Rotator cuff dysfunction
  - Older age
- Adequate compliance with postoperative rehabilitation programs and activity restrictions has been shown to influence outcomes following hemiarthroplasty.

Arthroplasty for Malunion

- Adaptability of third-generation implants is a potential technical advantage in the treatment of malunion.
- The ability to use variable inclination, retroversion, and offset allows one to reconstruct moderate deformities without the need to osteotomize the greater tuberosity or compromise on head size.
- Published studies with variable implants confirm that results are better in deformities that do not require osteotomy of the greater tuberosity.
- Unpredictable functional outcomes are common when treating complex deformities that require an osteotomy.
- A potential alternative for complex deformities with normal deltoid function is the use of the reverse implant.

Table 11–3   Outcomes of Proximal Humerus Fractures Treated With Hemiarthroplasty

AUTHORS	NUMBER OF PATIENTS	FOLLOW-UP (MONTHS)	OUTCOMES	FUNCTION	CONCLUSIONS
Demirhan et al.*	32	35	97% with no or mild pain; satisfactory Neer score in 75%	Average active elevation, 113 degrees	Preoperative delay, problems of tuberosity fixation, and the position of the tuberosities were parameters influencing outcome.
Tanner and Cofield†	48	38	93% satisfactory	Average active abduction, 101 degrees	Surgery should be performed early to avoid the scarring that engenders complications and limits functional recovery.
Hawkins and Switlyk‡	19	40	Pain relief satisfactory in 18/20 Patients satisfied with result in 16/20 shoulders	Average active forward elevation, 72 degrees; active external rotation, 16 degrees	Poor function appeared to be directly related to a lack of rotator cuff integrity. Surgical techniques securing tuberosity union are essential.
Zyto et al.§	27	39	Constant score of 51 for three-part fractures and 46 for four-part fractures	Average active forward elevation, 70 degrees; abduction; 70 degrees, external rotation; 45 degrees	Results following hemiarthroplasty for acute three- and four-part fractures are disappointing.
Boileau et al.‖	66	27	Average constant score of 56	Average active forward elevation, 101 degrees; external rotation, 18 degrees	Final tuberosity malposition correlated with an unsatisfactory result, superior migration of prosthesis, stiffness, weakness, and pain.

*Demirhan M, Kilicoglu O, Altinel L, et al. (2003). Prognostic factors in prosthetic replacement for acute proximal humerus fractures. *J Orthop Trauma* 17:181-188.
†Tanner MW, Cofield RH (1983). Prosthetic arthroplasty for fractures and fracture-dislocations of the proximal humerus. *Clin Orthop Relat Res* 179:116-128.
‡Hawkins RJ, Switlyk P (1993). Acute prosthetic replacement for severe fractures of the proximal humerus. *Clin Orthop Relat Res* 289:156-160.
§Zyto K, Wallace WA, Frostick SP, Preston BJ (1998). Outcome after hemiarthroplasty for three- and four-part fractures of the proximal humerus. *J Shoulder Elbow Surg* 7:85-89.
‖Boileau P, Trojani C, Walch G, et al. (2001). Shoulder arthroplasty for the treatment of the sequelae of fractures of the proximal humerus. *J Shoulder Elbow Surg* 10:299-308.

Complications

Introduction

- Common complications are as follows, in order of decreasing frequency (Hasan et al. 2002):
  - Loosening of glenoid component
  - Instability
  - Stiffness
  - Rotator cuff tear
  - Periprosthetic fracture
  - Nerve injury
  - Infection
  - Failure of the humeral implant
  - Deltoid muscle dysfunction
- The rate of revision probably underestimates the complication rate because it is estimated that almost 25% of unsatisfactory arthroplasties are not revised.
- Pain and weakness are common but are considered expressions of failure, not causes.

Glenoid Component Loosening

- Glenoid loosening is the most common prosthesis–related cause for revision surgery following TSA, with rates ranging from 0% to 12.5%.

- Causes are multifactorial and include the following:
  - Glenoid preparation
  - Soft tissue balancing
  - Wear debris triggering cellular mediators of osteoclastic bone resorption
  - Availability of glenoid bone stock for prosthetic fixation
  - Severe, irreparable cuff tears
  - Prosthetic design considerations, such as the articular surface geometry, glenohumeral conformity, biomaterials, and the glenoid keel or peg morphology (Fig. 11–21).

Instability

- Instability may occur in up to 22% of failed shoulder arthroplasties.
- Component positioning is most often the cause of instability; however, soft tissue abnormalities such as rotator cuff tears or subscapularis detachment are also potential causes.
- Anterior instability most commonly occurs in the early postoperative period and is usually the result of rupture of the subscapularis tendon or excessive humeral anteversion (Fig. 11–22).
- Posterior instability either may occur early or may develop late, and it is usually the result of combined

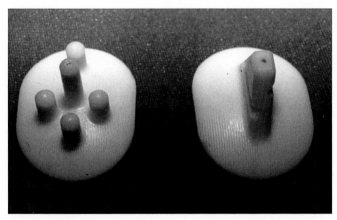

Figure 11–21: Distinction between a pegged glenoid and a keeled glenoid.
This figure demonstrates the design differences between a pegged glenoid *(left)* and a keeled glenoid *(right)*.

excessive retroversion of the humeral and glenoid components.
- Superior instability (anterior superior escape) most commonly occurs in patients with either massive cuff deficiency or failure of greater tuberosity repair after fracture in combination with failure of the coracoacromial arch.
- Inferior instability occurs most often following fracture and is the result of placing the humeral component too low, thus shortening the effective length of the deltoid.

Tuberosity Malunion or Nonunion

- This is a difficult complication following arthroplasty for fracture.

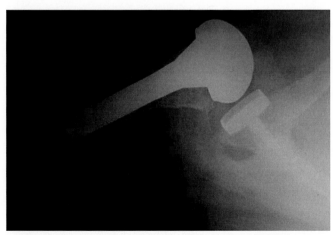

Figure 11–22: Anterior instability after total shoulder arthroplasty.
This axillary radiograph is of a patient who presented with anterior instability after total shoulder arthroplasty. This instability was found to be secondary to overstuffing of the joint with resultant subscapularis rupture and subsequent anterior instability and pain.

- No good, reliable solution to this problem exists.
- For proximal humeral fractures, every attempt should be made to recreate normal anatomy.
- Tuberosity reduction must be accurate, and the fixation must be secure.
- The surgeon should use all available anatomic landmarks to place the tuberosities as accurately as possible:
  - Bicipital tendon/groove
  - Fracture lines themselves
  - Fins on the stem
- An osteotomy of a nonfractured greater tuberosity fracture should be avoided if possible.
  - Adapting the procedures or the prostheses to the abnormal anatomy often allows the surgeon to avoid an osteotomy of the tuberosity.

Stiffness

- Stiffness ultimately results from soft tissue contracture or relative overtension because of large components or nonanatomic cuts.
- Excessive humeral stem height and excessive head size can place excessive tension on the rotator cuff, causing stiffness and pain.
- A 6-month period of supervised stretching exercises is recommended before consideration for operative release.
  - For isolated stiffness without other causes such as the prosthetic components, arthroscopic release is an option.
  - For postfracture stiffness, open release is generally required for patients desiring to regain motion.

Rotator Cuff Tears

- Problems with rotator cuff healing and subsequent rotator cuff tearing following arthroplasty are probably underreported.
- Rotator cuff repairs following TSA often yield poor results. A significant correlation exists among rotator cuff tearing, instability, and glenoid loosening (Iannotti and Norris 2003).

Deltoid Dysfunction

- This occurs for one of two reasons: denervation or detachment.
- Detachment is uncommon following the deltopectoral approach.
- The axillary nerve is vulnerable to injury, particularly in patients with distorted anatomy (e.g., trauma or previous surgery).

Nerve Injury

- The incidence among patients undergoing TSA is 1% to 4% (Boardman and Cofield 1999).
- Most injuries are localized to the plexus, with the upper and middle trunk most commonly affected.
- Return of nerve function is common (80%).

Heterotopic Ossification

- This complication can occur in up to 45% of patients.
- Although it is relatively common, it is rarely of functional consequence.

Subacromial Impingement

- This is rarely reported but can be a source of pain after arthroplasty.
- It can be treated arthroscopically with subacromial decompression when indicated.

Humeral Complications

- Humeral component malposition and excessive anteversion or retroversion can lead to anterior and posterior instability, respectively.
- Positioning the stem too low or too high, or oversizing the humeral head, can lead to inferior or superior instability or stiffness resulting from overstuffing. Attritional rupture of the rotator cuff can also occur under these conditions.

Loosening

- The incidence of radiographic lucencies around the humeral component is high, but this finding is rarely clinically significant.

Intraoperative and Periprosthetic Fracture

- Intraoperative fracture usually occurs while externally rotating the humerus during exposure of the humeral head, preparation of the humeral canal, or seating the prosthesis.
- Although rare, it is still the most common intraoperative complication (5%).
- Preferred treatment is with a long-stem humeral component and cerclage wiring.
- The stem should be extended distal to the fracture site by at least two cortical diameters from the fracture site.
- Postoperative periprosthetic fractures are classified as follows:
  - Type A: Fracture of the tuberosities
  - Type B: Fracture about the stem tip
  - Type C: Fracture distal to the stem tip
- Treatment is customized based on fracture location, alignment, and prosthetic fixation.

Hemiarthroplasty-Specific Complications

- Most common complications of hemiarthroplasty occur in 1% to 3% of cases, as follows, in descending order of frequency:
  - Instability
  - Glenoid arthritis
  - Tuberosity nonunion
  - Rotator cuff tears

- Nerve injury
- Infection
- Complications vary, depending on the preoperative diagnosis.
- Hemiarthroplasty has a higher early complication rate than TSA and approaches 16%.
  - Hemiarthroplasty for osteoarthritis is often complicated by glenoid surface degeneration.
  - Hemiarthroplasty for proximal humerus fractures is likely to result in tuberosity nonunion.
- When hemiarthroplasty alone is considered, the surgeon must confirm that the glenoid is concentric and noneroded.
  - Nonconcentric glenoids and glenoids with degenerative cartilage are replaced or reamed to a smooth concentric surface, if there is an indication (e.g., young age, heavy labor) to avoid glenoid replacement.
  - Patients with concentric glenoids can achieve about 85% satisfactory results, whereas patients with nonconcentric glenoids achieve only approximately 65% satisfactory results.
  - Most of the unsatisfactory results are caused by loss of forward elevation and external rotation.

General Complications of Arthroplasty

Pulmonary Embolism

- Little information exists regarding the incidence of this complication after shoulder replacement.
- Most of the literature consists of case reports of pulmonary embolism after TSA.

Infection

- The incidence is less than 1% in primary arthroplasty and 3% in revisions.
- Infection must be ruled out in any patient with a failed or painful arthroplasty.
- Plain radiographs may show bone resorption around the component, endosteal scalloping, or periosteal new bone formation.
- Aspiration and culture are useful when prior studies do not clearly indicate the status of the infection, as are sedimentation rate and C-reactive protein.
- Following the hip and knee literature, the current recommendation for treating infected shoulder arthroplasties consists of two-stage replantation in most cases.

Revision

Preoperative Evaluation

- Evaluation of a failed TSA begins with a careful history and physical examination, followed by appropriate diagnostic studies.

- Preoperative evaluation should determine the cause of failure and whether a correctable problem exists.
- Index diagnosis, details of prior surgical procedures, and the timing of failure of the primary arthroplasty all provide critical information.
- The differential diagnosis in the patient who fails to improve following an elective arthroplasty includes the following:
  - Instability, often resulting from a ruptured subscapularis repair
  - Error in component positioning
  - Failure to resurface an arthritic glenoid
  - Development of postoperative stiffness
  - Infection, which may occur early or late in the postoperative period
- Patients with unsuccessful arthroplasty for fracture may have problems with tuberosity position or healing or component malposition.
- Late failure after a period of satisfactory function most typically is the result of the following:
  - Glenoid loosening
  - Dissociation after TSA
  - Development of glenoid arthrosis following hemiarthroplasty
  - Humeral loosening (less common, but may occur typically in the setting of TSA, in which glenoid wear debris may induce humeral osteolysis)
- Physical examination begins with inspection of the shoulder for evidence of rotator cuff dysfunction and atrophy or detachment of the deltoid.
  - A standard shoulder examination should be carried out because more chronic problems such as impingement and acromioclavicular arthritis can also compromise the results of shoulder replacement.
  - Active and passive range of motion is recorded, as are the strength of the deltoid, strength of the rotator cuff, and the function of the peripheral nerves.
- Standard radiographs should include a true anteroposterior view in internal and external rotation, a scapular Y view, and an axillary view.
  - Serial radiographs should be reviewed for evidence of progressive radiolucent lines, osteolysis, or change in implant position.
- Most failed arthroplasties have two or more modes of failure (e.g., instability with associated glenoid loosening).
- Complexity of the technical aspects of revision arthroplasty is the result of the combination of bone loss, muscle weakness, scar, and increased risk of infection.
  - Even a well-executed revision arthroplasty can have an unsatisfactory outcome resulting from soft tissue limitations.

Surgical Considerations
Glenoid Bone Loss

- Glenoid bone loss is a significant problem with revision TSA, particularly in the setting of aseptic glenoid loosening.
- Causes of glenoid bone loss include the following:
  - Osteolysis (most common)
  - Macroscopically loose or displaced glenoid components
  - Excessive bone removal during the revision of a cemented or ingrowth component

Soft Tissues

- Soft tissues contribute to the success or failure of TSA.
- Abnormalities of the soft tissue include the following:
  - Laxity
  - Contractures
  - Paralysis
  - Adhesions
  - Tissue loss
- Adhesions make the exposure in revision TSA challenging.
  - The rotator cuff is commonly adhered to the undersurface of the acromion.
  - The more peripheral cuff and proximal humerus are often adhered to the overlying deltoid muscle.
- Contractures of the shoulder capsule and rotator cuff typically occur in the setting of instability where one side, anterior or posterior, is lax or deficient and the opposing side is contracted.
- Deltoid deficiency, from axillary nerve damage or dehiscence, can prevent a satisfactory result in revision arthroplasty.

Surgical Technique

- An extended, deltopectoral approach as described previously is used for all revision shoulder arthroplasties requiring prosthesis exchange.
  - Superficial exposure may be particularly difficult if the deltoid muscle is detached or fibrotic.
  - The coracoid tip is the most important landmark for the deep exposure.
- Dissection of the tissues medial to the coracoid puts the neurovascular structures at risk.
  - The subacromial and subdeltoid adhesions are released.
  - The subscapularis is identified, released, and mobilized.
- Attention must be paid to maintain the overall length of the subscapularis.
- In patients with more than 30 degrees of external rotation, the subscapularis tendon can be released 1 cm from its insertion on the lesser tuberosity and subsequently repaired primarily.
- In patients with less than 30 degrees of external rotation, the subscapularis is released right off the lesser tuberosity

and is subsequently reattached more medially on the glenoid neck to increase postoperative external rotation.

Management of Glenoid Bone Loss

- Central deficiency of the glenoid that is mild to moderate can be managed with cancellous bone graft and glenoid reimplantation.
- Cement fixation with supplemental bone graft is reasonable for minor deficiencies.
- In severe central and combined deficiencies, it is recommended to perform bone grafting of the glenoid vault without glenoid reimplantation.
- In patients with a deficient glenoid rim, concentric reaming of the glenoid without reimplantation of a glenoid component can be considered.

Management of Humeral Bone Loss

- Humeral prostheses need to be removed with attention to preserving bone stock.
  - Several options exist, including extended humeral osteotomies, bone windows, and ultrasonic cement removal.
- Absent or deficient tuberosities are best treated by repairing the available rotator cuff to the remaining proximal humeral bone or fracture stem or by using a reverse prosthesis.
- Several options exist for segmental bone loss:
  - Bulk allograft
  - Long-stem prosthesis
  - Impaction grafting

Management of Rotator Cuff Deficiencies

- Rotator cuff deficiencies should be carefully assessed, so appropriate decisions regarding type of component implantation can be made (Miller et al. 2003).
- In rotator cuff deficiencies (irreparable tears), the glenoid should not be reimplanted because of the risk of glenoid loosening.
  - In this situation, hemiarthroplasty or reverse prosthesis should be considered. As mentioned previously, the coracoacromial arch must be preserved at all costs because it is the only remaining restraint to proximal humeral migration.
  - If the rotator cuff is reparable without significant tension, then glenoid reimplantation can be considered.
- Isolated subscapularis deficiency can be treated with allograft reconstruction or a pectoralis major transfer.

Results

- Results vary depending on the initial diagnosis and the method of failure.

- Revision arthroplasty requiring either revision or removal of the glenoid component alone has a better outcome than other revision procedures.
- Patients who require only modular humeral head revision or arthroscopy with rotator cuff repair alone consistently have fair or poor results.
- Results of revision arthroplasty are better in patients who are able to undergo glenoid reimplantation.
- Results in the literature for revision shoulder arthroplasty to date clearly demonstrate inferior results for revision surgery when compared with primary shoulder arthroplasty.

References

Antuna SA, Sperling JW, Sanchez-Sotelo J, Cofield RH (2002a). Shoulder arthroplasty for proximal humeral malunions: Long-term results. *J Shoulder Elbow Surg* 11:122-129.

Fifty shoulders with proximal humeral malunions were treated with hemiarthroplasty or TSA and were followed-up for a mean of 9 years. At most recent follow-up, shoulder pain was more intense in patients who had initial operative treatment of their fracture, in those with osteonecrosis, and in those who had arthroplasty less than 2 years after their fracture. Postoperative motion was significantly less in those who had initial operative treatment of their fracture or who underwent tuberosity osteotomy. All shoulders with tuberosity nonunion or resorption had an unsatisfactory result.

Antuna SA, Sperling JW, Sanchez-Sotelo J, Cofield RH (2002b). Shoulder arthroplasty for proximal humeral nonunions. *J Shoulder Elbow Surg* 11:114-121.

Patients who have significant functional impairment from a nonunion of the humeral surgical neck with failed internal fixation, severe osteoporosis, cavitation of the humeral head, or secondary osteoarthritis may benefit from shoulder arthroplasty. Although function is not completely restored, pain relief and high levels of subjective satisfaction can be achieved.

Barrett WP, Thornhill TS, Thomas WH, et al. (1989). Nonconstrained total shoulder arthroplasty in patients with polyarticular rheumatoid arthritis. *J Arthroplasty* 4:91-96.

A retrospective review of 114 patients with polyarticular rheumatoid arthritis who had 140 TSAs revealed that 93% of the patients had excellent pain relief; however, improvement in active forward elevation averaged 34 degrees. Complications occurred in 7% of the shoulders, but no deep or superficial wound infections were noted.

Boardman ND 3rd, Cofield RH (1999). Neurologic complications of shoulder surgery. *Clin Orthop Relat Res* 368:44-53.

Nerve injuries are reported to occur in 1% to 2% of patients undergoing rotator cuff surgery, 1% to 8% of patients undergoing surgery for anterior instability, and 1% to 4% of patients undergoing prosthetic arthroplasty. Commonly, the nerve injuries occur secondary to traction or contusion. These injuries are avoided best by careful attention to patient positioning, retractor placement, and arm manipulation during surgery.

Boileau P, Trojani C, Walch G, et al. (2001). Shoulder arthroplasty for the treatment of the sequelae of fractures of the proximal humerus. *J Shoulder Elbow Surg* 10:299-308.

These authors concluded that a greater tuberosity osteotomy is the most likely reason for poor and unpredictable results after shoulder replacement arthroplasty for the treatment of the complex sequelae of proximal humerus fractures. Shoulder arthroplasty for the treatment of the sequelae of fractures of the proximal humerus should be performed without an osteotomy of the greater tuberosity when possible. If prosthetic replacement is possible without an osteotomy, surgeons should accept the distorted anatomy of the proximal humerus and adapt the prosthesis and their technique to the modified anatomy. A modular and adaptable prosthesis with both adjustable offsets and inclination may allow surgeons to adapt to a large number of malunions and may help to avoid the troublesome greater tuberosity osteotomy in a higher proportion of cases.

Bosch U, Skutek M, Fremerey RW, Tscherne H (1998). Outcome after primary and secondary hemiarthroplasty in elderly patients with fractures of the proximal humerus. *J Shoulder Elbow Surg* 7:479-484.

These authors concluded that the decision to perform prosthetic humeral head replacement in elderly patients should be made as early as possible after three- and four-part proximal humerus fractures.

Boulahia A, Edwards TB, Walch G, Baratta RV (2002). Early results of a reverse design prosthesis in the treatment of arthritis of the shoulder in elderly patients with a large rotator cuff tear. *Orthopedics* 25:129-133.

Results of shoulder arthroplasty in patients with a deficient rotator cuff often were suboptimal, with significant limitations in postoperative active mobility. Short-term results using a reverse design prosthesis in the treatment of the cuff-deficient arthritic shoulder were encouraging. This prosthesis compared favorably, particularly with regard to postoperative active anterior elevation, to other treatment options in this challenging patient population.

Cheng SL, Mackay MB, Richards RR (1997). Treatment of locked posterior fracture dislocations of the shoulder by total shoulder arthroplasty. *J Shoulder Elbow Surg* 6:11-17.

This report reviewed the surgical technique, postoperative rehabilitation program, and functional results of seven shoulders in five patients who had locked posterior dislocations of the shoulder.

Compito CA, Self EB, Bigliani LU (1994). Arthroplasty and acute shoulder trauma: Reasons for success and failure. *Clin Orthop Relat Res* 307:27-36.

Successful treatment of acute fractures of the proximal humerus with prosthetic replacement is a therapeutic challenge to the orthopaedic surgeon. Unsatisfactory results have been associated with tuberosity detachment, prosthetic loosening, inadequate or noncompliant rehabilitation, preoperative nerve injury, humeral malposition, dislocation, deep infection, and ectopic bone formation.

Demirhan M, Kilicoglu O, Altinel L, et al. (2003). Prognostic factors in prosthetic replacement for acute proximal humerus fractures. *J Orthop Trauma* 17:181-188.

This study investigated the effects of some epidemiologic and radiologic factors on the outcome of prosthetic replacement in acute proximal humerus fractures. This study concluded that preoperative delay, problems with tuberosity fixation, and position of

the tuberosities were parameters influencing the clinical outcome. Lateralization of the tuberosities resulted in better scores, whereas distal transfer of the tuberosities was sometimes related to a poorer outcome.

Gartsman GM, Roddey TS, Hammerman SM (2000). Shoulder arthroplasty with or without resurfacing of the glenoid in patients who have osteoarthritis. *J Bone Joint Surg Am* 82:26-34.

TSA provided superior pain relief compared with hemiarthroplasty in patients who had glenohumeral osteoarthritis, but it was associated with an increased cost per patient.

Hasan SS, Leith JM, Campbell B, et al. (2002). Characteristics of unsatisfactory shoulder arthroplasties. *J Shoulder Elbow Surg* 11:431-441.

Failure of shoulder arthroplasty is often defined as a complication or the need for revision, but it may also be viewed as a result that does not meet the expectations of the patient. The challenge of achieving patient satisfaction after arthroplasty may be greater than previously recognized. These authors suggested that greater attention to achieving proper component position, postoperative motion, and, in cases of fracture, fixation of the tuberosities may lead to increased patient satisfaction after shoulder arthroplasty.

Iannotti JP, Norris TR (2003). Influence of preoperative factors on outcome of shoulder arthroplasty for glenohumeral osteoarthritis. *J Bone Joint Surg Am* 85:251-258, 2003.

These authors recommended the use of a glenoid component in shoulders with glenoid erosion. Humeral head subluxation was associated with a less favorable result regardless of the type of shoulder arthroplasty. Severe loss of passive range of motion preoperatively was associated with decreased passive range of motion postoperatively. A reparable tear of the supraspinatus tendon was not a contraindication to the use of a glenoid component.

Levine WN, Djurasovic M, Glasson JM, et al. (1997). Hemiarthroplasty for glenohumeral osteoarthritis: Results correlated to degree of glenoid wear. *J Shoulder Elbow Surg* 6:449-454.

These authors stated that hemiarthroplasty could be an effective treatment for both primary and secondary arthritis but should be reserved for patients with a concentric glenoid, which affords a better fulcrum for glenohumeral motion.

Levy O, Funk L, Sforza G, Copeland SA (2004). Copeland surface replacement arthroplasty of the shoulder in rheumatoid arthritis. *J Bone Joint Surg Am* 86:512-518.

These authors concluded that the indications for surface replacement were the same as those for the conventional stemmed prostheses, but the surface replacement had the advantage of bone preservation as well as avoidance of the potential complications associated with a long humeral stem in rheumatoid bone. This procedure was not suitable for severely damaged joints in which the humeral head is insufficient or too soft.

Miller SL, Hazrati Y, Klepps S, et al. (2003). Loss of subscapularis function after total shoulder replacement: A seldom recognized problem. *J Shoulder Elbow Surg* 12:29-34.

Despite meticulous attention to subscapularis repair, suboptimal return of function was found on clinical examination and assessment of activities of daily living after TSA.

Parsch D, Lehner B, Loew M (2003). Shoulder arthroplasty in non-traumatic osteonecrosis of the humeral head. *J Shoulder Elbow Surg* 12:226-230.

Contrary to previously published retrospective studies, these authors recommended a more cautious prediction of midterm results for nontraumatic osteonecrosis of the humeral head treated with arthroplasty.

Rittmeister M, Kerschbaumer F (2001). Grammont reverse total shoulder arthroplasty in patients with rheumatoid arthritis and nonreconstructible rotator cuff lesions. *J Shoulder Elbow Surg* 10:17-22.

This study was undertaken to determine whether patients with severe rheumatoid arthritis and irreparable rotator cuff rupture could be treated successfully with the Grammont shoulder arthroplasty. The authors concluded that the data from the Grammont arthroplasty were encouraging with respect to restoration of stability and satisfactory function in rheumatoid, cuff-deficient shoulders.

Sneppen O, Fruensgaard S, Johannsen HV, et al. (1996). Total shoulder replacement in rheumatoid arthritis: Proximal migration in loosening. *J Shoulder Elbow Surg* 5:47-52.

This is a prospective study of 62 Neer Mark II total shoulder arthroplasties performed from 1981 to 1990 on 51 patients with rheumatoid arthritis. This study was undertaken to evaluate factors associated with component loosening and proximal humeral migration. It concluded that, in spite of progressive component loosening and progressive migration, good pain relief was demonstrated in 89% of the patients, and they experienced significant improvement in range of motion and function.

Stewart MP, Kelly IG (1997). Total shoulder replacement in rheumatoid disease: 7- to 13-year follow-up of 37 joints. *J Bone Joint Surg Br* 79:68-72.

These authors concluded that the Neer TSA provides a reasonable medium- to long-term outcome in rheumatoid arthritis, but they recommended that the humeral component should be routinely cemented.

Tanner MW, Cofield RH (1983). Prosthetic arthroplasty for fractures and fracture-dislocations of the proximal humerus. *Clin Orthop Relat Res* 179:116-128.

This study assessed 19 patients with 20 severe proximal humerus fractures who were treated with a Neer humeral prosthesis from 1979 to 1986. Complications consisted of one axillary nerve palsy, one postoperative posterior dislocation, one loosening of an uncemented humeral prosthesis, and one breakage of fixation wire requiring subsequent removal. Patients who could not comply with postoperative rehabilitation programs had poor results. Poor function appeared to be directly related to lack of rotator cuff integrity.

Torchia ME, Cofield RH, Settergren CR (1997). Total shoulder arthroplasty with the Neer prosthesis: Long-term results. *J Shoulder Elbow Surg* 6:495-505.

These authors determined the outcome of 113 TSAs performed with a Neer prosthesis between 1975 and 1981. The operations were performed for the treatment of osteoarthritis, rheumatoid arthritis, and old fractures or dislocations with traumatic arthritis. The probability of implant survival was 93% after 10 years and 87% after 15 years.

Zyto K, Wallace WA, Frostick SP, et al. (1998). Outcome after hemiarthroplasty for three- and four-part fractures of the proximal humerus. *J Shoulder Elbow Surg* 7:85-89.

This study reviewed 27 patients who had sustained displaced three- or four-part fractures of the proximal humerus and who were treated with a humeral hemiarthroplasty. The median range of movement for all the patients in flexion was 70 degrees, abduction 70 degrees, internal rotation 50 degrees, and external rotation 45 degrees. Nine patients still had moderate or severe pain. Eight patients had moderate or severe disability.

Elbow Arthroplasty

Bradford Parsons,* Sudheer Reddy,† and Matthew L. Ramsey‡

*MD, Assistant Professor, Department of Orthopaedics, Mt. Sinai School of Medicine,
New York, NY
†MD, Instructor, Department of Orthopaedic Surgery, University of Pennsylvania School of
Medicine, Philadelphia, PA
‡MD, Chief, Shoulder Study Group; Director, Shoulder and Elbow Fellowship; Associate
Professor, Department of Orthopaedic Surgery; and Chief, Shoulder and Elbow Service,
University of Pennsylvania School of Medicine, Philadelphia, PA

Introduction

- The predominant function of the elbow is to position the hand in space.
- Patients with elbow arthritis have difficulty using the affected limb because of pain and stiffness.
- Numerous advances in the techniques and instrumentation of elbow surgery, as well as improved understanding of pathologic elbow anatomy, have occurred in the past decade.
- A large range of options, both operative and nonoperative, is available to today's orthopaedic surgeon treating patients with elbow arthritis.
- This chapter is an overview of the predominant causes of elbow arthritis as well as a review of the current tools available to diagnose these conditions and manage these patients effectively.

Patient Selection

Etiology of the Arthritic Elbow and Patient Demographics

- Arthritis of the elbow falls into one of three main categories: primary osteoarthritis (OA), inflammatory arthritis (usually rheumatoid arthritis [RA]), and post-traumatic degenerative arthritis.
- Other, less common conditions that lead to degenerative elbow changes include comminuted periarticular fractures (including nonunions) and the chronically dislocated or unstable elbow.

Primary Osteoarthritis

- Primary OA of the elbow is uncommon, typically affecting less than 2% of the population.
- Although rare, primary OA of the elbow has a consistent presentation:
  - Most patients are male, heavy laborers, and middle aged (~50 years of age).
  - Primary OA is rare in women.
- The primary pathologic process of elbow OA involves loss of articular cartilage with osteophyte formation on the olecranon process, on the coronoid process, and in their respective fossae (Fig. 12–1).
- Secondary resultant changes involve osteophyte formation at the radial head margin and the formation of loose bodies.
- Patients with OA often have a stiff elbow, and most complain of pain at the extremes of motion.
  - Terminal extension pain can be a sign of impingement of olecranon osteophytes in the olecranon fossa.
  - Patients often present with a flexion contracture, often with greater than 30 degrees of extension loss.
  - Terminal flexion pain can result from impingement of coronoid process osteophytes in the coronoid fossa. This is seen less frequently than extension pain in primary OA of the elbow.
- Total elbow arthroplasty (TEA) is rarely needed in patients with primary OA.

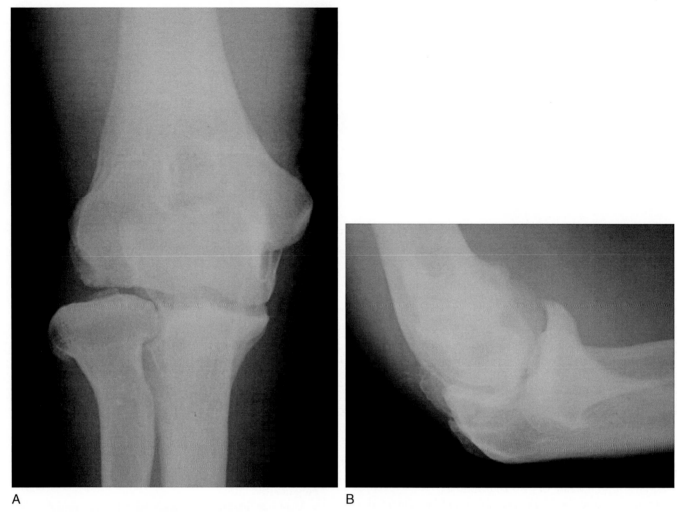

A   B

Figure 12–1: Osteoarthritis of the elbow.
The typical radiographic appearance of osteoarthritis of the elbow on anteroposterior (**A**) and lateral (**B**)
radiographs. Note the presence of rim osteophytes on the radial head and medial aspect of the coronoid on the
anteroposterior projection, as well as the large anterior coronoid and posterior olecranon fossa osteophytes on
the lateral projection.

Inflammatory Arthritis (Rheumatoid Arthritis)

- The most common inflammatory arthritis of the elbow is RA.
- Unlike primary OA, RA frequently affects the elbow, can be bilateral and is often polyarticular.
- RA affects approximately 1% to 2% of the population and involves the elbow in 20% to 50% of these patients. Patients are predominantly white women, and they often have a lower functional demand of their elbows relative to the population with OA because of systemic joint involvement.
- The underlying cause of elbow pain in RA is synovitis that leads to progressive destruction of the elbow joint.
- RA primarily involves the ulnohumeral joint early in the disease process, with the remaining segments of the elbow joint becoming involved as the disease progresses.

- Most patients with RA of the elbow have painful loss of motion and function.
- Patients often demonstrate mild, but persistent flexion contracture and synovitis.
- Pockets of inflamed synovium can invade the soft tissue envelope and cause compression of the radial and ulnar nerves, inducing neuropathy.
- With disease progression, ligamentous destruction can also occur, leading to instability.

Post-traumatic Arthritis

- Unlike RA or primary OA, post-traumatic arthritis of the elbow can affect patients of any age or sex. It is most commonly seen following intra-articular comminuted fractures of the elbow that heal with residual incongruity of the articular surface.
- Ligamentous insufficiency may also lead to articular wear and progressive arthritis in the post-traumatic elbow.

- Stiffness is often the main complaint in patients with post-traumatic arthritis of the elbow, followed by pain.
- Although treatment for OA and RA is more standardized, treatment in this case is individualized, depending on the functional demands, age, occupation, and degree of injury of the patient.

Chronic Dislocation

- Most acute dislocations are managed appropriately; therefore patients rarely have chronically dislocated or unstable elbows.
- This condition is mostly seen in developing countries.
- No standard patient demographic is recognized.
- The pathologic anatomy includes contracted or attenuated ligaments, anterior capsule, and muscles (triceps). Additionally, heterotopic bone may be seen. The joint surface is often spared but encased in fibrous tissue unless the distal humeral articular surface is perched on the coronoid. In this case, articular damage can be considerable.

Acute Periarticular Fracture or Fracture Nonunion

- This is a more recently identified indication for elbow arthroplasty.
- Arthroplasty is often reserved for elderly patients with acute, comminuted, periarticular fractures of the distal humerus.
- Periarticular nonunions, especially after attempted fixation, comprise another potential indication for elbow arthroplasty.

Evaluation of the Patient With Elbow Arthritis

History and Physical Examination of the Arthritic Elbow

- As with any condition affecting the musculoskeletal system, a detailed history and physical examination are important.

History

- The history should elicit symptoms of pain, instability, stiffness, or mechanical symptoms (catching, clicking, or locking) that could suggest loose bodies or osteochondral lesions.
- Additionally, any neurologic symptoms such as numbness, tingling, or weakness should be discerned.
- Previous trauma or surgery of the elbow should also be discussed.

Physical Examination

- Physical examination of the elbow should follow a structured, anatomic approach.
- Inspection of the elbow allows for visualization of the orientation of the resting extremity (aids in identifying malunion or nonunion) and evaluating for swelling and previous surgical scars.
- Active range of motion (ROM) should be evaluated.
  - Normal ROM varies, but it should be symmetric and include at least nearly full extension (may have

hyperextension) to 130 to 140 degrees of flexion (less in muscular patients, more in thin patients). Normal pronation and supination comprise an arc of 170 degrees, with slightly more supination than pronation.
  - Morrey and colleagues (1981) described the functional ROM as 30 to 130 degrees, with 50 degrees each of pronation and supination.
- Passive ROM is then assessed, to look for terminal impingement pain in both flexion and extension as well as forearm rotation.
- Palpation of the elbow can identify tenderness or swelling and should follow anatomic structures:
  - The medial epicondyle, lateral epicondyle, radiocapitellar joint, radial head, posterolateral gutter, olecranon, posteromedial gutter (including Tinel's of the cubital tunnel), and anterior cubital fossa are palpated.
  - Palpation medially during passive ROM can reveal a subluxatable ulnar nerve.
  - Posterolateral swelling along the infracondylar recess can indicate synovial inflammation.
  - Rheumatoid nodules may frequently be found on the subcutaneous border of the ulna posteriorly in patients with RA.
- Provocative examination of the elbow includes assessment of stability and muscle function.
  - Valgus instability (medial collateral ligament [MCL] deficiency) is best tested with the humerus externally rotated, the forearm in maximal supination, and valgus stress applied at the elbow in approximately 30 degrees of flexion.
  - The moving valgus stress test, recently described, is believed to be 100% sensitive in identifying patients with MCL injury (O'Driscoll et al. 2005). The test is performed by applying and maintaining a constant moderate valgus torque to the fully flexed elbow and then extending the elbow quickly. A positive test will elicit medial elbow pain at the medial collateral ligament and is maximal between 120 and 70 degrees.
  - Varus stress (lateral ulnar collateral ligament [LUCL] deficiency) is tested with the elbow in similar flexion, but with the humerus in full internal rotation and the forearm pronated.
  - The lateral pivot shift test can also be used to test for posterolateral rotatory instability (LUCL deficiency).
    - This test consists of extending the elbow, with valgus and axial stress while the elbow is being extended.
    - The test may be difficult to conduct in the awake patient and is best performed with the patient under anesthesia.
  - Muscle testing is used to evaluate extension strength (triceps integrity) primarily.
    - Extension strength is approximately 70% that of flexion strength and is best measured with the elbow at 90 degrees of flexion and with the forearm in neutral rotation.

- Pronation, supination, and grip strength are also best determined with the elbow flexed to 90 degrees and the forearm in neutral rotation. Supination strength is roughly 15% greater than pronation strength.

Radiographic Examination of the Arthritic Elbow

- Standard anteroposterior and lateral radiographs are the mainstays of radiographic evaluation of the arthritic elbow.
  - Radiographs can identify osteophytes, loose bodies, abnormal osseous anatomy, and loss of articular cartilage.
  - Lateral views help to reveal osteophytes on the olecranon and coronoid.
  - The anteroposterior view can reveal osteophytes in the olecranon fossa.
  - Stress radiographs are used to evaluate for instability.
  - More than 2 mm of joint gapping with varus or valgus loading is considered abnormal.
- Computed tomography scans may be helpful to evaluate patients with bone loss, malunion, nonunion, heterotopic bone, or ankylosis of the elbow.
- Magnetic resonance imaging is infrequently used in the evaluation of the patient with elbow arthritis, but it may help to visualize ligamentous anatomy or evaluate triceps integrity.
- The typical radiographic findings for each cause of elbow arthritis follow.

Osteoarthritis

- Radiographic features of the osteoarthritic elbow correlate strongly with clinical features and follow a defined pattern.
- Primary OA of the elbow typically follows a pattern involving initial preservation of joint space, with osteophyte formation in the olecranon and coronoid and their respective fossae.
- Table 12–1 correlates the clinical features with radiographic findings of OA of the elbow.

Rheumatoid Arthritis

- Radiographic signs of RA also follow a typical pattern (Fig. 12–2).
- These signs are categorized into grades by the Mayo classification (Table 12–2).

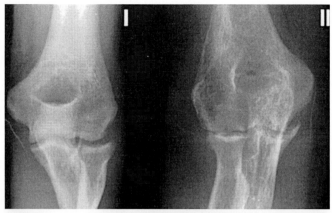
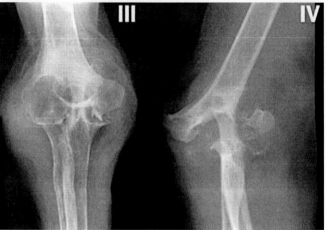

Figure 12–2: Rheumatoid arthritis.
These radiographs depict the progressive severity of elbow arthritis denoted in the Mayo classification of elbow involvement in patients with rheumatoid arthritis. Grade I elbows have a normal radiographic appearance. In grade II, a loss of articular cartilage is observed, but the subchondral bone remains intact. Grade III is characterized by subchondral bone loss that may progress to deformity (grade IIIb). Elbows that are grossly deformed are classified as grade IV. An ankylosed elbow has been added to the classification as grade V. (From Morrey BF, ed. [2000]. *The Elbow and Its Disorders*, 3rd ed. Philadelphia: WB Saunders.)

Table 12–1	Presenting Clinical and Radiographic Features of Elbow Osteoarthritis
CLINICAL FEATURES	**RADIOGRAPHIC FEATURES**
1. Extension loss, mild pain	1. Small olecranon spur
2. As for 1, limits activity	2. Larger olecranon/coronoid spurs
3. Locks, catches	3. Loose body formation
4. Pain with flexion/extension, motion restricted	4. Osteophyte: foramina, coronoid/olecranon
5. As for 1–4, with ulnar nerve symptoms	5. As above
6. Pain and motion loss over entire arc, marked restriction	6. Extensive osteophytic changes, joint narrowing

Table 12–2	Mayo Classification of Radiographic Grading of Rheumatoid Arthritis of the Elbow
GRADE	**DESCRIPTION**
I	Synovitis, but no radiographic changes other than osteoporosis
II	Synovitis persists with narrowing of the joint and intact architecture
III	Variable synovitis with architectural changes of the joint
IV	Gross destruction of the joint
V	Ankylosis of the elbow

Data from Morrey BF, ed. (2000). *The Elbow and Its Disorders*, 3rd ed. Philadelphia: WB Saunders.

Post-traumatic Arthritis

- Radiographic changes of post-traumatic arthritis typically reflect the underlying trauma to the joint.
- Evidence of malunion or articular incongruity can be observed on plain radiographs.
- Computed tomography scans may be helpful in these patients.

Nonoperative Treatment

- Nonoperative management of elbow arthritis centers on preserving ROM and alleviating stiffness and inflammation.
- Several available modalities are aimed at managing the pain and stiff elbow, including medications, physical therapy, dynamic or static adjustable splinting, and injections.

Physical Therapy

- Physical therapy is aimed at improving motion and decreasing pain and inflammation in the arthritic elbow.
- Physical therapy should be done cautiously because aggressive passive stretch of an arthritic, stiff elbow can worsen inflammation and increase pain.
- Modalities include active-assistive ROM exercises, as well as gentle passive stretch, coupled with modalities to reduce inflammation such as heat, cold treatments, or iontophoresis or phonophoresis.

Dynamic Splinting

- This is a popular method of treating elbow stiffness.
- Success is limited when the ulnohumeral articulation is significantly involved.
- The rationale behind this treatment is that because soft tissues about the elbow are viscoelastic, application of a constant force via a dynamic splint can lead to creep (progressive deformation of the soft tissues) that can help to combat stiffness (Bonutti et al. 1994).
- Similarly to physical therapy, dynamic splinting is done cautiously to prevent tearing and worsening of inflammation.
- Numerous prefabricated or custom splints can be used to provide stretch to stiff elbows.

Static Adjustable Splinting

- Force is applied as in dynamic splinting, but the force is not continuously applied.
- Compared with dynamic splinting, static splinting allows for stress relaxation of the soft tissues, which may reduce or even eliminate the potential rebound inflammation and stiffness.
- This often can be done around physical therapy (e.g., at night during sleep) to improve motion passively.
- In one study of 20 patients with elbow contractures managed with static splinting, the average increase in ROM was 30 degrees. No complications were found in this study at 1 year of follow-up, and all patients maintained their ROM gains.

Medications

- As in any arthritic condition, aspirin and other nonsteroidal anti-inflammatory drugs are commonly used to control pain.
  - Long-term use may increase the risk of gastrointestinal complications.
- More potent agents such as antimalarial drugs, gold salts, and immunosuppressives such as corticosteroids have proven beneficial, especially in the treatment of RA.
  - Newer antirheumatoid agents have been recently found very effective in the control of painful synovitis in these patients.
  - Prescription and administration of these medications should be left to the treating rheumatologist.

Corticosteroid Injections

- Corticosteroid injections can prove useful in alleviating symptoms of acute flare-up of arthritis or synovitis.
  - This often temporary intervention may be repeated every few months (no more than three times per year).
- For patients with RA, acute synovitis may respond to chemical synovectomy. Agents such as gold,[32] P-chromic phosphate, osmic acid, and yttrium-90 have all been used to treat synovitis in this condition.
  - Application of this technique has been limited because of concerns over articular cartilage damage or potential chromosomal mutation that could result in malignancy.

Implant Selection

Anatomy of the Elbow

- Familiarity and recognition of normal and pathologic anatomy of the arthritic elbow are critical to successful management of elbow arthritis.
- Additionally, anatomic features have direct implications on TEA design.

Osteology

- The distal humerus consists of two condyles (medial and lateral) that support the articular surfaces of the trochlea and capitellum.
- The articular surface of the distal humerus has a characteristic orientation in reference to the diaphysis of the humerus.
  - In the sagittal plane, the articular surface is flexed anteriorly 30 degrees from the long axis of the humerus.
  - In the transverse plane, it is rotated inwards by 5 degrees.
  - In the coronal plane, it is angulated in 6 degrees of valgus.
  - The *carrying angle* of the elbow refers to the angle formed by the long axes of the humerus and ulna with the elbow fully extended. In male patients, the angle is

approximately 11 to 14 degrees, and in female patients, it is between 13 and 16 degrees.
- The trochlea is shaped like a spool and articulates with the greater sigmoid notch of the ulna.
- The capitellum is hemispheroidal, articulating with the concave radial head.
  - The capitellotrochlear groove separates the capitellum from the trochlea.
  - The edge of the radial head articulates with the capitellotrochlear groove throughout the ROM of the elbow.
- Elbow stability is enhanced by the form and relationship of the articular surfaces of the elbow.
- The sigmoid notch has a longitudinal ridge that articulates with the central recess of the "spool" of the trochlea, whereas the medial and lateral slopes of the trochlea and sigmoid notch are conforming.
- Flexion stability is enhanced by the positioning of the coronoid and radial head in their respective fossae along the anterior surface of the distal humerus.
  - The olecranon tip similarly fits in the posterior olecranon fossa in extension, enhancing stability.
  - The concave, elliptical surface of the radial head articulates with the capitellum, whereas the circumferential aspect articulates with the ulna in the lesser sigmoid notch.
  - Approximately 240 degrees of the outside circumference of the head articulates with the ulna in the lesser sigmoid fossa, thus resulting in a sum total of 170 degrees of pronation and supination.
- The anterolateral third of the head is devoid of articular cartilage and is the part of the head most often fractured.
- The radial head and neck are also not collinear with one another because the head and neck form an angle of

15 degrees with the radial shaft, with the angle opposite the location of the radial tuberosity.
- The articular surfaces of the ulna, the greater sigmoid notch and the lesser sigmoid notch, articulate with the trochlea and radial head, respectively.
  - The anterior, distal aspect of the greater sigmoid notch is composed of the coronoid process.
  - The coronoid process provides an anterior buttress preventing posterior displacement of the ulna.
  - The proximal medial base of the coronoid is termed the *sublime tubercle*, which serves as the attachment site of the anterior band of the MCL.
  - Along the lateral aspect of the coronoid is the lesser sigmoid notch, which has an arc of approximately 70 degrees and articulates with the radial head.

Capsuloligamentous Anatomy

- The elbow joint is encased within the capsule.
- On the medial and lateral sides of the joint, thickenings of the capsule comprise the collateral ligament complexes.
- The anterior capsule originates proximal to the coronoid and radial fossae and inserts onto the distal aspect of the coronoid process (5 to 8 mm distal to the tip).
  - The anterior capsule is taut in extension.
- The posterior capsule encases the olecranon and the olecranon fossa and is taut in flexion.

Medial Collateral Ligament Complex

- The humeral origin of the MCL is on the broad anteroinferior surface of the medial epicondyle (Fig. 12–3*A*).
- The three distinct components of the MCL are the anterior, posterior, and transverse bundles.

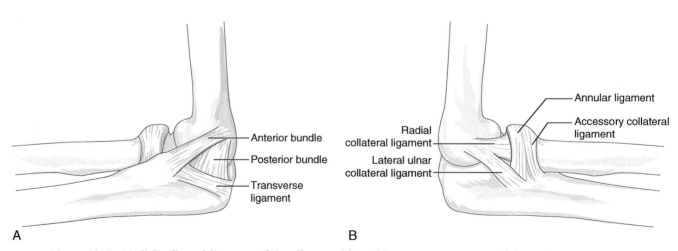

A   B

Figure 12–3: Medial collateral ligament of the elbow and lateral ligamentous anatomy of the elbow. **A,** Schematic representation of the orientation of the medial collateral ligament of the elbow. The anterior bundle of the medial collateral ligament has been found to be critical to elbow stability, especially against valgus loading. **B,** Schematic representation of the lateral ligamentous anatomy of the elbow. The lateral ulnar collateral ligament has been found to be an integral component of the lateral stability of the elbow, especially against posterolateral rotatory instability. (From Morrey BF, ed. [2000]. *The Elbow and Its Disorders,* 3rd ed. Philadelphia: WB Saunders.)

- The anterior bundle is the primary restraint to valgus stress and is the most discrete component.
- The posterior bundle is a thickening of the posterior capsule and is well defined at 90 degrees of elbow flexion.
  - The transverse component has no known contribution to elbow stability.
- The anterior bundle inserts onto the anteromedial base of the coronoid process on the sublime tubercle.

Lateral Collateral Ligament Complex

- The lateral collateral ligament complex is made up of four components: (1) the radial collateral ligament, (2) the annular ligament, (3) an accessory lateral collateral ligament that is variably present, and (4) the LUCL (See Fig. 12–3B).
- The radial collateral ligament originates from the lateral epicondyle and terminates in the annular ligament. It provides a source of origin for the supinator and is almost uniformly taut throughout the ROM of the elbow.
- The annular ligament attaches to the medial and lateral margins of the lesser sigmoid notch, thus creating a hammock around the radial head, and maintains its contact with the lesser sigmoid notch of the ulna.
- The *accessory lateral collateral ligament* refers to the ulnar insertion of discrete fibers onto the supinator crest of the proximal ulna. Proximally, it also merges with fibers of the annular ligament.
  - The primary function of this structure, when present, is to stabilize the annular ligament further during varus stress of the elbow.
- The LUCL is the primary lateral stabilizer of the elbow. It originates from the lateral epicondyle at its isometric point and inserts onto the supinator crest of the ulna.
- Deficiency of the LUCL has been found to result in posterolateral rotatory instability of the elbow.

Muscular Anatomy

- Numerous muscles cross the elbow joint and have a role in flexion, extension, or rotation of the forearm or a combination of these motions.
- This section affords a brief overview of the major muscles involved in motion of the elbow, as well as those that contribute to the dynamic stability of the elbow joint.

Elbow Flexors

- The brachialis, biceps, and brachioradialis are the primary elbow flexors.
- The brachialis has the largest cross-sectional area of these three muscles and inserts onto the proximal ulna just distal to the insertion of the anterior capsule.
- The biceps inserts onto the bicipital tuberosity of the radius.
  - Although the biceps has a smaller cross-sectional area than the brachialis, it has a greater moment arm and mechanical advantage.

- The biceps contributes substantially to supination of the forearm, particularly with the elbow in the flexed position.
- The brachioradialis originates from the lateral supracondylar ridge and inserts onto the base of the radial styloid, and it has the greatest mechanical advantage of any of the elbow flexors.

Elbow Extensors

- The triceps is the key muscle for elbow extension, whereas the role of the anconeus is still being elucidated.
- The triceps has three heads: long, lateral, and medial. The long and lateral heads are superficial to the deep head, and all three merge together in the midline of the humerus to form a common attachment into the tip of the olecranon.
- The anconeus is a short muscle that traverses the posterolateral aspect of the elbow joint. Although the exact role of the anconeus has been debated, its primary role is likely stabilization of the elbow joint.

Neurovascular Anatomy

- The elbow has complex neurovascular anatomy that requires a thorough understanding of anatomic relationships.
- This discussion of neurovascular elbow anatomy is limited to the ulnar nerve because it is the most frequent neurovascular structure that must be visualized and addressed in many of the surgical procedures performed on the elbow, especially during TEA.
- Many of the other neurovascular structures are rarely affected by the pathoanatomy of elbow arthritis and therefore are rarely visualized during surgery for elbow arthritis.
- The radial nerve, particularly the posterior interosseous nerve, can be affected by articular synovitis in patients with RA.
- The ulnar nerve is derived from the medial cord of the brachial plexus, passes posteriorly to the medial intermuscular septum, and then passes posteriorly to the medial epicondyle as it enters the cubital tunnel.
- In the cubital tunnel, the ulnar nerve rests against the posterior bundle of the MCL.
- The capacity of the cubital tunnel varies with elbow positioning; it flattens with flexion and expands with extension.
- The first motor branch of the ulnar nerve is to the flexor carpi ulnaris. Often, it gives a small sensory branch to the elbow joint that is proximal to the first motor branch.

Biomechanics

- This section discusses the relevant kinematics of the elbow and reviews the osseous and soft tissue structures that play a role in stabilizing the elbow.
- Additionally, the relevant joint forces exhibited across the elbow joint are reviewed.

Kinematics (London 1981, Morrey et al. 1981)

- The elbow is a trochoginglymoid joint, indicating that it possesses two degrees of freedom: flexion-extension and pronation-supination.

Flexion–Extension Motion

- The flexion-extension motion of the elbow has a range of roughly 0 to 140 degrees, with 30 to 130 degrees being the functional ROM.
- The axis of rotation for elbow flexion passes through the center of the arcs formed by the trochlear sulcus and capitellum, as seen on a lateral radiograph of the elbow.
- However, the flexion-extension motion of the elbow does not occur around a fixed axis, rather through a locus of instant centers of rotation.
  - The elbow has thus been termed a "loose" or "sloppy" hinge.
  - Biomechanical studies have revealed that the locus of the instantaneous center of rotation for flexion and extension is an area 2 to 3 mm in diameter at the center of the trochlea.
  - The axis is collinear with the anterior cortex of the humerus.
  - The actual locus moves less than 2 mm during the entire arc of elbow flexion and extension.
  - Additionally, the axis position is effected by pronation and supination of the forearm.

Pronation–Supination Motion

- The range of forearm rotation is approximately 170 degrees, with 90 degrees of supination and 80 degrees of pronation.
- Kinematic studies have shown that the radius moves proximally with pronation and distally with supination.

Stabilizers

- Static restriction to motion is conferred on the elbow by both the osseous congruity of the elbow joint and the ligamentous anatomy of the elbow.
- Muscle contraction results in compressive forces across the elbow, thus lending dynamic stability to the joint.

Osseous Structures

- Approximately 80% of valgus loading is resisted by the proximal part of the greater sigmoid notch, whereas the distal sigmoid notch resists 65% of varus loading.
- As previously discussed, the olecranon process–olecranon fossa articulation confers stability in terminal extension, while the coronoid–coronoid fossa and radial head–radial head fossa articulations confer stability in flexion.
- The coronoid process also plays a critical role in providing stability, particularly with increasing angles of elbow flexion.
- The radial head has historically been considered a secondary stabilizer to valgus stress, becoming a primary stabilizer in the MCL- and MCL-coronoid–deficient elbow.

- However, recent cadaveric studies have shown that elbow kinematics and stability are affected by excision of the radial head, even in the MCL-intact elbow (Schneeberger et al. 2004).
- These findings may indicate that radial head excision in vivo may have consequences for elbow stability and kinematics.

Capsuloligamentous Structures

- The anatomy of the MCL is discussed earlier.
  - The anterior bundle of the MCL has been found to be critical to valgus stability of the elbow.
  - The posterior bundle of the MCL contributes little to static stability of the elbow.
  - The anterior bundle of the MCL demonstrates lengthening as the elbow ranges from full extension to terminal flexion, a finding indicating that this ligament is not an isometric structure.
- The LUCL has been found to account for substantial varus stability, especially in resisting posterolateral rotatory instability, both clinically and experimentally.
  - The LUCL contribution to varus and rotational stability increases as the elbow is flexed.
  - However, recent studies have found contributions from both the annular ligament and radial collateral ligament components of the lateral collateral ligament complex in resisting varus and posterolateral stress (Schneeberger et al. 2004).
  - Unlike the anterior band of the MCL, the LUCL has been found to be isometric during flexion and extension of the elbow.
- The anterior capsule contributes to stability in elbow extension, whereas the posterior capsule tightens during flexion.

Dynamic Stabilizers

- Muscle force results in compression of the conforming articular surfaces of the elbow.
- These forces add to the dynamic stability of the elbow joint.

Joint Forces

- The elbow can experience substantial joint contact and reaction force with normal daily activities.
- The direction of joint reaction forces varies, depending on the position of the elbow in the flexion-extension arc.
- Nearly 60% of load transmitted across the elbow occurs at the radiocapitellar joint, whereas the other 40% crosses the ulnohumeral joint, when the elbow is loaded in extension.
- Strenuous activity, such as weight lifting, can result in joint reaction forces nearly three times body weight.

Design Considerations and Biomechanics of Elbow Arthroplasty

- The ideal prosthetic elbow should be adequately designed to allow for reliable replication of the flexion-extension axis of rotation.

- This not only serves to enhance stability and replicate normal motion, but also allows for replication of joint contact forces resulting from the dynamic activity of muscles.
- Additionally, the native stability of the elbow should be replicated by the prosthesis used.
  - Depending on the type of prosthesis implanted, this may require maintenance of the capsuloligamentous integrity of the elbow or may be reestablished by the inherent stability of the implant.
- Finally, the implant should be seated with appropriate cement mantle to fix the implant adequately.
  - Currently, most implantations utilize first-generation cement techniques because of limitations in implant plug design and difficulty with pressurization of the humeral-ulna canal.
  - However, one study has demonstrated the advantage of using a cement restrictor, low viscosity cement, and pressurization (Faber et al. 1997).
- One design parameter that has been found to resist the posterosuperior moment across the elbow with increasing flexion is an anterior flange on the prosthesis.
  - This flange further allows for improvement in the rotational stability of the implant.
- Early constrained prosthetic designs failed early as a result of aseptic loosening in part because they failed to replicate the normal "sloppy hinge" motion of the native elbow.
  - This resulted in excessive load at the bone-cement-prosthesis interface and early failure.
  - These early failures led to the advent of unlinked designs, as well as less constrained linked designs.
- Recent changes in the nomenclature of TEA prostheses have resulted in use of the terms *linked* and *unlinked* in preference to constrained, semiconstrained, and nonconstrained.
- Each of these design aspects is discussed in more detail in the following section.

Types of Implants

- This section is an overview of current design differences of available elbow prostheses.

Linked—Semiconstrained

- These "loose-hinged" (sloppy-hinged) prostheses were designed to maintain the stability seen with fully constrained prostheses as well as to decrease the stress transmitted to the bone-cement interface to reduce loosening.
- These implants have been shown to track within the limits of the "sloppy hinge," thus allowing the soft tissues to absorb some of the stresses across the elbow. However, without adequate soft tissue support, the semiconstrained implant behaves mechanistically as a more constrained implant (O'Driscoll et al. 1992).
- Three examples of linked-semiconstrained implants are the Coonrad-Morrey, Discovery, and GSB III designs.

Coonrad-Morrey Implant

- This implant is the prototypical linked prosthesis with a hollow cobalt-chrome pin that is used to articulate the ulnar and humeral components together.
- The hinge design allows for varus-valgus and internal-external rotational laxity of approximately 8 degrees.
- Lining the hinge are high-molecular-weight polyethylene bushings to prevent metal-on-metal contact.
- An anterior flange is present on the humeral component to resist posteriorly directed forces on the humeral component. The humeral stems also have 10-, 15-, and 20-cm lengths for use in revisions.
- The center of the ulnar ring is coincident with the center of the greater sigmoid fossa.
- A concern seen with the Coonrad-Morrey prosthesis is that it does not reproduce the normal anatomy of elbow joint; the flexion-extension axis of the prosthesis is anterior to the normal axis of elbow rotation.
- Ulnar loosening is the most common failure mode seen with this prosthesis.

Discovery Implant

- The humeral component of this implant has 5 degrees of varus-valgus angulation and 5 degrees of internal rotation with respect to the humeral shaft.
- Unlike the Coonrad-Morrey implant, the humeral design has an anatomic bow and lateral offset to replicate normal humeral anatomy more closely.
- The humeral component base is cylindric in profile to preserve bone with implantation and to minimize stress at the supracondylar columns.
- The ulnar component has an anterior neck angle of 23 degrees to approximate the flexion-extension axis of the normal elbow more closely. The articulating surface is spheric, with a polyethylene bearing that increases the contact surface area, potentially to reduce wear. This articulation allows for 7 degrees of varus-valgus laxity.

GSB III Implant

- The humeral component of the GSB III implant (Zimmer, Inc., Warsaw, IN) has large broad flanges that rest on the humeral condyles. The flanges are designed to reduce stress on the humeral stem and bone-cement interface.
- The humeral component has a polyethylene bearing into which the ulnar component inserts.
- The ulnar component can slide within the polyethylene bushing during flexion to reduce strain on the bone-implant interface.
- The varus-valgus and rotational laxity seen with this prosthesis is approximately 12 to 14 degrees.
- A potential disadvantage of this prosthesis is that if the soft tissue integrity is compromised, the ulnar component can potentially disassociate from the humeral component.

Unlinked—Minimally Constrained

- The unlinked series of implants resurface the elbow articulation and do not have a hinge.
- Stability is conferred by the soft tissues, rather than the actual articulation, to reduce stress on the bone-implant interface.
- Examples of this type of implant are the capitellocondylar, Sorbie-Questor, and Kudo implants.

Capitellocondylar Implant

- This has a cobalt-chrome humeral implant and a high-density polyethylene ulnar component that is encased in metal.
- The articular surface of the distal humerus has two grooves: one for the trochlea and the other inbetween the trochlea and capitellum. These grooves are shallower than in the normal elbow.
- The radial head is resected and is not replaced.
- The ulnar component has a stemmed metal-back design and a central trochlear ridge that guides joint motion. This ridge articulates with the trochlear groove of the humeral component.
- A disadvantage seen with this prosthesis (as seen with unlinked prostheses in general) is instability. Because the grooves between the humeral and ulnar components are shallower, the design places significant strain on the soft tissues to confer stability, and this can lead to instability.

Sorbie-Questor Prosthesis

- This unlinked implant was designed to duplicate the normal surface anatomy of the elbow joint.
- It is intended for use with a radial head component.

Kudo Implant

- The humeral component of this implant is made of cobalt-chrome alloy and has a central saddle-shaped distal articular surface that is similar to a trochlea.
- The ulnar component is composed of high-density polyethylene with a metal-backed support. The ulnar component shape reciprocates that of the distal humerus, with the radius of curvature of the ulnar component slightly larger than the humeral component, as in the normal elbow.
- The radial head is excised and is not replaced.
- The main shortcoming with this implant is that the articulation is radially offset, and this produces excess strain, especially on the medial soft tissue structures. Sacrificing the MCL is a common practice with this implant that can offset the soft tissue balance and can lead to gapping of the implant medially.

Unlinked—Semiconstrained

- The design strategy behind this implant was to improve the articulation from that seen with the minimally constrained implants but also to retain stability.

- An example of this type of implant is the Souter-Strathclyde prosthesis (Redfern et al. 2001).
- The humeral component is a cobalt-chrome alloy implant with a trochlear articular surface that is deeper than that seen in the minimally constrained implants. Side flanges are attached to the trochlea to insert into the capitellum and the medial epicondyle to resist torsional stress.
- The ulnar component is composed of high-density polyethylene and has an intramedullary stem. It articulates more closely with the distal humeral surface to confer additional stability.
- The prosthesis allows for approximately 6 to 8 degrees of varus-valgus angulation, depending on the degree of flexion.
- Disadvantages seen with this prosthesis are fractures of the medial and lateral epicondyles when inserting the flanges of the humeral component. Adequate bone stock must be present to utilize this prosthesis. There is also a tendency to lateralize the humeral component, thus increasing loosening rates.

Combined Linked and Unlinked

- Newer designs have been created to capture the benefits of both the linked and unlinked designs.
- The Acclaim total elbow system is a combined linked and unlinked design that retains the same humeral and ulnar components, but the modularity of the system allows either a linked or an unlinked articulation to be placed.

Surgical Approaches

- Various approaches are available to the orthopaedic surgeon operating on the elbow.
- Most arthroplasty procedures require wide exposure of the articular surface of the elbow.
- Most approaches utilize a posterior skin incision over the elbow that avoids (medial or lateral) the tip of the olecranon.
- The following section is an overview of the most common approaches used for exposure of the elbow and includes the Bryan-Morrey, triceps-reflecting anconeus pedicle (TRAP), extensile Kocher's, and triceps-splitting (Campbell's) approaches.

Bryan-Morrey (Triceps-Sparing) Approach

- This common approach is often used for TEA.
- This approach allows for exposure of the elbow articular surfaces using a laterally attached triceps reflection (Fig. 12–4).
- The main indications are for TEA, interpositional arthroplasty, and distal humerus fracture management.

Technique

- The patient is placed in the supine position, with a bump under the ipsilateral scapula.

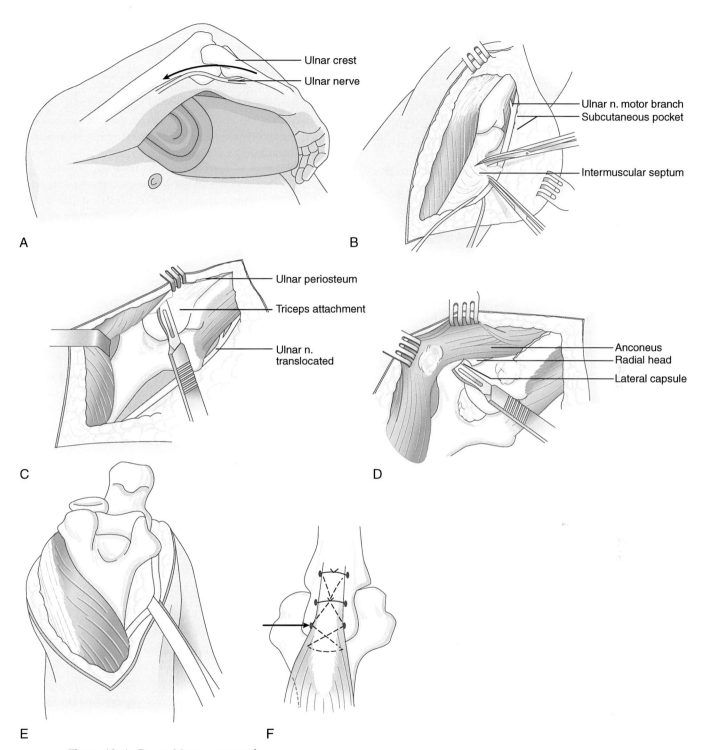

Figure 12–4: Bryan-Morrey approach.

The Bryan-Morrey approach is a medial reflection of the triceps and anconeus to the lateral side, maintaining a laterally based insertion. **A** and **B,** Before reflection, the ulnar nerve is identified, released from the cubital tunnel distally to the first motor branch, and then protected. **C** and **D,** The triceps is reflected starting at its medial insertion, subperiosteally off of the ulnar insertion, from medial to lateral, including the anconeus. **E,** Sufficient exposure is obtained when the lateral column and radial head are exposed. **F,** After completion of the procedure, the triceps insertion is repaired through bone tunnels, and the medial fascia is also repaired. (From Morrey BF, ed. [2000]. *The Elbow and Its Disorders*, 3rd ed. Philadelphia: WB Saunders.)

- Tourniquet control is used.
- A posterior skin incision is made slightly medial to the midline of the elbow, coursing approximately 9 cm proximal and 8 cm distal to the olecranon.
- Large subcutaneous skin flaps are made superficial to the posterior fascia.
- The ulnar nerve is identified proximally in the medial intermuscular septum and is either protected or transposed in front of the cubital tunnel.
- The medial aspect of the triceps is elevated distally to the level of the posterior capsule of the elbow, continuing through the capsule and posterior bundle of the MCL.
- The superficial fascia of the posteromedial forearm is obliquely incised to the posterior border of the ulna between the anconeus and the flexor carpi ulnaris.
- The periosteum of the proximal ulna is exposed, and the ulnar periosteum, posterior fascia, and proximal triceps are reflected *as one layer* from medial to lateral off the ulna and distal humerus.
  - This is performed with the elbow in 20 to 30 degrees of flexion to decrease tension on the tissue.
  - The medial periosteum and triceps insertion are the weakest portions of this flap, and care must be taken to preserve continuity at this point. The lateral aspect of the triceps mechanism and its attachment to the anconeus are more stable and less likely to rupture.
- Dissection is continued laterally, and the triceps and anconeus are subperiosteally raised off the distal humerus and proximal ulna.
  - This allows for exposure of the radial head.
  - The LUCL is released from the humeral attachment during this continuation from medial to lateral.
- Medial release of the anterior bundle of the MCL then allows the ulnohumeral joint to be dislocated, thus exposing the articular surfaces of the elbow.
  - If ligamentous integrity is necessary (i.e., unlinked arthroplasty), then the LUCL and MCL should be tagged with plans at reattachment via bone tunnels in the humerus during closure.
- The tip of the olecranon can be removed to visualize the trochlea more clearly.
- Following the procedure, the triceps mechanism is repaired through bone tunnels in the ulna. Cruciate tunnels are made, with each limb of No.5 nonabsorbable suture passing through the triceps in Bunnell's fashion. An additional horizontal tunnel in the ulna may be used to pass additional suture.
- The flexor carpi ulnaris fascia and anconeus are then repaired to surrounding tissue.
- Ulnar transposition, if desired, is then completed.
- The tourniquet is then deflated, hemostasis is obtained, and skin closure is completed.

Triceps-Reflecting Anconeus Pedicle (TRAP) Approach

- This approach offers increased exposure over the Bryan-Morrey approach and may be used for difficult fractures or TEA implantation (Fig. 12–5).
- Essentially, this approach combines the dissection discussed earlier for the Bryan-Morrey triceps-reflecting approach with a continuation via Kocher's interval.
- The initial steps of the approach are identical to those described earlier in the Bryan-Morrey approach.
  - After the triceps, anconeus, and ulnar periosteum are reflected off the olecranon, the distal attachment of the anconeus and periosteum is released.
  - This is performed by incising the lateral fascia through Kocher's interval.
  - The anconeus attachment is then raised off the proximal ulna, and the dissection is carried proximally along this interval to the lateral condyle.
  - Reflection of this triangular triceps-anconeus flap, with ulnar periosteum, allows for visualization of the entire distal humerus and proximal olecranon.
- Repair is performed much like described earlier for the Bryan-Morrey approach with reattachment of the triceps flap to the olecranon.
- Additionally, the lateral fascial incision along Kocher's interval is repaired.

Extensile Kocher's Approach

- The lateral extensile Kocher's approach allows for exposure of the lateral aspect of the elbow joint (Fig. 12–6).
- The approach utilizes the interval between the anconeus and the extensor carpi ulnaris.
- Indications for the extensile Kocher's posterolateral approach include joint replacement (with an unlinked prosthesis), débridement of the elbow (including synovectomy), and management of distal humerus fractures.

Technique

- Patients are positioned supine, with a bump under the ipsilateral scapula.
- Tourniquet control is used.
- A utilitarian posterior skin incision can be used (recommended), or an incision centered over the lateral column may also be used, extending proximal and distal to the elbow (it is less extensile and does not allow exposure of the medial side of the elbow).
- The interval between the extensor carpi ulnaris and the anconeus is identified (often by a fat stripe in the fascia). Development of these two intervals allows exposure of the capsule of the radiohumeral joint.
- Dissection is carried proximally along the lateral column of the humerus.
- The triceps-anconeus flap is reflected subperiosteally off the lateral distal humerus and ulna, including the origin of

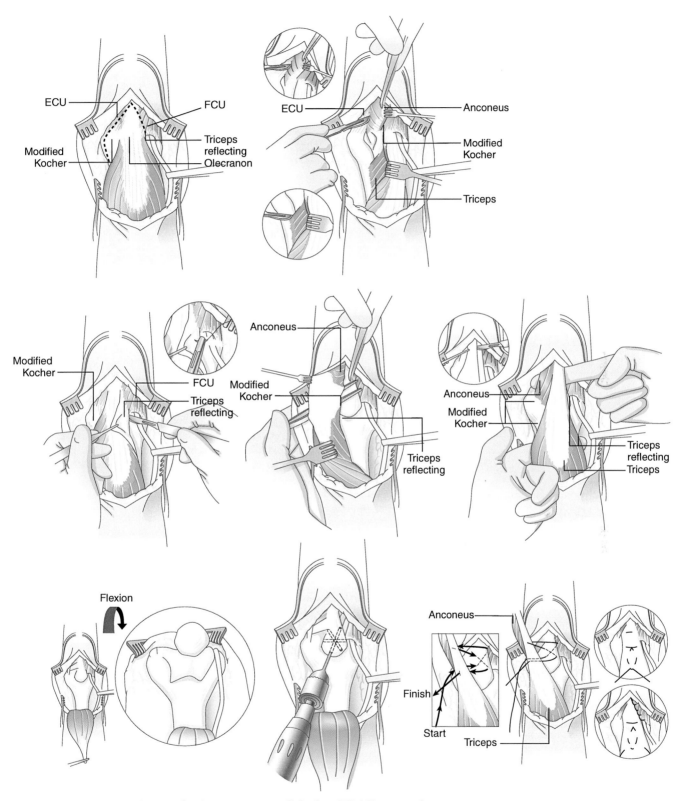

Figure 12–5: Triceps-reflecting anconeus pedicle flap (TRAP) approach.
The TRAP approach incorporates the medially to laterally based reflection of the triceps and anconeus performed in the Bryan-Morrey approach, but it adds a lateral release of the anconeus/triceps insertion through Kocher's interval, thus completely exposing the distal humerus and olecranon. Once the procedure is completed, the triceps insertion is repaired through bone tunnels in the olecranon, and the medial and lateral fascia is repaired. *ECU*, extensor carpi ulnaris; *FCU*, flexor carpi ulnaris.

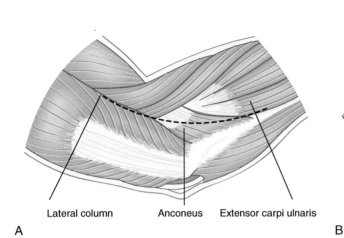

A

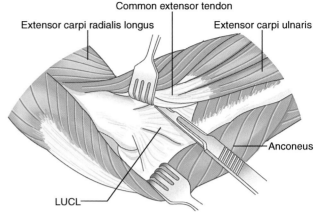

B

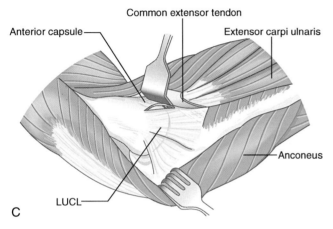

C

Figure 12–6: Kocher approach.
A, Kocher's approach exposes the lateral elbow through the interval between the extensor carpi ulnaris and the anconeus *(dotted line)*. Typically, a "fat stripe" in the fascia helps to identify the interval.
B and C, The common extensors are then reflected from their origin off the lateral column, with care taken to protect the lateral ulnar collateral ligament *(LUCL)*, thus exposing the capsule of the radio-capitellar joint. Although useful for laterally based procedures, this approach is limiting in that it is not extensile. (From Morrey BF, ed. [2000]. *The Elbow and Its Disorders*, 3rd ed. Philadelphia: WB Saunders.)

the LUCL (off the lateral epicondyle), extending medially behind the humerus.
  • Care must be taken to elevate the triceps subperiosteally off the olecranon, to maintain integrity for later repair.
• The elbow can then be dislocated to expose the articular surfaces.
• The distal anconeus insertion is left intact, along with the triceps insertion.
• If a posterior skin incision is used, the ulnar nerve can be released from the cubital tunnel and transposed anteriorly for protection during elbow dislocation.
• Following completion of the surgical procedure, the lateral collateral ligament is then reattached to the lateral epicondyle via bone tunnels using a Kessler-type stitch in the ligament (using No. 2 nonabsorbable suture).
• The triceps is also repaired through bone tunnels in the olecranon using No. 5 nonabsorbable sutures.
• Routine wound closure is then performed.

Triceps-Splitting (Campbell's) Approach

• This is a posterior approach to the posterior elbow (Fig. 12–7).
• Indications include ulnohumeral (Outerbridge-Kashiwagi) arthroplasty, TEA, and distal humerus fracture treatment.

Technique

• The patient is placed in the lateral decubitus position, with the arm over a support, or supine with the arm across the chest.
• Tourniquet control is used.
• A utilitarian posterior skin incision is made midline to the olecranon tip.
• Subcutaneous flaps are made at the level of the triceps fascia.
• The triceps fascia and muscle are split in the midline to the distal humerus, posterior joint capsule, and posterior ulna.
• The triceps-anconeus flap is elevated off the distal humerus and ulna laterally, and the triceps-flexor mass is elevated off the distal humerus and ulna medially.
• The ulnar nerve is protected or transposed as necessary.
• Exposure to the posterior elbow is thus obtained.
• Joint dislocation can be obtained with elevation (subperiosteally) or transection of the collateral ligaments at the level of the humeral epicondyles (which can later be repaired via bone tunnels to the humerus).
• At the cessation of the procedure, the medial and lateral triceps flaps are closed side to side through bone tunnels in the olecranon.
• Routine wound closure is then performed.

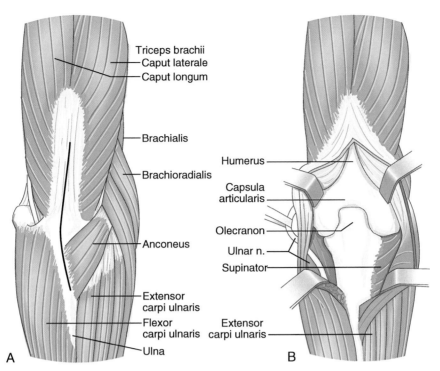

Figure 12–7: Campbell's approach.
A, Campbell's approach utilizes a triceps-splitting approach to the posterior elbow joint and distal humerus.
B, The triceps is split in the midline and is then reflected medially and laterally, thus leaving the peripheral insertions intact. The triceps insertion can then be repaired through bone tunnels in the olecranon at the end of the procedure. (From Morrey BF, ed. [2000]. *The Elbow and Its Disorders*, 3rd ed. Philadelphia: WB Saunders.)

Surgical Alternatives to Total Elbow Arthroplasty

- Patients in whom nonoperative treatment of a painful, arthritic elbow has failed are candidates for surgical intervention.
- Young patients (<60 years for OA and <40 years for RA), high-demand patients (laborers), or patients with early-stage arthritis (see earlier) are often candidates for procedures other than TEA.
- Often, these procedures offer temporary improvement because the underlying disease process is not ultimately treated with these options.
- Currently, the four main surgical alternatives to TEA are open débridement; open débridement, open synovectomy in patients with RA; arthroscopic débridement; and interpositional arthroplasty.
- Other (historical) options for treating painful arthritic elbows include resection arthroplasty and arthrodesis. These options are not discussed further because they are rarely indicated today (mostly in salvage situations following infected TEA).

Open Débridement Arthroplasty

- This procedure is performed to remove loose bodies, to remove osteophytes, and to reshape the articular portion of the humerus and ulna (and occasionally the radius) (Antuna et al. 2002, Wada et al. 2004).

- It is mostly indicated in younger patients (<60 years) with primary or post-traumatic OA.

Indications

- Painful elbow that has failed to improve with nonoperative measures
- Relief of end-ROM pain secondary to osteophyte impingement
- Resolution of painful locking or clicking secondary to entrapment of loose bodies
- Improvement in ROM in elbows with painful contractures

Contraindications

- Advanced arthritis with significant loss of motion and painful midarcs of motion, not end-range pain
- Arthritis in an unstable elbow, especially in patients with advanced RA
- Ulnar nerve symptoms that require a procedure or approach that allows for exposure of the ulnar nerve

Open Débridement (Column Procedure)

- This procedure is often used for capsulectomy in patients with extrinsic contractures; it may also be used for débridement of osteophytes, excision of loose bodies, and recontouring of the distal humerus and proximal olecranon.

- It is similar to the Outerbridge-Kashiwagi procedure but allows management of anterior capsular contracture and osteophytes.
- The objectives are to remove bony impingement, to improve ROM, and to reshape articular segments if necessary.
- It is most often indicated in patients with primary OA or post-traumatic OA.

Technique

- The anterior interval utilizes release of the extensor carpi radialis longus from the lateral supracondylar column with distal extension into the common extensors.
- The posterior interval utilizes an extended Kocher's approach on the lateral elbow.
- If wide exposure of the articular surface is needed, the triceps may need to be reflected.
- Anterior and posterior capsules are removed, as are osteophytes.
- Reshaping of the distal humerus is performed as necessary.
- When working on the medial column, it is often necessary to mobilize the ulnar nerve from the cubital tunnel, especially when dealing with a posteromedial osteophyte.
- This procedure allows for tricompartment (anterior ulnohumeral, posterior ulnohumeral, and radiocapitellar) débridement.
- Capsular contracture may be addressed by capsulectomy.
  - Care is taken to protect the radial and medial nerve during capsulectomy.
- The radial head is often not involved (especially in primary OA), and resection is rarely indicated or advised.

Results

- The procedure yields predictable improvements in ROM and relief of impingement pain.
- Oka reported an average of 24 degrees of improvement in motion and good pain relief in 50 laborers and athletes treated with open débridement. Twenty patients were available for long-term (>5 years) follow-up, and 90% had minimal pain (none or mild) and preservation of motion. All patients reporting minimal pain at latest follow-up had resumed their prior occupation or sport (Oka 2000).
- Tsuge and Mizuseki similarly reported a 34-degree improvement in motion and good pain relief in patients followed for 64 months (Tsuge and Mizuseki 1994).

Complications

- Recurrence of symptoms is the most frequent complication
- Ulnar nerve irritation does occur postoperatively in some patients (~15% of patients), especially in those with preoperative restriction in flexion motion (<90 degrees) or preoperative ulnar nerve irritation.
- Care must be taken to avoid compromise of collateral ligaments with wide débridement.

Arthroscopic Débridement

- Improved arthroscopic techniques have led to a tremendous increase in the use of arthroscopy for treatment of a variety of elbow disorders.
- Historically, the primary indications for arthroscopic débridement were removal of loose bodies and modest débridement of the elbow (olecranon and olecranon fossa).
- Surgeons with extensive expertise in elbow arthroscopy are performing more extensive débridements, including full synovectomy, capsular release, and modified ulnohumeral arthroplasty.

Indications

- Indications are similar to those for open débridement:
- They include painful impingement, loose bodies, contracture, and painful synovitis in patients with RA (Fig. 12–8).

Contraindications

- Prior elbow surgery or trauma that has resulted in distorted anatomy (especially neurovascular anatomy)
- Previous ulnar nerve transposition that may require open exposure of the nerve before establishing any medial portal
- Ankylosed elbow preventing cannula entry or joint distention.

Technique

- The patient is placed in the lateral decubitus position with the arm over a padded bolster, prone, or supine with the arm suspended.
- Tourniquet control is used.
- The joint is insufflated via posterolateral "soft spot" with 20 to 30 mL of normal saline solution.
- The arthroscope is introduced via proximal anteromedial portal for anterior joint inspection (Fig. 12–9).
- Working portals include a proximal anterolateral or an anterolateral portal, introduced under direct visualization, as well as accessory medial and lateral portals as necessary for retractors.
- After the anterior work is completed, the posterior joint is visualized via a midline posterior portal 3 cm above the level of the proximal aspect of the olecranon fossa.
- A posterolateral working portal is also established.
- Débridement, removal of loose bodies, reshaping of distal humerus, synovectomy, and capsulotomy all can be performed.

Results

- Overall results of arthroscopic débridement are similar to those of open procedures in terms of pain relief, ROM, and patient satisfaction.
- However, this procedure has the possible benefit of decreased perioperative pain and earlier onset of motion and therapy.

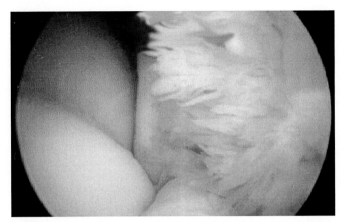

Figure 12–8: Arthroscopic view of synovitis.
This arthroscopic picture shows the anterior aspect of the elbow joint from the anteromedial portal. Exuberant synovitis is seen anterior to the coronoid process *(foreground)* and the radial head. Wide exposure of the articular surface of the elbow is obtainable with arthroscopic techniques, which allow for thorough débridement procedures, including full synovectomy in patients with inflammatory arthritis.

- Savoie and colleagues reported an average increase of 81 degrees motion and a significant decrease in pain in 24 patients (Savoie et al. 1999).
- A prospective study comparing the Outerbridge-Kashiwagi procedure with an arthroscopic variant found no difference in patient satisfaction between the two procedures. However, the authors noted that they performed more complete débridement and release in the open Outerbridge-Kashiwagi procedure, and as a result, found significantly more flexion in these patients (15 versus 4 degrees, $p < .05$).
- Arthroscopic synovectomy offers results comparable to those of open synovectomy, with the benefit of potentially faster rehabilitation and excellent exposure without radial head excision.
- Horiuchi and colleagues reported successful pain relief in 76% of 21 elbows with Mayo grade I or II status at 2-year follow-up. However, 5 of 21 elbows had recurrent synovitic pain at follow-up (Horiuchi et al. 2002).
- Lee and Morrey found that 93% had good or excellent subjective results initially, but these deteriorated to 57% at latest follow-up (average, 42 months) (Lee and Morrey 1997).
- Kelly and colleagues found that the *most significant risk factor* for development of postoperative nerve palsy after elbow arthroscopy was RA of the elbow with contracture (Kelly et al. 2001).

Open Synovectomy

- This procedure is primarily indicated in patients with painful synovitis refractory to nonoperative measures, often in patients with early grades of RA (Mayo I and II).

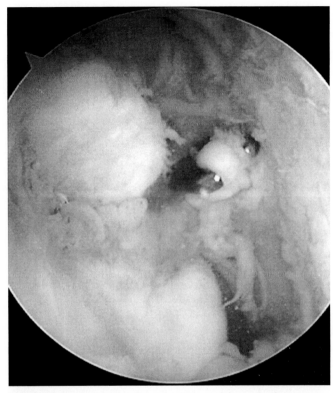

Figure 12–9: Arthroscopic osteophyte and loose body removal.
This arthroscopic image of the anterior aspect of an arthritic elbow from an anteromedial portal depicts a supracapitellar osteophyte and a loose body that is being removed with a grasper from the lateral portal. The supracapitellar osteophyte prevents terminal flexion because of bony impingement, whereas loose bodies can become interposed between the articular surfaces, causing locking of the elbow. Again, note the extensive synovitis.

- The primary goal is to relieve pain, not to improve motion.
- Improved medical management of RA has lessened the role of surgical synovectomy.

Technique

- This procedure is often performed via Kocher's approach. Historically, exposure involves resection of the radial head to allow access to medial synovium.
- The anterior and posterior synovium is then removed.
- The recent literature has found that radial head resection alters elbow kinematics and may lead to more rapid onset of ulnohumeral instability and degeneration (Kaufmann et al. 2003).
- Arthroscopic techniques may allow for improved exposure without resection of the radial head, but they are technically more difficult and require significant expertise.
- Most reports of open synovectomy yield good results in temporary pain relief.
- Many patients have recurrent symptoms in 5 years after surgical intervention.

Interpositional Arthroplasty

Indications

- This procedure is performed in patients with painful arthritic elbows who are too high demand (laborers) or too young for TEA and in whom nonoperative treatment has failed (Fig. 12–10).
- These patients usually have more advanced arthritis with extensive articular cartilage loss and not only end-ROM pain but also painful midarc motion.
- Often, these patients have significant loss of motion with concomitant pain.
- Historically, the primary indication has been post-traumatic OA, but it includes young (<40 years) patients with RA.

Contraindications

- Postseptic arthritis with residual infection
- Gross elbow instability (post-traumatic or end-stage RA)

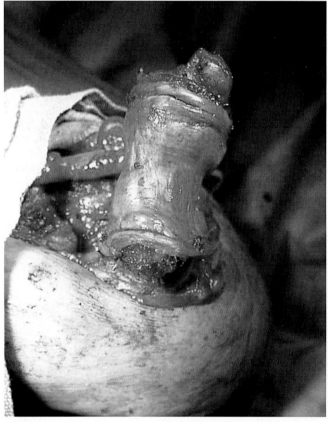

Figure 12–10: Interpositional arthroplasty. Intraoperative image of the distal humerus after fascial covering for interpositional arthroplasty. Various tissues can be used, such as autograft fascia lata or allograft tissues, including fascial tissue or dermal tissue. The articular surface of the distal humerus is denuded with a burr, and the interposition tissue is tightly sutured in place to cover the distal humerus completely.

- Inadequate bone stock
- Unwillingness or inability to follow postoperative guidelines including care of an external fixator
- Relative contraindication: a need for the elbow to bear weight or to assist with ambulation

Technique

- Allograft Achilles tendon or autogenous dermis and fascia (lata) are most often used.
- Allograft Achilles tendon offers the advantage of no donor site morbidity and can be fashioned to reconstruct collateral ligaments.
- Exposure is obtained through a posterior skin incision followed by an extensile Kocher's approach or through a triceps-reflecting approach such as the Bryan-Morrey or TRAP approach (see earlier).
- The ulnar nerve is isolated and protected.
- The shoulder is externally rotated and the elbow is flexed, thus exposing the distal humerus articular surface (especially in the ligament-deficient elbow).
- The osseous architecture of the distal humerus is reshaped into a smooth, single articular surface that conforms to the olecranon. The incisura of the olecranon is also smoothed into a conforming surface.
- The interposition tissue is then placed over the distal humerus and is secured with through-and-through sutures. Tails of tissue (especially when using Achilles tendon) can then be fashioned to reconstruct the collateral ligaments.
- The radial head is usually left intact.
- A distraction, dynamic (hinged) external fixator is then applied, following the precise center of rotation of the elbow.
- The triceps (if reflected) is then repaired through cruciate bone tunnels in the proximal ulna, followed by fascial and skin closure.
- Drains are routinely placed.

Postoperative Management

- ROM is started immediately and may be assisted with a continuous motion machine.
- Patients are seen at 1 week, at 4 weeks, at 8 to 10 weeks and finally at 6 months.
- The external fixator is left in place for approximately 4 weeks and then is removed in the operating room with assessment of elbow stability and motion while the patient is under anesthesia.
- Rehabilitation is continued, with concentration on obtaining functional ROM.

Results

- Most studies have reported a 70% satisfaction rate among patients with respect to pain relief, and 80% of patients regain functional ROM.
- Preoperative instability has been associated with an increased likelihood of postoperative instability and a poorer outcome.

- Cheng and Morrey found that 67% of patients treated for RA had satisfactory relief of pain, and 75% of patients treated for OA were satisfied at 5-year follow-up (Cheng and Morrey 2000).
- Ljung and associates found similar results but reported that the long-term results (>10 years) were inferior to those of TEA in patients with RA (especially those with instability) (Ljung et al. 1996).

Complications

- These include superficial pin tract infections as well as deep infections, progressive instability, ulnar nerve irritation, heterotopic bone formation, ankylosis of the elbow, and resorptive bone loss.
- Complications in the literature have been reported to occur in up to 25% of patients.
- Resorptive bone loss most commonly occurs at the distal humeral condyles and may make later TEA more difficult.
- Most complications reported involve long-term failure of the elbow with recurrence of pain.
- Interpositional arthroplasty is a technically demanding procedure with a substantial learning curve. It requires appropriate indications and proper patient selection for a successful outcome.

- The salvage procedure for failed interposition arthroplasty is TEA.

Ulnohumeral Arthroplasty (Outerbridge-Kashiwagi Procedure)

- This procedure is indicated in the patient with painful osteophyte impingement and subsequent loss of motion (Fig. 12–11).
- It is primarily performed in patients with primary OA or post-traumatic OA.
- Originally described by Outerbridge and reported in Japan in 1978 by Kashiwagi, this procedure allows for débridement of osteophytes on the olecranon, olecranon fossa, and coronoid. The procedure was modified by Morrey to include the use of a trephine and was termed *ulnohumeral arthroplasty* (Kashiwagi 1978, Morrey 1992).

Technique

- Posterior exposure of the elbow is accomplished via a triceps-splitting or medial triceps-reflecting approach.
- The tip of the olecranon, including osteophytes, is removed.
- A trephine, used to widen and deepen the olecranon fossa, eventually penetrates the anterior cortex of the distal humerus.

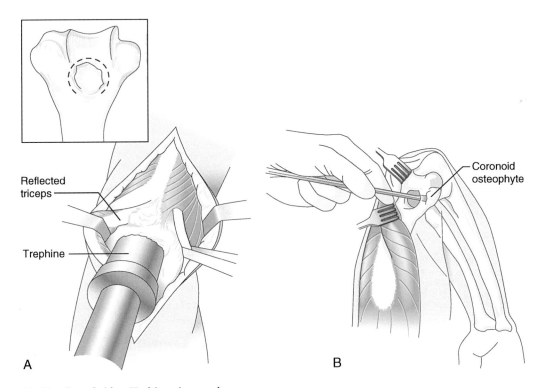

Figure 12–11: Outerbridge-Kashiwagi procedure.
During ulnohumeral arthroplasty or the Outerbridge-Kashiwagi procedure, a trephine can be used to fenestrate the distal humerus through the olecranon fossa posteriorly. **A,** Positioning of the trephine centrally, to prevent damage to either distal humeral column that could result in fracture. This effectively widens the area for the olecranon to articulate with posteriorly, as well as increasing room for the coronoid process anteriorly.
B, Additionally, resection of coronoid osteophytes is possible once the fenestration has been made.

- It is important to follow the contour of the trochlea and to aim the trephine proximally because the distal humerus is flared anteriorly.
  - Errant trephine placement can result in violation of the trochlea or capitellar cartilage or may excessively weaken the medial or lateral column, thus increasing the risk of fracture.
- Anterior débridement of coronoid osteophytes, the coronoid fossa, and the supracapitellar recess can then be performed through the trephinated hole in the distal humerus.
- Associated anterior capsular contracture is difficult to address through this exposure.

Results

- Most reports indicate substantial improvement in pain relief and improvement in painless ROM (especially terminal extension pain) in the short term.
- However, most long-term studies have found that the initial success wanes over time.
- Minami and colleagues reported that 90% of patients had marked pain relief in the early postoperative period after treatment with the Outerbridge-Kashiwagi procedure. However, only 55% of the 44 patients had no or mild pain at 10-year follow-up (Minami et al. 1996).

Complications

- Most complications are associated with recurrence of arthritic pain over time.
  - A 20% rate of recurrence of pain and progressive loss of motion can be expected over 10 years.
- Ulnar nerve irritation can occur as arthritis progresses and may occur after surgery.
  - Improvement in flexion postoperatively, especially in the elbow with a long-standing loss of flexion of less than 90 degrees, may stretch a tethered ulnar nerve.
  - In these situations, visualization of the ulnar nerve during flexion, with possible transposition, is recommended.
- Early complications, with perioperative fracture being the most concerning, are avoidable if technical guidelines are followed.

Surgical Technique of Total Elbow Arthroplasty

- Two main implant designs currently used:
  - Unlinked
  - Linked
- The choice of implant depends on the underlying cause, the patient's pathoanatomy, and the surgeon's preference.
- The primary indication for TEA is pain, with additional possibility of improvement of motion and function, as well as increased stability (using linked designs).

- The indications for TEA have broadened and currently include the following:
  - RA
  - Post-traumatic arthritis
  - Distal humerus fractures (comminuted acute fractures or nonunions)
  - Primary OA
- Contraindications for TEA include persistent infection and lack of functional motors with which to power the elbow.

Anatomic Considerations

- Understanding surgical anatomy, as well as normal anatomy, of the elbow is critical to success.
- Distal humeral anatomy can dictate the choice of implant
- Intact humeral condyles with intact ligamentous anatomy allow for a choice of an unlinked or a linked prosthesis.
- The absence of ligamentous integrity necessitates reconstruction of ligaments or replacement with a linked device.
- The absence of intact distal humeral condyles necessitates use of a linked TEA design.
- Experimental studies have shown that certain linked designs can be implanted with up to 8 cm of distal humeral loss before custom designs are needed.
- The flexion axis of elbow is collinear with the anterior humeral cortex.
- The rotational alignment of an implant is fixed by anterior humeral cortex proximally and the posterior ulnar cortex (proximal flat portion) distally.
- Flexion plane of the elbow is perpendicular to the proximal flat posterior ulna.

Surgical Approaches

- Various approaches are available for implantation.
- The choice of surgical approach depends on the surgeon's preference and the indication for elbow arthroplasty, as well as the choice of implant.

Key Elements of Success

- Regardless of approach used, certain key steps are critical to a successful outcome.
- Triceps function must be preserved by meticulous reconstruction after implantation of the prosthesis.
- Collateral ligament integrity is critical to a successful outcome when using unlinked implants.
- Routine transposition of the ulnar nerve is often recommended.

Technical Considerations of Unlinked Design Implantation

- At present, the following four unlinked designs are most frequently used:
  - Capitellocondylar prosthesis
  - Kudo
  - Souter-Strathclyde
  - Sorbie

- Tourniquet control is used on the upper arm.
- Various approaches are available.
- Dislocation of joint necessitates release of a collateral ligament, often the LUCL.
- Resection of radial head is performed.
- Humeral preparation is performed first.
  - The central portion of the trochlea is removed with a saw to gain access to the humeral canal.
  - Central reaming is then performed with maintenance of integrity of the osseous columns of the distal humerus.
  - Depending on the unlinked design being implanted, a variable amount of distal humerus articular surface is then resected.
- Trial implantation is performed with orientation to appropriate axis of rotation.
- Ulnar preparation is then performed.
  - A burr or an awl is used to gain entry into the ulnar canal.
  - The tip of the olecranon is often resected for easier canal entry.
  - The canal is then broached, and trial implantation is performed.
  - The posterior cortex of the proximal ulna is perpendicular to the flexion axis of the elbow and helps to guide the rotational orientation of the implant.
- Some unlinked designs resurface the radial head to match the corresponding capitellar resurfacing.
- Trial reduction assesses stability and soft tissue tension.
- The surgeon monitors for *pistoning* of implants.
  - This indicates that the flexion axis is "off."
- The stability of the elbow through ROM is checked.
- Proper alignment and contact of the humerus and ulna through the arc of motion are ensured.
- Cementing of components is performed, often with the humerus first.
- Some designs incorporate the use of a bone block placed between the anterior flange of the humeral component and the anterior humeral cortex.
- Reconstruction of collateral ligament takedown is performed.
- The triceps is then repaired.
- The wound is closed over a drain.

Technical Considerations of Linked Implantation

- Two main linked designs are currently used:
  - Coonrad-Morrey (Figs. 12–12 and 12–13)
  - GSB-III
- Various surgical approaches are available.
- The triceps mechanism may be left intact in some acute fracture or nonunion situations.
- The ulnar nerve is transposed.
- The collateral ligaments are resected.
- Humeral preparation is performed first.
  - Most TEA systems have jigs that direct bone cuts.

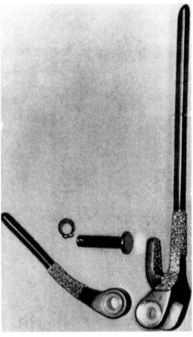

Figure 12–12: Coonrad-Morrey total elbow arthroplasty. The Coonrad-Morrey total elbow arthroplasty (Zimmer, Inc., Warsaw, IN) is a locked, semiconstrained implant that replicates the kinematics of a "sloppy hinge." The cobalt-chrome coupling pin allows for 8 degrees of varus-valgus laxity and internal-external rotation laxity. The anterior flange augments rotational stability and aids in preventing posterior drift of the humeral implant, which has helped to reduce the incidence of humeral implant loosening.

- The precision of bone cuts are not as critical in linked designs as in unlinked designs because stability is obtained via the linking mechanism of the implant, not by collateral ligaments.
- The humeral canal is reamed and broached, and trial implantation is performed.
- The anterior humeral cortex orients the implant to the appropriate flexion axis.
- Ulnar preparation is then performed.
  - The tip of the ulna is removed to gain access to the canal.
  - A burr or an awl is used to enter the ulnar canal.
  - The ulnar canal is reamed and broached, and a trial implant is placed.
  - The posterior proximal cortex (flat spot) orients the ulnar implant perpendicular to the flexion axis.
- Trial reduction is performed.
  - This assesses soft tissue balance, rotational orientation, and stability of the implant.
- The final components are cemented: the humerus first, then the ulna.

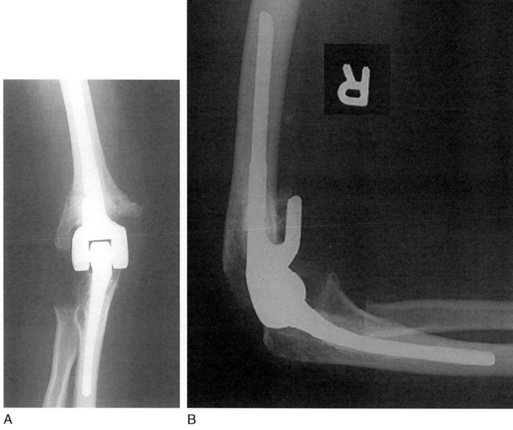

Figure 12–13: Coonrad-Morrey total elbow arthroplasty.
A and **B,** Anteroposterior and lateral radiographs of a Coonrad-Morrey total elbow arthroplasty after implantation. Radiographs reveal excellent cement mantles proximally and distally. A piece of cortical bone graft (usually obtained from the resected trochlea) has been interposed between the anterior flange of the humeral component and the anterior cortex of the distal humerus.

- The triceps is repaired through bone tunnels (if necessary).
- The wound is closed over a drain.

Postoperative Management After Total Elbow Arthroplasty

Splinting and Home Exercise

- The elbow is immobilized in full extension with a splint.
- The splint is removed after 24 to 48 hours, and gentle active ROM is begun.
  - If the integrity of the triceps repair is questionable, then flexion is limited for first few weeks.
- Patients are allowed to use their elbow for activities of daily living.
- Formal physical therapy is often not necessary.
- Many patients regain ROM and function with a home exercise program without formalized therapy.

Physical Therapy

- When necessary, physical therapy is aimed at wound healing, regaining ROM, and ultimately regaining strength and function of the extremity.
- Physical therapy can be broken down into the following phases:
  - Phase I (0 to 6 weeks): Protect soft tissue repair and begin active-assistive ROM; avoid active-assistive ROM in extension if the triceps was released from its insertion and repaired at the time of surgery.
  - Phase II (6 to 8 weeks): Improve ROM and begin strengthening exercises including isometrics.
  - Phase III (8 to 12 weeks): Pursue further strengthening, including isotonic exercises, and begin functional use of elbow.
  - Phase IV (12 to 16 weeks): Return to normal functional activities.
- Postoperative stiffness may be helped with splinting, either dynamic or static.

Restrictions

- Lifetime limitations of the operated extremity are 10-lb single-event flexion and 2- to 5-lb repetitive flexion.

Results of Total Elbow Arthroplasty

- Linked implants are used for most TEAs performed in the United States.
  - Historically, linked designs were fully constrained, and this ultimately caused excess strain across bone-cement-implant interfaces and led to early failure.
  - This situation, in part, led to the development and use of nonconstrained, unlinked designs.
  - Currently, unlinked implants are predominantly used outside the United States for mild to moderate RA of the elbow (Mayo grade II to III).
- Newer linked designs have less constraint than earlier, fully constrained implants, thus yielding lower early failure rates secondary to aseptic loosening.
- In addition, the inherent stability of a linked elbow is considered more versatile and therefore can be used for a greater variety of indications, including the following:
  - Fractures (both acute and nonunion)
  - Post-traumatic arthritis with more severe alteration of joint anatomy
  - Grossly unstable arthritic elbows (inflammatory arthritis or chronic dislocations).
- Most series of TEA (unlinked and linked) report greater than 90% pain relief and functional ROM of the elbow.
  - Functional improvement is frequently obtained, but not as reliably as pain relief.
- It is most accurate to analyze TEA results by pathologic origin.

Results in Rheumatoid Arthritis

- TEA in patients with RA in general yields superior results to those for TEA in other disorders.
- Unlinked designs have been found to have a 90% survivorship at 10 years.
- Early aseptic failure of unlinked designs often resulted from dislocation of the implant.
- Ewald and colleagues reported excellent results with the capitellocondylar prosthesis (Ewald et al. 1993):
  - A 1.5% dislocation or aseptic loosening rate at an average of 6 years of follow-up was noted.
- However, other series reported dislocation rates of up to 20%.
- Aseptic loosening rates have been reported up to 33%.
- Stemless designed implants perform poorly compared with unlinked designs with intramedullary stems.
- Linked designs yield similar results to unlinked implants in many series.

- In general, 90% pain relief and functional ROM are reported.
- However, newer linked designs (Coonrad-Morrey, GSB III) have been reported in some series to have lower loosening rates than unlinked designs at late (>10-year) follow-up.
- Dislocation rates of linked designs are lower than those of unlinked elbows in most series.
- Gill and Morrey reported follow-up results of the Coonrad-Morrey elbow at an average of 16 years (Gill and Morrey 1998): 92% survival at 16 years with 86% excellent pain relief and functional motion.

Results in Post-traumatic and Primary Osteoarthritis

- Results for post-traumatic or primary OA are not as predictable as for RA.
- They are often related to the severity of the underlying disease and the patient's activity level (Schneeberger et al. 1997).
- Patients with RA often have lower functional demand.
  - Best results seen in older patients (>60 years) who have lower functional demand of their elbows.
- Initial results of pain relief and function are comparable to those in a population with RA.
- Most of the differences in outcome between RA and post-traumatic arthritis have been observed in comparison of long-term results and survivorship of the implant.
- Survivorship has generally been lower in patients with OA, with an earlier rate of revision and a higher incidence of aseptic loosening.
- Hildebrand and colleagues reported increased subjective functional scores in patients with RA compared with patients with post-traumatic arthritis at average follow-up of 4.6 years (Hildebrand et al. 2000).
- Schneeberger and colleagues found 74% good to excellent pain relief with 21% loosening and 26% revision rate at a follow-up average of 9.8 years using both early and later linked-design elbows (Coonrad-Morrey I, II, and III) (Schneeberger et al. 1997).
  - The Coonrad-Morrey III design had the best long-term results in this series, with 88% good pain relief and an 8% aseptic loosening rate at average follow-up of 3.2 years.
- Kozak and colleagues reported the outcome of TEA in patients with primary OA and found that linked elbows may have better outcomes compared with unlinked designs. However, they also found a higher rate of complications following TEA for primary OA compared with other pathologic causes (Kozak et al. 1998).

Results in Acute Fracture Treatment

- This approach has been recently reported in the literature as an option for treatment of periarticular fractures, especially in comminuted, osteoporotic fractures in low-demand elderly patients (Kamineni and Morrey 2004).

- Cobb and Morrey reported their results of 21 TEAs performed for acute fractures with a minimum follow-up of 2 years (Cobb and Morrey 1997).
- All elbows had good to excellent results at short-term follow-up, including a functional arc of motion (25 to 130 degrees).
- Similar results were found in other series.
- Patients treated initially with TEA have been found to do better than those patients who have early failure of initial open reduction and internal fixation requiring conversion to TEA.
- This option is supported by the literature for patients with comminuted, intra-articular fractures, who are physiologically older than 65 years and have underlying joint arthrosis.

Complications of Total Elbow Arthroplasty

- TEA is associated with higher complication rates than total hip or knee arthroplasty.
- Complication rates as high as 57% have been reported in the literature.
- Major complications include the following:
  - Infection
  - Loosening
  - Instability
  - Periprosthetic fracture
  - Triceps insufficiency
  - Neurologic injury
  - Wound complications
- Each of these major complications is discussed further, including diagnosis, classification, and, in some cases, management. Much of the discussion concerning management of complications involving revision TEA is discussed later, under revision TEA.

Infection

- The current literature reports infection rates of 2% to 5% for primary TEA.
- This rate was historically as high as 11%.
- Inflammatory arthritis (RA), oral steroid use, post-traumatic arthritis, and a history of previous surgery of the elbow result in higher incidences of infected TEA.
- Once an infection is diagnosed, aggressive treatment is necessary.
- The diagnosis is made by clinical examination, radiographic signs of loosening (Fig. 12–14), and laboratory evaluation (sedimentation rate, C-reactive protein, and joint aspirate).
- Often, surgical intervention is necessary, as follows:
  - Irrigation and débridement
  - Primary exchange arthroplasty
  - Staged exchange arthroplasty

- Rarely, an infected prosthesis may be managed with chronic antibiotic suppression (usually in elderly patients too unstable for surgery).
- The pathogen involved has a major impact on the treatment and intervention.
  - *Staphylococcus epidermidis* infections (which can form a biofilm around implants) have been shown not to respond to irrigation and débridement; therefore removal of the infected prosthesis may be required.
  - Conversely, *Staphylococcus aureus* infections have been effectively treated by early, aggressive irrigation and débridement.
- Multiple irrigations and débridements are required if salvage of the implant is attempted.
- Primary exchange arthroplasty has limited indications in TEA.
  - It may be performed for early infections involving gram-positive pathogens (not including *S. epidermidis*).
  - Most infected prostheses are managed with staged exchange arthroplasty involving resection, culture-guided antibiotic treatment for 6 weeks, followed by reimplantation of new prosthesis.
  - Often, interval cultures are obtained between cessation of antibiotics and reimplantation.
  - Antibiotic cement is routinely used during reimplantation.
- Revision TEA is discussed further later.

Loosening

- Historically, this complication is most common with linked prostheses.
- Early constrained designs had loosening rates of up to 25%.
- Early loosening rates resulted in newer designs that were less constrained.
- Higher loosening rates are seen after TEA for post-traumatic arthritis, compared with inflammatory arthritis.
- Poor cement technique can result in higher loosening rates as well.
- Improper implant positioning resulting in maltracking can lead to early polyethylene wear, osteolysis, and loosening.
- Infection must be ruled out in the loose prosthesis.
- The diagnosis is made by clinical examination and radiography.
  - Radiographic signs of loosening include progressive radiolucent lines, subsidence of the implant, or change of position of the implant (Fig. 12–15).
- Loose TEA components have been classified by amount of bone loss and stability of elbow:
  - Type I: Intact metaphyseal bone and elbow stability
  - Type II: Loss of metaphyseal bone, potentially involving either column, resulting in elbow instability
- Planning for revision of loose components takes into consideration the osseous defect, the quality of the bone, the age of the patient, and the type of implant being removed.
- Revision TEA is discussed later.

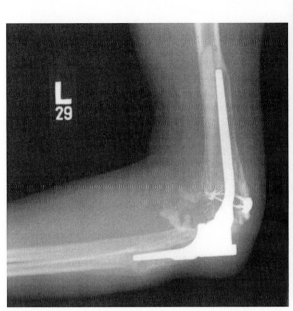

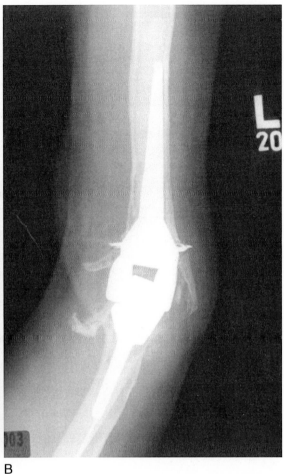

Figure 12–14: Infected total elbow arthroplasty.
A and **B,** Anteroposterior and lateral radiographs of an infected total elbow arthroplasty with characteristic loosening of the humeral and ulnar components. Lucency around the cement mantle is observed proximally around the humeral component and distally around the ulnar component.

Instability

- This is most often seen in unlinked prostheses (Fig. 12–16).
- The rate of instability ranges from 0% to 14% in the literature.
- The stability of a prosthesis is determined by the design of prosthesis (degree of constraint and linked versus unlinked), the capsuloligamentous integrity (static restraints), and the dynamic soft tissue (muscles) constraints.
- Certain factors are associated with an increased risk of TEA instability, as follows:
  - Inflammatory arthritis (leading to attenuation of ligamentous restraints)
  - Post-traumatic arthritis associated with ligamentous injury
  - Previous radial head resection or synovectomy
  - Improper implant selection

- Improper implant positioning resulting in maltracking and soft tissue attenuation or implant loosening
- TEA instability is classified as either early or late.
  - Early instability occurs within the first 6 weeks.
    - Causes include component malposition and soft tissue disruption (MCL, LUCL, or triceps).
  - Late instability occurs after 6 weeks.
    - It can be the result of component malposition, polyethylene wear, soft tissue attenuation, and trauma.
    - It is rarely the result of failure of the linking mechanism in linked TEA designs.
- Management of unstable implants is dependent on underlying cause. Options include the following:
  - Soft tissue reconstruction or repair
  - Revision TEA of unlinked to linked design (Figgie et al. 1997)
  - Revision linked TEA (i.e., for failure of linking mechanism)

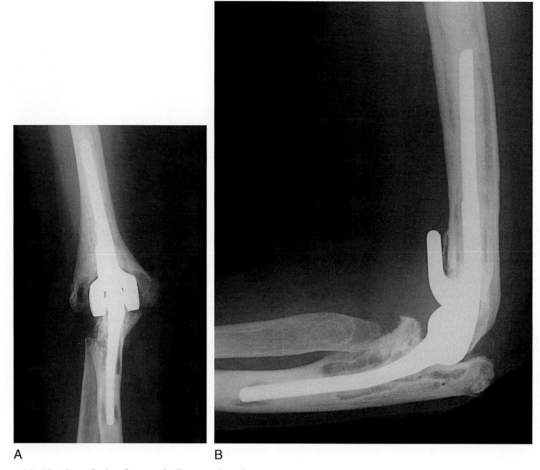

A   B

Figure 12–15: Osteolysis after total elbow arthroplasty.
A and **B,** Radiographic appearance of osteolysis following total elbow arthroplasty. "Pockets" of bone loss can be seen around both components and is most frequently a result of wear of the implant. As osteolysis increases, the implant may become loose.

Associated Fractures

- The incidence ranges from 1% to 23%.
- Fractures can be intraoperative or perioperative.

Intraoperative Fracture

- These fractures are associated with perforation of the humerus or ulna during reaming.
- Osteoporosis increases the risk of fracture.
- An unrecognized fracture is associated with a higher loosening rate.

Periprosthetic Fracture

- Management depends on location of the fracture and fixation of TEA components.
- Loose prostheses are managed differently from well-fixed prostheses associated with a periprosthetic fracture.

Management

- Management can be guided by classification (ulna and humerus are classified separately):

- Type I: Metaphyseal fracture with well-fixed implant
- Type II: Diaphyseal fracture with loose prosthesis, often involving fracture of cement mantle
  - Subdivided by A (good bone quality) and B (poor bone quality)
- Type III: Diaphyseal fracture not involving stem or cement mantle
- Management of type I fractures often involves splinting and rehabilitation.
- Management of type II fractures often involves revision TEA; type IIB fractures may require allograft augmentation.
- Type III fractures are managed by same criteria as standard diaphyseal fractures (irrespective of TEA); open reduction and internal fixation may require specialized plates or cerclage wires.

Triceps Insufficiency (Celli et al. 2005)

- Triceps insufficiency following TEA can involve partial or complete rupture or avulsion of the triceps tendon.

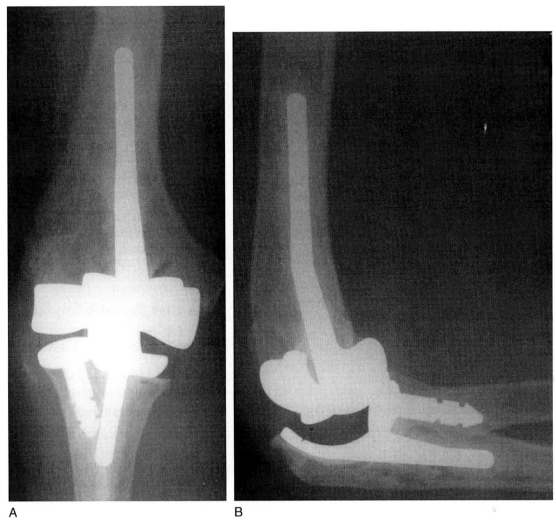

Figure 12–16: Instability of unlinked prostheses.
A and B, Unlinked total elbow arthroplasties can become unstable, resulting in dislocation of the implant, as shown in these radiographs. Patients with compromised stability of the elbow, whether from soft tissue compromise (ligamentous instability) or osseous compromise (bone loss), are not candidates for unlinked arthroplasty. This patient had rheumatoid arthritis and gradually attenuated her ligamentous structures around the elbow, with resulting prosthetic instability of this Sorbie unlinked arthroplasty.

- Triceps insufficiency most commonly occurs as a result of failed surgical reattachment, especially when tendon quality is poor.
- Patients will commonly complain of an inability to actively extend the elbow and of pain. They will have difficulty with overhead activities, in particular.
- When evaluating surgical options for triceps insufficiency, consider tissue quality, the degree of tendon retraction, and the status of the olecranon.
- Celli and associates evaluated three basic techniques: direct suture reattachment, anconeus rotation, and use of an Achilles allograft in a series of 15 patients.
- Of these 15 patients, 15 of 16 elbows regained the ability to extend against gravity, and 11 elbows were considered to have an excellent outcome.

Ulnar Neuropathy

- The incidence ranges from 0% to 10% for permanent neuropathy and from 0% to 26% for transient neuropathy.
- Multiple causes include trauma, postoperative scarring and hematoma, inadequate decompression or transposition, and postoperative swelling.
- Routine ulnar nerve transposition is recommended during TEA.
- Sensory deficits can be monitored, and most recover.
- Acute motor deficits, or progressive deficits, often require exploration.
- Symptoms may be associated or exacerbated with elbow flexion and therefore may require limitation of flexion until nerve irritation resolves.

Wound Complications

- These are often associated with previous surgery of the elbow.
- They may be associated with posterior incisions placed directly over the olecranon.
- Prevention is the best management:
  - Brief immobilization in extension with splinting and elevation after prosthetic implantation
  - Suction drain placement to avoid hematoma formation
- If a perioperative hematoma develops, it should be evacuated.

Revision Surgery for Failed Total Elbow Arthroplasty

Presentation

- In the failed TEA, symptoms are usually referable to the cause of failure.
  - For example, patients with a loose or unstable implant often complain of pain and report subluxation or frank dislocation of the implant.
  - In addition, they may report mechanical symptoms such as locking or clicking as the implant subluxates or catches.
- Failed TEA can be categorized broadly into four etiologic groups: septic failure, device failure, instability, and loosening.
- Many of the presentations and the diagnosis of these conditions are discussed earlier.

Septic Failure

- As mentioned previously, this cause of failure requires prompt attention.
- This condition is challenging to treat and often requires removal of the prosthesis, which may be difficult and fraught with complications.
- Removing a well-fixed prosthesis can result in a fracture of either the humerus or the ulna.
- Current recommendations for infected arthroplasty are removal of the prosthesis, culture-guided antibiotic management, and staged reconstruction.

Device Failure

- This complication can result from problems with the implant stems or the articular coupling elements (Fig. 12–17).
- In snap-fit designs, the articulation can dislocate, or the transhumeral axis pin can dislodge.
- In the semiconstrained designs, stem fracture has been reported following excessive activity.

Instability

- Most cases of instability after TEA are associated with unlinked prostheses.

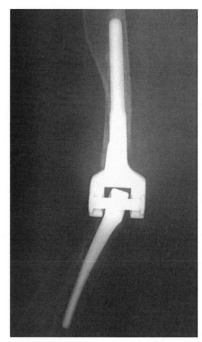

Figure 12–17: Signs of wear in a Coonrad-Morrey total elbow prosthesis.
This anteroposterior radiograph provides a characteristic example of asymmetric wear of the polyethylene bushings in the Coonrad-Morrey total elbow prosthesis. The normal varus-valgus laxity of 8 degrees is accentuated in this prosthesis, in which the bushings have worn, to allow nearly metal-on-metal contact.

- Instability can also result from implant malposition, which may lead to soft tissue attenuation and polyethylene wear with associated osteolysis (and loss of osseous support).
- Frank dislocation is a worrisome end point to instability; most dislocations of prostheses occur posteriorly.

Loosening

- Loosening of elbow implants occurred frequently with constrained implants because of the high stress transferred to the implant-cement interface.
- With the advent of semiconstrained implants, this became less of an issue.
- With the Coonrad-Morrey implants, loosening can be seen equally at the ulna and humerus implant interfaces, but it most frequently affects the ulnar component.
- Loosening of an implant can manifest in one of three ways:
  - A painful, loose implant with few or no radiographic changes
  - Gross instability and loosening owing to bone destruction
  - Acute fracture

Management (Surgical Options)

- Surgical options for the failed elbow arthroplasty depend on the adequacy of the available bone stock.

- Table 12–3 shows the options available for revision depending on the bone stock.
- A useful classification for distal humeral bone loss has been provided by Morrey.

Options With Adequate Bone Stock

Arthrodesis

- Generally, arthrodesis is a poor option in this situation, given the poor functional capacity of elbow arthrodesis.
- Additionally, if the available bone stock is adequate, revision TEA could be performed, thus providing stability and also maintaining functionality.

Resection

- Resection is indicated in the presence of infection, but it is limited to the setting in which adequate bone stock is available.
- Both supracondylar columns and competent ligamentous and soft tissue integrity are necessary to maintain some degree of stability.
- This is the easiest of all of the salvage options and has the potential of being a pain-relieving procedure.
- It requires a prolonged period of immobilization (≥ 8 to 10 weeks) and can result in instability in the long term.
- Resection may be performed with a distracting, dynamic external fixator for 6 to 8 weeks to allow for fibrous scarring and to improve stability.

Interposition Arthroplasty

- Interpositional arthroplasty is also an option to salvage a failed elbow replacement.
- This procedure requires adequate bone stock.
- The details of interposition arthroplasty are discussed earlier.

Revision Total Elbow Arthroplasty

- Ideally, this is the best option in a patient with a nonseptic, failed TEA in that it provides the patient the best chance of having a pain-free, functional elbow.

Table 12–3	Revision Options as a Function of Bone Stock	
BONE STOCK	**OPTIONS**
Adequate	Arthrodesis, resection, interposition, total elbow arthroplasty (semiconstrained prosthesis)
Inadequate	Resection, allograft, total elbow arthroplasty using a semiconstrained implant (long-flange), composite (total elbow with allograft), custom-made prosthesis

From Morrey BF, ed. (2000). *The Elbow and Its Disorders,* 3rd ed. Philadelphia: WB Saunders.

- In addition to considering the mode of failure, it is also important to take into consideration the anatomy of the remaining bone.
  - This includes not only the location of remaining bone, but also the quality.
  - Periprosthetic fractures should be identified.
- On the humeral side, evaluation should look at the integrity of the columns, determine the distal bone quality, and rule out the presence of fracture.
- On the ulnar side, the proximal bone of the olecranon is assessed, as is the diameter of the ulnar shaft (especially distally) because this may limit implantation of a revision stem.
  - As in the humerus, the quality (thickness) of the remaining ulnar bone is also assessed.
- The semiconstrained elbow is the ideal implant option for the resected elbow following a failed TEA implant.
  - Often, longer revision stems are necessary to bypass previous cemented mantles and osteopenic bone.
  - The ulna often limits the size and length of the revision implant in revision TEA.
  - Components with an anterior flange also allow for additional rotational stability, even in the presence of poor medial and lateral osseous column integrity.

Options With Inadequate Bone Stock

Osteoarticular Allograft Replacement

- Allograft replacement is rarely used to treat the arthritic elbow.
  - The justification for osteochondral allograft replacement is usually an unstable, arthritic elbow in physiologically young, active patients (usually secondary to trauma) with insufficient bone stock to allow for fascial covering or ligament reconstruction.
  - This may be used as a temporizing agent before TEA, especially when attempting to improve poor bone stock for later procedures.
  - For it to be effective, however, osseous union must occur by osteoconduction at the host-allograft interface in both the humerus and ulna.
  - Hemiosteochondral allografts may also be used, but they have the added complexity of attempting to match articular surface conformity.
  - Complications rates are high and include infection, allograft fracture, allograft resorption, and instability for TEA allografts.
  - High complication rates limit the usefulness of this method.
- The technical aspects of allograft replacement resemble those for TEA, with similar approaches used.
  - Ligamentous stability must be maintained.
  - Secure fixation of allograft bone to host diaphyseal bone is obtained and may be augmented with the use of polymethylmethacrylate in the canal of the allograft bone.

Allograft Augmentation With Revision Total Elbow Arthroplasty (Kamineni et al. 2004)

- This is more frequently used than osteoarticular allografts.
- The indication is usually extensive bone loss of either the humerus or ulna (or both), thus prohibiting implantation of revision TEA.
- Often this is seen in patients with substantial osteolysis or inflammatory arthritis.
- It is an alternative to a custom prosthesis
- Onlay allograft augmentation may be used to enhance preexisting bone stock, or in a very deficient situation, a prosthesis can be cemented into the allograft humerus or ulna or both, which is then secured to the native bone.
- As with osteoarticular allografts, secure fixation of host and allograft bone is required.

Custom Total Elbow Arthroplasty Implantation

- When bone loss is severe enough that it cannot be restored by allograft or by a longer-stem revision implant, a custom implant can be used that is tailored to the specific situation.
- However, its use is hindered by its cost and delay in manufacturing.
- Some implant systems have various features, including longer stems and extended anterior flanges on the humeral component, that allow noncustom implants to be used for difficult surgical cases.

Technique of Revision Elbow Replacement

- Wide exposure is often necessary.
- Previous incisions should be utilized, except when inadequate (i.e., a laterally based incision used for implantation of an unlinked prosthesis via Kocher's interval).
- The ulnar nerve is identified and protected. It may be necessary to decompress the nerve if it is encased in scar tissue. If was not previously transposed, it should be.
- Often, surgical planes are difficult to identify; therefore some of the triceps-sparing approaches may not be applicable.
- Often, revision exposure requires a Campbell-type midline incision through the triceps mechanism, to expose the olecranon and distal humerus.
- After exposure of the joint, the loose prosthesis is removed.
- This may require cortical "windows" to remove cement and extract the component.
- Uncontrolled cortical perforation, especially near neurovascular structures, should be avoided.
- In some situations, the cement mantle is adequate, and the prosthesis may be removed without disrupting the cement-bone interface.
  - In these situations, a new, smaller implant may be cemented in the previous mantle.

- This is contraindicated in the failed, septic TEA.
- It is also usually applicable to the humerus and is unlikely in the ulna, given the small canal size of the ulna.
- Exposure of the ulnar implant and cement mantle may be increased using an osteotomy analogous to a trochanteric osteotomy of the hip.
  - This is then reconstructed around the cemented ulnar implant using cerclage wires.
- After reimplantation of the new prosthesis, the triceps is repaired through bone tunnels and then in a side-to-side fashion.

Results of Revision Total Elbow Arthroplasty

- Early reports of revision TEA found a high incidence of complications, including infection, recurrent loosening, and fracture.
- Newer reports revealed improved results but still showed higher complication rates than with primary TEA.
- Most studies report reliable improvement in ROM, pain, and function of the failed TEA after revision.
  - ROM averages a functional arc of motion (30 to 130 degrees) in most studies.
  - Nearly 90% of patients report pain relief after revision.
  - Functional stability is improved with the use of a semiconstrained implant.
- King and colleagues reported on 41 patients treated with revision TEA with an average follow-up of 6 years (King et al. 1997).
  - Of these patients, 38 were able to perform activities of daily living, and 22 had complete relief of pain.
  - Fourteen patients sustained a fracture or cortical perforation at the time of implant removal, a finding highlighting the difficulties encountered with primary implant removal.
- Revision TEA for infected arthroplasty has had improved results with a staged approach.
- Yamaguchi and colleagues reported on the Mayo Clinic (Rochester, MN) experience of 25 infected TEAs with an average of more than 9 years of follow-up (Yamaguchi et al. 1998).
  - Seven of 14 well-fixed prostheses were well managed with aggressive débridement and component retention.
  - Six loose prostheses were managed with staged exchange, with four resulting in eradication of infection and improvement in symptoms.

Complications of Revision Total Elbow Arthroplasty

- The complication rate of revision TEA is higher than that seen in primary TEA; some studies report rates of 60%.
- Most frequent complications reported include intraoperative fracture, neurovascular injury, wound healing and infection problems, and loosening.

- Intraoperative fracture often occurs secondary to difficulty with implant extraction.
  - Fracture rates range from 6% to 27% in the literature.
- Cortical perforation rates vary from 14% to 69% in the literature.
  - Perforation may be associated with cement extrusion, which may result in neurovascular injury.
- King and colleagues found the rate of nerve injury to be 10% in their series of 41 revision TEAs (King et al. 1997).
  - Three of four nerve injuries were to the radial nerve and resulted from cement extrusion through cortical perforation and thermal injury to the nerve.
  - Ulnar neuropathy was found to be higher when the ulnar nerve was not transposed.
- Wound problems and skin infections occur in up to 10% of revision cases, and deep infection rates are as high as 11%, with recent studies reporting rates of approximately 3% to 4%.
- Finally, loosening of revision TEA occurs at a higher rate than in primary TEA.
  - Morrey and Bryan reported 21% aseptic loosening rates at 5.1 years of follow-up (Morrey and Bryan 1987).
  - More recent studies have shown lower rates, approximately 5% in short-term (5 years) follow-up.
  - Patients undergoing revision TEA for post-traumatic OA have higher aseptic loosening rates when compared with revision TEA in patients with RA.

Conclusions

- The management of patients with elbow arthritis has evolved over the past decade as advances in implant design and surgical technique have coincided with improved understanding of the normal and pathologic anatomy of the elbow.
- The surgeon treating these patients now has numerous options for managing the arthritic elbow.
- Recent reports of results of surgical management of the arthritic elbow, including both nonreplacement and prosthetic replacement, have shown improvements with respect to pain relief and restoration of function.
- Similar improvements have also been seen in newer reports of revision management of the arthritic elbow.

References

Antuna SA, Morrey BF, Adams RA, O'Driscoll SW (2002). Ulnohumeral arthroplasty for primary degenerative arthritis of the elbow: Long-term outcome and complications. *J Bone Joint Surg Am* 84:2168-2173.

This study reviewed the outcome of 46 elbows with primary OA treated with open débridement at an average of 80 months. The procedure involved resection of osteophytes, removal of loose bodies, and fenestration of the olecranon fossa. The arc of motion improved from an average of 79 degrees to 101 degrees. Of these

patients, 76% were not in pain or had only mild pain at latest follow-up. The authors concluded that ulnohumeral arthroplasty yields satisfactory long-term results but cautioned that patients with substantial preoperative contractures (<60 degrees of extension, <100 degrees of flexion) are at risk for postoperative ulnar nerve dysfunction, and transposition should be considered.

Bonutti PM, Windau JE, Ables BA, Miller BG (1994). Static progressive stretch to reestablish elbow range of motion. *Clin Orthop Relat Res* 303:128-134.

This study evaluated the use of an orthosis in developing patient-directed static progressive stretch. Twenty patients with elbow contractures in whom prior therapies, including serial casting, dynamic splinting, and surgery, had failed underwent static progressive stretch using the orthoses. There was an average increase in ROM of 31 degrees, with no complications and no loss of motion at 1-year follow-up.

Cheng SL, Morrey BF (2000). Treatment of the mobile, painful arthritic elbow by distraction interposition arthroplasty. *J Bone Joint Surg Br* 82:233-238.

This study reported the results of 13 patients treated for painful arthritic elbows with distraction interposition arthroplasty using fascia lata graft at an average follow-up of 63 months; 69% of patients had satisfactory relief of pain, and 62% had an excellent or good outcome based on the Mayo Elbow Performance score. Similar results were observed in patients with RA and post-traumatic arthritis. The authors concluded that interposition arthroplasty is an option in young, high-demand patients with elbow arthritis.

Celli A, Arash A, Adams RA, et al. (2005). Triceps insufficiency following total elbow arthroplasty. *J Bone Joint Surg Am* 87:1957-1964.

This is a retrospective study evaluating 14 patients (16 elbows) who had triceps insufficiency following total elbow arthroplasty. Three basic techniques were used to reconstruct the triceps mechanism, including direct suture reattachment, anconeus rotation, and Achilles allograft. Fifteen of 16 elbows regained the ability to extend against gravity, and 11 elbows were considered to have an excellent outcome.

Cobb TK, Morrey BF (1997). Total elbow arthroplasty as primary treatment for distal humeral fractures in elderly patients. *J Bone Joint Surg Am* 79:826-832.

Twenty-one elbows in 20 consecutive patients (mean age, 72 years) who had sustained an acute distal humerus fracture were reviewed at a mean follow-up time of 3 years. Fifteen elbows had an excellent result. The authors concluded that total elbow arthroplasty can be an effective option for treatment of comminuted distal humeral fractures in older patients.

Ewald FC, Simmons ED Jr, Sullivan JA, et al. (1993). Capitellocondylar total elbow replacement in rheumatoid arthritis: Long-term results. *J Bone Joint Surg Am* 75:498-507.

These authors evaluated the long-term (69 months) results of 202 capitellocondylar TEAs performed for RA. Improvement occurred in the areas of pain, functional status, and ROM, based on a 100-point scoring system. These improvements were maintained at latest follow-up, with no deterioration noted. Radiolucent lines were seen in 8 humeral and 19 ulnar components at latest follow-up, and 3 (1.5%) of the elbows required revision.

Faber KJ, Cordy ME, Milne AD, et al. (1997). Advanced cement technique improves fixation in elbow arthroplasty. *Clin Orthop Relat Res* 334:150-156.

> This is an in vitro study performed to assess the efficacy of advanced cementing techniques in the fixation of the humeral stem in elbow arthrosplasty. The development of an effective restrictor and application of advanced cement techniques should improve the initial fixation of the humeral component.

Figgie HE, Inglis AE, Ranawat CS, Rosenberg GM (1987). Results of total elbow arthroplasty as a salvage procedure for failed elbow reconstructive operations. *Clin Orthop Relat Res* 219:185-193.

> This study looked at the surgical technique and the clinical results of the use of a semiconstrained implant in a revision TEA situation in a series of 20 patients in whom prior elbow reconstructions had failed. TEA can be successful as a revision procedure, especially in cases of failed open reduction internal fixation and as a staged procedure for revision of previously infected elbows.

Gill DR, Morrey BF (1998). The Coonrad-Morrey total elbow arthroplasty in patients who have rheumatoid arthritis: A ten to fifteen-year follow-up study. *J Bone Joint Surg Am* 80:1327-1335.

> These authors reported the results of 78 elbows followed for a minimum of 10 years following TEA with a semiconstrained implant; 32 of the elbows were in patients who had either died or required revision before 10-year follow-up, yielding 46 elbows available for long-term follow-up. The rate of survival of the prosthesis in these patients was 92.4 %, with 86% good or excellent results based on their Mayo Elbow Performance scores.

Hildebrand KA, Patterson SD, Regan WD, et al. (2000). Functional outcome of semiconstrained total elbow arthroplasty. *J Bone Joint Surg Am* 82:1379-1386.

> Clinical results of total elbow arthroplasty (Coonrad-Morrey prosthesis) were reviewed in patients with inflammatory arthritis, acute fracture, and post-traumatic arthritis. Mayo elbow performance scores for those with inflammatory arthritis were significantly higher (90 points) than those with either a traumatic or post-traumatic condition (78 points). Ulnar nerve dysfunction was observed in 26% of patients, whereas 23% had an intraoperative fracture.

Horiuchi K, Momohara S, Tomatsu T, et al. (2002). Arthroscopic synovectomy of the elbow in rheumatoid arthritis. *J Bone Joint Surg Am* 84:342-347.

> The authors investigated the results of arthroscopic synovectomy for synovitis caused by rheumatoid arthritis. They reported successful pain relief in the majority of their patients, with 5 of 21 patients developing clinically apparent synovitis and recurrent synovitic pain. The authors concluded that arthroscopic synovectomy in a rheumatoid elbow is a reliable pain-relieving procedure.

Kamineni S, Morrey BF (2004). Distal humerus fractures treated with noncustom total elbow replacement. *J Bone Joint Surg Am* 86:940-947.

> These authors reviewed the outcome of 49 acute distal humerus fractures treated with TEA as the primary procedure. The average age of patients was 67 years, and patients were followed for a minimum of 2 years. The Mayo score averaged 93 (out of 100) at latest follow-up. ROM was 24 to 131 degrees on average; 65% of the elbows were functioning well without complications or revision at latest follow-up. The authors concluded that TEA is a viable option for the treatment of acute distal humerus fractures in which fixation is not feasible, especially in physiologically older, less demanding patients.

Kamineni S, Morrey BF (2004). Proximal ulnar reconstruction with strut allograft in revision total elbow arthroplasty. *J Bone Joint Surg Am* 86:1223-1229.

> This study reported the authors' experience with the use of strut allograft reconstruction of the proximal ulna as an adjunct to the revision TEA. Twenty-one patients were followed for an average of 4 years; the mean Mayo Elbow Performance score improved from 34 points preoperatively to 79 points at latest follow-up. The authors concluded that despite the high complication rate, most deficiencies of bone stock of the proximal ulna can be treated with allograft strut grafting.

Kashiwagi D (1978). Intraarticular changes of the osteoarthritic elbow, especially about the fossa olecrani. *J Jap Orthop Assn* 52:1367-1382.

> This article provides the original description of the ulnohumeral arthroplasty used to débride the osteoarthritic elbow.

Kauffman JI, Chen AL, Stuchin S, et al. (2003). Surgical management of the rheumatoid elbow. *J Am Acad Orthop Surg* 11(2):100-108.

> This review article describes the pathology of the rheumatoid elbow as well as surgical and nonsurgical treatment options. Controversies regarding the various treatment options are also discussed.

Kelly EW, Morrey BF, O'Driscoll SW (2001). Complications of elbow arthroscopy. *J Bone Joint Surg Am* 83:25-34.

> The authors retrospectively reviewed 473 elbow arthroscopies to determine the complication rate and attempt to determine risk factors for complications following elbow arthroscopy. Major complications (joint infection) occurred in 0.8% of patients. Minor complications included incisional drainage and infections, persistent minor contractures (<20 degrees), and transient nerve palsy (the ulnar nerve was most commonly affected) in 11% of patients. A diagnosis of RA and the presence of preexisting contractures were found to be risk factors for postoperative nerve palsy.

King GJW, Adams RA, Morrey BF (1997). Total elbow arthroplasty: revision with use of a non-custom semiconstrained prosthesis. *J Bone Joint Surg Am* 79:394-400.

> This case series presents the results of the use of the Mayo-modified Coonrad implant in 41 patients in a revision TEA situation. The average duration of follow-up was 6 years. Patients were evaluated clinically, by the Mayo Elbow Performance score, and radiographically. The average Mayo score was 87 ± 16 points at last follow-up compared with 44 ± 17 points preoperatively. This article presents the classification for distal humeral bone loss and also describes the technique of revision TEA.

Kozak TKW, Adams RA, Morrey BF (1998). Total elbow arthroplasty in primary osteoarthritis of the elbow. *J Arthroplasty* 13:836-842.

> This study is a case series of five patients, with a minimum follow-up of 3 years, who underwent total elbow arthroplasty for primary osteoarthritis of the elbow. Complications occurred in four patients, with two requiring revision of the implant. All had a satisfactory outcome at the most recent follow-up. However, the authors recommended that replacement should not be the first option for primary osteoarthritis of the elbow and should be considered only when other options are unacceptable.

Lee BPH, Morrey BF (1997). Arthroscopic synovectomy of the elbow for rheumatoid arthritis. *J Bone Surg Br* 79:770-772.

A short-term follow-up of patients who had undergone arthroscopic synovectomy for rheumatoid arthritis of the elbow revealed that 93% had good or excellent subjective results. However, this decreased to 57% of patients having a good or excellent result at latest follow-up (average, 42 months).

Ljung P, Jonsson K, Larsson K, et al. (1996). Interposition arthroplasty of the elbow with rheumatoid arthritis. *J Shoulder Elbow Surg* 5(2 Pt 1):81-85.

Radiographic and clinical outcomes were reviewed in a series of 35 patients with rheumatoid arthritis who underwent interposition arthrosplasty. Pain relief was rated as good, but joint mobility and stability were rated only as fair. Long-term results were inferior to those of total elbow arthroplasty in patients with rheumatoid arthritis. The authors recommended that total elbow replacement be the first choice in the surgical treatment of the painful rheumatoid elbow with cartilage destruction.

London JT (1981). Kinematics of the elbow. *J Bone Joint Surg Am* 63:529-535.

This cardinal article describes the kinematics of the elbow. Kinematic analyses of eight normal elbows (four in cadavers and four in living subjects) were conducted to determine motion at the joint surface and the axis of rotation. An important rule regarding TEAs, that the axis of flexion of the prosthesis should be the same as the flexion axis of the normal joint, is presented in this article.

Minami M, Kato S, Kashiwagi D (1996). Outerbridge-Kashiwagi's method for arthroplasty of osteoarthritis of the elbow—44 elbows followed for 8-16 years. *J Orthop Sci* 1:11-15.

The authors reported their results of the Outerbridge-Kashiwagi procedure for primary osteoarthritis of the elbow. They reviewed 44 elbows, with a mean follow-up period of more than 10 years. Approximately half of the patients had good pain relief and improvement in range of motion but there was a progression of osteoarthritic change for more than 10 years following the procedure.

Morrey BF (1992). Primary degenerative arthritis of the elbow. *J Bone Joint Surg Br* 74:409-413.

This is a classic article describing the use of ulnohumeral arthroplasty to treat primary degenerative arthritis of the elbow. Clinical outcomes on 15 patients at a mean of 33 months are described; the majority had good pain relief and improved range of motion of the elbow.

Morrey BF, Askew LJ, An KN, Chao EY (1981). A biomechanical study of normal functional elbow motion. *J Bone Joint Surg Am* 63:872-877.

This article analyzed 33 normal patients to determine required level of elbow motion for 15 activities of daily living. Most of the activities could be performed with 100 degrees of elbow flexion (30 to 130 degrees) and 100 degrees of forearm rotation (50 degrees of pronation and 50 degrees of supination).

Morrey BF, Bryan RS (1987). Revision total elbow arthroplasty. *J Bone Joint Surg Am* 69:523-532.

Thirty-three consecutive revision total elbow replacements were performed and assessed at a minimum follow-up of 3 years. Eighteen patients (55%) had good results and 15 (45%) had a poor result. The results of the study indicated that reimplantation is a viable option for the failed total elbow, although more than one revision may be required.

O'Driscoll SW, An KN, Korinek S, Morrey BF (1992). Kinematics of semi-constrained total elbow arthroplasty. *J Bone Joint Surg Br* 74:297-299.

Eleven cadaver elbows were analyzed with an electromagnetic tracking device to record elbow motion before and after implantation of a semiconstrained TEA prosthesis. The normal cadaver elbow and implanted prosthesis demonstrated less varus-valgus laxity during simulated motion than during directed varus-valgus stress. This finding indicates that the surrounding musculature helps to absorb stress in a semiconstrained prosthesis that otherwise would be transferred to the bone-implant interface.

O'Driscoll SWM, Lawton RL, Smith AM (2005). The "moving valgus stress test" for medial collateral ligament tears of the elbow. *Am J Sports Med* 33:231-239.

This article describes the "moving valgus stress test" and its applicability in the setting of medial elbow pain arising from the medial collateral ligament.

Oka Y (2000). Débridement arthroplasty for osteoarthrosis of the elbow. *Acta Orthop Scand* 71:185-190.

The results of débridement arthroplasty were investigated in athletes and manual laborers with osteoarthrosis of the elbow. Long-term outcomes at greater than 5 years showed recurrence of mild osteoarthrosis with minimal symptoms. The author concluded that débridement arthroplasty is an effective treatment in athletes and laborers with osteoarthrosis of the elbow.

Redfern DRM, Dunkley AB, Trail IA, Stanley JK (2001). Revision total elbow replacement using the Souter-Strathclyde prosthesis. *J Bone Joint Surg Br* 83:635-639.

The Souter-Strathclyde prosthesis was used in 52 revisions of TEAs. Fifty revisions in 45 patients were followed for an average of 53 months; the procedure provided a reliable relief of pain and preservation of ROM, but with a high rate of complications (30%). The authors concluded that revision is the procedure of choice for patients with failed aseptic primary arthroplasties.

Savoie FH 3rd, Nunley PD, Field LD (1999). Arthroscopic management of the arthritic elbow: Indications, technique, and results. *J Shoulder Elbow Surg* 8:214-219.

These authors reviewed 24 patients with elbow arthritis treated with an arthroscopic modification of the Outerbridge-Kashiwagi procedure. Patients were followed for an average of 32 months, and the average improvement of the arc of motion was 81 degrees. Pain improved from 8.2 to 2.2 on the visual analog scale. The authors found their complication rate to be comparable to that of open techniques and concluded that arthroscopic débridement yields satisfactory pain relief and improvement in motion.

Schneeberger AG, Adams R, Morrey BF (1997). Semi-constrained total elbow replacement for the treatment of post-traumatic osteoarthrosis. *J Bone Joint Surg Am* 79:1211-1222.

This study discussed the results of TEA for post-traumatic arthrosis of the elbow in 41 patients with an average age of 57 years. Patients were followed a minimum of 2 years (average, 5 years). By Mayo scoring, 39% of the results were excellent, 44% good, 5% fair, and 2% poor; 95% of patients were satisfied with the outcome. However, the authors that reported 11 elbows (27%) had major complications including fracture of the ulnar implant (5), bushing failure (2), and infection (2). The authors concluded that TEA can give satisfactory results in patients with post-traumatic arthrosis, but it needs to considered carefully in physiologically young or active patients because of the incidence of catastrophic failure.

Schneeberger AG, Sadowski MM, Jacob HAC (2004). Coronoid process and radial head as posterolateral rotatory stabilizers of the elbow. *J Bone Joint Surg Am* 86:975-982.

This study evaluates the role of the coronoid and radial head in preventing posterolateral rotatory laxity; both structures contribute significantly. Elbows with a defect greater than 50% of the coronoid along with a radial head resection are grossly unstable despite intact ligamentous structures and require both coronoid reconstruction and radial head replacement to achieve stability.

Tsuge K, Mizuseki T (1994). Débridement arthroplasty for advanced primary osteoarthritis of the elbow. Results of a new technique used for 29 elbows. *J Bone Joint Surg Br* 76:641-646.

The authors reported their results of débridement arthroplasty of the elbow at a mean follow-up of 64 months. The average increase in range of motion was 34 degrees, with improved pain relief and grip strength in the majority of patients.

Wada T, Isogai S, Ishii S, Yamashita T (2004). Debridement arthroplasty for primary osteoarthritis of the elbow. *J Bone Joint Surg Am* 86:233-241.

These authors described the long-term (average, 10 years) follow-up of 33 elbows with primary OA treated with open débridement. Débridement involved resection of osteophytes and removal of loose bodies. At latest follow-up, the arc of motion had improved 24 degrees, with an average flexion increase of 17 degrees; 19 elbows followed for longer than 10 years had progressive loss of extension (7 degrees) when compared with results 1 year postoperatively. Flexion improvement remained constant. The authors concluded that débridement arthroplasty offers reliable long-term results with regard to pain relief and improvement in motion.

Yamaguchi K, Adams RA, Morrey BF (1998). Infection after total elbow arthroplasty. *J Bone Joint Surg Am* 80:481-491.

Twenty-five patients who developed infection after primary TEA were reviewed to examine the indications for salvage of the prosthesis versus resection arthroplasty. The authors concluded that salvage of the prosthesis with extensive débridement can be successful if the offending organism is not S. *epidermidis* and if the implant was well fixed both radiographically and intraoperatively at the time of irrigation and débridement. Resection arthroplasty remains the procedure of choice in patients with low functional demand.

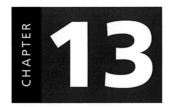
Total Wrist Arthroplasty

David J. Bozentka* and Robert B. Carrigan[†]

*MD, Chief, Hand Surgery, Penn Orthopaedic Institute; Associate Professor, Department of
Orthopaedic Surgery, University of Pennsylvania School of Medicine, Philadelphia, PA
[†]MD, Physician, Premier Orthopaedics and Sports Medicine, Ridley Park, PA

Introduction

- Total wrist arthroplasty (TWA) is an evolving surgical procedure with continued improvements in implant material, design, and function.
- Wrist arthrodesis has traditionally been considered the "gold standard" in treating the painful arthritic wrist.
  - Patients note improvement in their ability to perform activities of daily living, in spite of the limitation in motion following wrist fusion.
- TWA has a greater complication rate and requires appropriate patient selection, meticulous surgical technique, and effective treatment of complications.
  - As these parameters become better defined, the results of wrist arthroplasty will continue to improve.

Anatomy
Distal Radius

- The radial shaft flares distally into a metaphyseal region to articulate with the distal ulna and the proximal carpal row.
- Lister's tubercle is a dorsal prominence that redirects the extensor pollicis longus tendon and is a landmark in dorsal surgical approaches.
  - Lister's tubercle is also 1 cm proximal to the scapholunate joint.
- The distal articular surface is composed of two fossae, which are concave in the dorsal/palmar and medial/lateral planes (Fig. 13–1).
  - The smaller lunate fossa is ovoid, and the scaphoid fossa is more triangular (Fig. 13–2).
- The distal articular surface is tilted with a 22-degree radial inclination and an 11-degree palmar tilt (Fig. 13–3).

- The average radial height (longitudinal distance from the tip of the radial styloid to the ulnarmost aspect of the distal radius) is 11 mm.
- The sigmoid notch articulates with the ulnar seat at the distal radioulnar joint (DRUJ).

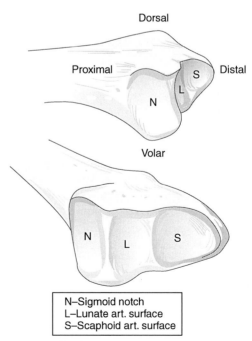

N–Sigmoid notch
L–Lunate art. surface
S–Scaphoid art. surface

Figure 13–1: Distal radius.
The distal radius is viewed from the ulnar aspect of the carpus (*bottom*) and from directly ulnar (*top*). Note the confluence of the lunate facet and the sigmoid notch. (From Bowers WH [1999]. The distal radioulnar joint. In: Green DP, Hotchkiss RN, Pederson WC eds. *Operative Hand Surgery*, 4th ed. New York: Churchill Livingstone, p 988.)

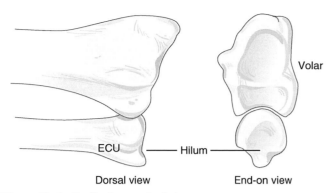

Figure 13–2: Radioulnar articulation.
The radioulnar articulation in neutral or zero rotation as viewed from the dorsum and from end on. The arc of the notch circumscribes a circle of greater diameter than that of the ulnar head. *ECU*, extensor carpi ulnaris. (From Bowers WH [1999]. The distal radioulnar joint. In: Green DP, Hotchkiss RN, Pederson WC eds. *Operative Hand Surgery*, 4th ed. New York: Churchill Livingstone, p 989.)

- Although the notch is classically described as concave, the shape can vary.
- The arc of curvature of the notch covered with articular cartilage averages 71 degrees.

Distal Ulna

- The distal ulna is the articular extension of the ulnar shaft into the carpus and the DRUJ.
- It is composed of the ulnar head (faces the undersurface of the triangular fibrocartilage complex [TFCC]), seat (articulates with the sigmoid notch), styloid, and fovea.
- The arc of curvature of the ulnar seat is 111 degrees.

Carpal Bones

- The eight carpal bones (scaphoid, lunate, triquetrum, pisiform, hamate, capitate, trapezoid, and trapezium) are arranged in two rows between the metacarpal bases distally and the distal radius and ulna (with the intervening TFCC) proximally (Fig. 13–4).
- Whereas the proximal and distal surfaces are articular, the dorsal and volar surfaces are primarily points of ligament attachment and vascular supply.
- The scaphoid occupies a position in both the proximal and distal row.
- The pisiform is a sesamoid bone within the tendon of the flexor carpi ulnaris that articulates with the volar surface of the triquetrum.

Radiocarpal Joint

- The radiocarpal joint is an ellipsoid biaxial joint.
- It allows flexion, extension, radial deviation, and ulnar deviation through a complex combination of muscle contraction, intrinsic and extrinsic ligament constraints, and intra-articular motion.

Intercarpal Joints

- The distal carpal row (trapezium, trapezoid, capitate, and hamate) articulates with the distal aspect of the scaphoid, lunate, and triquetrum.

Distal Radioulnar Joint

- The DRUJ is a trochoid or pivot joint.
- The bony components include the sigmoid notch of the distal radius and the ulnar head and seat.
- The TFCC also confers the primary stability of the joint.
- A mismatch in the radii of curvature of the articular surfaces of the radius and ulna leads to a combination of rolling, sliding, and gliding in pronosupination.

Ligaments

- A series of extrinsic (connect carpal bones to forearm bones) and intrinsic (connect carpal bones) ligaments binds the bones of the wrist.
- Dorsal wrist radiocarpal ligaments (Fig. 13–5)
  - These ligaments can be divided into the radioscaphoid and radiotriquetral ligaments.
  - The radiotriquetral ligament (dorsal radiocarpal ligament) originates from the dorsal rim of the lunate fossa of the distal radius and inserts into the dorsal triquetrum.
  - The dorsal intercarpal ligament originates from the dorsal triquetrum and largely inserts onto the dorsal ridge of the scaphoid and to a lesser extent the trapezium and trapezoid.
- Palmar wrist ligaments (Fig. 13–6)
  - The palmar radiocarpal and ulnocarpal ligaments are the primary stabilizing structures of the wrist joint.
- Ulnocarpal ligaments (Fig. 13–7)
  - The ulnocapitate ligament originates from the fovea of the ulnar head and reinforces the lunotriquetral interosseous ligament before its insertion, and before interdigitating with the radioscaphocapitate ligament at its insertion.
  - The ulnotriquetral and ulnolunate ligaments facilitate forearm rotation (stabilizing the DRUJ) while maintaining ulnocarpal stability.
- Distal radioulnar ligaments (Fig. 13–8)
  - The dorsal and volar radioulnar ligaments originate from the dorsal and palmar aspect of the sigmoid notch and insert in the base of the ulnar styloid. The superficial and deep components of these ligaments may act in opposite fashion to confer stability on the DRUJ during pronation and supination by increasing the area of joint contact.
  - The TFCC is the most important stabilizer of the DRUJ.
  - In a normal static load situation with neutral ulnar variance, 18% is transmitted to the ulnocarpal joint (82% radiocarpal).

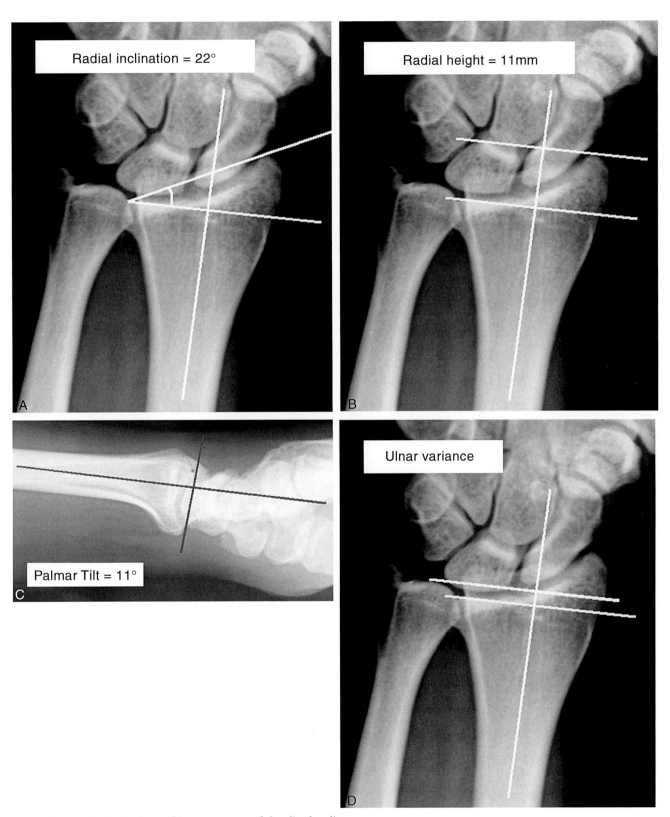

Figure 13–3: Radiographic parameters of the distal radius.
A, Radial inclination. **B,** Radial height. **C,** Palmar tilt. **D,** Ulnar variance. (From Chou KE, Savvis I, Papadimitriou NG, et al. [2004]. Fractures. In: Beredjiklian PK, Bozentka DJ, eds. *Review of Hand Surgery.* Philadelphia: WB Saunders, p 4.)

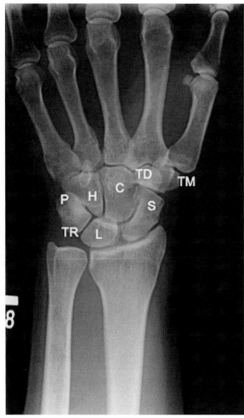

Figure 13–4: The carpal bones.
Posteroanterior radiograph of the wrist. *C*, capitate; *H*, hamate; *L*, lunate, *P*, pisiform; *S*, scaphoid; *TD*, trapezoid; *TM*, trapezium; *TR*, triquetrum. (From Monaghan BA [2004]. Anatomy. In: Beredjiklian PK, Bozentka DJ, eds. *Review of Hand Surgery*. Philadelphia: WB Saunders, p 4.)

Kinematics

- An overview of carpal kinematics is shown in Table 13–1.
- Several theories of carpal kinematics have been proposed.
- The capitate is the center of rotation of the wrist joint.
- The motors of the wrist attach to the metacarpals.
- Motion starts at the distal carpal row, which acts functionally as a single unit and is transmitted to the proximal carpal row through ligamentous attachments and compressive forces.
- There are no direct tendinous attachments to the proximal carpal row.
- Wrist flexion and extension occur equally through the radiocarpal and midcarpal joints.
- Radial and ulnar deviation occur 60% through the midcarpal and 40% through the radiocarpal joint.

Total Wrist Arthroplasty
Patient Selection

- TWA should be considered in patients with end-stage wrist degenerative changes.

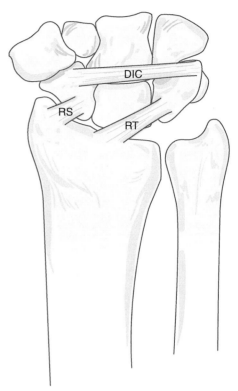

Figure 13–5: Dorsal wrist ligaments.
DIC, dorsal intercarpal ligament; *RS*, radioscaphoid ligament; *RT*, radiotriquetral ligament (dorsal radiocarpal ligament). (From Weber ER [1997]. Physiologic bases of wrist function. In: Lichtman DM, Alexander AH, eds. *The Wrist and Its Disorders*. Philadelphia: WB Saunders, p 50.)

- Patients with low functional demands and bilateral wrist disease are the best candidates for this procedure (Palmer et al. 1985).
- Most patients undergoing TWA have wrist degeneration resulting from inflammatory arthritides, most commonly rheumatoid arthritis (Fig. 13–9).
  - These patients typically have arthritis that affects multiple joints. Preservation of motion can be a distinct advantage

Table 13–1	Carpal Kinematics
Wrist flexion	Distal and proximal carpal rows flex and ulnar deviate
Wrist extension	Distal and proximal carpal rows extend and radially deviate
	Scaphoid rotates 80 degrees
	Lunate rotates 54 degrees
Radial deviation	Distal carpal row extends
	Proximal carpal row flexes
	Scaphoid flexion allows space for trapezium and radial styloid
Ulnar deviation	Distal carpal row flexes
	Proximal carpal row extends
	Palmar position of triquetral facet of hamate (hamate low position)

From Monaghan BA (2004). Anatomy. In: Beredjiklian PK, Bozentka DJ, eds. *Review of Hand Surgery*. Philadelphia, WB Saunders, p 4.

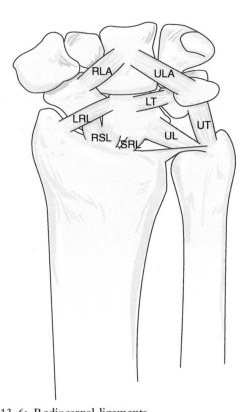

Figure 13–6: Radiocarpal ligaments.
Ligaments: Palmar aspect of the wrist, extrinsic. *LRL*, long
radiolunate ligament; *LT*, lunotriquetral ligament; *RLA*, radial
arm of the arcuate ligament; *RSL*, radioscapholunate ligament;
SRL, short radiolunate ligament; *UL*, ulnolunate ligament;
ULA, ulnar arm of the arcuate ligament; *UT*, ulnotriquetral
ligament. (From Weber ER [1997]. Physiologic bases of wrist
function. In: Lichtman DM, Alexander AH, eds. *The Wrist and
Its Disorders*. Philadelphia: WB Saunders, p 49.)

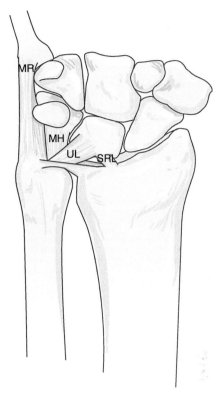

Figure 13–7: Ulnocarpal ligaments.
Palmar view: Ligaments of the ulnar side of the carpus.
MH, meniscus homologue; MR; meniscus reflection;
SRL, short radiolunate ligament; UL, ulnolunate ligament.
(From Weber ER [1997]. Physiologic bases of wrist function.
In: Lichtman DM, Alexander AH, eds. *The Wrist and Its
Disorders*. Philadelphia: WB Saunders, p 49.)

when elbow and shoulder motion is affected in the same
upper extremity or when bilateral disease is present
(Murphy et al. 2003).
- TWA is generally not considered in the treatment of
osteoarthritis and post-traumatic arthritis conditions such
as scapholunate advanced collapse and scaphoid-nonunion
advanced collapse (Fig. 13–10).
  - Although the bone stock is typically better in the
  osteoarthritic patients, their disease is monoarticular and
  can typically best be managed by arthrodesis rather than
  by arthroplasty.
  - Furthermore, these patients tend to have higher functional
  demands, a concern with regard to implant longevity.
- TWA is contraindicated in patients without active
wrist extension related to neurologic dysfunction or
unreconstructable wrist extensor tendons.
- Relative contraindications include nonfunctional digits,
failed metacarpal or interphalangeal arthroplasty, and laxity
related to lupus erythematosus.
- Remote history of septic arthritis is also a relative
contraindication.

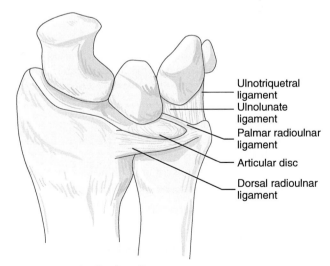

Figure 13–8: Radioulnar ligaments.
Schematic of the triangular fibrocartilage complex revealing
the radioulnar ligaments and the triangular fibrocartilage.
(Loftus JB, Palmer AK [1997]. Disorders of the DRUJ and
TFCC. In: Lichtman DM, Alexander AH, eds. *The Wrist and Its
Disorders*. Philadelphia: WB Saunders, p 388.)

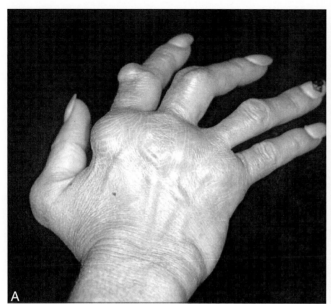

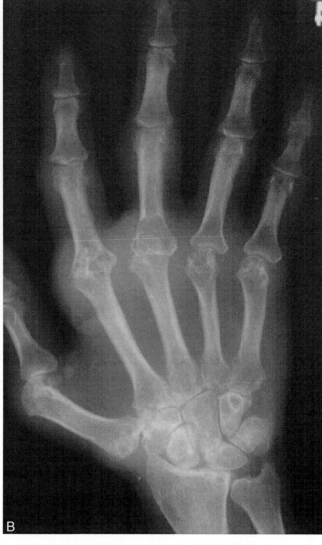

Figure 13–9: Rheumatoid arthritis.
Clinical photograph (**A**) and radiograph (**B**) of a patient with rheumatoid arthritis. Note the radial deviation deformity of the wrist and ulnar deviation of the digits. Soft tissue swelling is noted over the articulations. Note the rheumatoid nodule over the proximal interphalangeal joint of the index finger. (From Naidu S [2004]. Arthritis. In: Beredjiklian PK, Bozentka DJ, eds. *Review of Hand Surgery.* Philadelphia: WB Saunders, p 183.)

- Appropriate tests, including synovial aspirate, erythrocyte sedimentation rate, and C-reactive protein levels should be obtained before considering TWA.
- Severe deformities of the wrist and the need to weight bear through the wrist are also relative contraindications.

Nonoperative Treatment

- Treatment by a rheumatologist with appropriate medical management is initiated before consideration of surgical treatment.
- Splints for wrist immobilization provide pain relief.
- Occasional corticosteroid injections and therapy modalities can provide temporary relief.
- Surgical management is considered for the patient with symptomatic disease progression despite these modalities.

Alternative Surgical Options

- The surgical options in treating the rheumatoid wrist are classified as preventive, corrective, and salvage.
- Flexor or extensor tenosynovectomy and tendon reconstruction may prevent tendon rupture and progressive deformity with limited range of motion.
  - These soft tissue procedures are considered before more destructive salvage procedures such as TWA or arthrodesis.
- Wrist synovectomy and denervation are indicated for the painful rheumatoid wrist with limited articular bony destruction.
- Resection arthroplasty is unpredictable and proximal row carpectomy is contraindicated in patients with inflammatory arthritis.

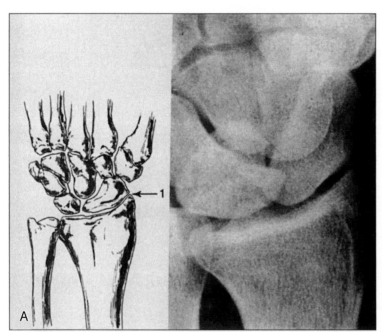

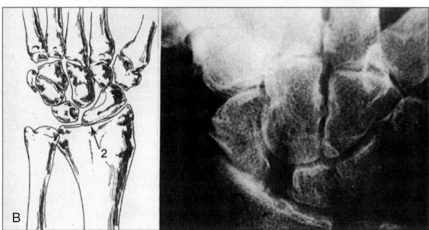

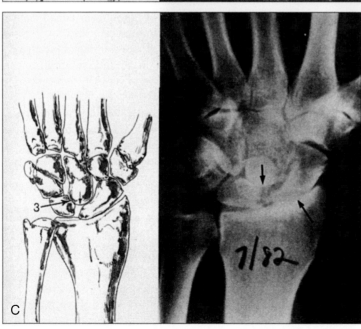

Figure 13–10: Scapholunate advanced collapse wrist.

The progression of scapholunate advanced collapse follows a predictable pattern. **A,** The early degenerative process is visualized at the tip of the radial styloid and distal scaphoid. **B,** Eventually, the entire radioscaphoid joint is involved in the degenerative process. **C,** The capitolunate joint becomes involved with the degenerative process and leads to proximal migration of the capitate. At this point, the radiolunate joint is still preserved. *Arrows* show proximal migration of the capitate and radioscaphoid joint arthritis. (From Watson HK, Ballet FL [1984]. The SLAC wrist: Scapholunate advanced collapse pattern of degenerative arthritis. *J Hand Surg Am* 9:358-365.)

- Limited arthrodesis, such as radiolunate and radioscapholunate arthrodesis, with or without midcarpal arthroplasty, is considered in the early stages of rheumatoid arthritis to prevent progressive deformity and to decrease pain (Fig. 13–11) (Adams 2000).
- Total wrist arthrodesis is considered for patients in whom wrist arthroplasty is contraindicated, such as patients with severe deformity, limited bone stock, need for weight bearing through the wrist, or failed TWA.

Implant Selection

- TWA implants have evolved significantly since the mid-1970s (Grosland et al. 2004, Sheperd and Johnstone 2002).

Swanson Implant

- Swanson first introduced the silicone elastomer, intramedullary, and flexible hinged implant for the wrist in 1967. This prosthesis bears his name.
- The Silastic prosthesis was indicated in patients who had advanced rheumatoid wrist arthritis.
  - It performed well in lower-demand patients with rheumatoid arthritis compared with younger patients with isolated post-traumatic radiocarpal arthritis.
- The intent of the Swanson implant was to act as a space-occupying device and to allow the body to create new capsule-ligamentous tissue to stabilize the wrist.
- Common complications involving the Swanson silicone wrist prosthesis included loosening, silicone synovitis, and implant fracture (Fig. 13–12) (Fatti et al. 1986, 1991).
- The original design consisted of only the silicone hinge; bony titanium grommets were added later to prevent implant subsidence.

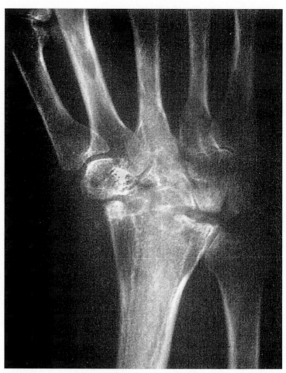

Figure 13–12: Swanson silicone implant.
Swanson silicone implant used for rheumatoid arthritis with implant breakage 5 years after surgery. (From Adams BD [2000]. Total wrist arthroplasty. *Semin Arthroplasty* 11:72–81.)

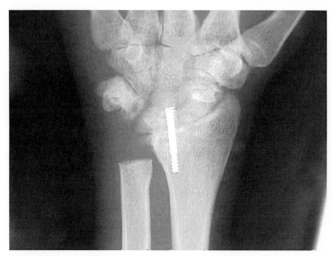

Figure 13–11: Rheumatoid arthritis: after fusion.
A patient with rheumatoid arthritis after radiolunate fusion and distal ulna excision. (From Naidu S [2004]. Arthritis. In: Beredjiklian PK, Bozentka DJ, eds. *Review of Hand Surgery.* Philadelphia: WB Saunders, p 183.)

Meuli and Volz Prostheses

- In the 1970s, both Meuli and Volz developed fixed-fulcrum TWA devices (Fig. 13-13).
- Both devices are ball-and-socket designs with differing amounts of constraint. Each of these devices can be placed with or without cement fixation.
- The Meuli design is a ball-in-socket unconstrained device that allows greater motion than other implants.
- The Volz prosthesis is an articulated nonhinged prosthesis that allows flexion and extension but little rotation.
  - The complications tend to be lower than those reported for the Meuli prosthesis.
- Balancing of these prostheses is difficult in that the center of rotation for the prostheses is slightly more radial than that of the normal wrist and may result in ulnar deviation of the hand with respect to the forearm.

Biaxial Total Wrist Arthroplasty

- In the 1980s, the scaphoid-nonunion advanced collapse biaxial prosthesis design (DePuy Orthopedics, Inc., Warsaw, IN) was developed.
- This prosthesis differed from the Meuli and Volz designs by way of an elliptic convex articulation that was more representative of the normal radiocarpal articulation.
- This prosthesis is an unconstrained device that aims to mimic the physiologic actions of the wrist by offsetting

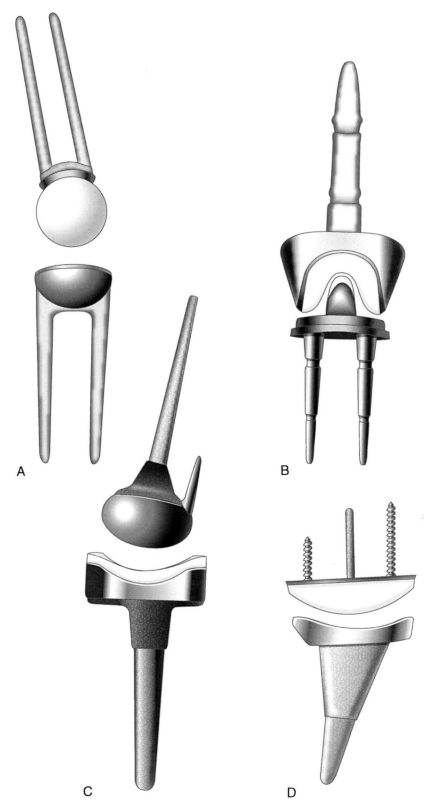

Figure 13–13: Diagrams of various total wrist arthroplasty designs.
A, Meuli. **B,** Volz. **C,** Biaxial. **D,** Universal.

the radial component in a more ulnar and volar direction (Fig. 13–14).
  • This offset is believed to provide better mechanical balance and to prevent the implant from becoming fixed in ulnar deviation.
• The carpal component is typically cemented, and the radial component has the option to be fixed in a cemented or an uncemented fashion.
• Early designs featured a shorter distal carpal component (Fig. 13–15).
• Later designs trended toward a longer metacarpal stem that was originally intended for revision surgical procedures.

Universal Total Wrist Implant

• The Universal Total Wrist implant (KMI, San Diego, CA) was designed to improve fixation of the distal component.

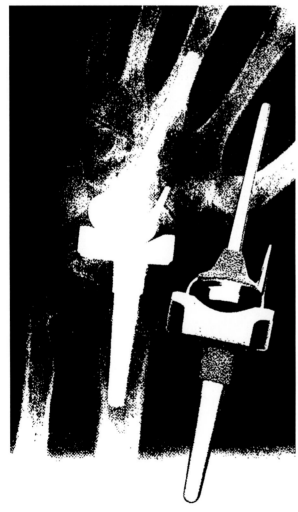

Figure 13–14: Biaxial total wrist arthroplasty.
The long-stem metacarpal component of biaxial total wrist arthroplasty superimposed on an anteroposterior radiograph of a wrist after wrist replacement. (From Rizzo M, Beckenbaugh RD [2003]. Results of biaxial total wrist arthroplasty with a modified (long) metacarpal stem. *J Hand Surg Am* 28:577-584.)

• The distal component is cemented into the capitate. Two osteointegrative screws are placed in the carpus. An intercarpal fusion of the capitate, hamate, and trapezoid theoretically provides greater bone stock for distal component fixation.
• The Universal Total Wrist implant radial component has a 20-degree radial inclination that mimics the normal radial inclination of the wrist.
• The geometry of the articulation is toroidal (Grosland et al. 2004).

Surgical Approaches

• Surgical approaches to the wrist for TWA vary by prosthesis selection.
• Proprietary differences in bony resection and implant insertion also vary from prosthesis to prosthesis.
• The size of the implant is estimated preoperatively using templates and patient radiographs.

Surgical Technique (Universal Total Wrist Arthroplasty) (Adams 2000)

• A longitudinal incision is made over the dorsum of the wrist along the axis of the third metacarpal.
• The skin and subcutaneous tissues are elevated sharply, with careful attention to handling of the tissue to prevent skin necrosis.
• The extensor retinaculum is split through the volar aspect of the fourth compartment. The retinaculum is elevated radially, leaving the septum between the first and second compartments intact.
• In patients with rheumatoid arthritis, complete extensor tenosynovectomy is performed.
• Extensor tendons are evaluated for rupture, possible repair, or transfer.
• The integrity of the extensor carpi radialis brevis tendon is confirmed.
• A distally based dorsal capsular flap is elevated along the medial and lateral aspect of the carpus along with 1 cm of the dorsal distal radius periosteum to lengthen the flap (Fig. 13–16).
• The head of the distal ulna is resected with a sagittal saw at the proximal edge of the sigmoid notch. The head is saved for bone graft.
• The brachioradialis and first dorsal compartment tendons are elevated subperiosteally, and retractors are placed on each side of the radius for exposure.
• The dorsal rim of the distal radius is resected using the cutting guide (Fig. 13–17).
• An osteotomy through the proximal aspect of the capitate is made with a sagittal saw perpendicular to the capitate and third metacarpal in the coronal and sagittal planes.
• Kirschner wires may need to be placed along the dorsal cortex of the residual distal scaphoid and triquetrum to the capitate and hamate if the carpal bones are loose.
• A guidewire is placed through the center of the capitate into the base of the third metacarpal and position checked by fluoroscopy.

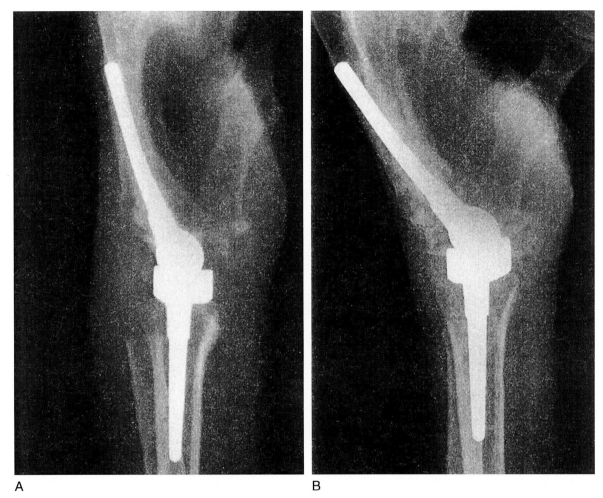

A   B

Figure 13–15: Biaxial total wrist arthroplasty.
A, Early postoperative lateral radiograph shows a stem that has penetrated the dorsal cortex of the metacarpal.
B, At 6 years after surgery, the component continues to show protrusion through the dorsal cortex of the
metacarpal. (From Rizzo M, Beckenbaugh RD [2003]. Results of biaxial total wrist arthroplasty with a
modified (long) metacarpal stem. *J Hand Surg [Am]* 28:577-584.)

- A cannulated drill is used to drill just longer than the distal component stem.
- A 3.5-mm drill bit may be used to open the hole further for the shoulder of the component.
- The distal trial component is inserted such that it covers the carpus but does not extend more than 2 mm beyond the margin of the bone.
- The radial screw hole is drilled at an angle slightly off the perpendicular across the residual scaphoid, the trapezoid, and into the base of the second metacarpal.
- The position and length are confirmed fluoroscopically, and a 4.5-mm self-tapping screw, often between 30 and 35 mm, is placed.
- The ulnar screw, often 20 mm long, is placed through the triquetrum and hamate but typically not into the mobile fourth and fifth carpometacarpal joints unless needed for fixation.
- The position is confirmed using image intensification.

- The canal of the radius is determined with a curette and image intensification. The canal is opened with a starter broach.
- The canal is prepared with successive broaches.
- The broach is placed parallel to the volar cortex but slightly dorsal to the midaxis to prevent volar angulation.
- The broaches are inserted at a valgus angle or radial tilt to limit ulnar deviation deformity.
- After the placement of the broach with the best fit, the second radius cutting guide is placed over the broach, thus allowing the radius to be cut matching the sloping contour of the radial component.
- The trial radius component is inserted, and a polyethylene component is placed in the carpal component (Fig. 13–18).
- The wrist should be positioned in a neutral resting alignment. Lengthening of the flexor carpi ulnaris and flexor carpi radialis in a step-cut fashion may be required to provide appropriate balance and motion.

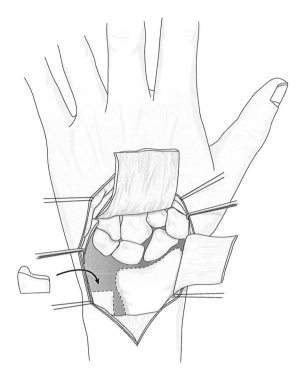

Figure 13–16: Exposure for wrist arthroplasty.
The retinaculum is reflected radially and the joint capsule raised distally based. The distal ulna has been resected. (From Adams BD [2000]. Total wrist arthroplasty. *Semin Arthroplasty* 11:72-81.)

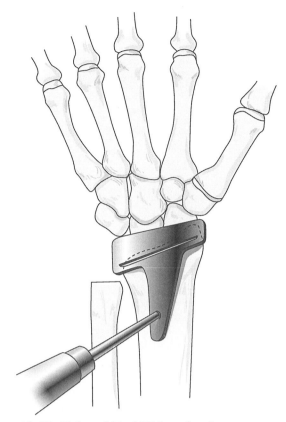

Figure 13–17: Universal Total Wrist arthroplasty.
The distal radius is resected using a template. (From Adams BD [2000]. Total wrist arthroplasty. *Semin Arthroplasty* 11:72-81.)

- A tight joint may require further radius bone resection.
- Looseness is avoided to prevent dislocation.
- The volar capsule is repaired to the volar cortex of the distal radius through drill holes, and any rents in the capsule are repaired.
- A thicker polyethylene component may also provide greater stability.
- The trials are removed, and the wrist is pulse lavaged and dried. A bone plug may be placed in the canal of the radius proximally to prevent excessive proximal injection of cement.
- Two or three sutures are placed in the dorsal cortex of the distal radius for later capsular repair.
- Cement is injected into the hole in the capitate, and the carpal component is inserted.
- Excess cement is removed, including the intercarpal spaces.
- The radial and ulnar screws are placed in the carpal component.
- Cement is injected into the canal of the radius, and the radius component is implanted, thus preventing varus or palmar tilt malalignment.
- The trial polyethylene component is placed, an axial load is applied on the wrist, and the cement is allowed to harden.
- The temporary pin fixation is removed. The final size of the polyethylene component is determined and is inserted to provide adequate stability and motion.

- Intercarpal arthrodesis is performed by excising the articular surfaces of the remaining carpus. The previously resected cancellous bone is placed in the intercarpal spaces.
- The capsular repair is performed.
- The capsule is closed over the distal ulna, and the dorsal capsular flap is sutured to the distal radius using the previously placed sutures.
- Half of the extensor retinaculum may be used to cover the prosthesis if the capsule is deficient.
- The retinaculum is repaired to prevent postoperative bowstringing of the extensor tendons. The extensor carpi ulnaris is maintained in a dorsal position using a sling from the retinaculum.

Postoperative Management

- The patient is placed in a bulky compressive dressing.
- A plaster splint is applied incorporating the elbow with the wrist in neutral.
- The forearm is placed in supination to prevent subluxation of the ulnar stump.
- Radiographs are obtained to confirm reduction of the prosthesis (Fig. 13–19).
- The dressings and splint are removed in 10 days to 2 weeks, along with the sutures.

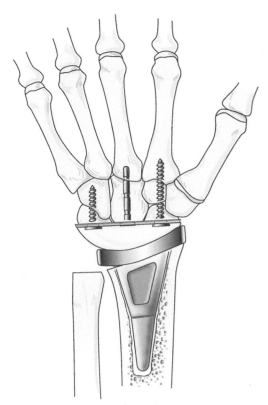

Figure 13–18: Universal Total Wrist arthroplasty.
Universal Total Wrist implants properly inserted. Minimal bone resection is required. The entire carpus is supported by the carpal component, which is not reliant on fixation in the metacarpal canal. (From Adams BD [2000]. Total wrist arthroplasty. *Semin Arthroplasty* 11:72-81.)

- Subsequent rehabilitation depends on wrist stability, determined at the time of surgery.
- If optimal stability is achieved, the patient is placed in a short arm cast for 2 more weeks. If there is any question of instability, the patient is immobilized in a short arm cast for several weeks longer.
- The patient is also given a removable volar wrist splint in 10 degrees of extension to wear when not engaging in therapy for an additional 2 to 4 weeks following cast removal.
- After removal of the cast, active wrist motion is started.
  - Passive motion is discouraged.
- Strengthening is not started until 8 to 10 weeks. At this time, passive range of motion can be started as well.
- Unrestricted use of the wrist can be started at approximately 2 to 3 months. Repetitive use and axial impact loading of the prosthesis are discouraged.

Results

- Several different outcome measurements have been used to evaluate the effectiveness of TWA.
  - These include quantitative measurements such as wrist motion, radiographic loosening, and implant failure rates, as well as subjective measurements of pain relief and patient satisfaction.
  - Several of these parameters have been combined into scoring systems to evaluate the effectiveness of wrist arthroplasty better.
- Swanson arthroplasty has been shown to provide good early results with improvements in pain and maintaining range of motion.
  - The longer-term results show unpredictable balancing of the wrist, with pain relief in only 52% of patients.
  - In addition, progressive radiographic deterioration in 70% and a rate of implant breakage of up to 52% have been reported.
- Meuli's series using 38 Meuli prostheses in 33 patients had an average follow-up of 5.5 years (Meuli 1997).
  - Excellent results were reported in 20, good in 10, fair in 2, and poor in 6.
  - Others have shown less optimal results with problems of loosening of the distal component and carpal tunnel syndrome.
- The Volz prosthesis, a partially constrained device allowing little rotation, was found to have a complication rate of 29%, with a problem with tendon imbalance in 22% and a revision rate of 12% (Volz 1984).
- The series by Cobb and Beckenbaugh using the biaxial prosthesis had an overall survival rate of 82% at 5 years, with an average range of motion of 36 degrees of extension and 29 degrees of flexion.
  - Of the 11 failures, 8 were related to distal loosening.
- Using the biaxial prosthesis modified with a longer stem for the metacarpal, Rizzo and Beckenbaugh had no failures in 17 implants with an average 6-year follow-up (Rizzo and Beckenbaugh 2003).
  - Four of the patients showed evidence of loosening.
  - Grip strength and pain were improved, and all patients were satisfied.
- In Menon's series of the Universal Total Wrist implant, no distal implant loosening occurred in 37 implants at a mean follow-up of 6.7 years (Menon 1998).
  - Pain relief was good in 88% of patients.
  - Twelve complications occurred, the most common being dislocation, which was reported in 5 implants.
- The early results of the series of Divelbiss and associates using the Universal Total Wrist prosthesis with 1-year follow-up in 8 patients and 2-year follow-up in 14 patients showed that 3 prostheses were unstable and required further treatment (Divelbiss et al. 2002).
  - All patients had improvements in range of motion, and Disabilities of the Arm, Shoulder, and Hand scores improved 14 points at 1 year and 24 points at 2 years.

Complications

- Long-term complications of TWA are often related to the progression of the disease and patient activity demands.

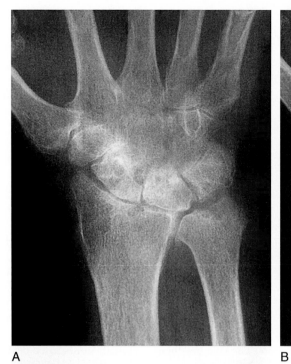

A

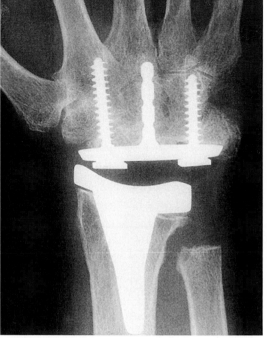

B

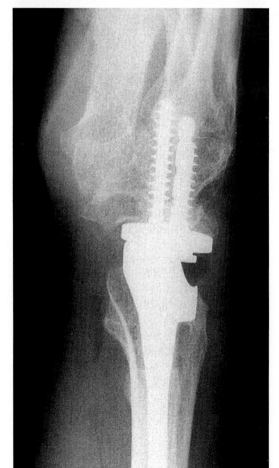

C

Figure 13–19: Universal Total Wrist arthroplasty.
A, Preoperative radiograph of a patient with rheumatoid arthritis. **B** and **C,** Universal Total Wrist arthroplasty at 3 years after surgery. (From Adams BD [2000]. Total wrist arthroplasty. *Semin Arthroplasty* 11:72-81.)

- The 5-year survivorship of wrist arthroplasty ranges from 74% to 83%.
- Component loosening is the most common complication seen following TWA.
  - At 5 years, 20% of prostheses show some evidence of loosening.
  - This is typically seen in the distal component.
- The distal component tends to migrate volarly and rotating, with the distal stem prominent dorsally when it becomes loose. This, in turn, may cause symptoms resembling those of carpal tunnel syndrome that require revision surgery and carpal tunnel release.
- Prosthetic instability and dislocation are common complications. They tend to occur in patients with highly active rheumatoid disease with ligamentous laxity.
- Wound dehiscence and superficial infections are reported, although deep infection is relatively uncommon.
- Tendon attritional rupture has been reported.

Revision Surgery

- The failure rate, as previously described, has been reported to be as high as 20% at 5 years.
- Failure is usually a result of implant loosening or dislocation.
- Implant loosening is typically seen with a large amount of bone stock loss.
- Revision to another wrist arthroplasty typically requires a custom prosthesis (Lorei et al. 1997).
- Revision surgery, in most cases, is typically managed as conversion to wrist arthrodesis.
  - Arthrodesis is accomplished by removing all the components and cement. The void is filled with a large iliac crest bone graft or allograft to maintain length and tendon balance (Carlson and Simmons 1998).
- Rigid fixation is accomplished by one of two methods.
  - Screw and plate fixation is applied to the dorsum of the wrist from the third metacarpal to the radius.
  - Rigid plate and screw fixation is preferable as it is a durable and stable construct. However, if skin and soft tissue coverage is an issue, intramedullary fixation, with Steinmann pins placed in retrograde fashion down the shafts of the second and third metacarpals through the bone graft and into the radius, is considered.
  - Similar fusion rates have been observed for both methods.

Distal Ulna Prosthetic Arthroplasty

Introduction

- The DRUJ is important in forearm stability in the longitudinal and transverse directions.
- The ulnar head prosthesis may prevent radioulnar convergence and can maintain the kinematics of the wrist during rotation.

- Loads experienced by the ulnar head prosthesis depend on position and contact with the radius articulation.
  - Neutral ulnar variance: 80% radius, 20% ulna
  - 1-mm positive ulnar variance: 30% ulna
  - 2-mm positive ulnar variance: 40% ulna
  - 1-mm negative ulnar variance: 10% ulna
  - 2-mm negative ulnar variance: 5% ulna

Patient Selection

- The main indication for ulnar head prosthetic replacement is symptomatic instability following partial or complete ulnar head excision.
- Other indications include the following:
  - Pain and weakness resulting from osteoarthritis or rheumatoid arthritis of the DRUJ not improved by nonoperative treatment (Fig. 13–20)

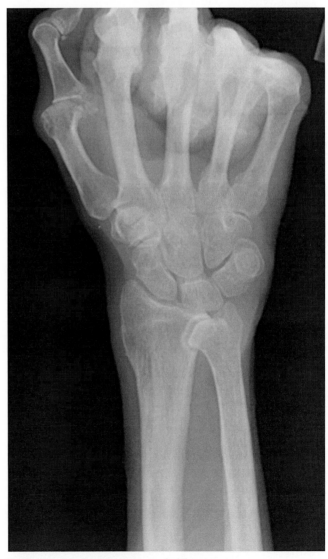

Figure 13–20: Primary osteoarthritis.
Primary osteoarthritis of the distal radioulnar joint. (From Naidu S [2004]. Arthritis. In: Beredjiklian PK, Bozentka DJ, eds. *Review of Hand Surgery.* Philadelphia: WB Saunders, p 183.)

- Pain and weakness resulting from post-traumatic arthritis of the DRUJ following a displaced fracture of the distal radius through the sigmoid notch
- Irreparable, severely comminuted fractures of the ulnar head and neck
- Correction of a deformity of the radius should be undertaken before ulnar head replacement or at the time of the procedure in cases of distal radius malunion.
- Contraindications include the following:
  - History of sepsis
  - Lack of adequate periarticular soft tissues required for restoration of stability after implantation of the prosthesis

Nonoperative Treatment

- Judicious use of a splint, nonsteroidal anti-inflammatory medication, and a short course of physical therapy are alternative nonoperative modalities.

Alternative Surgical Options

- Various nonprosthetic distal ulna arthroplasties have been described that may result in pain and weak grip strength related to forearm instability, particularly in the higher-demand patient.
- The Darrach procedure involves resection of the distal 1 inch of ulnar head.
- The altered mechanical function and load transmission following resection arthroplasty lead to difficulty in treating those patients having a failed procedure.
- Complications including instability of the ulnar stump can result if the tissues are not balanced or if an excessive amount of distal ulna is resected.
- Hemiresection with interposition and the matched resection techniques are partial excision procedures (Fig. 13–21).

- The Suave-Kapandji procedure is performed by fusing the head of the ulna to the sigmoid notch and developing an ulnar pseudarthrosis more proximally for forearm rotation (Fig. 13–22).
- Radioulnar fusion or one bone forearm is the ultimate salvage procedure, resulting in no forearm rotation and a high complication rate.

Implant Selection

- Silastic implants initially were found to provide pain relief, but implant failure has caused the procedure to fall out of favor.
- Several metallic ulnar head prostheses are available
  - The uHead ulnar head component (Avanta, San Diego, CA) is a modular system available in different sizes (Fig. 13–23).

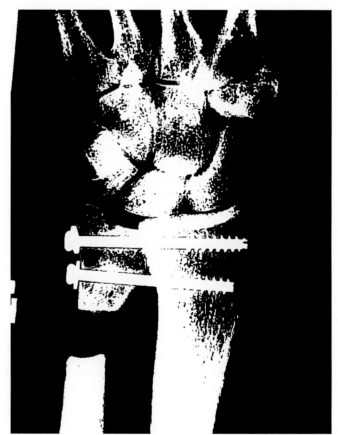

Figure 13–22: Suave-Kapandji procedure.
Patient treated with a Suave-Kapandji procedure for distal radioulnar joint arthrosis secondary to chronic instability from a radial shaft malunion. A segment of the distal ulnar shaft is removed to allow forearm rotation, and arthrodesis of the ulnar head to the sigmoid notch of the radius is performed with cannulated screws. (From Blazar P [2004]. Dislocations and instability. In: Beredjiklian PK, Bozentka DJ, eds. *Review of Hand Surgery*. Philadelphia: WB Saunders, p 150.)

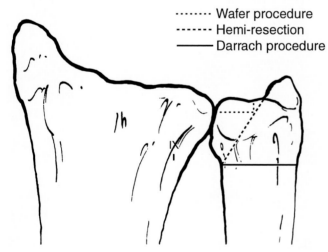

········· Wafer procedure
------- Hemi-resection
——— Darrach procedure

Figure 13–21: Distal ulna excision.
Surgical margins of distal ulna excision. (From Naidu S [2004]. Arthritis. In: Beredjiklian PK, Bozentka DJ, eds. *Review of Hand Surgery*. Philadelphia: WB Saunders, p 183.)

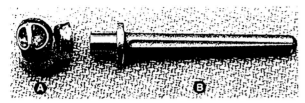

Figure 13–23: Ulnar head endoprosthesis.
Exploded view of an ulnar head endoprosthesis (Avanta Orthopedics) showing distal *(A)* and proximal *(B)* components. (From Sauerbier M, Hahn ME, Fujita M, et al. [2002]. Analysis of dynamic distal radioulnar convergence after ulnar head resection and endoprosthesis implantation. *J Hand Surg Am* 27:425-434.)

- Cement is considered for patients with rheumatoid arthritis, whereas a press fit is often used for patients with degenerative arthritis.
  - The E-centrix ulnar head prosthesis (Wright Medical, Arlington TN) is also a modular system.

Surgical Approach and Surgical Technique

- The approach depends on the specific prosthesis used.

- In general, a curvilinear dorsal ulnar incision is made. Care should be taken to protect the dorsal ulnar cutaneous nerve branch that lies distal to the ulnar styloid.
- An ulnarly based capsular-retinacular flap is elevated from the radius at the base of the fifth extensor compartment.
- The capsule and retinaculum with the extensor carpi ulnaris tendon are elevated from the dorsal TFCC and the distal ulna.
- The neck of the ulna is cut using an oscillating saw at a length according to the template.
- Any bone spurs from the sigmoid notch are removed, and the TFCC is inspected and repaired if required.
- The canal is reamed to the appropriate stem size.
- The trial stem and head are placed and are evaluated for providing adequate stability and length.
- The size of the head should be large enough for support but should not stretch the soft tissue repair.
- The length of the prosthesis should result in approximately 2 mm ulnar negative variance.
- The final stem is placed in the shaft.
  - The ulnar head replacement may require suturing of the distal soft tissues and TFCC through holes in the prosthesis.

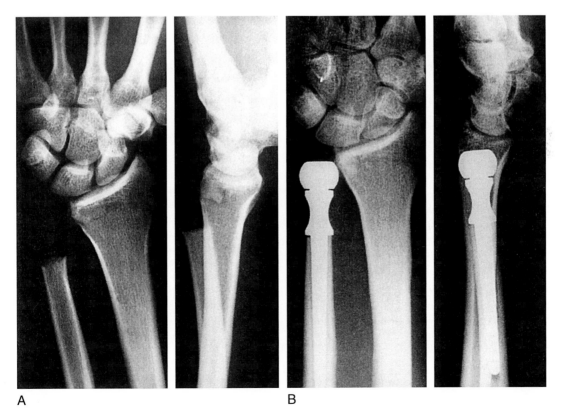

A   B

Figure 13–24: Results of ulnar head arthroplasty.
A, Radiographs showing the instability of the distal end of the ulna following ulnar head resection. **B,** Radiographs obtained 11 months after implantation of the ulnar head prosthesis demonstrate a 2-mm ulnar minus situation at the wrist level and a stable joint. (From van Schoonhoven J, Fernandez DL, Bowers WH, Herbert TJ [2000]. Salvage of failed resection arthroplasties of the distal radioulnar joint using a new ulnar head prosthesis. *J Hand Surg Am* 25:439-446.)

- The ulnar head is impacted on the neck of the stem.
- The capsule is repaired to the TFCC and radius in the appropriate tension for stability.

Postoperative Management

- An above-elbow splint is worn for 2 weeks
- The sutures are removed, and physical therapy is started allowing 30 degrees of supination and pronation to protect the soft tissue repair.
  - While the patient is not exercising, the wrist is protected in a sugar-tong or above-elbow ulnar gutter splint.
- The splint is discarded at 6 weeks, and the patient progresses to normal daily activities.
- Patients with inadequate soft tissues such as in rheumatoid arthritis may require immobilization for 6 weeks.

Results

- Few series in the literature have documented the results of metallic ulnar head replacements.
- Symptomatic improvement was noted in all patients reported by Von Schoonhoven and associates (Von Schoonhoven et al. 2000). In this series, 23 patients were treated with a mean follow-up of 27 months (Fig. 13–24).

Complications

- Recurrent instability and pain may follow ulnar head prosthesis implantation.
- Infection may require removal of the prosthesis.
- Early results of Von Schoonhoven and colleagues showed loosening of the stem in only 1 of 23 patients, and it may have been related to inappropriate sizing.

References

Adams BD (2004). Surgical management of the arthritic wrist. *Instr Course Lect* 53:41-45.
This is a review of procedures performed for the wrist affected by rheumatoid arthritis. Surgical procedures are discussed for end-stage wrist deformity to alleviate pain and to reduce progression of deformity at earlier stages. Available procedures including arthroscopic synovectomy, partial and complete arthrodesis, and implant arthroplasty are reviewed.

Adams BD (2000). Total wrist arthroplasty. *Semin Arthroplasty* 11:72-81.
A historical perspective of TWA is included with a literature review. A through description of the operative technique for the Universal Total Wrist implant arthroplasty is provided. The results with high patient satisfaction are discussed.

Carlson JR, Simmons BP (1998). Wrist arthrodesis after failed wrist implant arthroplasty. *J Hand Surg Am* 23:893-898.
The authors reviewed their experience in revising a wrist implant arthroplasty to an arthrodesis with a block graft of fresh-frozen allograft femoral head or iliac crest bone graft. Ten patients with 12 failed wrist implants required wrist arthrodesis, and an intramedullary Steinmann pin was used for fixation. Seven had wrist arthrodesis with a bulk allograft femoral head, 4 with an iliac crest

bone autograft, and 1 without a bone graft. Patients were followed for an average of 5 years. All patients went on to a fusion and were pain free. Complications included 1 patient with acute carpal tunnel syndrome, 2 patients with nonunions required secondary bone grafting procedures, and 2 patients who required revision of their intramedullary pins. The two patients with a nonunion had iliac crest bone graft for the initial arthrodesis. All the patients were satisfied.

Cobb TK, Beckenbaugh RD (1996). Biaxial total-wrist arthroplasty. *J Hand Surg Am* 21:1011–1021.
This is a review of 64 biaxial total wrist arthroplasties. Overall survival rate was 82% at 5 years. There were 11 failures, 8 of which were related to loosening of the distal implant.

Divelbiss BJ, Sollerman C, Adams BD (2002). Early results of the Universal Total Wrist arthroplasty in rheumatoid arthritis. *J Hand Surg Am* 27:195-204.
Twenty-two Universal Total Wrist prostheses (KMI, San Diego, CA) were implanted in 19 patients for the treatment of severe rheumatoid arthritis. Two-year follow-up results of 8 wrists and 1-year follow-up results of 14 wrists were reviewed. Total arcs of motion all improved postoperatively. Disabilities of the Arm, Shoulder, and Hand outcome scores improved 14 points at 1 year and 24 points at 2 years. Three patients (14%) with severe wrist laxity and highly active disease had unstable prosthesis requiring further treatment.

Fatti JF, Palmer AK, Mosher JF (1986). The long-term results of Swanson silicone rubber interpositional wrist arthroplasty. *J Hand Surg Am* 11:166-175.
Fifty-three Swanson silicone rubber interpositional wrist arthroplasties in 42 patients were reviewed. The most common operative indication was a painful wrist with rheumatoid arthritis; 90% of the wrists had significant pain relief in early follow-up. In the group of wrists followed-up for more than 2.5 years, only 61% had good or excellent results, with a reoperation rate of 25%. Complications included prosthetic breakage (9.4%), ulnar cap breakage (71%), and progressive radiographic deterioration (70%).

Fatti JF, Palmer AK, Greenky S, Mosher JF (1991). Long-term results of Swanson interpositional wrist arthroplasty: Part II. *J Hand Surg Am* 16:432-437.
This is a continuation of the previously published study in which 58 Swanson silicone interpositional wrist arthroplasties in 47 patients between 1974 and 1984 were reviewed. Thirty-nine of the original wrists were available for follow-up at an average of 5.8 years. Progressive deterioration of clinical results was noted. With a follow-up of less than 2.5 years, 75% had relief of pain. After a follow-up of 4.8 years, 67% had relief of pain. Finally, with an average follow-up of 5.8 years, only 51% had relief of pain. Cystic changes were noted in a significant proportion of the wrists radiographically, and silicone synovitis was documented histologically in several cases.

Grosland NM, Rogge RD, Adams BD (2004). Influence of articular geometry on prosthetic wrist stability. *Clin Orthop Relat Res* 421:134-142.
Ellipsoid and toroid articulations for total wrist prostheses were evaluated using computer modeling. An ellipsoid design was found to result in better capture and prosthetic stability than a toroid shape. An ellipsoid articulation also provides greater contact area through the available arc of motion. It was recommended that an ellipsoid design should be considered for TWA.

Lorei MP, Figgie MP, Ranawat CS, Inglis AE (1997). Failed total wrist arthroplasty: Analysis of failures and results of operative management. *Clin Orthop Relat Res* 342:84-93.

The authors reviewed a series of nine metal-on-polyethylene TWAs revised for failure. Causes of failure included sepsis in one patient, progressive wrist flexion contracture in two patients, and mechanical failure in six patients. Mechanical failure most commonly was related to loosening of the distal component in the metacarpal with dorsal perforation of the stem. The patient with an infected wrist was managed with resection arthroplasty. Follow-up averaged 3.3 years. The five patients undergoing arthrodesis were without pain, required one operation, and had wrists considered fused at an average of 4.8 months. The three patients treated with revision arthroplasty with custom trispheric components were pain-free, functional, and had no evidence of loosening. The authors concluded that a failed TWA could be salvaged successfully with either fusion or revision arthroplasty.

Menon J (1998). Universal Total Wrist implant: Experience with a carpal component fixed with three screws. *J Arthroplasty* 13:515-523.

Thirty-one patients (37 wrists) with pancarpal arthritis were treated with the Universal Total Wrist implant. The mean age of the patients was 58.1 years. There was a mean follow-up of 79.4 months (6.7 years), ranging from 48 to 120 months. Removal of the prosthesis was required in three patients because of infection and persistent dislocation. Patients with the other 34 wrists achieved excellent pain relief. Complications occurred in 12 cases (32%). The most common complication was dislocation.

Meuli HC (1997). Total wrist arthroplasty: Experience with a noncemented wrist prosthesis. *Clin Orthop Relat Res* 342:77-83.

Meuli reported his series of 38 Meuli prostheses implanted in 33 patients without cement. At an average of 5.5 year follow-up, there were 20 excellent results, 10 good, 2 fair, and 6 poor.

Murphy DM, Khoury JG, Imbriglia JE, Adams BD (2003). Comparison of arthroplasty and arthrodesis for the rheumatoid wrist. *J Hand Surg Am* 28:570-576.

The outcomes of wrist arthrodesis and arthroplasty in the treatment of rheumatoid arthritis were evaluated using validated outcome patient surveys. Forty-six patients with 51 operated wrists (24 arthrodeses and 27 arthroplasties) were reviewed with a follow-up of 1 to 5 years. The Disabilities of the Arm, Shoulder, and Hand inventory, the Patient-Rated Wrist Evaluation, and a questionnaire designed specifically for this study were used for outcome assessment. Although there were no statistical differences in the survey scores between the two groups, patients in the arthroplasty group reported a trend toward greater ease with personal hygiene and fastening buttons. The authors reported similar complication rates between the two groups with a 56% complication rate in the arthrodesis group (22% major, 35% minor) and a 52% complication rate in the arthroplasty group (11% major, 41% minor). It was concluded that the Disabilities of the Arm, Shoulder, and Hand inventory and the Patient-Rated Wrist Evaluation may not be designed to measure impairment related to the wrist in patients with generalized arthritis appropriately. The authors noted that patients with rheumatoid arthritis accommodate to wrist arthrodeses, although may prefer and obtain greater benefit from wrist arthroplasty.

Palmer AK, Werner FW, Murphy D, Glisson R (1985). Functional wrist motion: A biomechanical study. *J Hand Surg Am* 10:39-46.

The authors used a triaxial electrogoniometer to measure functional wrist motion in 10 normal subjects. The subjects performed 52 standardized tasks. The normal functional range of wrist motion was noted to be 5 degrees of flexion, 30 degrees of extension, 10 degrees of radial deviation, and 15 degrees of ulnar deviation.

Rizzo M, Beckenbaugh RD (2003). Results of biaxial total wrist arthroplasty with a modified (long) metacarpal stem. *J Hand Surg Am* 28:577-584.

The authors presented a retrospective review of 17 long-stem metacarpal components for the biaxial (DePuy Orthopedics, Inc., Warsaw, IN) TWA. Postoperatively, pain and grip strength improved significantly. Overall wrist range of motion improved, but a significant difference was found only in radial deviation. All the patients were satisfied. Four wrists showed evidence of radiographic lucency about the cement mantle, although no gross loosening or settling was noted. No failures were reported following a 6-year average (4-year minimum) follow-up. Complications included two cases of intraoperative third metacarpal fracture and one case of dorsal metacarpal component placement that did not affect the outcomes. It was concluded that the survivorship of the biaxial TWA with the long stem is favorable compared with the standard biaxial distal component.

Shepherd DE, Johnstone AJ (2002). Design considerations for a wrist implant. *Med Eng Phys* 24:641-650.

The anatomy and biomechanics of the normal wrist are reviewed. The various designs of current and prior wrist prostheses are discussed. The design factors for a successful wrist implant in the future are recommended not to attempt to recreate the natural wrist, but to permit a limited functional range of motion. A recommendation is given for different materials and methods of fixation of the wrist prosthetic joints to improve implant durability.

Volz RG (1984). Total wrist arthroplasty: A clinical review. *Clin Orthop Relat Res* 187:112-120.

Volz reported that the single most common problem with the semiconstrained total wrist prosthesis was ulnar deformity. A modification of the prosthesis was made to the original prosthesis to replicate the instant center of motion of the wrist more precisely.

Von Schoonhoven J, Fernandez DL, Bowers WH, Herbert TJ (2000). Salvage of failed resection arthroplasties of the distal radioulnar joint using a new ulnar head prosthesis. *J Hand Surg Am* 25:438-446.

This was a multicenter series of 23 patients undergoing ulnar head replacement for failed distal radioulnar arthroplasty with a mean follow-up of 27 months. All patients had improvements in pain. One patient was noted to have loosening of the stem likely related to improper sizing. One patient had the prosthesis removed for infection.

CHAPTER 14

Arthroplasty in the Joints of the Hand

Pedro K. Beredjiklian,* Virak Tan,† and Sanjiv Naidu‡

*MD, Assistant Professor, Department of Orthopaedic Surgery, University of Pennsylvania
School of Medicine, Philadelphia, PA
†MD, Associate Professor, Department of Orthopaedics, University of Medicine and
Dentistry of New Jersey, Newark, NJ
‡MD, Professor, Orthopaedic Surgery and Rehabilitation, Penn State College of Medicine,
Hershey, PA

Distal Interphalangeal Joint

Introduction

- The distal interphalangeal (DIP) joint is most often affected by degenerative conditions, but it can also be affected in patients with inflammatory arthritis.
- It is the most common joint of the hand affected by osteoarthritis.
- In spite of significant degenerative changes, the DIP joint can remain only mildly symptomatic.
- Furthermore, loss of motion is very well tolerated from a functional standpoint.
  - As a result, arthrodesis is generally the procedure of choice for patients with painful degenerative changes of the DIP joint.
  - Nevertheless, a silicone prosthetic implant is available if motion retention is necessary.

Anatomy

- The DIP joint is a uniaxial hinge joint.
- The major soft tissue constraints are the capsule and the terminal extensor tendon dorsally, the collateral ligaments laterally, and the volar plate and flexor digitorum profundus tendon (or flexor pollicis longus tendon in the thumb) volarly (Fig. 14–1).
- The primary stability of the joint is conferred by articular congruity and the collateral ligaments and volar plate.

- The collateral ligaments arise from fossae on the lateral aspect of the middle phalangeal heads and insert into the volar third of the distal phalangeal base (proper collateral ligament) and the volar plate (accessory collateral ligament) (Fig. 14–2).
- The collateral ligaments are the primary restraints to radial and ulnar deviation of the joint.

Etiology of Degenerative Changes

- The DIP joints experience the greatest amount of longitudinal stresses of any joints in the hand.
- The most common cause of degeneration of the DIP joint is primary osteoarthritis.
- Degenerative changes at the DIP joints can also have several other possible causes, including trauma and systemic inflammatory conditions such as rheumatoid arthritis.

Evaluation

- Patients with symptomatic arthritis of the DIP joints often describe pain diffusely about the tip of the fingers.
- These symptoms often have an insidious onset and are frequently made worse with hand use, particularly pinching and gripping activities.
- Patients may relate a history of trauma.
- On physical examination, swelling with localized tenderness of the joints is common.
  - Osteoarthritis is characterized by enlargement of the joint (Heberden's nodes) (Fig. 14–3).

Figure 14–1: Distal interphalangeal joint. Midsagittal representation of the distal interphalangeal joint.

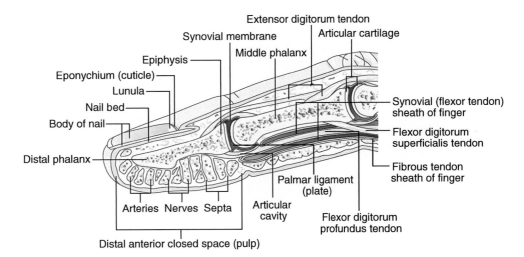

Extensor digitorum tendon
Synovial membrane
Articular cartilage
Middle phalanx
Epiphysis
Eponychium (cuticle)
Lunula
Nail bed
Body of nail
Distal phalanx
Synovial (flexor tendon) sheath of finger
Flexor digitorum superficialis tendon
Fibrous tendon sheath of finger
Arteries Nerves Septa
Articular cavity
Palmar ligament (plate)
Flexor digitorum profundus tendon
Distal anterior closed space (pulp)

- Nodular involvement and bone spurs lead to formation of cysts termed *mucous cysts* that are often associated with an osteophyte.
- Nail plate involvement may occur with loss of normal gloss, splitting, and deformity.
- Grip and pinch strength is often noted to be decreased.
- Radiographic assessment includes the following:
  - Plain radiographs should include posteroanterior, lateral, and oblique views of each finger.

- These radiographs typically reveal the presence of joint narrowing, osteophyte formation, and subchondral cyst formation (Fig. 14–4).
- Further diagnostic studies are often unnecessary.

Treatment

- Initial treatment should include nonoperative modalities.
  - Custom-molded Orthoplast fingertip splints maintaining the DIP joint in extension can be of benefit.

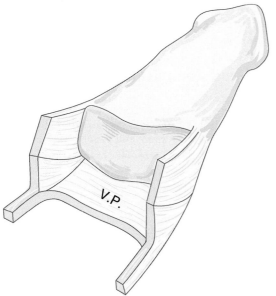

Figure 14–2: Interphalangeal joint.
Schematic of an interphalangeal joint without the more proximal phalanx, revealing the volar plate *(V.P.)* and the collateral ligaments. (From Glickel S, Barron AO, Eaton RG [1999]. Dislocations and ligament injuries in the digits. In: Green DP, Hotchkiss RN, Pederson WC, eds. *Operative Hand Surgery,* 4th ed. New York: Churchill Livingstone.)

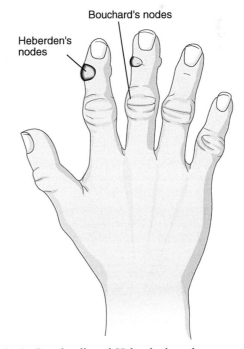

Bouchard's nodes
Heberden's nodes

Figure 14–3: Bouchard's and Heberden's nodes.
Clinical appearance of Bouchard's nodes.

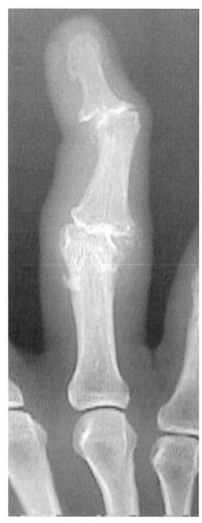

Figure 14–4: Osteoarthritis of the distal and proximal interphalangeal joints of the long finger.
Note the destruction of the articular surface and osteophyte formation. (From Naidu S [2004]. Arthritis. In: Beredjiklian PK, Bozentka DJ, eds. *Review of Hand Surgery.* Philadelphia: WB Saunders, 2004, p 174.)

- Modification of activities, nonsteroidal anti-inflammatory medications, and corticosteroid injections can also be helpful in providing pain relief.
- Surgical intervention should be considered for those patients with severe pain and functional disability refractory to nonoperative treatment.

Arthrodesis

- Fusion is the mainstay of treatment for patients with degenerative changes at the DIP joint.
- Various techniques have been used for arthrodesis, including tension band wire, Kirschner wires, interosseous 90-90 wires, and intramedullary Herbert screws (Fig. 14–5).

Technique

- The joint is approached dorsally via an H- or Y-shaped incision, with care taken to preserve the germinal matrix of the nail bed.
- The terminal extensor tendon is identified and is bisected sharply at or just proximal to the level of the joint.
- The collateral ligament origin and insertions are elevated sharply off the middle and distal phalanges, respectively.
- The volar plate insertion is elevated off the distal phalanx.
- The articular surface is denuded to subchondral bone using a curette, and all prominent osteophytes are removed (Fig. 14–6).
- The DIP joint is fused in approximately 0 to 10 degrees of flexion.
- The interphalangeal joint of the thumb can be fused at 15 to 20 degrees of flexion.
- The extensor tendon and skin are repaired.
- Postoperatively, the joint is maintained in a splint until bony consolidation is achieved.

Arthroplasty

- This procedure is rarely performed at the DIP joint.
- Indications may include situations in which motion at the DIP joint is critical for function (e.g., in musicians).
- The literature supports similar function and pain relief from arthroplasty as compared with arthrodesis.
- The Swanson double-stemmed silicone implant is most commonly used in clinical practice.
- The surgical approach is similar to the technique described earlier for arthrodesis (Fig. 14–7).
- The joint is maintained in extension for 8 weeks postoperatively.

Results and Complications

Arthrodesis

- DIP joint fusion is associated with a high degree of pain relief, functional restoration, and patient satisfaction.
- Nonunion is the most common complication of DIP joint arthrodesis.
  - The incidence ranges from 0% to 20%
  - Herbert screw fixation has the highest union rate.
  - Poor bone stock is the major reason for DIP joint nonunion after attempted arthrodesis.
- Other complications include wound breakdown, hardware prominence, and pin tract infections.

Arthroplasty

- Because it is rarely performed at the DIP joint, data in the literature regarding results of this procedure are scarce.
- Published reports suggest that the procedure is effective in eliminating pain while retaining motion and stability.
  - An average arc of motion of approximately 30 degrees has been described in these patients.

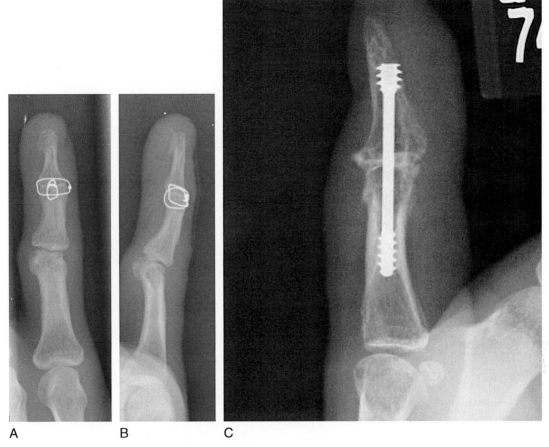

A B C

Figure 14–5: Distal interphalangeal joint arthrodesis.
Anteroposterior (**A**) and lateral (**B**) radiographs of a patient treated with distal interphalangeal joint arthrodesis using 90-90 cerclage wiring. **C**, Arthrodesis of the interphalangeal joint of the thumb with a compression (Herbert) screw. (From Naidu S [2004]. Arthritis. In: Beredjiklian PK, Bozentka DJ, eds. *Review of Hand Surgery.* Philadelphia: WB Saunders, 2004, p 173.)

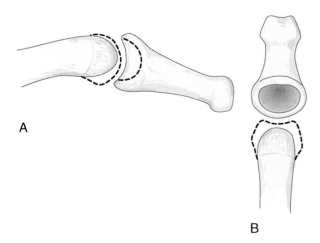

A

B

Figure 14–6: Distal interphalangeal joint arthrodesis.
A and B, Preparation of articular surfaces for distal interphalangeal joint arthrodesis.

- Authors have reported an average extension lag measuring 13 degrees.
- Complications include instability, wound breakdown, and fracture of the prosthesis.

Proximal Interphalangeal Joint

Introduction

- The proximal interphalangeal (PIP) joint is commonly affected by inflammatory arthritides, but it can also be affected in patients with degenerative or post-traumatic conditions.
  - In patients with inflammatory processes, soft tissue imbalances can occur in addition to the articular surface degeneration.
  - Common deformities include boutonnière and swan-neck deformities.
  - These soft tissue disturbances must be corrected at the time of joint reconstruction.

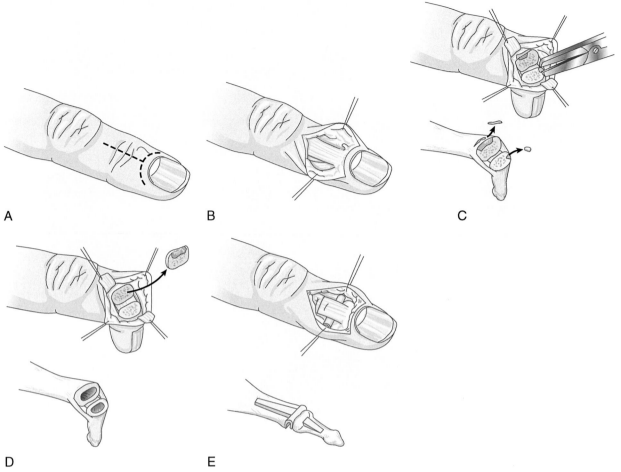

A   B   C

D   E

Figure 14–7: Distal interphalangeal joint arthrodesis.
A to E, Surgical approach for arthrodesis or arthroplasty of the distal interphalangeal joint.

- In contrast to the DIP joint, loss of motion at the PIP joint is poorly tolerated from a functional standpoint.
  - Stiffness at the PIP joint inhibits the patient's ability to make a fist and leads to significant weakness and disability.
  - As a result, reconstructive procedures allowing for retention of motion are ideal.
  - Arthrodesis, although very effective in eliminating the symptoms of pain, is less than ideal because of the inherent loss of motion.
- Silicone prosthetic implants are available and provide adequate pain relief and good functional outcomes and patient satisfaction.
  - Because of concerns with lack of lateral stability of these implants, prosthetic replacement has been favored for the middle fingers (long, ring), whereas arthrodesis has been recommended for the border digits, particularly the index finger.
  - In patients with multiple joint involvement resulting from a systemic inflammatory process, PIP joint arthrodesis in combination with metacarpophalangeal (MP) joint silicone arthroplasty is generally favored.

- Implant arthroplasty for the PIP joint is more commonly performed for an isolated digital degenerative process in which preservation of motion is of critical importance.
- Newer-generation, minimally constrained total joint replacements have generated interest and are in the process of being evaluated for widespread clinical use

Anatomy

- The base of the middle phalanx has a smooth facet to articulate with the proximal phalangeal head (Fig. 14–8).
- The head of the proximal phalanx is pulley shaped to form the hinge joint.
  - The PIP joint is a uniaxial hinge joint.
- The major soft tissue constraints are the capsule and the central slip dorsally, the collateral ligaments laterally, and the volar plate and flexor tendons volarly.
- The primary stability of the joint is conferred by articular congruity and the collateral ligaments and volar plate.
- The collateral ligaments arise from fossae on the lateral aspect of the proximal phalangeal head and insert into the volar aspect of the middle phalangeal base

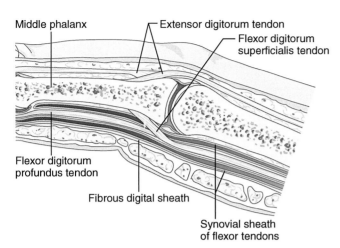

Figure 14–8: Proximal interphalangeal joint.
Midsagittal representation of the proximal interphalangeal joint.

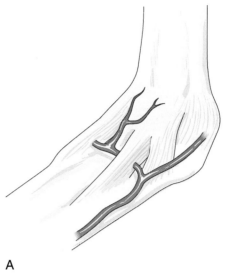

A

(proper collateral ligament) and the volar plate (accessory collateral ligament).
  • The collateral ligaments are the primary restraints to radial and ulnar deviation of the joint.
• *Check-rein ligaments* are fibrous connections between the proximal aspect of the volar plate and the volar bony ridges of the proximal phalanx in the PIP joint (Fig. 14–9).
  • These are implicated in flexion contractures of the PIP joint.

Evaluation

• Patients with symptomatic arthritis of the PIP joints often describe pain directly over the affected area.
• These symptoms often have an insidious onset and are frequently made worse with hand use, particularly lifting and gripping activities.
• On examination, swelling with localized tenderness of the joints is common.
  • Osteoarthritis is characterized by enlargement of the joint (Bouchard's nodes) (see Fig. 14–3).
  • Bone spurs lead to formation of cysts termed *mucous cysts* that are often associated with an osteophyte.
• Grip strength is often noted to be decreased.
• Significant loss of motion of the digits occurs, with significant flexion contractures and loss of composite flexion of the fingers.
• Radiographic assessment includes the following:
  • Plain radiographs should include posteroanterior, lateral, and oblique views of each finger.
  • These radiographs typically reveal the presence of joint narrowing, osteophyte formation, and subchondral cyst formation (Fig. 14–10).
• Assessment of deformities of adjacent joints is vital in the evaluation of these patients
• In patients with systemic inflammatory processes and multiple joint involvement, the timing of hand surgery,

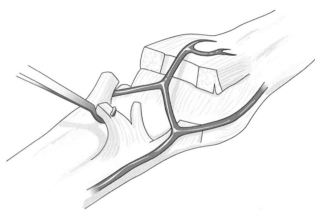

B

Figure 14–9: Check-rein pathologic bands.
A, The check-reins attach proximally to the assembly line and distally to the volar plate on both the radial and ulnar sides. The transverse communicating vessels traverse the collagen band approximately 2 mm proximal to the volar plate.
B, Complete excision of the check-reins often requires resection dorsal as well as volar to the transverse communicating vessels. These vessels should be preserved. (From Watson HK, Weinzweig J [1999]. Stiff joints. In: Green DP, Hotchkiss RN, Pederson WC, eds. *Operative Hand Surgery,* 4th ed. New York: Churchill Livingstone, p 554.)

if indicated, must also be staged with respect to other planned surgical procedures.
  • Correction of wrist and MP joint deformities should take place before the treatment of the PIP joints.
• Cervical spine instability and neural impairment are common in patients with inflammatory arthritis.
• Several other factors must also be evaluated, particularly in patients with systemic inflammatory processes.
  • Evaluations of the shoulder and elbow are critical in the assessment of the upper extremity.

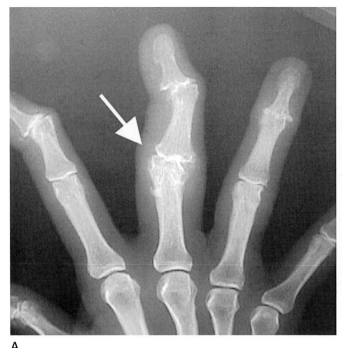

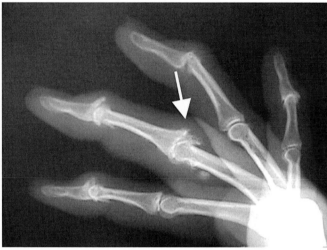

A   B

Figure 14–10: Osteoarthritis of the proximal interphalangeal joint.
Anteroposterior **(A)** and lateral **(B)** radiographs revealing a severely osteoarthritic proximal interphalangeal joint with loss of joint space and osteophyte formation *(arrows)*.

- In addition, careful assessment of any wrist joint deformity caused by the inflammatory process must be elicited.
  - Distal radioulnar joint instability can result in attritional extensor tendon ruptures to the ulnar digits.
- Correction of this deformity can minimize the incidence of extensor tendon insufficiency.
- *Swan-neck deformities* of the PIP joints are common in patients with inflammatory arthritis and occur in approximately 15% of patients.
  - This deformity is characterized by hyperextension of the PIP joint and flexion of the DIP joint (Fig. 14–11).
  - The functional loss resulting from this deformity is directly related to the loss of PIP joint motion.
  - The imbalance between the digital joints can originate at any of the three digital articulations and can result in a reciprocal deformity at the adjacent joints.
  - The PIP joint is often the site of primary deformity.
    - Loss of the static (volar plate, collateral ligaments) and dynamic (flexor digitorum superficialis tendon) restraints resulting from synovial proliferation allow the extensor mechanism to act unopposed and lead to PIP joint hyperextension.
    - With progression of PIP joint hyperextension, a reciprocal DIP joint flexion deformity can develop.
    - Because the extensor mechanisms of the PIP and DIP joints are linked, PIP joint hyperextension will result in a functional lengthening of the extensor mechanism.

- This relative lengthening creates an extension lag at the DIP joint. Decreased extension force of the DIP joint allows the flexor digitorum profundus to flex the DIP joint unopposed, resulting in a flexion (mallet) deformity of the DIP joint.
- The DIP joint can also be the site of initial involvement.
  - Because the extensor mechanism no longer extends the distal joint, the entire extensor tension force is concentrated on the PIP joint.
  - As the intrinsic palmar restraints of the PIP joint (volar plate and collateral ligaments) become attenuated, the increased extensor tension on the joint will result in a PIP hyperextension deformity.
- Swan-neck deformities have been classified by Nalebuf:
  - Type I: This deformity is characterized by full PIP joint flexibility in all positions, independent of MP joint position.
  - Type II: Type II deformities are characterized by limited PIP joint flexion dependent on MP joint position.
    - The limitation of motion is directly related to intrinsic muscle tightness.
    - The pattern of PIP joint motion limitation is typical of digits affected with intrinsic tightness: With the MP joint in extension, passive flexion of the PIP joint is limited; when the MP joint is in flexion, passive flexion in the PIP joint is increased.

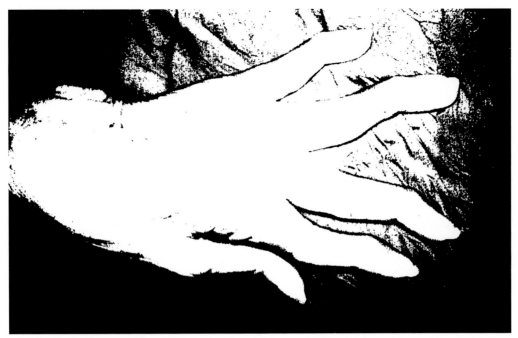

Figure 14–11: Rheumatoid arthritis.
This patient with rheumatoid arthritis displays swan-neck deformities of multiple digits. (From Naidu S [2004]. Arthritis. In: Beredjiklian PK, Bozentka DJ, eds. *Review of Hand Surgery.* Philadelphia: WB Saunders, 2004, p 183.)

- Type III: These deformities are characterized by limitation of PIP joint flexion independent of the position of the MP joint.
- Type IV: These deformities are characterized by a fixed limitation of PIP joint flexion with associated destruction of the articular surfaces.

- *Boutonnière deformities* are also common in patients with inflammatory arthritis, occurring in 36% of cases.
  - This deformity is characterized by flexion of the PIP joint and hyperextension of the DIP joint (Fig. 14–12).
  - The functional loss resulting from this deformity is related to the loss of PIP joint motion.

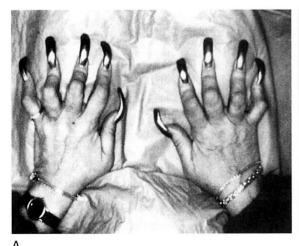
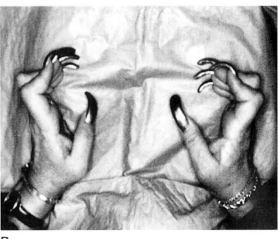

A   B

Figure 14–12: Boutonnière deformities in rheumatoid arthritis.
A and **B,** Clinical photographs of a patient with severe bilateral boutonnière deformities of all digits secondary to rheumatoid arthritis. Note the flexion deformities of the proximal interphalangeal joints and hyperextension of the distal interphalangeal joints. (From Deirmengian CA, Beredjiklian PK [2000]. Boutonniere deformities in rheumatoid arthritis. *Semin Arthroplasty* 11:115-120.)

- DIP joint hyperextension limits active digital flexion, another important factor in the functional deficit displayed by patients affected with this pathologic process.
- The boutonnière deformity always results from pathologic processes at the PIP joint.
- The joint capsule, the central slip of the extensor mechanism, and the transverse retinacular and triangular ligaments become attenuated and weakened as a result of the inflammatory process.
- The laxity of the soft tissue restraints about the joint eventually allows migration of the lateral bands volar to the axis of rotation of PIP joint motion.
- As the lateral bands migrate to this new position, the vector of force transmission is changed, and they act to flex rather than extend the PIP joint.
- In addition to the deformity at the PIP joint, the shift in the line of pull of the extensor mechanism creates hyperextension of the DIP joint.
- Boutonnière deformities have been classified by Nalebuf:
  - Stage I: In this type of deformity, the flexion posture of the PIP joint is passively correctable.
  - Stage II: The flexion deformity of the PIP joint is not passively correctable, but the articular cartilage and joint surface remain intact.
  - Stage III: This stage is characterized by a fixed flexion contracture of the PIP joint that cannot be extended passively. In addition, incongruity of the articular surface and malalignment of the PIP articular segment secondary to the degenerative process often contribute to the fixed deformity.

Treatment

- Initial treatment should include nonoperative modalities.
  - Custom-molded Orthoplast fingertip splints maintaining the PIP joint at rest can be of benefit.
  - Nonsteroidal anti-inflammatory medications and corticosteroid injections can also be helpful in providing pain relief.
- Patients in whom nonoperative treatment fails and who experience significant functional disability are candidates for surgical treatment.

Arthrodesis

- Fusion is the mainstay of treatment for patients with the following:
  - Inflammatory arthritis involving multiple joints requiring MP joint arthroplasty
  - Any arthritic process involving the PIP joint of the index finger
- Various techniques have been used for arthrodesis, including tension band wires, Kirschner wires, interosseous 90-90 wires, compression screws, and miniplates and screws (Fig. 14-13).

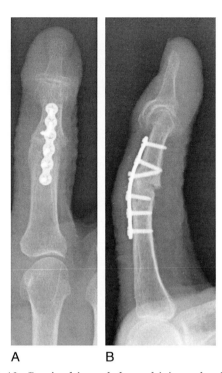

A   B

Figure 14-13: Proximal interphalangeal joint arthrodesis. Anteroposterior (**A**) and lateral (**B**) radiographs of a proximal interphalangeal joint after arthrodesis with a mini-titanium plate and screws.

Technique

- The PIP joint is accessed through a curvilinear or transverse dorsal approach (Fig. 14-14).
- The extensor mechanism is identified, and the central slip is bisected transversely proximal to the PIP joint.
- The collateral ligaments are exposed and released from their origin on the proximal phalangeal neck with a No. 69 Beaver blade.
- A small rongeur can be used to remove proliferative synovium, thus enhancing articular exposure.
- At this point, the PIP joint is flexed maximally, and an osteotomy is used to remove the distal end of the proximal phalanx.
- The osteotomy is made at an angle to allow eventual fixation of the joint in flexion.
- The functional angle of PIP joint fixation varies incrementally in a radial-ulnar direction, from 25 degrees at the index finger to 45 degrees at the small finger (Table 14-1).
- Using a rongeur and curettes, the articular cartilage is removed from the base of the middle phalanx until subchondral bone is identified.
- Fixation can be established and checked fluoroscopically.
- Postoperatively, a molded external splint is used to protect the patient until radiographs reveal evidence of consolidation, usually by 6 weeks.

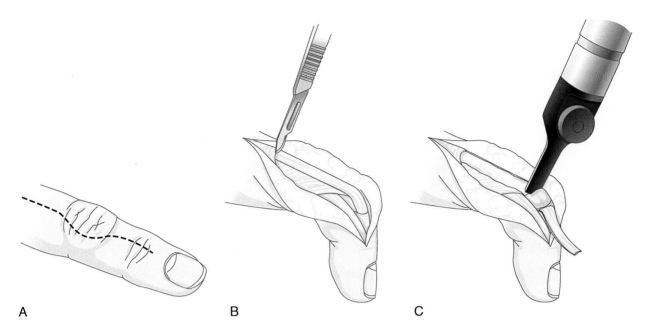

A   B   C

Figure 14–14: Proximal interphalangeal joint.
A to C, Surgical approach to the proximal interphalangeal joint.

Arthroplasty

Implant Designs

- Flexible silicone rubber
  - The flexible silicone rubber implants used for PIP joint arthroplasty differ from other prostheses commonly used in the larger joints.
  - Silicone rubber implants serve as dynamic spacers to maintain the joint alignment following resection of the joint.
  - Adequate soft tissue balance is critical for the success for the surgical procedure and should be achieved at the time of arthroplasty to improve outcomes.

Table 14–1	Optimal Position for Arthrodesis
DIP	10–20 degrees of flexion
PIP	30–45 degrees of flexion, cascading from the index to the small fingers in 5-degree increments
Thumb MP	15 degrees of flexion
	10 degrees of pronation
Thumb CMC	30–40 degrees of palmar abduction
	35 degrees of radial abduction
	15 degrees of pronation
Wrist	10 degrees of extension
	Neutral deviation (one side should be in neutral extension in bilateral cases)

DIP, distal interphalangeal; CMC, carpometacarpal; MP, metacarpophalangeal; PIP, proximal interphalangeal.
From Naidu S (2004). Arthritis. In: Beredjiklian PK, Bozentka DJ, eds. *Review of Hand Surgery.* Philadelphia: WB Saunders, p 173.

- The silicone implant design developed by Swanson is the most commonly used and the one with the greatest clinical experience.
- Swanson silicone implant arthroplasty technique
  - The PIP joint is accessed through a curvilinear dorsal approach with preservation of the dorsal veins.
  - Lateral and volar approaches for silicone arthroplasty have been described, but the dorsal approach remains the most commonly performed.
  - The extensor mechanism and central slip are identified, and the central slip is bisected transversely proximal to the PIP joint, to resect attenuated tendon tissue.
  - The collateral ligament origins on the proximal phalangeal neck are released subperiosteally from their origin on the proximal phalanx and are preserved for reattachment.
  - The distal aspect of the proximal phalangeal neck is excised with an osteotome.
  - The articular surface of the middle phalanx is denuded to subchondral bone with a curette.
  - The medullary canals of the phalanges are accessed using a curette, and the medullary canals are incrementally reamed by hand until adequate fit is achieved.
  - The implants are then placed in position using smooth forceps without manually handling the prosthetic implants.
  - Once the implants are placed, the collateral ligaments are reattached to the proximal phalanx using nonabsorbable sutures placed through the drill holes on the bone.
  - The central slip is advanced and repaired using 4-0 braided absorbable suture.

- In cases with severe central slip attenuation, a reconstruction of the central slip with one of the adjacent lateral bands (Matev procedure) should be performed.
- If DIP joint hyperextension remains following implant placement, a tenotomy of the terminal tendon can be performed.
- A splint holding the digits in full extension is applied.
- Active and passive range-of-motion exercises are started 1 week postoperatively.
- Custom-made static PIP extension splints are fabricated by a therapist and should be worn at all times (between therapy sessions) for 6 weeks following surgery.
- A protocol of night splinting is then started and is maintained for 3 to 6 months following the procedure.
- Minimally constrained designs
  - Minimally constrained designs have generated recent interest to address the limitations of large amount of bone resection required, loosening, osteolysis, and longevity of the silicone implants.

- Conservation of periarticular bone allows for the preservation of ligamentous structures and thereby confers added stability to these implants.
- These implants behave as true joint replacements, in contrast to the silicone implants, which act primarily as spacers.
- Available implants include pyrolytic carbon implants and hybrid implants consisting of a chromium-cobalt alloy proximal component and an ultrahigh-molecular-weight polyethylene component distally (Fig. 14–15).
- Widespread clinical experience is limited, and the use of these implants is primarily investigative.

Results

- Initial treatment should include nonoperative modalities.
- The Swanson silicone implant is the most widely studied prosthesis for reconstruction of the PIP joint, mostly in patients with rheumatoid arthritis.
  - In one study, pain was absent in 67% of joints at an average follow-up of 5.8 years. Implant survivorship

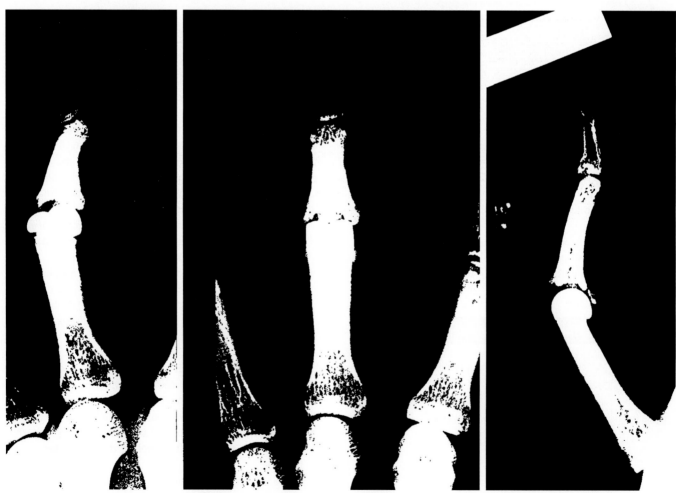

Figure 14–15: Proximal interphalangeal joint arthroplasty.
Radiographs demonstrate proper implantation of the proximal interphalangeal surface replacement prosthesis. (From Berger RA, Beckenbaugh RD, Linscheid RL [1999]. Arthroplasty in the hand and wrist. In: Green DP, Hotchkiss RN, Pederson WC, eds. *Operative Hand Surgery,* 4th ed. New York: Churchill Livingstone, p 154.)

was 81% at 9 years. The mean postoperative arc of motion was 29 degrees, compared with a preoperative mean of 38 degrees. The patients in this series experienced a minimal amount of complications.
- In a similar study, the authors reported on 69 silicone spacers; 48 underwent the procedure for degenerative changes. At a mean follow-up of 3.4 years:
  - Mean range of motion was 46 degrees after surgery compared with 44 degrees preoperatively.
  - Pain relief was obtained in 67 of 69 fingers.
  - Twelve complications, including loosening and infection, were reported in this group.
  - Five of the implants had fractured at latest follow-up.

Metacarpophalangeal Joint

Introduction

- MP joint arthroplasty is the most commonly performed and successful joint replacement surgical procedure of the hand.
- Although MP joint replacement is occasionally performed for osteoarthritic joints, most arthroplasties performed are for rheumatoid arthritis and other inflammatory arthropathies.
- The MP joint is essential for proper finger function and is the most common area of involvement in the rheumatoid hand.
- A thorough understanding of the anatomy, pathoanatomy, and pathomechanics of the MP joint is a prerequisite to the evaluation and treatment of any patient.
- Follow-up studies reveal that these patients experience significant functional improvement and correction of deformity following surgical intervention, although long-term follow-up reveals a decrease in the rate of successful results.
- MP joint arthroplasty is associated with a high degree of patient satisfaction.

Anatomy

- The normal MP joint is a diarthrodial, condylar-type joint that allows flexion, extension, radial and ulnar deviation, and circumduction (Fig. 14–16).
- The metacarpal head is asymmetric in both the coronal and sagittal planes.
- The radial condyle of the metacarpal head is larger than the ulnar condyle, and this causes the metacarpal head to slope ulnarly and proximally in the coronal plane, particularly in the index and long metacarpals.
- The metacarpal head has a longer and broader surface volarly compared with dorsally.
  - This shape of the metacarpal head accounts for the cam effect, which tightens the collateral ligaments with flexion of the joint (Fig. 14–17).

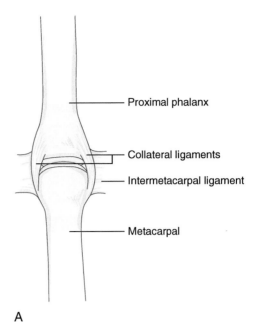

A

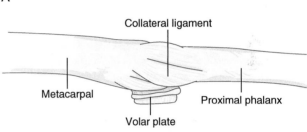

B

Figure 14–16: Metacarpophalangeal joint.
A and B, Bony and ligamentous anatomy of the metacarpophalangeal joint.

- The anatomic contour of the articular segment results in a mobile center of rotation for the MP joint, which moves volarly with flexion.
- The normal synovial membrane of the MP joint is attached around the periphery of the articular cartilage with volar and dorsal synovial reflections.
- The synovial fold is largest dorsally on the neck of the metacarpal.
- The volar plate supports the MP joint volarly.
  - The membranous portion of the volar plate attaches to the metacarpal neck and has more laxity compared with the distal insertion.
  - The cartilaginous portion of the volar plate is distal and attaches firmly to the base of the proximal phalanx.
  - The volar plates of the adjacent digits are interconnected by the fibers of the deep intermetacarpal ligament.
- The radial and ulnar collateral ligaments reinforce the MP joint.
  - These ligaments lie dorsal to the center of rotation of the MP joint, traversing from the metacarpal head dorsally to the base of the proximal phalanx volarly.

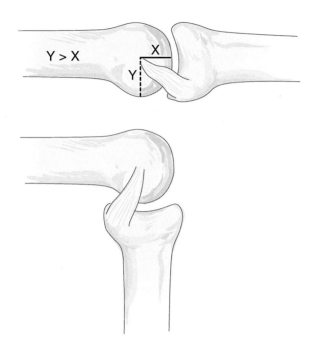

Figure 14–17: Metacarpophalangeal joint.
The distance from the center of rotation of the metacarpal head to the articular surface of the metacarpophalangeal joint is greatest at the most volar aspect of the joint *(Y)* and smallest at the most distal aspect of the head *(X)*. For this reason, the collateral ligaments are relaxed in full extension but become taut with metacarpophalangeal joint flexion. (From Monaghan BA [2004]. Anatomy. In: Beredjiklian PK, Bozentka DJ, eds. *Review of Hand Surgery.* Philadelphia: WB Saunders, p 4.)

- There is laxity in the ligaments when the joint is extended.
- The ligaments become taut when the joint is flexed because they lie on the dorsal aspect of the central axis.
- In addition, the shape of the metacarpal head also contributes to the tightness in flexion.
- The ulnar collateral ligament is more parallel with the longitudinal axis of the index finger compared with the radial collateral ligament, which lies in a more oblique fashion.
- When the joint is flexed, supination of the finger unwinds the radial collateral ligament allowing the ligament to run a less oblique course.
- Therefore, the index and long fingers allow more ulnar deviation of the MP joint with the joint in flexion and supination. The accessory collateral ligaments lie volar to the radial and ulnar collateral ligaments.
- They extend from the collateral ligament at the metacarpal head to the volar plate and are believed to be stabilizers of the volar plate.
- The extensor mechanism extends the MP joint through the sagittal bands and has variable attachments to the proximal phalanx through the dorsal capsule (Fig. 14–18).
  - The ulnar sagittal bands are considered to be stronger and denser than on the radial side.

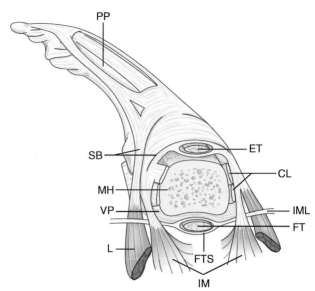

Figure 14–18: Metacarpophalangeal joint.
Normal anatomy of the metacarpophalangeal joint. *CL,* collateral ligament; *ET,* extensor tendon; *FT,* flexor tendon; *FTS,* flexor tendon sheath; *IM,* interosseous muscle or tendon; *IML,* intermetacarpal ligament; *L,* lumbrical; *MH,* metacarpal head; *PP,* proximal phalanx; *SB,* sagittal band; *VP,* volar plate. (From Wilson RL, Carlblom ER [1989]. The rheumatoid metacarpophalangeal joint. *Hand Clin* 5:223-237.)

- The intrinsic musculature provides flexion, abduction, and adduction of the MP joints.
- The dorsal interossei, with the exception of the third, have superficial and deep muscle bellies.
  - In general, the superficial belly becomes the medial tendon, which travels deep to the sagittal band and inserts onto the lateral tubercle of the proximal phalanx.
  - The deep muscle belly becomes the lateral tendon, which continues to form the lateral band.
  - The three volar interossei do not have separate muscle bellies.
  - They insert almost exclusively through the lateral band on the adductor side of the index, ring, and small fingers.
- The normal range of motion of the MP joint is from neutral to 90 degrees of flexion, although many individuals display hyperextension ($\leq \sim 20$ degrees).
- Some radial and ulnar deviation is present at the MP joint, which is decreased with flexion of the joint and the associated tightening of the collateral ligaments.

Evaluation

- MP joints in patients with rheumatoid arthritis typically assume a position of flexion and ulnar deviation (Fig. 14–19).
  - The rheumatoid process cause an imbalance of static and dynamic forces across the MP joint that leads to deformities.
  - Factors normally acting on the hand that have been implicated include gravitational pull on the fingers,

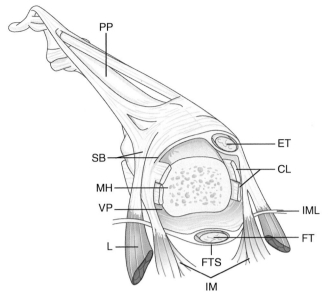

Figure 14–19: Metacarpophalangeal joint in rheumatoid arthritis. Metacarpophalangeal joint deformities from rheumatoid arthritis. *CL,* collateral ligament; *ET,* extensor tendon; *FT,* flexor tendon; *FTS,* flexor tendon sheath; *IM,* interosseous muscle or tendon; *IML,* intermetacarpal ligament; *L,* lumbrical; *MH,* metacarpal head; *PP,* proximal phalanx; *SB,* sagittal band; *VP,* volar plate. (From Wilson RL, Carlblom ER [1989]. The rheumatoid metacarpophalangeal joint. *Hand Clin* 5:223-237.)

force exerted on the radial side of the index finger by the thumb during pinch, and ulnar deviation of the fingers in power grip.
- Rheumatoid synovitis leads to destructive changes of the bone, particularly in the areas of synovial attachment.
- Erosive changes and softening of the metacarpal head prevent effective support for the proximal phalanx, thereby causing a static imbalance in the joint
  - Synovitic MP joint distension stretches the accessory collateral ligaments and the membranous portion of the volar plate and causes the proximal portion of the flexor sheath to be displaced from the midline of the MP joint.
  - In turn, the flexor tendons and flexor sheath shift ulnarly and volarly.
  - Normally, the volar forces of the flexor tendons are transmitted to the MP joint through the collateral ligaments, but the abnormal forces produced by the displaced flexor tendons pull the proximal phalanx volarly and ulnarward and contribute to deformities of the MP joint.
- Distension of the MP joint and direct synovial invasion also causes attenuation of the sagittal bands and deep fibers of the joint capsule.
  - This allows the extensor tendon to subluxate ulnarly into the intermetacarpal sulcus and causes a pull in the ulnar direction.
- Subluxation or rupture of the extensor mechanism allows an unopposed flexion force of the intrinsic and flexor tendon and results in volar subluxation of the proximal phalanx.

- Rheumatoid synovitis also produces diffuse changes in the interosseous muscles.
- These intrinsic muscles become contracted as a result of perivascular round cell infiltration, increased collagen deposition, and muscle fiber degeneration.
- Without the normal dorsal support of the proximal phalanx through the extensor tendons and collateral ligaments, the interosseous muscle contractures also lead to a volarly directed force on the MP joint, again contributing to volar subluxation.
- In addition to understanding the pathoanatomy of the MP joint, an assessment of the global function of the patient, particularly the deformities of the adjacent joints, is critical in the evaluation of these patients.
- In patients with systemic inflammatory processes and multiple joint involvement, the timing of hand surgery, if indicated, must also be staged with respect to other planned surgeries.
  - In general, lower extremity and more proximal upper extremity procedures should be performed before hand surgery.
  - Correction of MP deformities is usually undertaken before the treatment of the PIP joints.
- Cervical spine involvement is common in patients with inflammatory arthritis (≤90% of patients with rheumatoid arthritis) and is more common with long-standing disease and multiple joint involvement.
  - Significant instability is present in almost one third of patients, with atlantoaxial subluxation most common.
  - Radiculopathy and myelopathy secondary to cervical spine instability must be differentiated from peripheral compression neuropathy such as carpal tunnel syndrome.
  - Although compression neuropathies are common in rheumatoid arthritis, the presence of cervical instability must be determined before surgical intervention in the upper extremity, especially if general anesthesia with endotracheal intubation is being considered.
- Several other factors must also be evaluated, particularly in patients with systemic inflammatory processes.
  - Evaluations of the shoulder and elbow are critical in the assessment of the upper extremity.
  - In addition, careful assessment of any wrist joint deformity resulting from the inflammatory process must be elicited.
  - The presence of carpal collapse and the resultant radial deviation of the wrist can potentiate ulnar deviation in the digits (Fig. 14–20).
    - Failure to recognize this wrist joint imbalance will lead to poor outcome.
  - Distal radioulnar joint instability can result in attritional extensor tendon ruptures to the ulnar digits.
    - Correction of this deformity can minimize the incidence of extensor tendon insufficiency.
  - Involvement of the PIP and DIP joints must be assessed because their function is coupled with the mechanical properties of the MP joint.

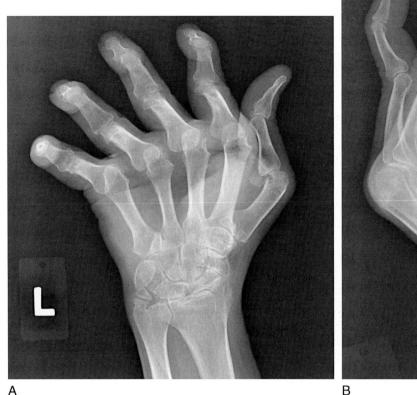
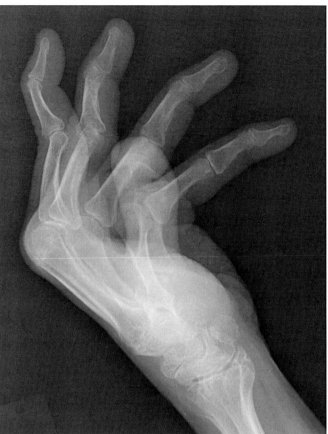

A   B

Figure 14–20: Rheumatoid arthritis.
Anteroposterior (**A**) and lateral (**B**) wrist and hand radiographs of a patient with rheumatoid arthritis. Note the carpal collapse with radial deviation of the wrist and ulnar deviation of the metacarpophalangeal joints.

- Swan-neck and boutonnière deformities are common in patients with rheumatoid arthritis, and they occur in 14% and 36% of patients, respectively.
  - The preference is to retain motion at the MP joints while gaining stability and adequate position at the PIP level.
  - Implant arthroplasties of both the MP and PIP are rarely indicated.
  - A preferred approach is to perform MP implant arthroplasties and to correct the PIP joint problems with either tendon reconstruction for flexible deformities or arthrodesis for fixed deformities.

Treatment

- The treatment goals should be based on the following priorities: pain relief, functional improvement, retardation of local disease progression, and cosmesis.
- Management of the MP joint depends on the severity of joint involvement in the disease process (Abboud et al. 2003) (Fig. 14–21).

- The determination about whether medical or surgical management is appropriate in each patient should be made on the basis of degree of synovial lining proliferation, articular surface derangement, and articular segment malalignment.

Indications for Arthroplasty

- Advanced arthritis of the MP joint requiring surgical intervention is uncommon except in the rheumatoid hand.
- The literature on MP joint arthroplasty in osteoarthritic or posttraumatic arthritis is very limited; therefore specific indications have not been well established.
- The general indications for MP joint arthroplasty in rheumatoid arthritis are painful deformities with destruction or subluxation of the joint and fixed deformity that cannot be corrected with soft tissue reconstruction alone.
- Implant arthroplasty is indicated in patients with (1) decreased arc of motion (40 degrees or less), (2) marked flexion contractures with the joint fixed in poor functional

Figure 14–21: Rheumatoid arthritis.
A and **B,** Clinical photographs of rheumatoid hand demonstrating characteristic deformities of volar subluxation and ulnar drift of the digits at the metacarpophalangeal joints. (From Abboud J, Beredjiklian, PK, Bozentka DJ [2003]. Metacarpophalangeal joint arthroplasty in rheumatoid arthritis. *J Am Acad Orthop Surg* 11:184-191.)

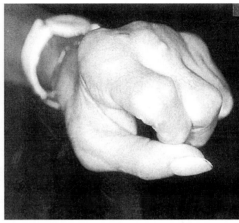

A B

position, (3) MP joint pain with associated radiographic abnormalities, and (4) severe ulnar drift (>30 degrees).
- In a relatively young patient with a functional range of motion of the MP joint (an active arc of motion of 60 to 70 degrees), careful consideration should be given to surgical intervention because there may be little functional improvement.

Contraindications to Arthroplasty

- Contraindications for MP joint arthroplasty include the presence of vasculitis, poor skin condition, or inadequate bone stock.
  - Excessive erosion of the metacarpal head and proximal phalanx or excessive fatty replacement of the cancellous bone may make prosthesis unstable, and rotation of the implant may occur.

Implant Designs

- Flexible silicone rubber
- The flexible silicone rubber implants used for MP arthroplasty differ (in fixation, articulation, and motion) from other prostheses commonly used in the larger joints.
- Silicone implants do not function as true prostheses, but serve as dynamic spacers to maintain the joint alignment following resection of the joint.
- The pistoning or gliding of the implant within the medullary canal is thought to add to the range of motion achieved by the arthroplasty and to disperse the forces along the implant-bone interface.
- Several silicone implant designs are available commercially.
- The design developed by Swanson in the 1960s is most commonly used (Fig. 14–22).
- More recently, the creation of the Sutter (Avanta Orthopaedics, San Diego, CA) and NeuFlex (DePuy Orthopaedics, Warsaw, IN) designs has provided alternatives to the Swanson implant.

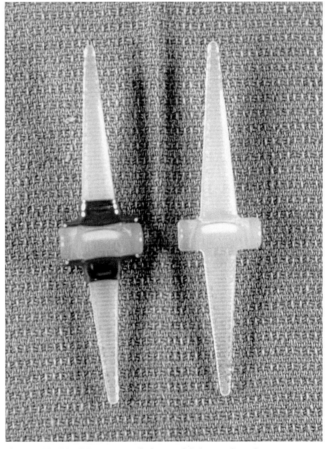

Figure 14–22: Metacarpophalangeal joint arthroplasty. Swanson Silastic implants used for metacarpophalangeal joint arthroplasty. The component on the left has titanium grommets in place. (From Naidu S [2004]. Arthritis. In: Beredjiklian PK, Bozentka DJ, eds. *Review of Hand Surgery.* Philadelphia: WB Saunders, 2004, p 182.)

- The track record of these newer devices has not been well established, and long-term follow-up will be necessary before any advantages or disadvantages of these components can be ascertained.
- Despite some drawbacks, the modified Swanson silicone implant remains the most reliable and accepted form of replacement arthroplasty in the hand.
- Swanson silicone implant arthroplasty technique
  - The dorsal approach is usually performed through a transverse incision (Fig. 14–23).
  - The incision is typically placed on the metacarpal head-neck junction.
    - Care should be taken to avoid a deep skin incision to prevent disruption of dorsal veins and the extensor tendon complex.
  - Dissection of the subcutaneous tissues reveals the presence of the dorsal veins in the interdigital spaces.
    - These veins should be dissected carefully and protected during the procedure; their preservation is important to avoid deleterious postoperative digital swelling.
  - The extensor mechanism is identified, and a longitudinal incision is made along the radial or ulnar border of the extensor tendon, to divide the radial or ulnar sagittal band, respectively.
  - In patients with rheumatoid arthritis, the radial sagittal band is almost always attenuated, and thus the incision is often made at the junction of the radial sagittal band and the extensor tendon.
  - The tendon is then retracted, and a longitudinal capsulotomy is made.
  - The collateral ligament origins on the metacarpal neck are identified and released subperiosteally with a blade.
  - Any synovial proliferation can be removed at this time with a small rongeur by flexing or distracting the joint.

- Using the motorized microsagittal saw, the metacarpal head is osteotomized and excised.
  - This osteotomy is typically made just distal to the origin of the collateral ligaments and perpendicular to the axis of the metacarpal shaft.
- Once the metacarpal head and proliferative tissue are excised, the volar plate and the base of the proximal phalanx are easily visualized.
- At this point, a soft tissue release including the ulnar intrinsics and volar plate can be performed if necessary to balance the joint and to allow access to the base of the proximal phalanx.
- The articular surface of the proximal phalanx is denuded with a motorized burr or a small curette, and any osteophytes are removed with a rongeur.
- The medullary canal of the proximal phalanx is accessed with a motorized burr or a curette.
- Using the reamers in the Swanson set, the medullary canals of the metacarpal and proximal phalanx are incrementally reamed by hand until a tight fit is achieved.
- For the index finger, the proximal phalanx is reamed in a supinated position to allow better tip pinch postoperatively.
- In contrast, the proximal phalanx of the small finger is reamed in a slight pronation to allow better grip.
- An adequately sized trial implant is then placed in each joint, and further soft tissue balancing or bone resection is performed as necessary.
  - The largest implant that does not buckle with full MP extension should be used.
- The trials are then removed, and two small (0.035-mm) drill holes are made on the dorsoradial aspect of the metacarpal neck for subsequent reattachment of the radial collateral ligament.

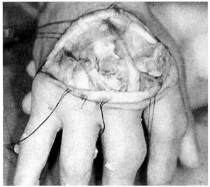 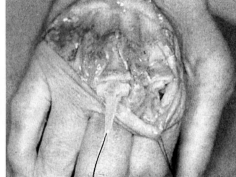 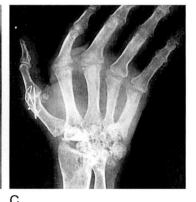

A   B   C

Figure 14–23: Metacarpophalangeal joint arthroplasty.
A, Dorsal transverse incision over the metacarpophalangeal joint with careful retraction of soft tissue and preservation of dorsal veins. **B,** An appropriately sized prosthesis shown here fitting comfortably into the metacarpal while the transverse midportion of the implant rests against the cut surface of the bone.
C, Postoperative radiograph after a metacarpophalangeal arthroplasty. (From Abboud J, Beredjiklian, PK, Bozentka DJ [2003]. Metacarpophalangeal joint arthroplasty in rheumatoid arthritis. *J Am Acad Orthop Surg* 11:184-191.)

- The medullary canals of the metacarpal and proximal phalanx are irrigated and sponge-dried carefully.
- The implants are then placed in position with smooth forceps without manually handling the implants (Fig. 14–24).
- The radial collateral ligament is then reattached to the metacarpal using 4-0 nonabsorbable, braided sutures placed through the drill holes on the bone.
- The dorsal hood is repaired by imbricating or reefing the radial sagittal band, which, in turn, should realign the extensor tendon.
- Also if deemed necessary, crossed intrinsic transfer can be performed.
- The skin is closed over a small Penrose drain with 5-0 nylon suture.
  - Care should be taken to avoid unnecessary trauma to the skin during closure.
- A soft, bulky dressing is applied, and a splint holding the digits in mild radial deviation with the MP joints in the extended position is placed before the patient leaves the operating suite. The drain can be removed on the first postoperative day.
  - The dressings are removed on postoperative day 2 or 3, and range-of-motion exercises are started 1 week postoperatively.
- A dynamic extension splint and a static nighttime resting splint are used for the first 6 weeks.

- These splints should help to maintain neutral or slightly radial deviation of the digits.
- Concomitantly, the patient is enrolled in a therapy protocol to encourage active range of motion of all digital joints.
- The dynamic splint is discontinued after 6 weeks, but the resting splint can be used for 3 to 4 months postoperatively.
- Total MP joint arthroplasty
  - These implants are typically nonconstrained and consist of two components that are fixed into the medullary canals.
  - Two of the available prostheses are the Steffee prosthesis (made of metal and polyethylene components) and the Ascension MCP (pyrolytic carbon components; Ascension Orthopedics, Austin, TX) (Fig. 14–25).
  - Because of the intrinsic morphology of the implants, there is increased inherent stability, particularly when a significant amount of bone resection is necessary to restore motion.
  - The pyrolytic carbon implants are still under investigation, and no long-term are data available to evaluate the results.

Results

- The results after MP arthroplasty are well documented, and function appears to be improved in appropriately selected patients.

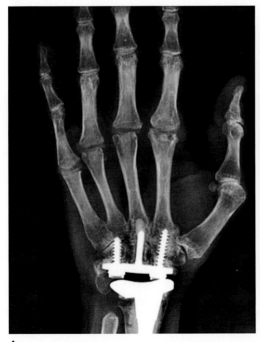 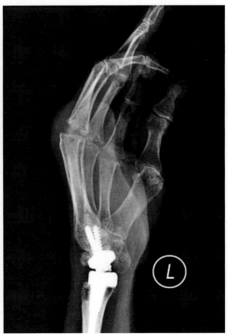

A   B

Figure 14–24: Metacarpophalangeal joint arthroplasty.
Anteroposterior (**A**) and lateral (**B**) postoperative radiographs in a patient treated with a total wrist arthroplasty and Silastic metacarpophalangeal joint arthroplasties for end-stage rheumatoid arthritis. Note the improvement of the digital alignment and correction of the ulnar deviation.

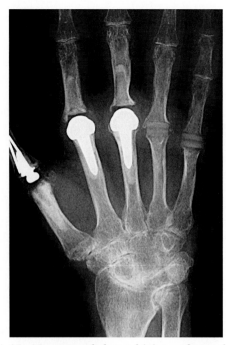

Figure 14–25: Metacarpophalangeal joint surface arthroplasty. Radiograph of properly implanted metacarpophalangeal surface replacement arthroplasty components. (From Berger RA, Beckenbaugh RD, Linscheid RL [1999]. Arthroplasty in the hand and wrist. In: Green DP, Hotchkiss RN, Pederson WC, eds. *Operative Hand Surgery,* 4th ed. New York: Churchill Livingstone, p 162.)

- The variables reported in the literature include range of motion, ulnar deviation, pain relief, and patient satisfaction (Table 14–2).
- Realistic expectations are important because patients are not expected to achieve full range of motion of the MP.
  - In patients with a substantial extensor lag or ulnar deviation, the arc of motion may only be minimally increased, but this will be in a more functional extended position.
  - Key and tip pinch will also be improved as the index is brought over into radial position.
  - Reported postoperative arcs vary from 38 to 60 degrees.
  - Extension lags also vary from 9 to 22 degrees.
  - A loss of approximately 12 degrees of active motion has been documented from an early postoperative arc of motion of 51 on long-term follow-up.
- The correction of the deformity has been documented as one of the major contributors to a patient's subjective sense of improvement.
  - Ulnar deviation reliably corrected to within a few degrees of neutral is reported in most series, although a tendency exists for some ulnar drift to recur with long-term follow-up.
  - Recurrence of ulnar drift has been reported in up to 43% of patients, but the magnitude of the recurrent ulnar deviation is usually less than 10 degrees.
  - Goldfarb and Stern reported that ulnar drift improved from 26 degrees preoperatively to less than 5 degrees immediately postoperatively (Goldfarb and Stern 2003).
  - However, ulnar drift then recurred to 16 degrees at average follow-up of 14 years.

Table 14–2 Long-term Follow-up of Swanson Metacarpophalangeal Implant Arthroplasty

STUDY	NO. OF IMPLANTS	FOLLOW-UP (MONTHS) MEAN (RANGE)	MEAN POSTOPERATIVE ARC OF MOTION (DEGREES)	RECURRENT DEFORMITY
Swanson	358	— (6–60)	60	<10-degree ulnar drift
Beckenbaugh et al.	186	32 (12–65)	38	11% mixed deformities
Madden et al.	92	>24 —	57	<10-degree ulnar drift
Blair et al.	115	54 (24–125)	43	43% ulnar drift
Bieber et al.	210	63 (24–96)	39	12-degree mean ulnar drift
Kirschenbaum et al.	144	102 (60–195)	43	7-degree mean ulnar drift
Hansraj et al.	348	64 (24–120)	27	NA
Gellman et al.	901	96	50	15-degree mean ulnar drift

NA, not available.
Adapted from Stirrat CR (1996). Metacarpophalangeal joints in rheumatoid arthritis of the hand. *Hand Clin* 12:515-529. In: Abboud J, Beredjiklian PK, Bozentka DJ (2003). Metacarpophalangeal joint arthroplasty in rheumatoid arthritis. *J Am Acad Orthop Surg* 11:184-191.

- Only 9 (18%) of the 50 joints reported had ulnar drift of greater than 30 degrees at the time of final follow-up.
- A positive correlation between the recurrence of deformity and a more severe disease course has also been noted.
- Pain relief has been consistently documented in most patients after MP arthroplasty.
  - For this reason, overall patient satisfaction rates are consistently high.

Complications

- Complications following silicone implant arthroplasty are generally uncommon.
- The most frequently reported complication involves osteolysis at the bone-implant interface, found in approximately 4% of cases.
  - The bone resorption is in all likelihood related to the immunogenic response of human macrophages to Silastic particulate debris.
  - Metacarpal midshaft cortical bone density has been found to be consistently decreased postoperatively.
  - Bone remodeling also results in thickening of the bony surfaces at the metacarpal and phalangeal metaphyses.
- Implant fracture has been found in approximately 2% of cases, ranging from 0% to 63%.
  - In most cases, however, implant fracture does not require revision of the prosthetic component.
  - The low morbidity of fractured prosthesis has been related to the function of the implant as a spacer rather than as an articulated prosthesis, and thus it still allows some motion and continued pain relief.
  - Several changes have been made in the implants to address this problem. The original silicone rubber has been replaced by high-performance silicone rubber, which has improved resistance to fracture and tear propagation.
- Infection is rare and seen in less than 1% of cases.
  - The organism most commonly isolated is *Staphylococcus aureus*.
  - Infections manifest in the early postoperative period and can be treated with implant removal and antibiotic.
  - Particulate synovitis and silicone-induced lymphadenopathy have received substantial attention. Both these complications were reported in less than 0.1% of cases.

Thumb Trapeziometacarpal Joint

Introduction

- The trapeziometacarpal (TMC) joint is the cornerstone of thumb and hand function.
- Its unique anatomy provides excellent mobility allowing for prehension at the expense of stability.
- Patients with TMC joint arthritis have difficulty using the affected limb because of pain leading to significant weakness in pinching, prehension, and thumb opposition.
- Multiple surgical options are available for the treatment of the persistently symptomatic joint.
- This section reviews treatment alternatives with prosthetic implants.

Anatomy

- The thumb carpometacarpal (CMC) joint is biconcave and is considered a saddle joint.
- The contour of the joint surface allows range of motion in flexion, extension, abduction, adduction, and rotation. Circumduction occurs during opposition and is a combination of these motions.
- The little constraint by the bony contours provides the joint with significant mobility and underscores the importance of the ligamentous structures for stability.
- Seven ligaments are directly involved in the stabilization of the thumb CMC joint. They are the deep anterior oblique, superficial anterior oblique, dorsoradial, posterior oblique, ulnar collateral, intermetacarpal, and dorsal intermetacarpal ligaments.
  - The deep anterior oblique ligament is also termed the *beak ligament* and is an important stabilizing structure. It originates at the base of the thumb metacarpal just ulnar to the volar tubercle and inserts on the volar tubercle of the trapezium centrally just ulnar to the ulnar aspect of the trapezial ridge. The ligament becomes taut in pronation with lateral pinch and limits dorsal translation of the joint (Fig. 14–26).
  - The dorsoradial ligament is the primary restraint for acute dorsal instability.

Etiology of Degenerative Changes

- Degenerative changes at the TMC joint can have several possible origins, including trauma, systemic inflammatory conditions such as rheumatoid arthritis, and idiopathic causes (most common).
- The development of idiopathic osteoarthritis of the thumb CMC joint is related to joint laxity.
  - An inverse correlation exists between the presence of degenerative changes and the integrity of the beak ligament in cadaveric thumb TMC joint specimens.
- Hyperextension of the thumb MP joint may also be related to the development of thumb CMC osteoarthritis.
- Articular incongruity after fractures may also lead to degenerative changes, but the extent of the degree of incongruity leading to arthritic changes remains controversial.

Evaluation

- Patients with symptomatic arthritis of the thumb TMC joint often describe pain diffusely about the base of the thumb in the thenar region as well as the first web space.

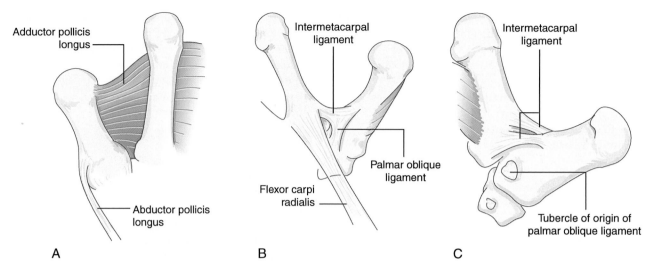

Figure 14–26: Anatomy and biomechanics of the basal joint of the thumb.
A, The adductor pollicis longus spans the "V" between the thumb and index metacarpals. The abductor pollicis longus inserts at the base of the thumb metacarpal and causes dorsal subluxation in the absence of sufficient ligamentous stability. **B,** The intermetacarpal ligament is an extracapsular tether between the two metacarpals. The palmar (anterior) oblique ligament is eccentrically positioned and tightens with thumb metacarpal pronation. The flexor carpi radialis tendon (either the entire tendon or only the radial half) is left anchored at its insertion on the base of the second metacarpal and is utilized for volar ligament reconstruction and tendon interposition. **C,** Palmar-to-dorsal view depicts the two arms of the intermetacarpal ligament and the tubercle of origin of the palmar oblique ligament. (From Stirrat CR [1996]. Metacarpophalangeal joints in rheumatoid arthritis of the hand. *Hand Clin* 12:515-529.)

- These symptoms often have an insidious onset and are frequently made worse with hand use, particularly pinching activities.
- Although idiopathic thumb TMC joint degenerative changes can affect any age group, this condition is most commonly seen in middle-aged women.
- Patients may also relate a history of trauma.
- On examination, swelling with localized tenderness of the thumb TMC joint (particularly at the radiovolar aspect of the joint) is common.
  - The thumb CMC grind test is a provocative maneuver that is helpful in confirming the diagnosis.
    - The thumb metacarpal is held by the examiner's thumb and index finger. The thumb metacarpal is rotated on the trapezium while evaluating for crepitation and pain that reproduces the patient's symptoms.
  - Grip and pinch strength is often noted to be decreased.
  - In the early stages of disease, some laxity can be elicited. Laxity is quantitated as the shaft is stressed radially. In general, a joint shift of 1 mm is considered 1+ laxity, 2 mm of joint shift corresponds to 2+ laxity, and so forth.
- Differential diagnoses include the following:
  - de Quervain's tenosynovitis
  - Flexor carpi radialis tendinopathy
  - Stenosing tenosynovitis (trigger thumb)
  - Intercarpal or radiocarpal arthrosis

- Associated diagnoses include the following:
  - Carpal tunnel syndrome (28%)
  - de Quervain's tenosynovitis (5%)
- Radiographic assessment includes the following:
  - Plain radiographs should include posteroanterior, lateral, and oblique views of the thumb (Fig. 14–27).
  - The Roberts view is an anteroposterior radiograph with the hand in hyperpronation. This view also allows visualization of all four trapezial articulations.
  - Stress views are obtained by having the patient push the tip of the thumbs together to apply a radial stress to the thumb CMC joint. Laxity of the joint will manifest a lateral subluxation in the posteroanterior radiograph.
- Eaton and Littler classified the extent of thumb CMC arthritis using radiographic criteria (Fig. 14–28).
  - Stage I is considered the synovitis phase. There is a normal joint contour with some widening of the joint space resulting from synovitis and less than one-third joint subluxation.
  - Stage II is characterized by significant joint laxity with instability on stress views with greater than one-third joint subluxation. Arthritic changes of mild joint space narrowing or sclerosis and osteophytes smaller than 2 mm in diameter are found.
  - Stage III is characterized by significant joint space narrowing, sclerosis, and cystic degenerative changes of

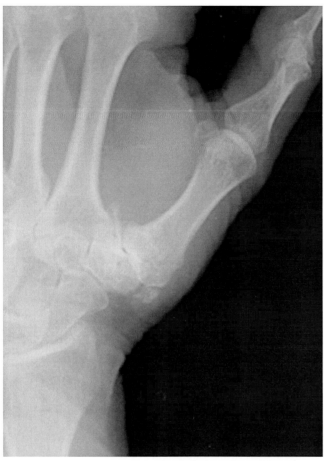

Figure 14–27: Osteoarthritis of the carpometacarpal joint of the thumb.
Note the destruction of the articular surface and osteophyte formation. (From Stirrat CR [1996]. Metacarpophalangeal joints in rheumatoid arthritis of the hand. *Hand Clin* 12:515-529.)

the subchondral bone. Osteophytes larger than 2 mm are found with sparing of the scaphotrapezial joint.
- Stage IV involves pantrapezial arthritis with significant joint space narrowing, sclerosis, and osteophytes of both the TMC joint and the scaphotrapezial joint.
- Arthroscopy of the thumb CMC joint has been used for further evaluation and minimally invasive treatment.
  - In addition, arthroscopy provides the opportunity for certain treatment modalities such as débridement, synovectomy, ligament shrinkage, hemitrapeziectomy, or complete trapeziectomy.
  - Few data are available in the literature regarding indications or results for these procedures.

Treatment

- Initial treatment should include nonoperative modalities.
  - Custom-molded Orthoplast thumb spica splints are of benefit, particularly in the early stages of the disease. Hand-based thumb spica splints are well tolerated for

day use, whereas forearm based splints are more limiting and are often prescribed for night use.
  - Modification of activities, nonsteroidal anti-inflammatory medications, and corticosteroid injections also are helpful in providing pain relief.
- Surgical intervention should be considered for those patients with severe pain and functional disability refractory to nonoperative treatment.
- The many different surgical procedures described in the treatment of thumb CMC arthritis range from synovectomy and joint débridement to arthrodesis or arthroplasty.
- The choice of procedure should depend on the extent of the arthritic changes and status of the MP joint.
- Procedures performed for stage I arthritis include synovectomy, débridement, metacarpal osteotomy, and ligament reconstruction.
- Synovectomy and débridement of the TMC joint (open or arthroscopic) can lead to symptom relief, but a paucity of data in the literature exists regarding outcomes for this procedure.
- Thumb metacarpal osteotomy has also been used in the treatment of the early stages of thumb CMC arthritis.
  - A dorsally based 30-degree wedge of bone is removed from the thumb metacarpal 1 to 2 cm from the base.
  - The osteotomy site is stabilized using various types of fixation including Kirschner wires or a plate and screws.
  - The exact mechanism for pain relief is not known, but a shifting of the arthritic contact areas in the joint provide a plausible explanation
- Ligament reconstruction is considered a treatment option because joint laxity, particularly disruption of the deep anterior oblique ligament, is considered a precursor to thumb CMC joint arthritis.
  - Various techniques have been described for stabilization of the thumb CMC joint using extensor tendon, abductor pollicis longus, or flexor carpi radialis tendon for stabilization.
  - The goal of these procedures is to restore ligament stability, to relieve pain, and to prevent or retard progressive joint degeneration (Fig. 14–29).
- More advanced arthritic changes (stages II to IV) about the thumb TMC joint require arthroplasty or arthrodesis.
- Soft tissue TMC joint arthroplasty can be performed using various techniques including trapeziectomy (partial or complete) with or without ligament reconstruction or joint replacement arthroplasty.

Partial or Total Trapezium Excision With Ligament Reconstruction With Tendon Interposition

- Partial or total trapezium excision with ligament reconstruction with tendon interposition (LRTI) is commonly used and represents the "gold standard" in the treatment of thumb TMC joint arthritis.

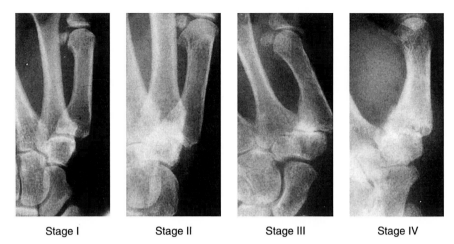

Stage I   Stage II   Stage III   Stage IV

Figure 14–28: Radiographic staging system for basal joint disease.
Stage I shows no degenerative changes. Cartilage space widening or mild subluxation may be present. Stage II is characterized by narrowing of the cartilage space and the presence of osteophytes less than 2 mm in diameter. Stage III displays more narrowing and subchondral sclerosis and osteophytes measuring more than 2 mm in diameter. Stage IV is characterized by advanced degenerative changes involving both the trapeziometacarpal joint and the scaphotrapezial joint. (From Stirrat CR [1996]. Metacarpophalangeal joints in rheumatoid arthritis of the hand. *Hand Clin* 12:515-529.)

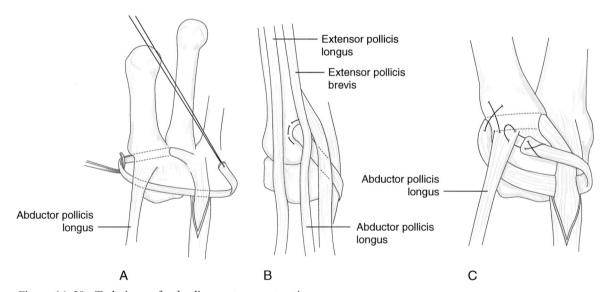

Figure 14–29: Technique of volar ligament reconstruction.
A, The radial half of the flexor carpi radialis tendon is passed through a hole in the thumb metacarpal base, deep to the abductor pollicis longus tendon, and then deep to the intact, undisturbed flexor carpi radialis tendon. **B,** A dorsal view shows the tendon strip passing deep to the extensor pollicis brevis and the abductor pollicis longus tendons. **C,** The final anchor point of the reconstruction is the abductor pollicis longus tendon. (From Stirrat CR [1996]. Metacarpophalangeal joints in rheumatoid arthritis of the hand. *Hand Clin* 12:515-529.)

- The trapezium is excised to remove the arthritic joints.
- The beak ligament is reconstructed to prevent shortening of the thumb and to provide stability during pinch.
- The tendon interposition may prevent further shortening of the thumb should the ligament reconstruction fail.

Technique

- The procedure is performed through an incision at the base of the thumb (Fig. 14–30).
- The radial sensory nerve branches are protected.

- The dissection is taken between the extensor pollicis brevis and abductor pollicis longus tendons, and the radial artery is dissected and retracted.
- A longitudinal capsular incision is made, and the capsule is dissected from the trapezium volarly and dorsally.
- The trapezium is excised, and a hole is made 1 cm from the base of the metacarpal on the extensor surface or thumbnail side to the volar beak region.
- The flexor carpi radialis is harvested through a separate incision in the forearm.

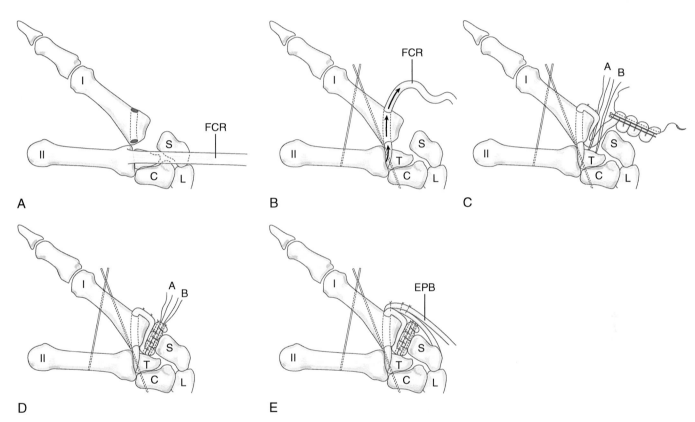

Figure 14–30: Ligament reconstruction and tendon interposition arthroplasty.
Technique of ligament reconstruction and tendon interposition arthroplasty. **A,** Through a dorsoradial skin incision and longitudinal capsulotomy, the entire trapezium is excised piecemeal with a sagittal saw and small osteotome. The oblique gouge hole through the base of the first metacarpal is made beginning on the lateral cortex 1 cm distal to the metacarpal base. **B,** The FCR tendon, anchored at its insertion on the second metacarpal base, is divided proximally at its musculotendinous junction, freed of adhesions at the carpal level, and then passed through the gouge channel. A nonabsorbable suture is used to repair any rent in the deep capsule of the arthroplasty space, with long tails to secure the interposed FCR tendon. After these steps, ideal positioning of the metacarpal is maintained with two Kirschner wires. **C,** The taut FCR tendon is secured to the periosteum and capsular tissue at the metacarpal base and is then sutured to itself in the depth of the arthroplasty space. The remaining FCR tail is threaded onto two Keith needles and is reinforced with corner sutures. **D,** The wad of tendon is passed into the arthroplasty space and is secured with sutures. **E,** The capsulotomy is then closed. The EPB tendon is divided distally and is sutured with appropriate tension to the FCR tendon exiting the lateral metacarpal and to the adjacent periosteum. The incision is closed, and a thumb spica plaster shell is placed, to remain for 4 to 5 weeks. *A,* distal suture limbs; *B,* proximal suture limbs; *C,* capitate; *EPB,* extensor pollicis brevis; *FCR,* flexor carpi radialis; *I,* first metacarpal; *II,* second metacarpal; *L,* lunate; *S,* scaphoid; *T,* trapezoid. (From Stirrat CR [1996]. Metacarpophalangeal joints in rheumatoid arthritis of the hand. *Hand Clin* 12:515-529.)

- The thumb metacarpal should be coaxial with the scaphoid and pronated so the thumb pulp faces the radial quadrant of the index finger pulp.
- The flexor carpi radialis graft is woven through the hole in the base of the metacarpal and is sutured to the adjacent periosteum and capsule dorsally. The tendon graft is then folded back on itself and is sutured to resurface the base of the thumb metacarpal.
- The remainder of the tendon graft is woven on itself and is sutured to the deep capsule as the interposition.
- The patient is immobilized for approximately 4 weeks, and a physical therapy exercise program is started.
- Variations of the procedure include the following:
  - Harvesting of one half versus the entire flexor carpi radialis tendon
  - Utilizing the extensor carpi radialis brevis to reconstruct the ligament
  - Temporary pinning of the thumb metacarpal for 4 weeks after trapeziectomy and ligament reconstruction
  - Partial trapeziectomy in the earlier stages of disease (stages II to III)
  - Complete trapeziectomy in combination with:
    - Ligament reconstruction without tendon interposition
    - Tendon interposition without ligament reconstruction (free palmaris longus tendon graft "anchovy")
    - Temporary pinning of the thumb metacarpal without tendon interposition or ligament reconstruction ("hematoma" technique)

Thumb Metacarpophalangeal Joint Deformity in Arthritis

- If hyperextension deformity is present, the MP joint must be surgically addressed to diminish stress across the CMC joint.
  - Less than 10 degrees of MP hyperextension: Pin the joint in flexion.
  - From 10 to 20 degrees: Use volar plate advancement and pinning of the MP joint.
  - More than 25 degrees of MP hyperextension: Consider arthrodesis, especially if radiographic osteoarthritis is visible in the MP joint. The optimal position for MP joint fusion is 15 degrees of flexion and 10 degrees of pronation. Other options include extensor pollicis brevis transfer and sesamoid fusion.

Principles of Implant Arthroplasty

- Implant arthroplasty in combination with trapezium excision has also been used as a treatment option for pantrapezial arthritis.
- Problems with particulate synovitis, implant fracture, and erosive changes in bone have caused silicone implants to fall out of favor. Other joint replacements including metallic and polyethylene components are still in the developmental stages.
- The more recent generation of prostheses employs varying designs and materials aimed at hemiarthroplasty

or interpositional arthroplasty of the basal joint rather than total joint replacement.

Hemiarthroplasty/Prosthetic Interpositional Arthroplasty

- The central theme of hemiarthroplasty is to save the trapezium.
- It is indicated for Eaton stage II and III disease.
- It requires minimal bony resection and it does not preclude conversion to trapeziectomy and LRTI.
- In the case of stage IV disease without excessive adduction contracture of the first metacarpal, and excessive compensatory hyperextension deformity at the MCP joint, hemiarthroplasty may be used in combination with soft tissue interposition arthroplasty of the scaphotrapezial joint.
- For patients with severe adduction contracture of the first metacarpal, and metacarpal subluxation, total trapezial excision and LRTI still comprise the gold standard.

Titanium Basal Joint Hemiarthroplasty (Wright Medical, Arlington, TN)

- The titanium basal joint implant resembles the Swanson convex condylar implant (Fig. 14–31).
- The stem is smooth and is centrally placed on the articulating hemisphere. The centrally placed stem/peg of the titanium implant restores the center of rotation at the trapezium.
- It is designed for use without cement, and the implant relies on fibrous fixation within the metacarpal medullary canal, along with a hemispherical fit into the trapezium.
- The implant is indicated for Eaton stage II to III disease in a patient with good bone stock.
- For optimum outcome, preoperative subluxation at the TMC joint should be absent, and compensatory MCP hyperextension deformity should be less than 5 degrees.
- Technique
  - The basal joint is exposed through a straight longitudinal incision along the dorsolateral aspect of the thumb metacarpal.
  - The terminal branches of the superficial radial nerve must be preserved. It is best to isolate the radial artery in the snuff box and to dissect and retract it distally and ulnarly away from the capsule while making sure to ligate all the small branches.
  - The TMC joint is exposed in the interval between the first extensor compartment tendons and the extensor pollicis longus.
  - The proximal 3 mm of metacarpal articular surface perpendicular to the metacarpal shaft and the medullary canal are broached to size.
  - The trapezial surface is reamed with spheric reamers to create a crater in the trapezium to seat the titanium hemisphere adequately, without causing impingement between the metacarpal shaft and the trapezial rim.

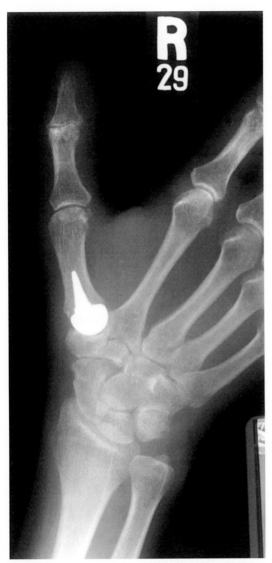

Figure 14–31: Hemiarthroplasty for end-stage basal joint osteoarthritis.
Anteroposterior radiograph of a patient with end-stage basal joint osteoarthritis treated with a titanium hemiarthroplasty.

- Inadequate reaming will lead to implant subluxation or dislocation; on the contrary, too much reaming will lead to metacarpal trapezial rim impingement and may cause trapezial rim fracture in osteopenic bone. The implant should be stable, without a tendency to subluxate dorsoradially.
- Postoperatively, a thumb spica cast/splint is applied for 6 weeks, and nighttime splinting is used for 1 more month. Formal hand therapy is started at 1 week.

Cobalt-Chrome Basal Joint Hemiarthroplasty (Biopro, Port Huron, MI)

- The rationale and indications for this implant are similar to those for the titanium basal joint implant.

- The mechanics of the implant are significantly different from the titanium implant, even though it is designated as a hemiarthroplasty.
- The stem is offset dorsally on the hemispheric surface to ensure that the center rotation is at the metacarpal base and not in the center of the trapezium.

Ceramic Spheric Interpositional Arthroplasty (Orthosphere, Wright Medical, Arlington, TN)

- The Zirconia ceramic sphere has superior wear properties (Fig. 14–32).

Silicone Interposition Arthroplasty

- Swanson silicone prosthesis
  - The original design of the implant had a solid convex head that articulated with the scaphoid. The design evolved into a prosthesis that had a concave head to form a better fit with the distal pole of the scaphoid.
- Eaton silicone prosthesis
  - Eaton designed a perforated implant so that a slip of tendon (a slip of abductor pollicis longus or part of extensor carpi radialis longus) could be passed through the implant and anchored to an adjacent carpal bone for stability.
- Niebauer silicone prosthesis
  - The implant has a Dacron mesh coating the intramedullary stem to promote bony ingrowth, and heavy Dacron ties extend from the prosthesis into either the flexor carpi radialis or the index metacarpal for fixation.

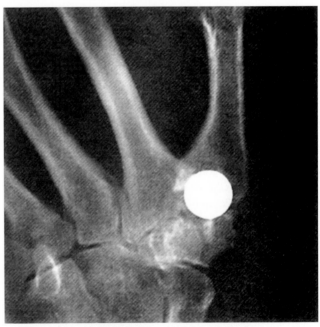

Figure 14–32: Arthroplasty for end-stage basal joint osteoarthritis.
Anteroposterior radiograph of a patient with end-stage basal joint osteoarthritis treated with a Zirconia ceramic sphere.

- Despite the novel method of transfixing the prosthesis and the added stability of the Dacron mesh, instability remains problematic.

Total Joint Replacement Arthroplasty

De la Caffiniere Prosthesis (Francobal, HowMedica, Rutherford, NJ)

- This cemented implant consists of a polyethylene cup fixed into the trapezium and a cobalt-chromium stem fixed into the shaft of the first metacarpal.
- This design is very similar to that used in total hip arthroplasty.
- The design has been plagued by early failure resulting from aseptic loosening, primarily of the trapezial component.
- Other cemented total joint designs such as the Braun (Zimmer, Warsaw, IN), Lewis (Howmedica, Rutherford, NJ), and Mayo (Depuy Orthopaedics, Warsaw, IN) prostheses have also demonstrated early failures as in the de la Caffiniere design.

Ledoux Prosthesis

- Ledoux introduced an uncemented prosthesis consisting of a ball-and-socket design with the center of rotation in the trapezium.
- The trapezial component is made of a titanium ring that is conical on the inside and cylindric on the outside, with a cylindric polyethylene lining.
- The metal cup has six longitudinally arranged wings that expand as the polyethylene element is introduced into the cup to produce an interference fit between the metal cage and the trapezium.
- The titanium stem reproduces the anatomic shape of the medullary canal, and its introduction allows for immediate mechanical fixation in the first metacarpal.

Arthrodesis

- This is considered primarily for the young (<50 years of age), active patient in whom nonoperative treatment has failed.
- The procedure is considered particularly for the heavy manual laborer who requires strong grip and pinch strength.
- Arthrodesis is also indicated as the ultimate salvage procedure for the failed excisional arthroplasty.
- Various techniques have been used for fusion fixation, including tension band wire, Kirschner wires, Herbert screws, power staples, and plate fixation.
  - The thumb is positioned with the metacarpal in 20 to 30 degrees of radial abduction, and 35 to 45 degrees of palmar abduction with the thumb slightly pronated.
- Despite the benefits of fusion, it has several main drawbacks compared with arthroplasty, as follows:
  - Limited range of motion with inability to flatten the hand fully

- Difficulty in activities requiring fine manipulation such as sewing, picking up small objects, and cutting
- Clumsiness and fatigue with sustained grip and pinch
- Longer postoperative immobilization
- 13% risk of nonunion
- Pain and degenerative changes of the joints adjacent to the trapezium

Results and Complications

Soft Tissue Trapeziometacarpal Joint Arthroplasty

- This procedure is associated with a high degree of pain relief, functional restoration, and patient satisfaction (>90%) regardless of the type of procedure.
- Motion is similar to that of the uninvolved side in long-term follow-up studies.
- Although significant improvement in grip strength is reported postoperatively, tip and pinch strength is less reliably improved. In spite of this limitation, the functional status of the patient is significantly improved in light of the reduction of symptoms.
- Radiographically, proximal migration of the thumb metacarpal can be observed in most cases. Nevertheless, radiographic subsidence is not related to clinical outcome.
- Complications include symptomatic proximal migration of the thumb metacarpal, neuroma or irritation of the radial sensory nerves, injury to the radial artery, and a "Z" deformity of the thumb related to a lack of correction of MP joint hyperextension.

Hemiarthroplasty/Prosthetic Interpositional Arthroplasty

- Although the track record of these implants is not clearly established, there appears to be a high rate of subsidence of the implant into the trapezium leading to pain and weakness.
- These early failures necessitate revision to a soft tissue arthroplasty.
- Currently, hemiarthroplasty appears to be indicated only for low-demand patients.

Silicone Interposition Arthroplasty

- Early outcome studies reported the presence of a stable, pain-free mobile thumb.
- In addition, patients experienced significant improvement of strength (grip and pinch strength) and postoperative pain relief, with a satisfaction rate reaching 90%.
- Longer-term studies, however, noted a high incidence of implant instability and subluxation, and early enthusiasm for silicone replacement was mitigated by difficulty in obtaining implant stability.
- In some studies, postoperative subluxation was not painful or symptomatic unless the implant had a complete dislocation.

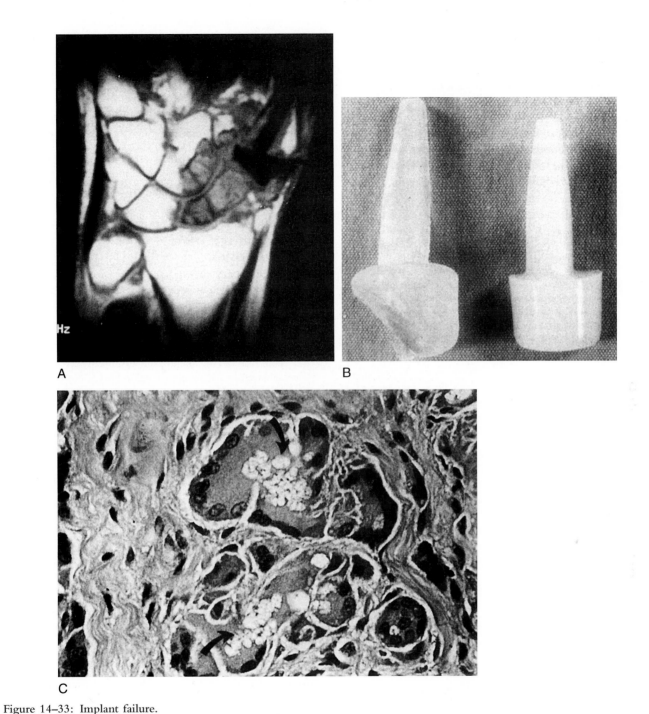

Figure 14–33: Implant failure.
A, Magnetic resonance image of a wrist with a failed silicone trapezial implant. Abundant silicone synovitis is present, and a silicone granuloma has replaced the scaphoid and part of the capitate and lunate. **B,** Retrieved implant *(left)* revealing significant surface wear compared with a new trapezial implant *(right).* **C,** Micrograph of synovial tissue from the wrist in **A** revealing a silicone granuloma displaying multinucleated giant cells containing silicone fragments and wear debris within the cells. (From Naidu S [1997]. Silicone elastomers and silicone synovitis: Materials and basic science. *Semin Arthroplasty* 8:195.)

- Other studies have noted that the instability becomes symptomatic in patients with high-grade subluxations.
- Later reports also began to note bony resorption, multiple carpal cysts, and collapse in patients with silicone implants.
  - This process later became known as *silicone synovitis*.
  - One study demonstrated that more than 50% of patients had cysts within the scaphoid, and almost 75% had cysts within the first metacarpal.
  - Histologically, this silicone synovitis showed foreign body giant cells associated with bony changes about a foreign nonbirefringent material consistent with silicone (Fig. 14–33).

Total Joint Replacement Arthroplasty

De la Caffiniere Prosthesis (Francobal)

- Good results are seen in about two thirds of patients at 2 years after surgery.
- Results are more encouraging in low-demand patients such as those with severe rheumatoid arthritis.
- Nearly 15% showed trapezial loosening of the implant.

Ledoux Prosthesis

- This implant has been associated with a high degree of early failure requiring revision surgery.

Arthrodesis

- This procedure is associated with pain relief, functional restoration, and patient satisfaction.
- Traditionally, this procedure has been traditionally reserved for younger, high-demand patients who were believed to be poor candidates for soft tissue or implant arthroplasty.
  - Some authors have noted outcomes similar to those of soft tissue arthroplasty in older patients.
- Complications include nonunion, malunion, and hardware irritation (worse in patients treated with plates and screws versus Kirschner wire fixation).

References

Abboud J, Beredjiklian PK, Bozentka DJ (2003). Metacarpophalangeal joint arthroplasty in rheumatoid arthritis. *J Am Acad Orthop Surg* 11:184-191.

> This article is a review of concepts related to MP joint arthroplasty in patients with rheumatoid arthritis.

Ashworth CR, Hansraj KK, Todd AO, et al. (1997). Swanson proximal interphalangeal joint arthroplasty in patients with rheumatoid arthritis. *Clin Orthop Relat Res* 342:34-37.

> One hundred thirty-eight Swanson PIP replacements were implanted in patients with rheumatoid arthritis. The average preoperative active arc of motion was 38 degrees, and postoperatively it was 29 degrees. Ten fractures were found and were revised. Sclerosis of bone was noted around 78% of the implants, and resorption was found adjacent to 12% of the implants. Survivorship analysis showed that 81% of implants were not revised at 9 years.

Barron OA, Glickel SZ, Eaton RG (2000). Basal joint arthritis of the thumb. *J Am Acad Orthop Surg* 8:314-323

> This article is a review of concepts related to soft tissue arthroplasty in patients with degenerative and inflammatory conditions of the basal joint of the thumb.

Beckenbaugh RD, Dobyns, JH, Linscheid RL, et al. (1976). Review and analysis of silicone-rubber metacarpophalangeal implants. *J Bone Joint Surg Am* 58:483-487.

Bieber EJ, Weiland AJ, Volenec-Dowling S (1986). Silicone-rubber implant arthroplasty of the metacarpophalangeal joints for rheumatoid arthritis. *J Bone Joint Surg Am* 68:206-209.

Blair WF, Shurr DG, Buckwalter JA (1984). Metacarpophalangeal joint implant arthroplasty with a Silastic spacer. *J Bone Joint Surg Am* 66:365-370.

Burton RI, Pellegrini VD Jr (1986). Surgical management of basal joint arthritis of the thumb. Part II: Ligament reconstruction with tendon interposition arthroplasty. *J Hand Surg Am* 11:324-332.

> The authors reviewed 25 procedures with an average follow-up of 2 years. LRTI arthroplasty more consistently improved pinch strength, increased grip strength endurance, and restored thumb web space than did silicone implant arthroplasty. Excellent results were achieved in 23 thumbs or 92% of cases. No deterioration of function or stability was noted over time, and no revision procedures were necessary.

Cook SD, Beckenbaugh RD, Redondo J, et al. (1999). Long-term follow-up of pyrolytic carbon metacarpophalangeal implants. *J Bone Joint Surg Am* 81:635-648.

> One hundred and fifty-one pyrolytic carbon MP implants were inserted in 53 patients. Eighteen implants (12%) in 11 patients were revised. The implants improved the arc of motion of the fingers by an average of 13 degrees and elevated the arc by an average of 16 degrees. No adverse remodeling or resorption of bone was seen. Survivorship analysis demonstrated an average annual failure rate of 2.1% and a 16-year survival rate of 70.3%. No evidence of intracellular particles or particulate synovitis was found.

Gellman H, Stetson W, Brumfield RH Jr, et al. (1997). Silastic metacarpophalangeal joint arthroplasty in patients with rheumatoid arthritis. *Clin Orthop* 342:16-21.

Goldfarb CA, Stern PJ (2003). Metacarpophalangeal joint arthroplasty in rheumatoid arthritis: A long-term assessment. *J Bone Joint Surg Am* 85:1869-1878.

> The results of a total of 208 arthroplasties in 52 hands of 36 patients were evaluated at an average of 14 years postoperatively. The mean arc of motion of the MP joints improved from 30 degrees preoperatively to 46 degrees immediately after the surgical procedure but decreased to 36 degrees at the time of final follow-up. One hundred thirty implants (63%) were broken and 45 (22%) more were deformed at the time of final follow-up. The patients expressed satisfaction with the function of only 38% of the hands, and only 27% of the hands were pain-free at the time of final follow-up. A greater degree of ulnar drift was associated with decreased patient satisfaction and a decreased score for the cosmetic appearance ($P \leq .01$). The outcome after silicone MP joint arthroplasty in patients with rheumatoid arthritis worsens with long-term follow-up.

Hansraj KK, Ashworth CR, Ebramzadeh E, et al. (1997). Swanson metacarpophalangeal joint arthroplasty in patients with rheumatoid arthritis. *Clin Orthop* 342:11-15.

Hartigan BJ, Stern PJ, Kiefhaber TR (2001). Thumb carpometacarpal osteoarthritis: Arthrodesis compared with ligament reconstruction and tendon interposition. *J Bone Joint Surg Am* 83:1470-1478.

> In a retrospective review, 42 patients (58 thumbs) treated with arthrodesis and 29 patients (44 thumbs) treated with arthrodesis were evaluated. The average duration of follow-up was 69 months. Subjective evaluation of pain, function, and satisfaction demonstrated no significant difference between the two groups, and more than 90% of patients were satisfied following either procedure. Although grip strength did not differ between the groups, the arthrodesis group had significantly stronger lateral pinch ($P < .001$) and chuck pinch ($P < .01$). The group treated with LRTI had a better range of motion with regard to opposition ($P < .05$) and the ability to flatten the hand ($P < .0001$). There was a higher complication rate in the arthrodesis group; nonunion of the fusion site accounted for the majority of the complications.

Kirschenbaum D, Schneider LH, Adams DC, et al. (1993). Arthroplasty of the metacarpophalangeal joints with use of silicone rubber implants in patients who have rheumatoid arthritis: Long-term results. *J Bone Joint Surg Am* 75:3-12.

Madden JW, DeVore G, Arem AJ (1997). A rational postoperative management program for metacarpophalangeal joint implant arthroplasty. *J Hand Surg Am* 2:358-366.

Nicholas RM, Calderwood JW (1992). De la Caffiniere arthroplasty for basal thumb joint osteoarthritis. *J Bone Joint Surg Br* 74:309-312.

> Twenty patients were treated with de la Caffiniere TMC arthroplasty for CMC joint osteoarthritis. Eighteen arthroplasties were satisfactory postoperatively, although all 20 patients had a satisfactory range of motion, and only one experienced postoperative pain such that it impeded normal function. Failure occurred in two patients and resulted from overreaming of the trapezium during surgery and a traumatic dislocation. Radiolucency between the prosthesis and bone was observed in one arthroplasty, although this patient was asymptomatic.

Sotereanos DG, Taras J, Urbaniak JR (1993). Niebauer trapeziometacarpal arthroplasty: A long term follow up. *J Hand Surg Am* 18:560-564.

> A retrospective review of long-term follow-up of Niebauer TMC arthroplasty for treatment of disabling arthritis of the basal joint was performed. Thirty implants in 27 patients were reviewed, with an average follow-up of 9 years (minimum, 4 years). Eighty-eight percent of the patients were subjectively pleased and would undergo the procedure again. Postoperative subluxation occurred in 83% of the patients. In 24 of 27 patients, pain was relieved, and satisfactory motion and stability were achieved.

Swanson AB (1972). Flexible implant arthroplasty for arthritic finger joints: Rationale, technique, and results of treatment. *J Bone Joint Surg Am* 54:435-455.

Swanson AB, Poitevin LA, Swanson GDG, et al. (1986). Bone remodeling phenomena in flexible implant arthroplasty in the metacarpophalangeal joints. *Clin Orthop Relat Res* 205:254-267.

> The purpose of this study was to evaluate the long-term bone response to silicone implants at the MP joint level in a series of 133 digits with a minimum of 5 years of follow-up evaluation. Bone remodeling resulted in the formation of a newly formed cortical bony shell around the implant stems. A postoperative decrease of the metacarpal midshaft cortical bone thickness was related to the surgical reaming and remained permanently. The shape of the cortical bone in implant resection arthroplasty was maintained, and the bone thickness increased.

Takigawa S, Meletiou S, Sauerbier M, Cooney WP (2004). Long-term assessment of Swanson implant arthroplasty in the proximal interphalangeal joint of the hand. *J Hand Surg Am* 29:785-795.

> A retrospective review of 70 silicone implants of the PIP joint in 48 patients was performed with an average follow-up period of 6.5 years. No significant change was seen in the active range of motion before and after PIP arthroplasty (26 versus 30 degrees). Correction of swan-neck and boutonnière deformities was difficult, usually leading to poor results. Pain relief was present in 70% of replaced PIP joints with residual pain, and loss of strength was noted in 30%. Radiographic analysis showed abnormal bone formation (cystic changes) in 45%. Eleven implant fractures occurred, and nine joints required revision surgery.

Wilgis EF (1997). Distal interphalangeal joint silicone interpositional arthroplasty of the hand. *Clin Orthop Relat Res* 342:38-41.

> This is a review of this procedure done in 38 digits. The average age of the patients at the time of operation was 58.3 years. The implants had been in place for a mean period of 10 years. Fewer than 10% of the implants had to be removed. Compared with arthrodesis, silicone interpositional arthroplasty appears to offer the advantage of retained motion while preserving stability.

Zimmerman NB, Zimmerman SI, Wilgis EF (1991). Distal interphalangeal joint silicone interpositional arthroplasty: Surgical technique and functional outcome. *Semin Arthroplasty* 2:153-157.

> Silicone interpositional arthroplasty was performed in 31 digits of patients whose mean age was 58.3 years. The patients were evaluated at an average of 72.2 months (range, 12.6 to 123.1 months) after surgery. All patients reported that their primary preoperative symptom of pain was effectively eliminated by the procedure. At reevaluation, the active range of motion of the DIP joint averaged 32.2 degrees, and the extension lag averaged 12.7 degrees. Two implants were removed 3 months postoperatively for wound problems and one at 31 months because of prothesis fracture.

CHAPTER 15

Limb Salvage Techniques in Lower Extremity Segmental Bone Defects

Harish S. Hosalkar,* Kristofer J. Jones,† and Richard D. Lackman‡

*MD, MBMS (Orth), FCPS (Orth), DNB (Orth), Clinical Instructor and Resident, Department of Orthopaedic Surgery, University of Pennsylvania School of Medicine, Philadelphia, PA
†BA, Medical Student, University of Pennsylvania School of Medicine, Philadelphia, PA
‡MD, Chairman and Professor, Division of Orthopaedic Surgery, Pennsylvania Hospital, Philadelphia, PA

Introduction

- Before the 1970s, no good solutions existed for large segmental bone defects, particularly when they involved adjacent joint surfaces. Regardless of whether the defect was the result of tumor or other causes, most of these patients were treated by amputation.
- With regard to patients with bone sarcoma, another challenge during the 1970s and earlier was that no effective adjuncts were available, thereby leaving amputation as the standard treatment.
- During the late 1970s, two primary advances generated surgeons' interest in limb salvage for at least a limited number of patients. First, early chemotherapy results demonstrated that the drugs of that day could have a positive effect on bone sarcomas. Second, some early limb salvage techniques became available for clinical use. Using osteosarcoma as an example, the 5-year survival rate in the early 1970s was approximately 20%. With the advent of neoadjuvant chemotherapy and advances in radiation therapy techniques, the 5-year survival rate has improved to approximately 60% to 70% (Zeegen et al. 2004). These limb salvage techniques included bone turn-up or turn-down procedures, as originally described by Enneking (Enneking 1987).
- The turn-down and turn-up procedures were described for tumors about the knee and involved resection of either the distal femur or the proximal tibia, followed by a sagittal split through either the remaining proximal tibia or the distal femur. The split piece was rotated up or down to span the gap and was then fixed in place and augmented with an intramedullary rod from the hip to the ankle with bone graft inserted at the junctions. Fig. 15–1 demonstrates such a procedure performed in a patient with a large giant cell tumor of the proximal tibia. Although this procedure was technically considered limb salvage, the limitations of knee fusion prevented this surgical option from becoming a popular operation with patients.
- Another technical advance that occurred during the late 1970s was the availability of primitive segmental replacement prostheses. These included proximal femoral replacement bipolar or total hip prostheses and segmental replacement Guepar-style total knee prostheses. The proximal femoral prostheses were one-piece units with varying body lengths and typically one stem option, which was a fixed diameter and length. The Guepar prostheses were fixed-hinge (Fig. 15–2), completely constrained versions of the standard Guepar knee prosthesis, which had been modified for segmental replacement. Because of their fixed "door hinge" design, these prostheses were subject to a high rate of loosening and breakage and did not constitute a viable long-term solution.
- Since the early 1980s, segmental replacement prostheses have evolved significantly and have become available for

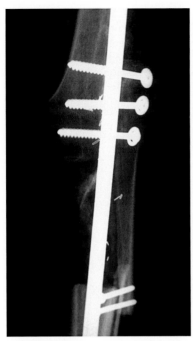

Figure 15–1: Turn-down procedure.
Postoperative anteroposterior radiograph of a turn-down procedure performed on a patient with a large giant cell tumor of the proximal tibia.

many anatomic locations, including the humerus, femur, and tibia, to provide functional shoulder, elbow, hip, and knee prostheses. Total bone replacement has also become a possibility for the femur and humerus, although these procedures are rarely indicated.

- The other major segmental replacement reconstructive option that arose in the 1980s was the use of osteoarticular allografts (Fig. 15–3). These grafts were met with initial

early enthusiasm because they represented a "biologic" alternative to massive metallic prostheses. The use of these grafts paralleled the evolution of bone banking techniques along with the availability of these grafts from a number of bone banks. Their use for tumor reconstruction in the United States was pioneered by various people, but it was extensively studied by Dr. Henry Mankin and his associates (Mankin et al. 1996).

- These osteoarticular allografts demonstrated early positive results with good joint function and a reasonable complication rate. Over time, however, the complications of fracture, nonunion, infection, dislocation, and arthritis rose to a level that decreased the overall enthusiasm for this technique in the lower extremity, where weight-bearing stresses made it difficult for the grafts to survive. However, osteoarticular grafts remain a popular option for non–weight-bearing applications such as the proximal humerus and distal radius, which are sites of frequent tumor involvement. In these locations, the stresses to which the grafts are subjected are much less than those experienced in weight-bearing applications, thereby increasing the longevity of the graft.

- Research by Mankin and colleagues demonstrated a fourfold increase in the number of endoprosthetic reconstructions performed at their institution from the mid-1980s to the mid-1990s compared with a concomitant 50% decrease in the use of allograft reconstructions for limb preservation surgery. In perhaps the largest published series of allografts (718 total, 386 of which were osteoarticular), these authors reported a 19% fracture rate, a 17% nonunion rate, an 11% infection rate, and a 6% rate of joint instability, with most of these complications occurring within the first 3 years of implantation (Mankin et al. 1996). If the allograft managed to survive the first 3 years, osteoarthritis typically became a problem for the osteoarticular allografts at around 6 years postoperatively. Even though 16% of the osteoarticular allografts ultimately required conversion to total joint arthroplasty, approximately 75% of the grafts were retained by the patient and were considered successful for more than 20 years following implantation (Mankin et al. 1996).

- In our experience at a tertiary level orthopaedic oncology university referral center, we have found endoprosthetic reconstruction to be a very reliable technique for restoration of segmental defects following wide resection of sarcomas. We recently reviewed the long-term survival of 139 endoprosthetic reconstructions performed over an 8-year period to achieve a better understanding of the factors affecting endoprosthetic survival (Torbert et al. 2005). Kaplan-Meier event-free survivorship analysis revealed that endoprosthetic survival was 86%, 80%, and 69% at 3, 5, and 10-year follow-up, respectively. The location and periprosthetic infection had a statistically significant effect on survival. The patient's age or type of reconstruction (primary versus revision) did not affect survival outcomes.

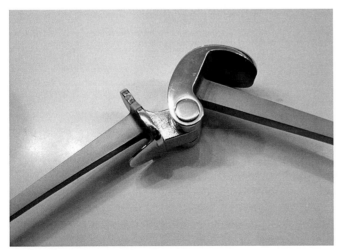

Figure 15–2: Guepar knee prosthesis.
Completely constrained standard Guepar knee prosthesis.

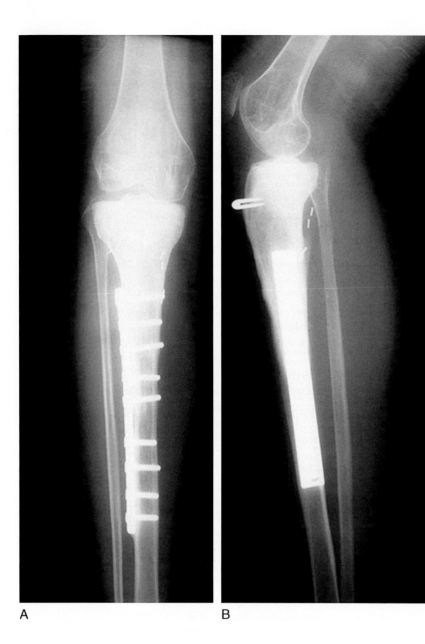

A   B

Figure 15–3: Osteoarticular allograft in segmental tibial reconstruction.
A and **B,** Postoperative anteroposterior and lateral radiographs demonstrating segmental reconstruction of the proximal tibia utilizing osteoarticular allograft.

There was a low early wound complication rate (3 of 129 patients; i.e., 2.3% developed early infections), and all these complications followed proximal tibia replacements (Torbert et al. 2005). These studies help to substantiate the evolution of this procedure and demonstrate the reliability of current techniques.

Categorization Based on Anatomic Zones
Proximal Femur

- Probably the simplest site for segmental replacement early designs was the proximal femur. In light of the early success of hemiarthroplasty and total hip replacement, the only necessary development was the longer body component and a stem to fit the diaphyseal location because that is where most of these stems were placed, given the common segmental replacement lengths of 60 to 160 mm.

- Initially, early models were one-piece femoral components that could be utilized for treatment with either total hip arthroplasty or hemiarthroplasty (Fig. 15–4). Cemented stems were used most commonly. The most difficult engineering challenge was the design of the attachment site for the greater trochanter. Early designs used a metal loop for trochanteric attachment, which was not optimal. The most common surgical technique utilized multistrand cables or thick nonmetallic sutures around the trochanter and through the prosthetic loop. The acute turn of the wire or suture around the loop compounded with the stress concentration and wear characteristics of this design caused cable or suture breakage and subsequent proximal migration of the trochanter.

- Most modern designs have replaced the prosthetic loop with holes through the prosthesis for use with wire or

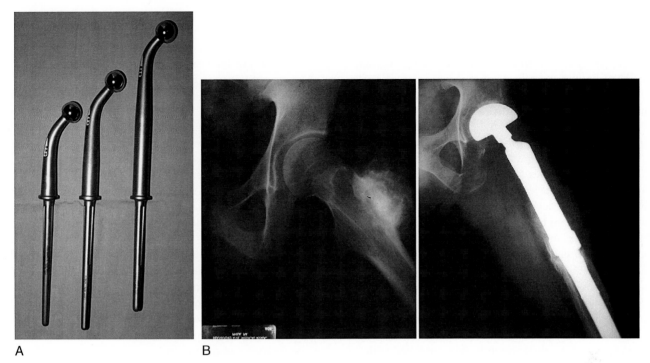

A   B

Figure 15–4: Proximal femoral segmental replacement.
A, Early proximal femoral segmental replacement prostheses. **B,** Preoperative anteroposterior pelvis radiographs of a patient who underwent proximal femoral segmental replacement.

heavy suture. Further accommodations for trochanteric reattachment vary among manufacturers.

- All current designs are modular with varying body sizes and stem diameters (Fig. 15–5). Several studies document the early success and long-term durability of these prostheses. The most common application for tumor replacements has been the use of these prostheses in association with a hemi-arthroplasty and a cemented stem. The rationale for the use of a hemiarthroplasty has been that, in most of these patients, the acetabulum is normal with regard to subchondral bone and articular cartilage. Another advantage of the hemiarthro-plasty was the increased inherent stability of a large ball in a deeper socket when compared with a total hip prosthesis.

- Several authors have discussed the efficacy of these prostheses in the context of massive bone loss involving the proximal femur associated with multiple hip revision operations. In these cases, many of the structures that normally aid hip joint stability have been destroyed or compromised, including the hip capsule and the trochanteric attachment.

- As such, meticulous surgical technique is needed to optimize performance and to minimize complications, including prosthetic failure. It is probably critical in these reconstructions that there be little or no toggle between the femoral and acetabular components because this may lead to instability and dislocation. As such, technical options include insertion of the prosthesis with no toggle and perhaps considering the use of a constrained liner to avoid instability. For the same reasons, proper version of the acetabular and femoral components is mandatory.

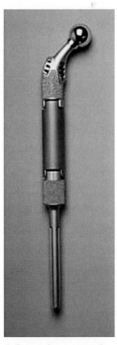

Figure 15–5: Proximal femoral segmental replacement prosthesis. A current modular proximal femoral segmental replacement prosthesis demonstrating a variety of body sizes and stem diameters.

Both closure of the capsule or pseudocapsule (if present) and advancement of the greater trochanter may help to secure fixation and to prevent dislocation.

- The use of an abduction brace is useful during the early phases of healing and rehabilitation. Since the mid-1980s, in the United States, most of the components on the market have utilized cemented stems. Several authors have reported on the issue of stem loosening, and this is probably the single largest reason for eventual revision. The revision rate for sterile loosening of these prostheses has varied from 10% to 33% at 10 years (Choong et al. 1996, Horowitz et al. 1993, Mittermayer et al. 2001). Although this rate is reasonable, more recent attempts have been made to develop noncemented stems to help avoid this complication.

- In Europe, Kotz and associates reported on the use of a bone ingrowth stem with an associated side plate (Fig. 15–6) (Kotz et al. 1989). Complications with this system have included stress shielding and bone-collar resorption secondary to particulate debris (Donati et al. 2001). A novel spring-loaded, titanium-alloy uncemented implant was recently developed to address the problem of loosening secondary to stress-shielding in patients managed with tumor prostheses (Bini et al. 2000).

- More recently, the United States market has seen the introduction of other cementless stem designs, although no data on the potential long-term success of these cementless designs are available to date. The answer as to whether these particular designs will eventually perform better or worse than cemented stems remains to be seen. As always, surgeons should carefully consider integrating any novel technology unsupported by long-term data into their practice.

Surgical Tips for Proximal Femoral Replacement Prostheses

- The main issues with proximal femoral replacement prostheses include stability and leg-length inequality.
- In terms of stability, several considerations are important. Whenever possible, it is advisable to repair any available capsule or pseudocapsular tissue to improve immediate postoperative stability.

- Similarly, retention and firm fixation of the greater trochanter to the prosthesis are invaluable in avoiding laxity and subsequent dislocation. To achieve successful reattachment, either multistrand cable or 5-mm suture tapes are acceptable. Most of these sutures eventually break, and the cable has the disadvantage of being visible on radiographs. In most cases, however, the trochanter is already scarred down to the prosthesis before suture failure and so the trochanter rarely migrates far cephalad.

- When the proximal femoral replacement prosthesis is performed for metastatic involvement of the proximal femur, it is reasonable to preserve the trochanter, if mechanically sound, despite the presence of tumor in the trochanter. Adjunctive radiation or chemotherapy will usually handle the tumor load in this limited area, and maintenance of the trochanter will greatly aid postoperative stability. One exception to this approach is planned wide resection of metastatic renal cell carcinoma, in which obtaining wide margins may be important for subsequent local control of the tumor.

- In addition to closing the capsule and advancing the greater trochanter, it is important to put the prosthesis in tightly with no toggle and correct anteversion, usually 15 to 20 degrees (Fig. 15–7).

- Assessing correct anteversion in the absence of normal anatomic proximal femoral landmarks may be difficult (Lackman et al. 2006). Moreover, proximal femoral replacement prostheses do not include lateral offset options because they would not be effective given that there is no intact capsule for the lateral offset to tighten. Ultimately, it may be necessary to lengthen the extremity beyond the length of the contralateral limb, and patients should be advised preoperatively that although this procedure is designed to reestablish a stable, painless hip, subsequent limb-length inequality may occur.

- When there is no capsule or trochanteric tissue to repair, joint stability depends solely on a tight fit and correct version of components. In these cases, it may be necessary to place the patient in an abduction cast around both the waist and one thigh, with the involved limb in mild abduction and slight flexion. Such casts can be maintained for a 6-week period, after which most patients will be stable on the basis of scar formation around the joint.

- In terms of the articulation, constrained liners may be beneficial in the context of revision total hip surgery. In cases performed for proximal femoral tumors where the acetabulum is not affected, bipolar articulations have a good long-term track record and have more intrinsic stability than total hip prostheses.

Distal Femur and Proximal Tibia

- Probably the most common use of segmental replacement prostheses has involved the knee. The distal femur has

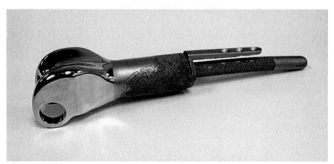

Figure 15–6: Segmental replacement prosthesis. **Segmental replacement prosthesis with associated compression side plate to facilitate prosthetic fixation about the hip and knee.**

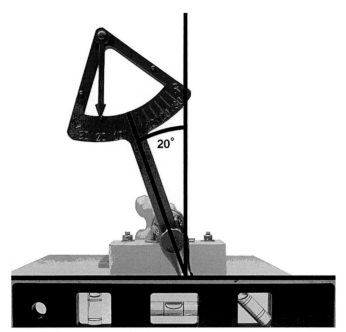

Figure 15–7: Anteversion jig.
Anteversion jig as designed by Richard Lackman.

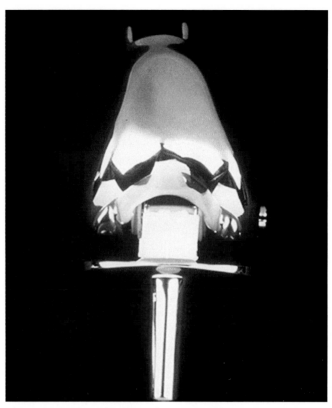

Figure 15–8: Rotating-hinge knee assembly.
Standard segmental rotating-hinge knee assembly.

accounted for the largest share of these procedures because it is a common site for primary and metastatic tumors.

- The real success of these designs dates back to the invention of the rotating-hinge total knee, which was a fixed-hinge knee prosthesis introduced by Walldius in 1953 for use in primary total knee arthroplasty (Barrack et al. 2000). As mentioned previously, initial hinged knee designs utilized constrained door hinge technology. This design, which transmitted tremendous stresses to the prostheses and the bone-cement interfaces, made early failure inevitable. The Walldius design utilized a hinge in the femoral component but was connected to the tibia with a rotating bearing component (Fig. 15–8). As such, the bearing component could toggle up and down within the tibial component and also allowed rotation. Thus, varus and valgus stresses were relieved by flexion and rotation and distraction forces were relieved by slight pistoning of the bearing component. This design allowed far less stress to be delivered to the prosthetic components themselves, as well as to the bone-cement interfaces. This design has been altered to some extent by a variety of manufacturers, but all current designs remain true to the basic plan of the original rotating hinge.

- Several design evolutions have occurred over the past 2 decades since segmental replacement designs became available. These changes have involved modularity, stem design, patellofemoral joint mechanics, patellar tendon attachment, prosthetic size, bearing component geometry, and jig improvements.

- With regard to modularity, initial designs were one-piece, custom-ordered items with primitive stem designs that afforded no intraoperative flexibility (Fig. 15–9). Current systems are completely modular with varying stem, body, and joint component sizes (Fig. 15–10). This variety affords the surgeon myriad intraoperative choices, which can optimize prosthetic placement, function, and stability. Body sizes that are inserted between the stem and the articular components replace lost bone stock and usually vary every 1 to 2 cm, depending on the manufacturer (Fig. 15–11). These are simple shafts with Morse tapers, and design differences are typically not an issue.

- Stem design is probably an important consideration, although no studies have investigated which parameters of individual designs are most effective. It is reasonable to assume that avoiding stems with very small diameters will decrease stem breakage. As such, stems used for lower extremity reconstructions should probably be at least 13 mm in diameter, although surgical judgment for individual cases is always essential, and excessive reaming of normal bone is not desirable.

- Similar to proximal femoral segmental replacement prostheses, both cemented and noncemented stem designs exist. Certainly, more data are available regarding the long-term survival of cemented stems than regarding

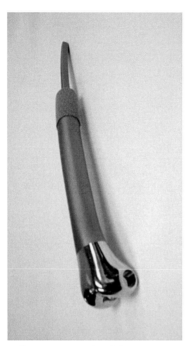

Figure 15–9: Early one-piece distal femoral replacement prosthesis.

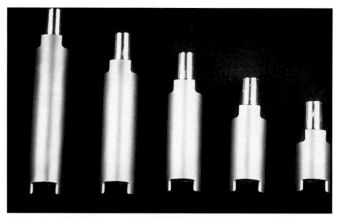

Figure 15–11: Segmental replacement prostheses. Varying body segments that allow for varying the length of segmental replacement at 2-cm increments.

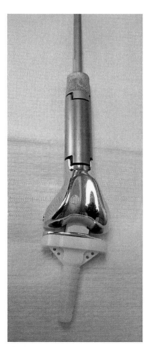

Figure 15–10: Distal femoral segmental replacement modular-hinge prosthesis.
A distal femoral segmental replacement modular-hinge prosthesis with the tibial component.

noncemented designs. As such, it is up to each surgeon to review design and outcome parameters before making implant decisions. Beyond that, the stem designs used for the proximal femur are usually the same provided by most manufacturers for the distal femur and proximal tibia as well.

- One of the most critical areas of concern with any knee design is patellofemoral articulation. This is an area of extreme stress concentration and a site where misalignment can result in pain and instability. Two important issues are inherent patellofemoral design stability and proper component insertion. In terms of design, several products on the market have developed improved patellofemoral stability by widening and deepening the trochlear notch on the distal femoral component. This has gone a long way toward making the articulation less precarious and has also added significant inherent stability to the patellar component as it rides in the trochlear notch.

- The other factor that remains important to proper function is proper version on the femoral and tibial components. In terms of the distal femur, the components are usually placed in anatomic position with neutral version, or they may have jigs to impart slight external rotation. The more critical prosthetic position involves the tibial component. This is usually placed in slight external rotation so during flexion, the tibia is slightly rotated internally, thus bringing the patella up on top of the femoral component and preventing lateral patellar dislocation. Typically, about 10 to 15 degrees of external rotation of the tibial component will be adequate, although individual situations may call for more, especially in the context of a failed standard total knee replacement.

- Patellar tendon reattachment and soft tissue coverage are the major challenges inherent in proximal tibial segmental replacement total knees. In terms of patellar tendon reattachment, no clear solution exists at present.

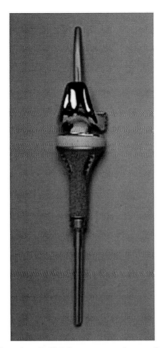

Figure 15–12: Proximal tibial segmental prosthesis.
Proximal tibial segmental prosthesis demonstrating a sintered anterior surface to facilitate soft tissue ingrowth.

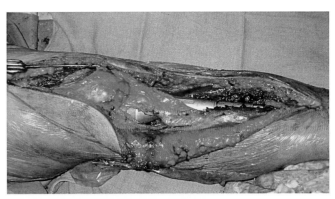

Figure 15–13: Primary wound closure.
Primary closure of the surgical wound overlying the proximal tibia is typically feasible with appropriate soft tissue dissection and use of proper endoprosthetic design as discussed.

Several designs are available, most of which utilize a sintered surface on the anterior aspect of the tibial component to facilitate soft tissue ingrowth (Fig. 15–12). This process aids in scar formation and adhesion of the patellar tendon to the surface of the prosthesis. Usually, this is performed in association with holes in the tibial component to allow insertion of large sutures to help stabilize the patellar tendon repair during healing. Protection of this repair is achieved by keeping the knee in extension in a knee immobilizer or a cylinder cast for 5 to 6 weeks following surgery. Most patients treated in this manner regain greater than 90 degrees of flexion with the help of gentle physical therapy. Many patients eventually develop an extensor lag, although this is usually less than 20 degrees and may be absent altogether. Rarely does this lag cause knee instability, but if it does, a drop-lock brace can be used to maintain the knee in extension during ambulation.

- In terms of soft tissue coverage for the proximal tibia, there are two important rules:

1. Be mindful to handle the soft tissue flaps with care to avoid necrosis.
2. Never close the wound with the tissues in tension.

- In many cases, flap coverage is unnecessary because primary closure over the tibial component is possible (Fig. 15–13) (Abboud et al. 2003). When the soft tissue is not adequate for primary closure, a medial gastrocnemius flap with or without a split-thickness skin graft provides adequate coverage.

- The other factor that facilitates ease of closure is the use of a downsized tibial component. Some manufacturers include regular and small versions of the rotating-hinge tibial component in their sets. This may make closure much simpler and helps to avoid the need for flap coverage. Finally, appropriate jigs will facilitate proper prosthetic insertion, especially in the hands of the occasional user. As such, it may be helpful for the occasional surgeon to review the techniques involved by using a "saw bones" knee and closely review all jigs along with their proper use and placement.

Distal Femoral Replacement: Illustrative Example

- A patient with metastatic hypernephroma sustained a pathologic fracture above a previously placed total knee arthroplasty. Before the injury, the patient had an intramedullary rod inserted for prophylactic treatment of a lytic lesion localized to the midshaft of the femur (Fig. 15–14). This lesion was approximately 10 cm proximal to the supracondylar fracture. The patient consented to undergo distal femoral replacement in an attempt to salvage the limb.
- Preparation and draping (Fig. 15–15) included the use of a sterile tourniquet to facilitate access to the proximal thigh. Anterior exposure of the knee was achieved utilizing a medial parapatellar incision similar to the type used in total knee arthroplasty (Fig. 15–16). The incision extended far enough to allow clear visualization and access to both the bony pathologic features and the preexisting instrumentation. On extending the longitudinal incision, the femoral intramedullary rod was noted to be protruding from the fracture (Fig. 15–17).
- In removing the distal femur, careful attention was paid to stay in the subplane. The protruding rod was further visualized with subperiosteal dissection, and following removal of the femoral rod, the incision was carried

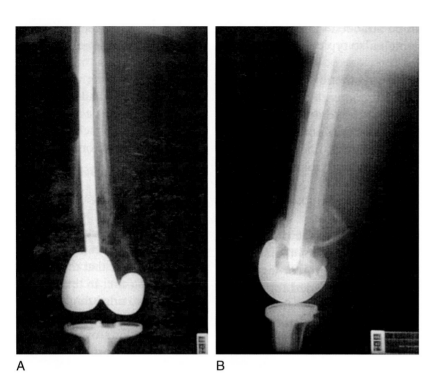

A

B

Figure 15–14: Pathologic supracondylar femoral fracture.
Anteroposterior (**A**) and lateral (**B**) radiographs demonstrating a pathologic supracondylar femoral fracture in a patient with metastatic hypernephroma that was prophylactically treated with an intramedullary rod.

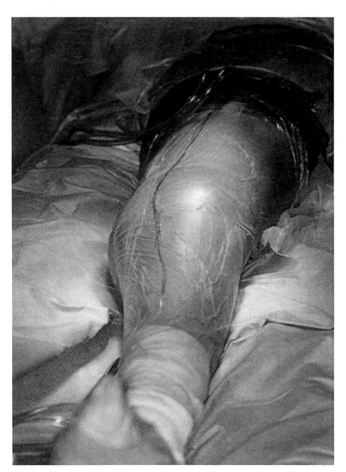

Figure 15–15: Distal femoral replacement.
Initial preparation and draping demonstrating far proximal placement of the sterile tourniquet.

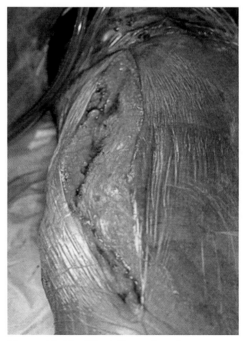

Figure 15–16: Distal femoral replacement.
Initial medial parapatellar incision.

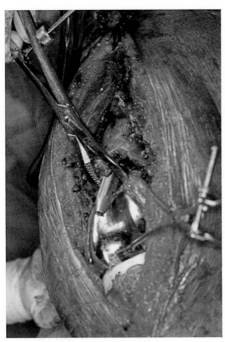

Figure 15–17: Distal femoral replacement. Further proximal exposure reveals an intramedullary rod protruding from the fracture.

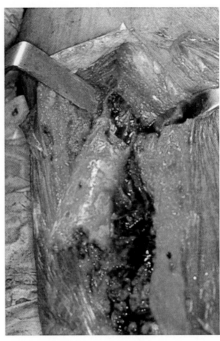

Figure 15–18: Distal femoral replacement. Adequate anterior exposure demonstrates a large lytic lesion of the femoral shaft.

proximally to expose the large lytic lesion in the midshaft of the femur, which was resected (Fig. 15–18).

Surgical Tips for Segmental Distal Femoral Replacement Prostheses

- This procedure has several key points that can facilitate trouble-free insertion of the femoral components.
- It is often difficult to identify the direct anterior surface of the femur once it has been osteotomized because the proximal fragment often externally rotates when these cuts are made. In our experience, we have found that marking the anterior aspect of the femur located proximally to the planned site of osteotomy can assist the surgeon in maintaining proper orientation of the femoral fragments.
- To maintain proper leg length on the operative side, it may prove useful to assemble the bone fragments that have been removed on a back table. Reconstruction of these fragments allows accurate measurement of the amount of bone that has been removed, thereby serving as a way to ensure that the same length of bone is reconstructed during surgery.
- In comparison with routine total knee arthroplasties, hinged knee prostheses require a thicker tibial cut to accommodate the insertion of both the tibial component and the medullary bearing component. These dimensions vary according to manufacturers, and thus one should review preoperatively the specifications of the particular system to be used.

- A particularly challenging area of distal femoral replacement hinged prostheses is maintaining appropriate patellofemoral tracking and stability. Marking the anterior aspect of the femur and externally rotating the tibial component approximately 15 degrees can prove useful in this regard. In our experience, we have found no apparent difference in stability between patients who had patellar resurfacing with a patellar button and those who did not receive resurfacing. Following insertion of the trial components, it is extremely important to note the patellar tracking within the trochlear notch. The patella should track well, with no evidence of lateral instability. If lateral tracking is noticed, it should be remedied by altering rotation of the tibial and, occasionally, femoral components. Furthermore, it is important to ensure that the patella does not impinge on the anterior aspect of the tibial occasionally component when the knee is in full flexion. Ultimately, this can become a problem if the tibial cut is not the proper thickness because it can cause patellotibial impingement.
- When utilizing cement, we favor cementing the tibial components first. Before cementing the femoral component, we recommend assembling the axle and bearing components so once the femoral component is placed into the cement filled femoral canal, subsequent reduction of the prosthesis can occur by insertion of the tibial bearing component into the tibial stem with the knee placed in full flexion. We then cycle the knee through flexion and extension to check the alignment and stability of the components before the cement hardens around the femoral stem.

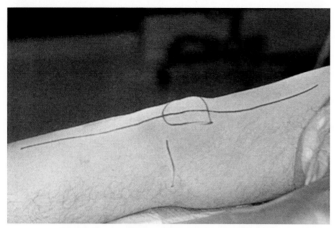

Figure 15–19: Proximal tibia replacement.
Preparation and draping utilized for proximal tibia replacement.

As the cement hardens, we can make last-minute modifications of the femoral component rotation and patellofemoral stability.

- To check rotational alignment of the knee, one can observe the tibial bearing component in relation to the tibial tray. Ultimately, the tibial component should remain in line with the edges of the tray, with no evidence of rotational shift during flexion and extension maneuvers. If it is clear that the femoral component rotated on the tibial component during flexion and extension of the knee, then proper rotational alignment has not been achieved, and modifications to tibial or femoral rotation should be made.

Proximal Tibial Replacement: Illustrative Example

- Routine preparation and draping are performed and are followed by a medial parapatellar incision (Fig. 15–19). It is important to be wary of the common peroneal nerve, which should be exposed as large medial and lateral flaps are dissected (Fig. 15–20).

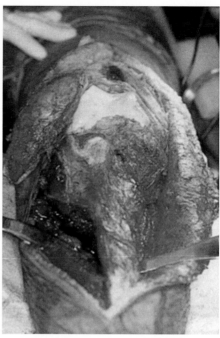

Figure 15–21: Proximal tibia replacement.
Extraperiosteal exposure of the proximal tibia for sarcoma.

- Once again, the dissection should remain in the subperiosteal plane, unless underlying tumor requires an extraperiosteal-wide resection (Fig. 15–21). The proximal tibia is subsequently excised (Fig. 15–22).
- The distal femur, as well as the origins of the medial and lateral collateral ligaments, should be adequately exposed to facilitate an accurate cut of the posterior femur.

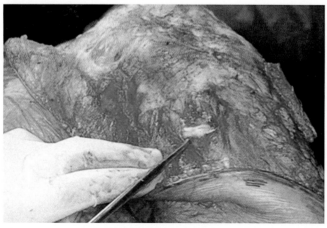

Figure 15–20: Proximal tibia replacement.
Large medial and lateral flaps facilitate exposure of the common peroneal nerve.

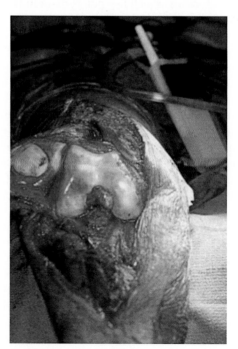

Figure 15–22: Proximal tibia replacement.
Surgical bed following excision of the proximal tibia.

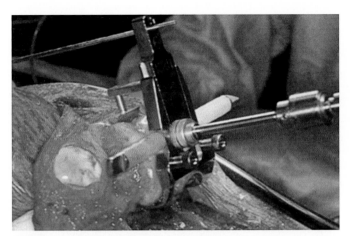

Figure 15–23: Proximal tibia replacement.
A sizing jig is applied to the distal femur. (Courtesy of
Howmedica, Rutherford, NJ.)

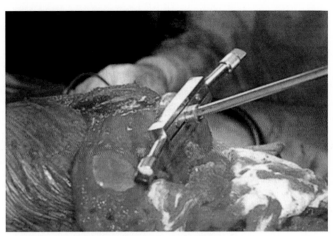

Figure 15–25: Proximal tibia replacement.
Distal femoral cuts in the anterior and posterior planes.
(Courtesy of Howmedica, Rutherford, NJ.)

The femoral jigs and cuts are similar to those made for the
nonsegmental rotating-hinge knee prosthesis because they
include a distal femoral sizing jig (Fig. 15–23), a transverse
distal femoral cut (Fig. 15–24), and anterior and posterior
femoral cuts (Fig. 15–25). When all the distal femoral cuts
have been made (Fig. 15–26), trial placement of the
femoral component can occur (Fig. 15–27).

- Flexible reamers are utilized to ream the tibial shaft
(Fig. 15–28), and a trial tibial stem and component are
then inserted to find the appropriate fit (Fig. 15–29). The
final prosthesis appears as shown following cementation of
the tibial and femoral components (Fig. 15–30). Finally,
No. 2 nonabsorbable sutures are used to reattach the
patellar tendon to the loop on the tibial component and
the retinaculum to provide additional support to the final
tendon repair (Fig. 15–31).

Surgical Tips for Segmental Proximal
Tibial Replacement Prostheses

- Typically, proximal tibial replacement utilizes routine distal
femoral cuts to facilitate placement of the nonsegmental
femoral component.
- The surgeon must be careful to keep the flap as thick
as possible and avoid unnecessary medial or lateral dissection, to preserve the native blood supply to the flaps.
To achieve adequate anterior coverage, it may prove useful
to use a gastrocnemius flap and skin graft at the time of
the initial procedure. This may help avoid having to do so
if flap necrosis occurs several days postoperatively, a situation that significantly increases the risk of infection.
- As mentioned earlier, the development of prosthetic
systems with downsized tibial components has facilitated

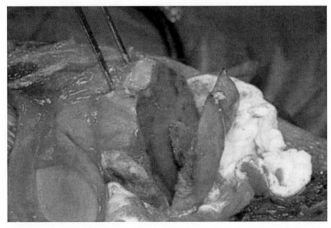

Figure 15–24: Proximal tibia replacement.
Transverse cut of the distal femur. (Courtesy of Howmedica,
Rutherford, NJ.)

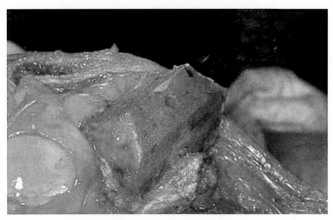

Figure 15–26: Proximal tibia replacement.
Distal femur following all cuts with a sizing jig. (Courtesy of
Howmedica, Rutherford, NJ.)

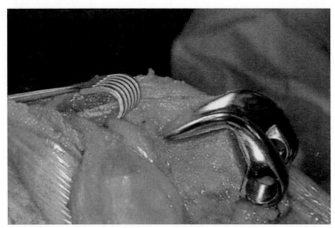

Figure15-27: Proximal tibia replacement.
A trial prosthesis is applied to the distal femur. (Courtesy of Howmedica, Rutherford, NJ.)

primary wound closure and has significantly relieved pressure from adjacent tissue flaps.
• Preservation of the patellar tendon attachment on the tibial tubercle is now possible. Many prosthetic systems have developed tibial components that can compensate for defects of 1 or 2 cm, thereby precluding the need for resection of longer segments of the tibia. In cases that involve significant proximal tibial segmental replacement, the tendon must be reattached to the prosthesis. By keeping the initial dissection in the subperiosteal plane when the

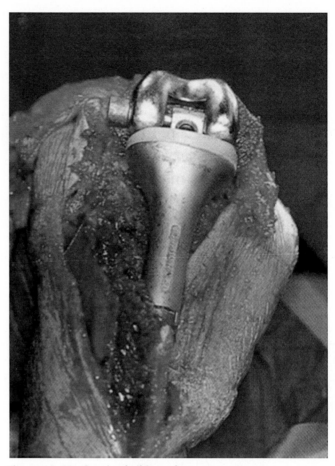

Figure 15–29: Proximal tibia replacement.
Trial components are inserted to ensure the proper size and position of the final prosthesis.

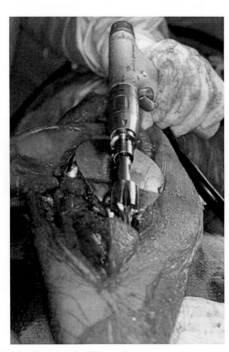

Figure 15–28: Proximal tibia replacement.
Flexible reamers are utilized to ream the tibial shaft followed by a chamfer reamer, as shown.

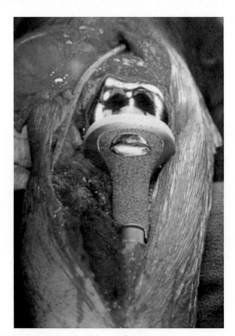

Figure 15–30: Proximal tibia replacement.
Following cementation of the tibial and femoral components, the final prosthesis is placed in proper position.

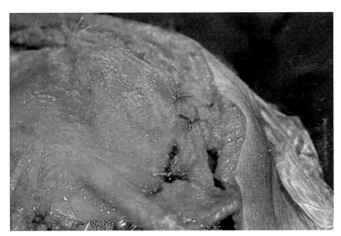

Figure 15–31: Proximal tibia replacement.
The patellar tendon is repaired to the prosthesis and the medial retinaculum to secure the repair.

patellar tendon is removed from its insertion on the tibial tubercle, it is sometimes possible to maintain the patellar tendon in continuity with the deep fascia of the anterior compartment of the leg. Ultimately, this preserves the distal anchoring of the patellar tendon and, perhaps, its native blood supply. Furthermore, this type of dissection helps to maintain the normal length of the tendon, thereby precluding estimation of appropriate length and tension when reestablishing the distal tendon attachment. If for some

reason this technique is not feasible, the patellar tendon should be incised from the tibia to maintain maximum length, which facilitates subsequent reattachment.

- To facilitate tendon reattachment, most prosthetic systems currently provide holes through the prosthesis itself for suture fixation with nonabsorbable No. 2 suture. We have found it useful to repair the sides of the patellar tendon to the medial or lateral edges of the anterior retinaculum to support the stability and length of the repair further.

Total Femoral Replacement Prostheses

- Occasionally, it becomes necessary to resect and replace the entire femur with a new articulation at the hip and the knee (Fig. 15–32). This is most commonly indicated in patients with extensive tumor involvement of the femur, but also occasionally in patients with multiple hip and knee prosthesis revision on the involved side.
- Extendable reconstruction devices (Fig. 15–33) for replacing all or part of the femur offer skeletally immature patients with malignant bone tumors the opportunity of a nearly normal leg length by overcoming an expected leg-length discrepancy.
- In patients undergoing total femur replacement, the hip and knee considerations are similar to those involved with segmental replacement of either end of the bone. Hip stability can be a major issue, and a constrained liner is a worthwhile consideration.

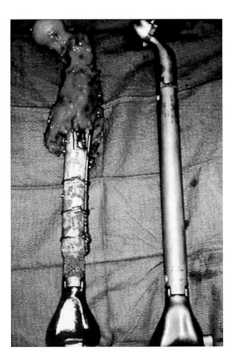

Figure 15–32: Femoral prosthesis replacement.
Prior tumor endoprosthesis is resected and replaced with total femoral replacement prosthesis.

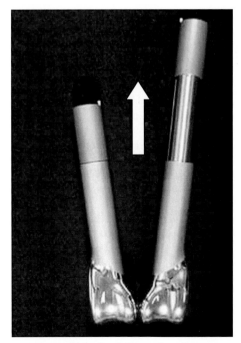

Figure 15–33: Extendable distal femoral replacement prosthesis.
Extendable prostheses facilitate segmental replacement in skeletally immature patients.

- Total femur replacements are less functional than proximal or distal femoral replacements individually, but they still can be a major improvement over high-level amputations in these patients.
- With regard to future trends for these prostheses, several avenues of research are currently in progress. One of the most promising of these studies is metal foam, which will facilitate and enhance soft tissue attachment to metallic components. This will likely improve the outcome with regard to abductor attachment to the proximal femur and patellar tendon attachment to the proximal tibia.
- The other area that will likely see further advancement relates to bone ingrowth into noncemented stems. We hope that biologic solutions will become available to enhance fixation and decrease sterile loosening of prosthetic stems.

References

Abboud JA, Patel RV, Donthineni-Rao R, Lackman RD (2003). Proximal tibial segmental prosthetic replacement without the use of muscle flaps. *Clin Orthop Relat Res* 414:189-196.

In this study, 22 patients with bone tumors had proximal tibial segmental prosthetic replacement using direct reattachment of the patellar tendon to the prosthesis without the use of a muscle flap. Two of 19 patients required reoperation in the postoperative period for hematomas. Both were free of infection or other complications at 24 months mean follow-up. No other wound complications occurred despite initiation of chemotherapy 2 to 3 weeks after surgery in patients with high-grade malignant tumors (15 of 19). The mean follow-up was 38.6 months (range, 13 to 99 months). The patients ranged in age from 15 to 74 years (mean, 39 years). The range of motion achieved postoperatively showed a mean of 97 degrees (±16.3 degrees). All patients had full passive extension with a mean extensor lag of 7.5 degrees. The mean Musculoskeletal Tumor Society score was 27.6 (±2.0). These results of patients without muscle flaps compare favorably with published results advocating gastrocnemius flaps for the attachment of the patellar tendon to the prosthesis.

Barrack RL, Lyons TR, Ingraham RQ, Johnson JC (2000). The use of a modular rotating hinge component in salvage revision total knee arthroplasty. *J Arthroplasty* 15:858-866.

This is a retrospective review of revision total knee arthroplasty using a second-generation modular rotating-hinge design performed on 16 knees in 15 patients over a 5-year period. Indications for revision were aseptic loosening of a hinged prosthesis (8 knees), loosening and bone loss associated with chronic extensor mechanism disruption (2 knees), component instability with chronic medial collateral ligament disruption (3 knees), and comminuted distal femur fracture (1 knee). Clinical and radiographic results were reviewed and compared with 87 patients who underwent revision total knee arthroplasty using a standard condylar revision design during the same period. Early results showed comparable postoperative knee scores and range of motion between the two groups despite the use of the rotating-hinge component in more complex revision cases. Short-term clinical and radiographic results were encouraging and suggest that a second-generation modular rotating-hinge component can be used successfully in selected salvage revision cases.

Bini SA, Johnston JO, Martin DL (2000). Compliant prestress fixation in tumor prostheses: Interface retrieval data. *Orthopedics* 23:707-712.

This article reported the first available human retrieval data following the use of a new fixation system for tumor prostheses. The compliant prestress fixation system obviates the need for long intramedullary stems. The compliant prestress system was designed to provide a stable, high-pressure, motion-free bone-implant interface that would prevent aseptic loosening and allow osseointegration at the bone-implant interface. At 10 months, the fourth patient in the human trial required amputation. Backscatter electron microscopy revealed a buttress of new bone had formed along 70% of the bone-metal interface, with excellent bony ingrowth (average, 42%) into the transverse, porous-coated titanium interface.

Choong PF, Sim FH, Pritchard DJ, et al. (1996). Megaprostheses after resection of distal femoral tumors. *Acta Orthop Scand* 67:345-351.

This is a retrospective review of 32 Kinematic Rotating-Hinge Knee tumor prostheses in 30 patients, of which 2 concerned revisions of the same type of prosthesis. The median age was 25 years (range, 12 to 60 years), and the median follow-up for survivors was 3.5 years (range, 2 to 6.6 years). Twenty knees had excellent Musculoskeletal Tumor Society (MSTS) scores for motion (median flexion, 120 degrees), 8 had good (84 degrees), and 4 had fair (45 degrees). The overall function was excellent in 6 cases, good in 14, fair in 9, and poor in 3. The radiographic assessment International Society of Limb Salvage (ISOLS) gave "excellent" or "good" scores in 27 knees for bone remodeling, 31 for the interface, 28 for the anchorage, 31 for the implant body, and 30 for the articulation.

Donati D, Zavatta M, Gozzi E, et al. (2001). Modular prosthetic replacement of the proximal femur after resection of a bone tumour: A long-term follow-up. *J Bone Joint Surg Br* 83:1156-1160.

This is a retrospective review of 25 patients who underwent proximal femur resection and replacement with an uncemented, bipolar, modular prosthesis. When followed up after more than 10 years, 4 prostheses (16%) had required revision. The most obvious feature in the bone-stem relationship was stress shielding, seen as osteoporosis of the proximal part of the femur around the stem in 68%. Functional activity was satisfactory in 68% of the patients.

Enneking WF (1987). Modification of the system for functional evaluation of surgical management of musculoskeletal tumors. In: Enneking WF, ed. *Limb Salvage in Musculoskeletal Oncology.* New York: Churchill Livingstone, pp 626-639.

This is an excellent review of functional evaluation after limb salvage surgery for musculoskeletal tumors.

Horowitz SM, Glasser DB, Lane JM, et al. (1993). Prosthetic and extremity survivorship after limb salvage for sarcoma: How long do the reconstructions last? *Clin Orthop Relat Res* 293:280-286.

This is a retrospective review of 93 consecutive prosthetic reconstructions performed for limb salvage after the resection of sarcomas of the lower extremity. Reconstruction was of the proximal femur in 16, the distal femur in 61, and the proximal tibia in 16 patients. Minimum follow-up time was 24 months, with a median of 66 months and mean of 80 months. Limb survival at 5 years was significantly better, with the proximal femur at 88%, the distal femur at 88%, and the proximal tibia at 78% intact. Aseptic loosening survival was better than the event-free prosthetic survival, a finding that demonstrates the influence of factors such as sepsis (hematogenous) or wound necrosis that lead to prosthetic removal. Prosthetic, extremity, and patient survival differed depending on the site.

Kotz R, Pongracz N, Fellinger EJ, Ritschl P (1989). Uncemented hinge prostheses with reinsertion of the ligamentum patellae. In: Yamamuro T, ed. *New Developments for Limb Salvage in Musculoskeletal Tumours.* New York: Springer Verlag, pp 605-610.

This is an excellent review of uncemented hinge prostheses with reinsertion of the ligamentum patellae.

Lackman RD, Torbert JT, Finstein JL, et al. (In press). Inaccuracies in the assessment of femoral anteversion in proximal femoral replacement prostheses. *University of Pennsylvania Orthopaedic Journal.*

This article outlines the use of a novel jig used to determine accurately the femoral anteversion intraoperatively as designed by Richard Lackman.

Mankin HJ, Gebhardt MC, Jennings LC, et al. (1996). Long-term results of allograft replacement in the management of bone tumors. *Clin Orthop Relat Res* 324:86-97.

This is a retrospective review of more than 870 massive frozen cadaveric allografts mostly for the treatment of defects after tumor resection. The results show that only stage and type of graft affected outcome predictably. Specifically, grafts for a stage 2 or stage 3 tumor had a poorer outcome than those for stages 0 and 1. The results for allograft arthrodeses were considerably poorer than osteoarticular, intercalary, and allograft plus prosthesis.

Mittermayer F, Krepler P, Dominkus M, et al. (2001). Long-term follow-up of uncemented tumor endoprostheses for the lower extremity. *Clin Orthop Relat Res* 388:167-177.

This is a retrospective review of 100 primary lower limb reconstructions using the Kotz Modular Femur Tibia Reconstruction System after resection of a malignant tumor. In 32 patients a proximal femur prosthesis was implanted, in 40 patients a distal femur prosthesis was implanted, in 19 patients a proximal tibia component was implanted, in 4 patients a total femur prosthesis was implanted, and in 5 patients a total knee prosthesis was implanted. The Kaplan-Meier estimate of the overall survival rate of the prostheses was 85% after 3 years, 79% after 5 years, and 71% after 10 years. The most common reason for implant failure was aseptic loosening in 27% of patients (11 patients; range, 10 to 121 months) after the initial operation.

Torbert JT, Fox EJ, Hosalkar HS, et al. (2005). Endoprosthetic reconstructions: Results of long-term follow-up of 139 patients. *Clin Orthop Relat Res* 438:51-59.

This was a retrospective study to determine the effect of prosthesis location, patient age, periprosthetic infection, and primary versus revision placement on endoprosthetic survival; 139 endoprosthetic reconstructions performed between 1984 and 2002, including 57 distal femur, 27 proximal femur, 26 proximal tibia, 17 proximal humerus, 4 distal humerus, 3 total scapula, 3 total femur, and 2 total humerus reconstructions, were reviewed. Overall, Kaplan-Meier event-free endoprosthetic survival was 86%, 80%, and 69% at 3, 5, and 10-year follow-up, respectively. The trend for endoprosthetic survival from best to worst was proximal femur, proximal humerus, distal femur, proximal tibia, and distal humerus. Reasons for failure included mechanical failure (8 patients), tumor recurrence (8 patients), aseptic loosening (6 patients), dislocation (2 patients), periprosthetic infection (2 patients), and endoprosthetic malalignment (1 patient). Periprosthetic infection rate was 2.2%.

Zeegen EN, Aponte-Tinao LA, Hornicek FJ, et al. (2004). Survivorship analysis of 141 modular metallic endoprostheses at early follow-up. *Clin Orthop Relat Res* 420:239-250.

This retrospective review of 141 patients who had a modular endoprosthesis implanted used Kaplan-Meier survival analysis, clinical scoring, and a multivariate regression analysis to identify independent risk factors. Based on Kaplan-Meier estimates, the endoprosthetic survival rate was 88% at 3 years and 76% at 5 years; per location, it was 100% for the proximal humerus, 100% for the proximal femur, 87% for modular knees, and 53% for total femoral implants at 3 years. The clinical scores were good to excellent in 74% of the patients. Multivariate analysis showed that only location and infection were independent risk factors for prosthesis failure. Loosening, infection, and dislocation were independently predictive of a fair or poor clinical score. Age, gender, diagnosis, length of implant, dislocation, and failed prior allograft had no independent effects on implant survival or clinical outcome. The proximal humeral and proximal femoral implants had greater survival rates than modular knee and total femoral implants. Conversion of failed allografts to modular endoprostheses had a trend for a higher failure rate, but after a multivariate analysis, it did not prove to be an independent risk factor for failure.

Outcomes Assessment

Norman A. Johanson* and Douglas L. Cerynik†

*MD, Chairman, Department of Orthopaedic Surgery, Hahnemann University Hospital/
Drexel University College of Medicine, Philadelphia, PA
†MD, Research Fellow, Department of Orthopaedic Surgery, Hahnemann University
Hospital/Drexel University College of Medicine, Philadelphia, PA

Introduction

- *Outcomes assessment* involves developing outcome measures to assess treatment effectiveness.
- *Outcomes research* is a patient-centered process that measures the result of care as perceived by the patient (pain, function, satisfaction, quality of life) (Keller 1993).
- Outcomes research is less focused on measures of process care (radiographic findings, range of motion, laboratory results).
- These assessments are driven by the health care community's desire to improve quality and effectiveness.
- Historically, orthopaedic surgeons have used outcome measures to study the effectiveness of treatments for total joint arthroplasty and lower back pain.

Brief History

- E. A. Codman and F. B. Harrington were the first to implement an outcomes-based system, known as the *End Result System*, into their surgical practice in the early 1900s (Codman 1934).
- Codman was unable to convince the hospital board that systematic and unbiased outcome evaluations be studied, so he left Massachusetts General Hospital in Boston in 1911.
- In 1914, Codman formed the Committee on the Standardization of Hospitals, which later became part of the American College of Surgeons.
- The Committee on the Standardization of Hospitals was instrumental in standardizing hospital care in the United States and later gave rise to the Joint Commission on Accreditation of Hospitals.

- The 1950s and 1960s saw a boom in health care services with a distorted distribution of physicians and services.
- The 1980s were a time of cost containment and competition for diminishing resources that revived the study of outcome measures (Relman 1988).
- Outcomes assessment now focuses not only on the true benefit to patients from a given procedure, but also on the cost-effectiveness of that treatment and the quality of evidence by which any treatment is justified.

Outcomes and Managed Care

- In the 1990s, there was the appearance of interest in outcomes by managed care and other payers.
- The reality became evident that few resources would be committed to measuring patient-centered outcomes in favor of outcomes involving cost and resource utilization.
- Managed care has implemented a cost-conscious policy that utilizes more easily obtained measures of quality that often have little relationship with outcomes that are important to the patient and that offer questionable relevance to the physician interested in evidence-based performance improvement.

Instrument Assessment and Validation

- Outcomes assessment must be accurate, reliable, and precise in describing the clinical state of a stable patient and responsive in showing quantitative change that corresponds with an observed change clinically (Johanson et al. 1992).
- Face validity

- This ensures that the study will measure what it is supposed to measure.
- A panel of experts decides that the instrument contains the essential elements or questions that define the expected outcomes of a treatment.
- Questions in the instrument must have an array of responses that are clearly defined, mutually exclusive, and ordered in hierarchic progression.
- Criterion validity
  - This compares the responses of the new instrument with a "gold standard" for the characteristics being measured.
- Construct validity
  - This complex analysis demonstrates how the various responses correlate with one another in describing a common health concept.
- Reliability
  - This measures the reproducibility or precision of an instrument.
  - It is tested by administering the instrument twice to a stable patient and analyzing the changes in response.
  - The reproducibility of each individual question must be verified.
- Responsiveness
  - This refers to an instrument's ability to detect clinically relevant changes that determine treatment effectiveness.

Modern Instruments Utilized for Outcomes Assessment

- Thirty-Six Item Short-Form Health Survey (SF-36)
  - Developed at multiple sites by the Medical Outcomes Study between 1986 and 1990 (Ware and Sherbourne 1992)
  - Measures three major health attributes containing eight health concepts that give a well-rounded assessment of physical function (Table 16–1)
  - Not a valuable measure for surgical indications by itself
  - Aids in evaluating the quality of life improvements from surgery

- Used successfully in conjunction with other orthopaedic-related outcomes instruments
- Western Ontario and McMaster University Osteoarthritis Index (WOMAC)
  - Developed for patients with hip and knee osteoarthritis (Bellamy et al. 1988)
  - Often used by orthopaedic surgeons for outcomes assessment
  - Overlaps with the SF-36
  - Measures three domains: Pain (5 questions), stiffness (2 questions), physical function (17 questions)
- Hip Rating Questionnaire
  - Developed solely for evaluating the outcomes of total hip arthroplasty in patients with arthritis (Johanson et al. 1992)
  - Equal weight given to overall impact of arthritis (1 question), pain (4 questions), walking (2 questions), and function (7 questions)
  - Maximum score, 100
- American Academy of Orthopaedic Surgeons (AAOS) Lower Limb Outcomes Assessment Instruments
  - Comprehensive measure of outcomes in patients with lower limb conditions (Johanson et al. 2004)
  - Focuses on the effects of interventions on symptoms and function
  - Contains Lower Limb Core Scale and Hip and Knee Core Scale
  - Each core scale containing seven portions focusing on pain, function, and stiffness and swelling
  - Complementary to the SF-36 and correlated with the WOMAC
- American Knee Society Knee Score
  - Developed by consensus of the Knee Society (Insall et al. 1989)
  - Focuses solely on the knee in question (independent of any other factors)
  - Consisting of two parts: Knee Score and Function Score
  - Knee Score
    - Parameters: Pain, stability, and range of motion
    - Deductions: Flexion contractures, extension lag, and malalignment
    - Maximum score, 100
  - Function Score
    - Parameters: Walking distance and stair climbing
    - Deductions: Use of walking aids
    - Maximum score, 100
- British Orthopaedic Association Score
  - Includes subjective and objective variables (Aichroth et al. 1978)
  - Multiple parameters are given four or five grades (equally weighted variables)
  - Assesses: Pain, walking ability, use of walking aid, gait, flexion deformity, maximal flexion, extension lag, valgus and varus angles on stressing, stair climbing, and the ability to rise from a chair

Table 16–1	Thirty-Six Item Short-Form Health Survey (SF-36) Consisting of One Multiple-Item Scale Measuring Eight Health Concepts	
SUMMARY MEASURES	**PHYSICAL HEALTH (PCS)**	**MENTAL HEALTH (MCS)**
Scales	Physical Functioning	Social Functioning
	Role (physical)	Role (emotional)
	General Health	Mental Health
	Bodily Pain	Vitality

MCS, mental component summary; PCS, physical component summary. Adapted from Ware JE Jr, Snow KK, Kosihski M, et al. (1993). *SF-36 Health Survey: Manual and Interpretation Guide.* Boston: The Health Institute, New England Medical Center.

- Patients also questioned regarding satisfaction with treatment and general disability resulting from the affected joint
  - Maximum score, 47; minimum score, 9
- Oxford 12-Item Questionnaire
  - Developed only for use with total knee arthroplasty (Dawson et al. 1998)
  - 12 subjective questions on knee function
  - Each question graded 1 to 5
  - Pain and disability weighted more heavily
  - Minimum score, 12 (normal function); maximum score, 60 (poor function)
- Quality-adjusted life year (QALY)
  - Accounts for the quantity and quality of life generated by a health care intervention (Rissanen et al. 1995)
  - Arithmetic product of life expectancy and a measure of the quality of the remaining life years
  - 1 year of perfect health = 1, less than perfect health <1, death = 0
  - Establishes a common value to assessing the extent of benefits gained from interventions as associated with health-related quality of life and patient survival
  - Combined with the costs of providing the interventions gives cost-utility ratios
  - Best used for determining resource allocation

Orthopaedic Total Joint Registries

- Registries have been established to monitor and improve the outcomes of total joint replacements by following prosthesis outcomes and allowing access to the data by physicians and other related parties (Malchau et al. 2005).
- A successful, statistically significant, registry will have close to 95% participation of all hospitals that perform total joint replacements, with roughly 95% of all surgical procedures reported.
- Most registries are owned by the government or the national orthopaedic association.
- Common sources of funding include government, membership fees, and mandated implant levies.
- Major international registries
  - Swedish Knee Registry
    - Established in 1975 (hips included in 1979)
    - First population-based national registry
  - Other countries with national registries (noninclusive list)
    - Finland, Norway, Denmark, New Zealand, Australia, Romania, Canada, United Kingdom
    - German registry discontinued in 2003 secondary to funding issues
- Data collection
  - All registries record hips and knees (primary and revision).
  - Some registries collect other major joints (e.g., shoulders, elbows, ankles).

- Few registries record minor joints and hemiarthroplasties.
- Most registries are paper-based, with data entry at registry.
- The Swedish Hip Registry and the United Kingdom National Joint Registry are Web-based.
- Most registries seek to validate data against inpatient data held by the government.
- Data analysis
  - Registries differ in methods of data analysis or in reporting.
  - These differences make comparisons among registries difficult.

Conclusions

- Modern outcomes assessment instruments are valid, responsive, and reliable in detecting clinically important patient change in modest-sized populations.
- Evidence-based practice standards should be founded on results of studies utilizing instruments and registries that collect appropriate and reliable data in large populations.
- By supporting a cooperative effort in measuring outcomes that matter to patients and surgeons, true quality improvement will be possible.

References

Aichroth P, Freeman MAR, Smillie IS, Souter WA (1978). A knee function assessment chart. *J Bone Joint Surg Br* 60:308-309.

This paper describes the development and application of the British Orthopaedic Association Score.

Bellamy N, Buchanan WW, Goldsmith CH, et al. (1988). Validation study of WOMAC: A health status instrument for measuring clinically important patient relevant outcomes to antirheumatic drug therapy in patients with osteoarthritis of the hip or knee. *J Rheumatol* 15:1833-1840.

This study was conducted to establish the validity of the WOMAC Osteoarthritis Index. The test was administered to 70 patients with osteoarthritis of the knee at baseline and at 12 weeks in a double-blind, randomized, controlled manner. Analysis of the results confirmed that this was a valid test.

Codman EA (1934). *The Shoulder*. Boston: EA Codman (self-published), pp v-xl.

This early work describes Codman's rationale and practices leading to early outcomes assessments during the early 1900s in Boston.

Dawson J, Fitzpatrick R, Murray D, Carr A (1998). Questionnaire on the perceptions of patients about total knee replacement. *J Bone Joint Surg Br* 80:63-69.

This paper reported on a prospective study of 117 patients who were administered the questionnaire before and 6 months after surgery. Comparisons were made with the SF-36, Stanford Health Assessment Questionnaire, and American Knee Society clinical score. The new questionnaire was proven to provide a measure of outcome for total knee replacement that is short, practical, reliable, valid, and sensitive.

Insall JN, Dorr LD, Scott RD, Scott WN (1989). Rationale of the knee society clinical rating system. *Clin Orthop Relat Res* 248:13-14.

This paper details the total knee rating system developed by the Knee Society. The scoring system is subdivided into a knee score that rates only the knee joint itself and a functional score that rates the patient's ability to walk and climb stairs. The dual rating system eliminates the problem of declining knee scores associated with patient infirmity.

Johanson NA, Charlson ME, Szatrowski TP, Ranawat CS (1992). A self-administered hip-rating questionnaire for the assessment of outcome after total hip replacement. *J Bone Joint Surg Am* 74:587-597.

This paper describes the development and validation of the self-administered hip rating questionnaire. Ninety-eight patients were enrolled in the prospective study and were followed for at least 3 months. The questionnaire was found to be reproducible, valid, sensitive, and responsive when compared and analyzed with other tests, including a 6-minute walking-distance test, arthritis impact-measurement scales, and clinical evaluations. This questionnaire was demonstrated to be a useful instrument for assessment of outcomes after surgery.

Johanson NA, Liang MH, Daltroy L, et al. (2004). American Academy of Orthopaedic Surgeons lower limb outcomes assessment instruments. *J Bone Joint Surg Am* 86:902-909.

This paper details the development and analysis of the AAOS lower limb outcomes assessment instruments; 290 subjects were tested, and 71 were followed for up to 1 year. All the scales correlated with other measures of pain and function and were found to be reliable and sensitive. Combined with the SF-36, the AAOS outcomes assessment instruments comprehensively and efficiently measure outcomes in orthopaedic patients with lower limb conditions.

Keller RB (1993). Outcomes research in orthopaedics. *J Am Acad Orthop Surg* 1:122-129.

This paper seeks to define what outcomes research is and what it involves. Time is spent detailing methods and analysis.

Malchau H, Garellick G, Eisler T, et al. (2005). Presidential guest address. The Swedish Hip Registry: Increasing the sensitivity by patient outcome data. *Clin Orthop Relat Res* 441:19-29.

This paper describes the establishment and validity of the Swedish Hip Registry and cites other known national registries.

Relman AS (1988). Assessment and accountability: The third revolution in medical care. *N Engl J Med* 319:1220-1222.

This paper looks at the how market factors such as cost containment have affected health care and have resulted in outcomes assessments that will affect utilization decisions.

Rissanen P, Aro S, Slatis P, et al. (1995). Health and quality of life before and after hip or knee arthroplasty. *J Arthroplasty* 10:169-175.

This study looked at subjective health outcomes after total joint arthroplasty in relation to quality-adjusted life years.

Ware JE Jr, Sherbourne CD (1992). The MOS 36-item short-form health survey (SF-36). *Med Care* 30:473-483.

This paper summarizes the history of the development of the SF-36, the origin of specific items, and the logic underlying their selection. The content and features of the SF-36 are compared with the 20-item Medical Outcomes Study short form and are proven to be valid and reliable.

Particle Disease and Implant Allergy

Nadim J. Hallab[*] and Joshua J. Jacobs[†]

[*]PhD, Associate Professor and Director, Materials Testing Laboratory, Department of Orthopaedic Surgery, Rush University Medical Center, Chicago, IL
[†]MD, Crown Family Professor of Orthopaedic Surgery, Rush University Medical Center, Chicago, IL

Introduction

- Excessive biologic reactivity to implant debris is commonly referred to as *particle disease* or *implant allergy*. However, the less popular terms *particle-induced osteolysis* and *implant debris hypersensitivity* are more accurate for the following reasons.
- *Particle disease* generally refers to the processes of peri-implant osteolysis, implant loosening, and inflammation resulting from implant particulate debris. However, the term *particle disease* is inappropriate largely because it misrepresents a normal and generally desirable response to particle challenge in vivo that is part of a necessary healthy innate immune response.
- *Implant allergy* generally implies an antibody-mediated type I immediate immune response (e.g., bee stings and hay fever). Thus *hypersensitivity* to implant debris is a more accurate characterization.
- Particle-induced osteolysis and hypersensitivity to implant debris are two sides of the same coin in which each represents the two basic categories of immune responses:
  - *Particle-induced osteolysis:* The *innate nonspecific immune system responses* mediated by the phagocytic responses of macrophages to particles
  - *Hypersensitivity to implant debris:* The *adaptive specific immune system responses* mediated by the responses of conditioned lymphocytes to antigenic stimuli
- Implant hypersensitivity has been predominantly characterized as specific and of the type IV delayed-type hypersensitivity (DTH) response.

Particle Disease: Debris-Induced Osteolysis

Local Tissue Effects: Aseptic Osteolysis

- Implant loosening resulting from aseptic osteolysis generally accounts for more than 90% of total joint arthroplasty (TJA) implant failure and is considered the predominant factor limiting the longevity of current TJAs.
- In large studies of implant longevity with multivariable analysis, the only predictive factor of implant loosening was wear rate. More specifically, a 15% revision rate at 20 years was predicted only by a wear rate of the ultra-high-molecular-weight, polyethylene (UHMWPE) acetabular cup of greater than 0.1 mm/year (Kerboull et al. 2004).
- The general consensus in the orthopaedic research community is that increased debris will result in decreased longevity and implant performance.
- Conversely, it is generally accepted that decreased wear and corrosion debris will lead to increased longevity of orthopaedic implants (i.e., <15% revision after 20 years of service). This latter axiom has yet to be determined with the relatively new development or redesign of alternative bearings such as ceramic-on-ceramic, new-generation metal-on-metal, and metal-on-highly cross-linked polyethylene.
- Osteolysis attributed to particulate wear debris is typically observed as diffuse cortical thinning or as a focal cystlike lesion.
  - Particle-induced focal lesions can involve diaphyseal cortical bone or metaphyseal trabecular bone.

- This form of aseptic osteolysis was first recognized as endosteal osteolysis in cemented total hip arthroplasty (THA), which was initially described as an "alteration in the texture of the cortex."
  - The incidence of radiographically evident osteolysis in stable implants has been reported as high as 8% at 5-year follow-up, and it increases to approximately 15% at 8 years postoperatively (Martell et al. 1993).
- The incidence of radiographically evident focal femoral osteolysis can be as high as 10% to 20% at 2- to 9-year follow-up with uncemented implant systems composed of both cobalt (Co)- and titanium (Ti)-base alloy (Gautam et al. 1992).
- Particle osteolysis can be associated with both cemented and uncemented acetabular components, in which radiologically recognizable lesions are *periacetabular* (identified primarily in the periphery of the acetabulum) and *retroacetabular* (identified centrally infiltrating the body of the ilium and/or, sometimes, the body of the ischium).
- Debris-induced osteolysis around total knee arthroplasties is less than in hips.
- Investigators reported an incidence of osteolysis as high as 16% in less than ideal cementless Co alloy devices at less than 3 years postoperatively. In this case series, the most common site for bone resorption was the medial aspect of the proximal tibia where the screw-bone interface provided a preferential pathway for progression of this particle-induced osteolysis process (Fig. 17–1). This finding points to accelerated polyethylene and metal wear-induced osteolysis (Blumenthal and Cosma 1989).
- It remains unclear why particle-induced osteolysis is reported more frequently about the hip than about the knee.

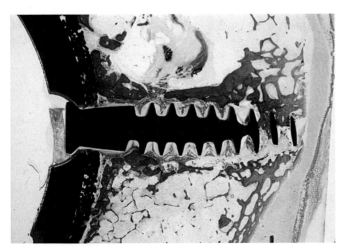

Figure 17–1: Granuloma.
Granuloma surrounding an acetabular fixation screw, a common site for bone resorption because of the preferential pathway for progression of particle-induced osteolysis processes.

Differences between total knee arthroplasty and THA environments include the following:
- Loading and stress environments between hip and knee prostheses
- Mechanisms of hip and knee wear
- Joint volume
- Interfacial barriers to migration of debris

Biology of Particle-Induced Osteolysis

- Normal bone maintenance relies on the balance of bone formation and bone resorption, which mainly involves the coordinated function of osteoblasts and osteoclasts. Thus either a decrease in osteoblastic bone formation or an increase in osteoclastic bone resorption can result in net bone loss and osteolysis.
- Bone loss (i.e., osteolysis) around an implant is directly associated with the local effects of orthopaedic implant degradation.
  - It was initially thought that only reactions to particulate polymethylmethacrylate bone cement produced osteolytic lesions in loose implants, based on histologic studies demonstrating cement debris associated with macrophages, giant cells, and vascular granulation tissue.
  - However, osteolysis is now well recognized in association with loose and well-fixed cemented and uncemented implants alike, a finding demonstrating that the absence of bone cement does not preclude the occurrence of osteolysis (Jacobs et al. 2001).
- Numerous secretory products created by peri-implant cells can negatively affect bone turnover (Fig. 17–2, Table 17–1).
  - The pro-inflammatory cytokines interleukin-1 (IL-1), IL-6, and tumor necrosis factor-α (TNF-α) are thought to be some of the most important to this process.
  - In addition, anti-inflammatory cytokines such as IL-10 may also modulate this process.
  - Other major factors involved in tipping the balance of bone homeostasis toward resorption are likely the enzymes responsible for catabolism of the organic component of bone. These include matrix metalloproteinases, collagenase, and stromelysin.
  - Prostaglandins, in particular prostaglandin E_2 (PGE_2), are also known to be important intercellular messengers in the osteolytic cascade produced by implant debris.
  - More recently, several mediators known to be involved in osteoclast differentiation and maturation, such as RANKL (also referred to as osteoclast differentiation factor) and osteoprotegerin, respectively, have been suggested as key factors in the development and progression of bone loss (osteolytic lesions) produced from implant debris. However, it was shown that fibroblasts exposed to particulate wear debris could regulate the

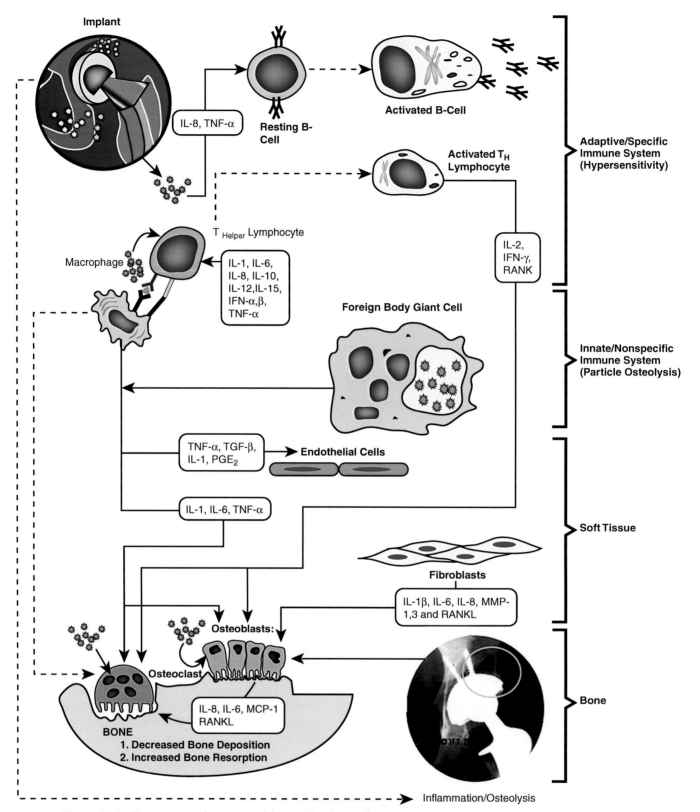

Figure 17–2: Secretory products created by peri-implant cells.
This schematic shows the numerous secretory products created by peri-implant cells reacting to implant debris, which can negatively affect bone turnover (the pro-inflammatory cytokines interleukin-1 *(IL-1)*, interleukin-6 *(IL-6)*, and tumor necrosis factor-α *(TNF-α)* are thought to be some of the most important to this process). *IFN*, interferon; *MCP*, monocyte chemotactic protein; *MMP*, matrix metalloproteinase; *PGE₂*, prostaglandin E_2; *RANKL*, osteoclast differentiation factor.

Table 17–1	Cytokines Relevant to Peri-implant Immune Responses, Their Source Cells, and Mechanisms of Action	
CYTOKINE	**PRINCIPAL SOURCE**	**PRINCIPAL ACTIVITIES**
IL-1	Macrophages	T-cell, B-cell activation, inflammation
IL-2	T_H1 cells	T-cell proliferation
IL-4	T_H2 cells	B-cell and T_H2 cell growth and differentiation
IL-6	Macrophages, T cells	B-cell stimulation, inflammation
IL-8	Macrophages	Neutrophil (PMN) attraction
IL-10	T cells	Inhibition of T_H1 cytokine production
IL-12	APCs	Stimulation of T cells, NK cells
IL-13	T_H2	Inhibition of macrophage activation
IFN-γ	T_H1, NK cells	Inflammation, activation of macrophages
TGF-β	Macrophages, lymphocytes	T-cell, B-cell, and macrophage inhibition
TNF-α	Macrophages, $T_H.1$ cells	Inflammation, tumor killing
TNF-β	T cells	Inflammation, enhancement of phagocytosis
MIF	T cells	Inhibition of T-cell and macrophage migration
MCP-1	Monocytes, endothelial cells	Chemotactic for monocytes but not neutrophils

APC, antigen-presenting cells; IFN, interferon; IL, interleukin; MCP, monocyte chemotactic protein; MIF, migration inhibitory factor; NK, natural killer; TGF, transforming growth factor; T_H cells, helper T cells; TNF, tumor necrosis factor.

expression of the bone-resorbing metalloproteinases collagenase and stromelysin (Jacobs et al. 2001).

- Particulate debris may suppress the osteoblast synthetic function of collagen type I and type III precursors.
- Goldring and associates were among the first to describe the synovial-like character of the bone–implant interface in patients with loose THAs and determined that the cells within the membrane have the capacity to produce large amounts of bone resorbing factors such as PGE_2 and collagenase (Goldring et al. 1983). (These studies typically can document only the end stage of the loosening process, rather than those initiating processes.)
- Polyethylene particles are generally recognized as the most prevalent particles in the periprosthetic metal-on-polyethylene TJA milieu.
- Metallic and ceramic particulate species are also produced by modular junctions and alternate bearing surfaces in variable amounts and may affect fixation over the long term. When present in sufficient amounts, particulates generated by wear, corrosion, or a combination of these processes can induce the formation of inflammatory, foreign body granulation tissue with the ability to invade the bone–implant interface (Fig. 17–3).
- Particle-induced osteolysis remote from the articulation surfaces has shown substantial particle migration between the joint space and the distal regions of the THA implant space. Autopsy specimens of retrieved implants have demonstrated the presence of particles in connective tissue macrophages (histiocytes) in cavities surrounding regions of the femoral component.
  - Femoral osteolysis associated with THA tends to be proximal in the initial stages; over time, it tends to progress distally.

- The volume of debris generated from THA polyethylene is related to certain variables, including the following:
  - The smoothness of the concave metallic surface of the acetabular component
  - The tolerance between polyethylene and metal shell
  - The relative stability of the insert
- The relative contribution of specific particulate compositions and sizes to the overall process of periprosthetic bone loss remains incompletely characterized.
  - In vitro cell culture studies have demonstrated that the macrophage and fibroblast response to particulate debris is a function of particle size, composition, and

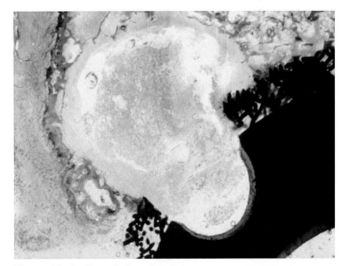

Figure 17–3: Granulation tissue.
Particulates generated by wear, corrosion, or a combination of these processes can induce the formation of an inflammatory, foreign body granulation tissue with the ability to invade the bone-implant interface, as shown in this photomicrograph (5×) of an expanding granuloma in an unfilled screw hole.

dose, although particles of different materials likely exhibit differential reactivity and cytotoxicity.
  - Polyethylene particles are believed to be the most biologically active, by virtue of their overwhelmingly greater numbers (relative to metallic debris) and small size that give rise to an enormous surface area for interaction with the surrounding tissues (Jacobs et al. 2001).
- Several major factors have been associated with particle-induced osteolysis and are purported to tip bone homeostasis at the bone-implant interface toward osteolysis, including the following:
  - Pressure
  - Stress shielding
  - Osteoclastogenesis
  - Hydrodynamic pumping (Fig. 17–4)
- The role of elevated intra-articular pressure and fluid access in the development of osteolysis also has been considered (Schmalzried et al. 1997). Computer simulations and direct measurements have found fluid pressures in the hip or knee to be elevated to as high as 700 mm Hg with activity. One study found that a pressure of 200 mm Hg applied for 2 weeks in a rabbit bone chamber model caused massive bone resorption under the pressurized area (Van der Vis et al. 1998).

Characterization of Particle Debris

- Evaluating particulate implant debris in the joint pseudocapsule and interfacial membranes from patients

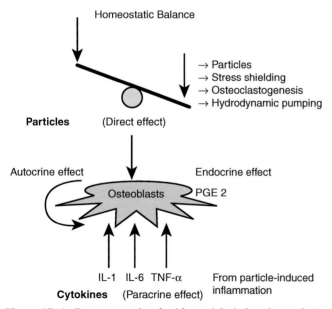

Figure 17–4: Factors associated with particle-induced osteolysis. Schematic showing several major factors associated with particle-induced osteolysis that are purported to tip bone homeostasis at the bone-implant interface toward osteolysis. These include stress shielding, osteoclastogenesis, and hydrodynamic pumping. *IL*, interleukin; *PGE₂*, prostaglandin E₂; *TNF-α*, tumor necrosis factor-α.

with osteolysis requires the use of techniques such as electron microprobe analysis, analytic electron microscopy, and Fourier transform infrared spectroscopy.
  - Metallic particles in tissues range in size from less than 1 to 20 μm.
  - Polymeric particles around implants have been chemically identified as UHMWPE at sizes as small as 5 μm. Despite the observance of polymeric particles in the micron and submicron range, these lie beyond the range of typical quantitative analytic techniques, such as Fourier transform infrared spectroscopy, thus complicating compositional qualitative identification.
  - Metal and ceramic particles are more easily identifiable using x-ray diffraction and have been readily identified in the submicron range.
- In vivo studies of UHMWPE wear debris in peri-implant tissues have shown that 70% to 90% of recovered particulates were submicron, with a mean size of approximately 0.5 μm (Campbell et al. 1995).
- Studies of in vivo particles have typically been conducted using "number-based" analysis; however, more accurate analysis methods include "volume" or "mass" analysis.
  - In number-based analysis, particles are counted, and each is assigned an equivalent spheric diameter based on an idealized spheric particle volume.
  - Volume or mass analysis displays particle distribution as percentages of total volume or mass in which the contribution of larger particles to the total volume or mass of debris is observable (Fig. 17–5).
- Past reliance on number-based analysis alone led to the unsupported assumption that all wear debris particles are small because it is difficult if not practically impossible to find the few large particles hidden in tissues.
- To date, the osteolytic potential of implants has been largely characterized using number analysis of simulator fluid and histology of retrieved tissue.
- Techniques that cannot detect large but rare debris particles misrepresent an implant's potential for debris-induced osteolysis.
  - The ability to size debris accurately is critically important to the new generation of alternate bearing surfaces in which weight loss from the implant after a year or so of use (e.g., <0.2 mm³ volume loss after a million cycles of use) could be attributed to the loss of 200 particles that are 100 μm diameter or, equivalently, 200 million particles only 1 μm in diameter (for reference, a typical lymphocyte is 20 μm in diameter).
  - This phenomenon is illustrated in Figure 17–5, in which similar number distribution characterizations of two sets of particles are not mirrored by similar volume distribution characterizations.

Histologic Features

- There is a high latent capacity for cells of the interfacial membrane to produce IL-6 and IL-1β. Cells closest to a

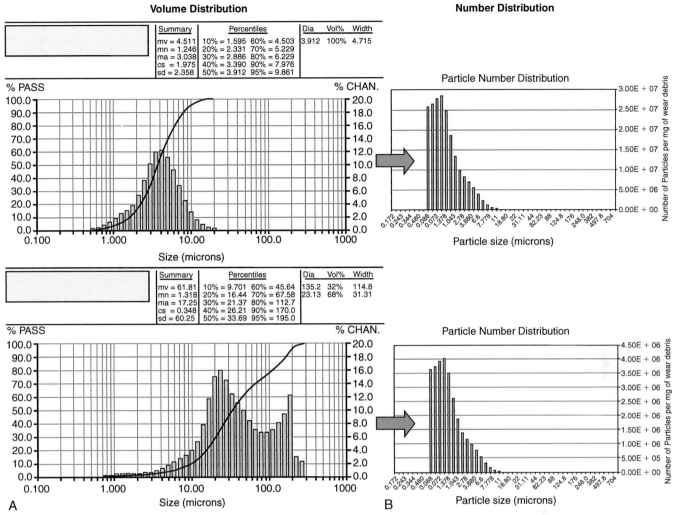

Figure 17–5: Volume and number distribution analyses.
These analyses of volume (**A**) and number (**B**) distributions of two debris samples demonstrate how similar number distributions can result from very different actual size distributions, as evident in A, the volume distributions. The *x*-axis represents increasing particle diameter, and the *y*-axis is the percentage of total particle debris (**A**) and the number per milligram of particle debris (**B**). The volume lost in 0.2 mm^3 of implant bearing surface can be attributed to the loss of 200 particles that are 100 μm diameter or equivalently 200 million particles only 1 μm in diameter.

failed implant tend to be associated with highest levels of IL-1β.
- The tissues surrounding modern implants may include areas of osseointegration, fibrous encapsulation, and a variable presence of the foreign body response to polyethylene and cement debris in joint replacement devices.
- Accelerated corrosion and a tissue response that can be directly related to identifiable corrosion products can be demonstrated in the tissues surrounding multipart devices.

Stainless Steels

- Histologic sections of the tissues surrounding stainless steel internal fixation devices generally show two types of corrosion products.
  - The first consists of iron (Fe)-containing granules.

- The second, termed *microplates*, consists of relatively larger particles of a chromium (Cr) compound. X-ray diffraction has indicated that the granules consist of a mixture of two or more of the Fe oxides, αFe_2O_3 and σFe_2O_3, and the hydrated iron oxides, $\alpha Fe_2O_3 \cdot H_2O$ and $\sigma Fe_2O_3 \cdot H_2O$.

Cobalt-Base Alloys

- The corrosion products found at modular Co alloy–containing connections are similar whether modular heads are mated with Co-Cr alloy or Ti-6Al-4V alloy femoral stems.
  - The principal corrosion product is Cr-phosphate $(Cr(PO_4)4H_2O)$ hydrate–rich material termed *orthophosphate*.

- Particles of the orthophosphate material have been found at the bearing surface of the UHMWPE acetabular liners, a finding suggesting their participation in three-body wear and an increased production of polyethylene debris.
- Cr orthophosphate particles range in size from submicron to aggregates of particles up to 500 μm.

Titanium-Base Alloys

- The degradation products observed in histologic sections of tissues adjacent to Ti-base alloys have the same elemental composition as the parent alloy, as opposed to precipitated corrosion products that occur with stainless steel and Co-Cr alloys.

Remote and Systemic Effects

- The effects of implant debris are not only local, but they may also be transported in the bloodstream or lymphatics to remote organs.
- Co, Cr, and possibly nickel (Ni) and vanadium (V) are essential trace metals in that they are required for certain enzymatic reactions. In excessive amounts, however, these elements may be toxic.
  - Excessive Co may lead to polycythemia, hypothyroidism, cardiomyopathy, and carcinogenesis.
  - Excessive Cr can lead to nephropathy, hypersensitivity, and carcinogenesis.
  - Ni can lead to eczematous dermatitis, hypersensitivity, and carcinogenesis.
  - V can lead to cardiac and renal dysfunction, and it has been associated with hypertension and depressive psychosis.
- At this time, the association of metal release from orthopaedic implants with any metabolic, bacteriologic, immunologic, or carcinogenic toxicity is conjectural because cause and effect have not been well established in human subjects.

Metal Release

- Implants, or wear debris generated from implants, may release chemically active metal into the surrounding tissues.
- Although this metal may stay bound to local tissues, soluble metal may also bind to protein moieties that are then transported in the bloodstream or lymphatics to remote organs (Jacobs et al. 1994, 1999).
- Normal human serum levels of prominent implant metals are approximately as follows: 1 to 10 ng/ml aluminum (Al), 0.15 ng/ml Cr, less then 0.01 ng/ml V, 0.1 to 0.2 ng/ml Co, and less than 4.1 ng/ml Ti.
- Following TJA, levels of circulating metal (Al, Cr, Co, Ni, Ti, and V) have been shown to increase (Table 17–2).
- Chronic elevations in serum and urine Co and Cr occur following successful primary TJA.
  - Transient elevations of urine and serum Ni have been noted immediately following surgery.

- This hypernickelemia or hypernickeluria may be unrelated to the implant itself because there is such a small percentage of Ni within implant alloys. This may be related to the use of stainless steel surgical instruments or the metabolic changes associated with the surgery itself.
- Long-term elevations in serum Ti and Cr concentrations are found in subjects with well-functioning Ti- or Cr-containing THR components without measurable differences in urine and serum Al concentrations.
- Concentrations of V have not been found to be greatly elevated in patients with TJA (see Table 17–2).
- Factors affect soluble metal levels within the serum and urine of TJA patients.
  - Up to 100 times normal control values of serum Ti elevations have also been reported in patients with failed metal-backed patellar components in whom unintended metal-on-metal articulation was possible. However, even among these patient populations with TJA, no elevation in serum or urine Al, serum or urine V levels, or urine Ti levels has been noted (Jacobs et al. 1999).
  - Mechanically assisted crevice corrosion in patients with modular femoral stems from THA has been associated with elevations in serum Co and urine Cr.
- Recent studies suggest that disseminated Cr can predominantly come from fretting corrosion of the modular head-neck junction.
- However, wear of the articulating surface remains the purported predominant source of metallic implant debris (Jacobs et al. 1998).
- Homogenates of remote organs and tissue obtained post mortem from subjects with Co-base alloy TJA components have indicated that significant increases in Co and Cr concentrations occur in the heart, liver, kidney, spleen, and lymphatic tissue (see Table 17–2).
- Ti-base alloy implants demonstrated elevated Ti, Al, and V levels in joint pseudocapsules with up to 200 ppm of Ti (six orders of magnitude greater than that of controls), 880 ppb of Al, and 250 ppb of V.
- Spleen Al levels and liver Ti concentrations can also be markedly elevated in patients with failed Ti alloy implants (Jacobs et al. 1998).

Particle Distribution

- Component loosening, duration of implantation, and the modular designs of contemporary THA and knee replacement increase the generation of metallic and polymeric debris.
- Wear particles found disseminated beyond the periprosthetic tissue are primarily submicron.
- Metallic, ceramic, or polymeric wear debris particles from TJA are found in regional and pelvic lymph nodes (Fig. 17–6), along with the following:
  - Lymphadenopathy
  - Gross pigmentation resulting from metallic debris
  - Fibrosis (buildup of fibrous tissue)

Table 17–2 Approximate Concentrations of Metal in Human Body Fluids and in Human Tissue With and Without Total Joint Replacements

BODY FLUIDS (ng/ml or ppb)		Ti	Al	V	Co	Cr	Mo	Ni
Serum	Normal*	0.06	0.08	<0.02	0.003	0.001	NA	0.007
	TJA	0.09	0.09	0.03	0.007	0.006	NA	<0.16
Urine	Normal	<0.04	0.24	0.01	NA	0.001	NA	NA
	TJA	0.07	0.24	<0.01	NA	0.009	NA	NA
Synovial fluid	Normal	0.27	4.0	0.10	0.085	0.058	0.219	0.086
	TJA	11.5	24	1.2	10	7.4	0.604	0.55
Joint capsule	Normal	15.0	35	2.4	0.42	2.6	0.177	69
	TJA-F	399	47	29	14	64	4.65	100
Whole blood	Normal	0.35	0.48	0.12	0.002	0.058	0.009	0.078
	TJA	1.4	8.1	0.45	0.33	2.1	0.104	0.50
Body Tissues (µg/g)								
Skeletal muscle	Normal	NA	NA	NA	<12	<12	NA	NA
	TJA	NA	NA	NA	160	570	NA	NA
Liver	Normal	100	890	14	120	<14	NA	NA
	TJA	560	680	22	15200	1130	NA	NA
Lung	Normal	710	9830	26	NA	NA	NA	NA
	TJA	980	8740	23	NA	NA	NA	NA
Spleen	Normal	70	800	<9	30	10	NA	NA
	TJA	1280	1070	12	1600	180	NA	NA
Pseudocapsule	Normal	<65	120	<9	50	150	NA	NA
	TJA	39400	460	121	5490	3820	NA	NA
Kidney	Normal	NA	NA	NA	30	<40	NA	NA
	TJA	NA	NA	NA	60	<40	NA	NA
Lymphatic Tissue	Normal	NA	NA	NA	10	690	NA	NA
	TJA	NA	NA	NA	390	690	NA	NA
Heart	Normal	NA	NA	NA	30	30	NA	NA
	TJA	NA	NA	NA	280	90	NA	NA

*Normal: Subjects without any metallic prosthesis (not including dental).
Al, aluminum; Co, cobalt; Cr, chromium; Mo, molybdenum; NA, data not available; Ni, nickel; Ti, titanium; TJA, total joint arthroplasty; TJA-F, total joint arthroplasty in women; V, vanadium.
Data from Dorr LD, Bloebaum R, Emmanual J, Meldrum R (1990). Histologic, biochemical and ion analysis of tissue and fluids retrieved during total hip arthroplasty. *Clin Orthop Relat Res* 261:82-95; Jacobs JJ, Gilbert JL, Urban RM (1998). Corrosion of metal orthopaedic implants. *J Bone Joint Surg Am* 80:268-282; Jacobs JJ, Skipor AK, Urban RM, et al. (1994). Systemic distribution of metal degradation products from titanium alloy total hip replacements: An autopsy study. In: *Transactions of the Annual Meeting of the Orthopaedic Research Society.* New Orleans: Orthopaedic Research Society, p 838; and Michel R, Nolte M, Reich M, Loer F (1991). Systemic effects of implanted prostheses made of cobalt-chromium alloys. *Arch Orthop Trauma Surg* 110:61-74.

- Lymph node necrosis
- Histiocytosis (abnormal function of tissue macrophages, including complete effacement of nodal architecture)
- Metallic wear particles have been detected in the para-aortic lymph nodes in up to 70% of patients with TJA components (Urban et al. 2000).
- The inflammatory response to metallic and polymeric debris in lymph nodes has been demonstrated to include immune activation of macrophages and associated production of cytokines.
- Wear particles migrate via perivascular lymph channels as free or phagocytosed particles within macrophages, in which most disseminated particles are submicron in size; however, metallic particles as large as 50 µm and polyethylene particles as large as 30 µm have also been identified (Urban et al. 2000).
- Particles may further disseminate to the liver or spleen, where they are found within macrophages or, in some cases, as epithelioid granulomas in organs.

- Within liver and spleen, the maximum sizes of histologically observed metallic wear particles are nearly an order of magnitude less than in lymph nodes, a finding indicating that additional stages of filtration may precede the lymphatic system or alternate routes of particle migration. In the liver and spleen, as in the lymph nodes, cells of the mononuclear phagocyte system may accumulate small amounts of a variety of foreign materials without apparent clinical significance. However, accumulation of exogenous particles has been shown capable of inciting granulomas or granulomatoid lesions in the liver and spleen (Fig. 17–7).
- It is likely that the inflammatory reaction to particles in the liver, spleen, and lymph nodes is modulated similarly to other tissues by such factors as the following:
- Material composition
- Number of particles
- Rate of accumulation
- Duration
- Inherent biologic reactivity of cells to debris challenge

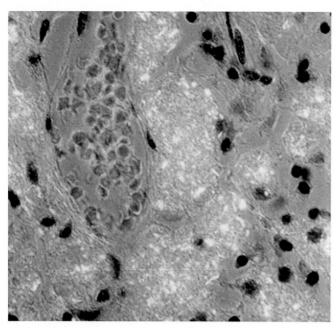

Figure 17–6: Birefringent polyethylene particles.
Abundant birefringent polyethylene particles within macrophages are shown here in a polarized light micrograph (190×) of a para-aortic lymph node as identified by infrared spectroscopy.

- Metallic particles in the liver or spleen have been more prevalent in patients with previously failed arthroplasties when compared with well-functioning primary joint replacements.
- Metal particles, unlike polyethylene debris, can be characterized using an electron microprobe, which allows identification of individual, submicron metallic wear particles against a background of particulates from environmental or sources other than the prosthetic components.
- The smallest identifiable disseminated particles are approximately 0.1 μm in diameter. However, metallic wear debris particles likely extend into the nanometer range (Urban et al. 2000).
- Polyethylene particles comprise the major fraction of the disseminated wear particles in patients with revision and primary TJAs. Although the presence of these polyethylene particles in lymph nodes can be confirmed by Fourier transform infrared spectroscopy microanalyses, polyethylene particulates in liver and spleen have so far precluded unequivocal identification.
- Diseases that obstruct lymph flow through lymph nodes, such as metastatic tumor, or that cause generalized disturbances of circulation, such as chronic heart disease or diabetes, may be expected to decrease particle

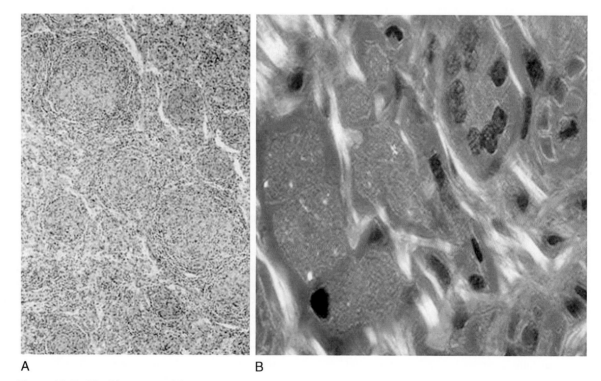

A   B

Figure 17–7: Birefringent particles.
Epithelioid granulomas within liver tissue within the portal tract of the liver (40×) **(A)** and a polarized light micrograph (190×) **(B)** demonstrating the abundance and morphology of birefringent particles. These findings demonstrate that the accumulation of exogenous particles is capable of producing granulomas or granulomatoid lesions.

migration to remote organs. Other diseases, such as acute or chronic active inflammation in the periprosthetic tissues, may increase particle migration.

Pharmacotherapy

- Novel therapeutic strategies are currently being developed to address the potential pharmacologic modification of the adverse host response to particulate debris.
- The effects of indomethacin, anti–TNF-α antibody, and disodium pamidronate on bone resorption induced by macrophages exposed to bone cement particles were found effective in inhibiting the release of calcium, a finding indicating decreased bone resorption in rat calvaria and macrophage coculture models (Horowitz et al. 1996).
- The efficacy of an oral bisphosphonate to inhibit THA wear debris–mediated bone resorption has been used in a canine model to show a reduction in radiographic periprosthetic radiolucencies, whereas levels of PGE_2 and IL-1 remained elevated in tissue cultures from these implants (Shanbhag et al. 1997).
- Human studies have also shown promising results of bisphosphonates for what will likely be a subset of particularly susceptible patients, but definitive studies are still needed.
- Before any of these pharmacologic treatments are recommended for general clinical use, extensive long-term human clinical trials will be needed.

Hypersensitivity to Implant Debris: Metal Allergy

- Some adverse responses to orthopaedic biomaterials are subtle and continue to foster debate and investigation.

One of these responses is "metal allergy" or hypersensitivity to implant debris.

- Released ions, although not sensitizers on their own, can activate the immune system by forming complexes with native proteins.
- Polymeric wear debris is not easily chemically degraded in vivo and thus has not been widely implicated as a source of allergic-type immune responses (Hallab et al. 2001).
- Dermal hypersensitivity to metal is common, affecting approximately 10% to 15% of the population. Dermal contact and ingestion of metals have been reported to cause immune reactions, which most typically manifest as hives, eczema, redness, and itching (Hallab et al. 2001).
- Degradation products of metallic biomaterials include particulate wear debris, colloidal organometallic complexes (specifically or nonspecifically bound), free metallic ions, inorganic metal salts and oxides, and precipitated organometallic storage forms.
- Metals accepted as sensitizers (haptenic moieties in antigens) include beryllium, Ni, Co, and Cr, whereas occasional responses have been reported to tantalum, Ti, and V (the amounts of these metals found in medical-grade alloys are shown in Table 17–3).
  - Ni is the most common metal sensitizer in humans, followed by Co and Cr.
  - Cross-sensitivity reactions among metals are common. Ni and Co are reportedly the most frequently cross-reactive.

Mechanisms of Metal Hypersensitivity in Orthopaedic Populations

- Implant hypersensitivity reactions are generally associated with type IV DTH. Metal antigen–sensitized T_{DTH} lymphocytes release various cytokines that result in the accumulation and activation of macrophages.

ALLOY	Ni	N	Co	Cr	Ti	Mo	Al	Fe	Mn	Cu	W	C	Si	V
Stainless Steel (ASTM† F138)	10–15.5	<0.5	*	17–19	*	2-4	*	61-68	*	<0.5	<2.0	<0.06	<1.0	*
CoCrMo Alloys (ASTM F75)	<2.0	*	61–66	27–30	*	4.5-7.0	*	<1.5	<1.0	*	*	<0.35	<1.0	*
(ASTM F90)	9–11	*	46–51	19–20	*	*	*	<3.0	<2.5	*	14–16	<0.15	<1.0	*
(ASTM F562)	33–37	*	35	19–21	<1	9.0-11	*	<1	<0.15	*	*	*	<0.15	*
Ti Alloys CPTi (ASTM F67)	*	*	*	*	99	*	*	0.2-0.5	*	*	*	<0.1	*	*
Ti-6Al-4V (ASTM F136)	*	*	*	*	89–91	*	5.5–6.5	*	*	*	*	<0.08	*	3.5–4.5
45TiNi	55	*	*	*	45	*	*	*	*	*	*	*	*	*
Zr Alloy (97.5% Zr, 2.5% Nb)	*	*	*	*	*	*	*	*	*	*	*	*	*	*

Table 17–3 Approximate Weight Percent of Different Metals Within Popular Orthopedic Alloys

* Indicates less than 0.05%.
†Alloy compositions are standardized by the American Society for Testing and Materials (ASTM vol. 13.01).
Al, aluminum; C, carbon; Co, cobalt; Cr, chromium; Cu, copper; Fe, iron; Mn, manganese; Mo, molybdenum; N, nitrogen; Nb, niobium; Ni, nickel; Si, silicon; Ti, titanium; V, vanadium; W, tungsten; Zr, zirconium.

- In a classic DTH response, most DTH participating cells are macrophages; only 5% of the participating cells are antigen-specific T lymphocytes (T_{DTH} cells) within a fully developed DTH response. This is important because the distinction between this and an innate (macrophage only) response is difficult to determine histologically.
- The effector phase of a DTH response is initiated by contact of sensitized T cells with antigen and the release of a variety of cytokines, including the following:
  - IL-2, which promotes T cell growth and activation
  - IL-3 and granulocyte-macrophage colony-stimulating factor, which promote hematopoiesis of granulocytes
  - Monocyte chemotactic activating factor, which promotes chemotaxis of monocytes toward areas of activation
  - Interferon-γ (IFN-γ) and TNF-β, which affect local endothelial cells that facilitate infiltration
  - Migration inhibitory factor, which inhibits the migration of macrophages away from the site of a DTH reaction
- Activation, infiltration, and eventual migration inhibition of macrophages comprise the final phase of a classic DTH response.
- Activated macrophages, because of their increased ability to present class II major histocompatibility complex (MHC) and IL-2, can trigger the activation of more T cells. This, in turn, activates more macrophages, which activate more T cells, and so on, such that this self-perpetuating response creates extensive tissue damage.
- The specific T-cell subpopulations, the cellular mechanism of recognition and activation, and the antigenic metal-protein determinants created by these metals remain incompletely characterized.
- The subsets of participating lymphocytes of Ni-sensitive individuals have been reported to be primarily CD4+, whereas CD8+ lymphocytes were shown to be underrepresented (Silvennoinen-Kassinen et al. 1992).
- The dominant antigen-presenting cells (APCs), if any, responsible for mediating implant-related hypersensitivity responses remain unknown.
- Candidate APCs in the periprosthetic region include macrophages, endothelial cells, lymphocytes, dendritic cells, and, to lesser extent, parenchymal tissue cells.
- Although there is general consensus implicating the T-cell receptor (TCR) in metal-induced activation, reports conflict regarding which region or receptor specificity is responsible for dominating metal reactivity.
  - Some investigators report no preferential receptor selection (Silvennoinen-Kassinen et al. 1992), whereas others have shown the CDR3B region of the VB17+ TCR to be critical in the sense that without this region, metal reactivity is abrogated (Vollmer et al. 1999).
  - Metals have also been shown to act as facilitating agents in the cross-linking of receptors (e.g., VB17 of CDR1 TCR) to create superantigen-like enhancement of TCR-protein contact (Vollmer et al. 1999), whereby metalloproteins or metal-peptide complexes that would

not otherwise be antigenic are able to provoke a response.
- However, despite reports of non–hapten-related mechanisms of metal-induced lymphocyte activation, type IV DTH remains the dominant mechanism associated with implant-related hypersensitivity responses.

Case Studies in Metal Implant–Related Metal Sensitivity

- Implant degradation products have been shown in case studies to be temporally associated with severe dermatitis, urticaria, vasculitis, and nonspecific immune suppression (Hallab et al. 2001).
- Generally, more case reports of hypersensitivity reactions have been associated with stainless steel and Co alloy implants than with Ti alloy components (Hallab et al. 2001).
- In one of the earliest case studies, an orthopaedic implant was implicated as a source of metal sensitivity (Barranco and Solloman 1972).
  - A 20-year-old woman was examined for extensive eczematous dermatitis on her chest and back 5 months after she received stainless steel screws to treat chronic patellar dislocation.
  - Treatment with topical corticosteroids abrogated her condition for 1 year, after which it worsened, with further generalized dermatitis.
  - Additional topical corticosteroid application yielded poor results.
  - The stainless steel screws were removed.
  - The day after screw removal, her eczema subsided with complete disappearance within 72 hours.
  - "The orthopaedist still doubted that the steel screws could be the cause of her dermatitis and applied a stainless steel screw to the skin of her back. In a period of a 4 hours, generalized pruritus and erythema developed" (Barranco and Solloman 1972). On patch testing, she showed reactions to Ni, Ni sulfate, and the steel screw.
- Hypersensitivity responses are not to the implant but to the dissolution and corrosion products.
- Skin testing remains problematic. There may be false-positive results from mechanical irritation or false-negative results from lack of readily available corrosion products.
- The time between implantation and a developed reaction does not generally fit that of a classic type IV response.

Cohort Studies of Implant-Related Metal Sensitivity

- Cohort studies generally indicate a correlation between the presence of a metal implant and metal sensitivity (Hallab et al. 2001). Data (from these different investigations) regarding the prevalence of metal sensitivity are compiled in Figure 17–8. Unfortunately, these studies include heterogeneous patient populations and testing methodologies and consequently reach a disparate variety of conclusions.

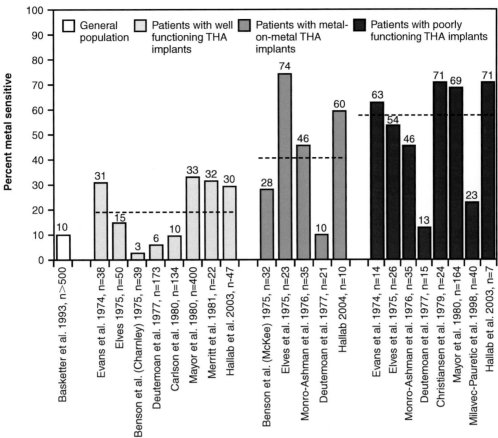

Figure 17–8: Incidence of metal sensitivity.
This compilation of investigations shows the averaged incidence percentages of metal sensitivity for nickel, cobalt, or chromium among the general population, in patients after receiving metal-containing total hip arthroplasty *(THA)*, in patients with metal-on-metal bearing arthroplasty, and in patient populations with significant osteolysis or those who are scheduled for revision surgery. Studies by Hallab and associates used lymphocyte transformation testing to measure hypersensitivity, and all others used dermal patch testing.

- The prevalence of metal sensitivity among patients with well-functioning implants is approximately 25%, roughly twice as high as that of the general population. This approximation was obtained using a weighted average based on the numbers of subjects in each study.
- The average prevalence of metal sensitivity among patients with a failed or poorly functioning implant (as judged by a variety of criteria) using the investigations shown in Figure 17–8 is approximately 60% (Hallab et al. 2001).
- Similar association of sensitivity to polymeric materials among patients with well-functioning implants has not been demonstrated.
- The association of metal release from implants with adverse immunologic response remains conjectural because cause and effect have not been established in symptomatic patients.
- The identification of implant-referable hypersensitivity processes depends on the ability to perform multiple tests on

individual patients before implantation, during device service and, in the case of adverse outcome, before and after device removal. Such intensive studies have not been performed to date, in large part because standardized effective testing methodologies have not been established.
- Specific types of implants with greater propensity to release metal in vivo may be more prone to induce metal sensitivity.
  - Failures of total hip prostheses with metal-on-metal bearing surfaces have been associated with greater prevalence of metal sensitivity than similar designs with metal-on-UHMWPE bearing surfaces.
  - New alternative orthopaedic metal alloys purported to be less allergenic have been put forward by orthopaedic companies to address these growing concerns (e.g., zirconium alloy; Oxinium, Smith and Nephew, Inc., Memphis TN).
- One study in 1980 indicated that after TJA with metallic components, some patients show an induction of metal

tolerance; that is, a case of previously detected metal sensitivity abated after implantation of a metal-containing prosthesis.

- Rooker and Wilkinson reported that of 67 patients patch tested both preoperatively and postoperatively, 6 tested positive for metal sensitivity preoperatively, and of these 6, 5 lost their sensitivity on retesting at 3 to 19 months postoperatively (Rooker and Wilkinson 1980). None of the remaining 49 patients available for postoperative retesting showed indications of metal sensitivity.

- An additional factor obscuring a clear connection between metal sensitivity and implant failure is the lack of any reported correlation between the prevalence of metal sensitivity and implant residence time, infection, reason for removal, or pain.

  - Painful articulation was reportedly the same among metal-sensitive patients undergoing revision as in metal-insensitive patients undergoing revision procedures. However, this lack of clear causality is largely the result of a history of inadequate testing methods.

Lymphocyte Transformation Testing for Quantifying Metal Hypersensitivity

- Dermal patch testing limitations: Although general patch testing protocols and commercial kits do exist for a variety of commonly antigenic substances, concern is mounting about the applicability of dermal testing to the study of immune responses to orthopaedic implants.

  - Knowledge about appropriate APCs and metal challenge agents is lacking.

  - The haptenic potential of metals using dermal contact (in which dermal Langerhans' cells are the primary effector cells) is likely different from a more closed peri-implant in vivo environment. This difference is highlighted by characteristics such as the antigen-processing/endosomal-recycling organelles called *Birbeck's granules*, which are unique to Langerhans' cells (the primary APC of the dermis) and are not found in APCs around implants.

  - The relatively subjective and nonquantitative nature of grading a dermal reaction generally precludes detection of more subtle but statistically different reactivity levels in orthopaedic research group studies.

  - The diagnostic utility of patch testing to predict implant reactivity may be affected by possible immunologic tolerance (i.e., suppression of dermal response to metals).

  - Induction of metal hypersensitivity is possible in a previously insensitive patient.

  - The uncontrolled environment required in a patch test both is uncomfortable for the patient and incorporates an additional degree of variability, depending on an individual's adherence to testing protocol, such as keeping the patch test area dry for at least 48 hours.

- Current methods of patch testing lack standardized dosing and challenge agents for potentially allergenic orthopaedic alloy metals (e.g., Al, Co, Mo, V, and Zr; see Table 17–3).

- In vitro lymphocyte transformation testing (LTT) involves measuring the proliferative response of lymphocytes (obtained from peripheral vasculature) following exposure to antigen (the incorporation of radioactive $[H^3]$-thymidine into cellular DNA on mitosis facilitates the quantification of a proliferation response through the measurement of incorporated radioactivity after a set time period).

  - After 6 days of challenge (with 0.01 to 1.0 mM Al^{+3}, Co^{+2}, Cr^{+3}, Mo^{+5}, Ni^{+2}, V^{+3}, and Zr^{+4} chloride solutions) and 12 to 24 hours of $[^3H]$-thymidine exposure, proliferation is measured by harvesting cells onto a membrane and measuring radiation in counts per minute (cpm).

  - A normalized proliferation or stimulation index is calculated as follows: Proliferation Index (Factor) = (mean cpm with challenge agent)/(mean cpm without challenge agent).

- The use of LTT has been established as a method for testing sensitivity in a variety of clinical settings, including drug allergy (Hallab 2004).

- The use of LTT for correlating implant performance with related metal reactivity has been limited.

- However, the few investigations that have been conducted indicate that metal sensitivity may be more readily detected by LTT than by dermal patch testing (Hallab 2004).

- LTT addresses some of the concerns associated with dermal testing for implant alloy metal sensitivity.

  - Relevant cells: Peripheral mixed mononuclear cell fractions are used for exposure to a metal challenge agent, which may more closely approximate that of the in vivo environment.

  - Challenge agents: Metal used in LTT consists of well-defined concentrations of soluble metal chlorides available for in vivo–like, ion-to-serum protein interactions when using autologous serum.

  - Quantitative: LTT is highly quantitative. A stimulation index is generated using multiwell replicates that facilitate a stimulation index average and standard deviation.

  - Facilitates dose response: LTT can test for many metals (e.g., >10) at several concentrations (e.g., 0.01, 0.1, and 0.5 mM) in replicate in culture plate wells (e.g., in triplicate or quadruplicate). This incorporates a means to assess those individuals who may be sensitive only at relatively low concentrations of metal challenge. This situation is illustrated in Figure 17–9, in which typical LTT results of a metal-sensitive individual versus a nonsensitive individual demonstrate reactivity to Ni at 0.1 mM but not at 0.01 or 0.5 mM.

  - Sensitivity: LTT may be inherently more sensitive when compared with dermal patch testing (Hallab 2004).

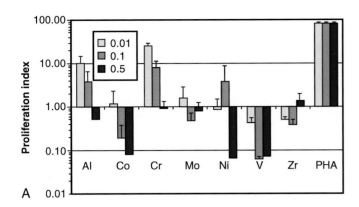

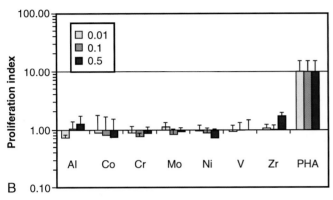

Figure 17–9: Metal reactivity results.
Case examples of typical results generated from lymphocyte transformation testing demonstrate high and low metal reactivity results. **A,** High reactivity to aluminum *(Al)* and chromium *(Cr)* in which lymphocyte activation was greater than 10 for Al and Cr at 0.01 mM. **B,** The typical results of lymphocyte transformation testing in an individual with no metal hypersensitivity. *Co,* cobalt; *Mo,* molybdenum; *Ni,* nickel; *PHA,* phytohemagglutinin; *V,* vanadium; *Zr,* zirconium.

Although this may increase the likelihood of false-positive results, it may also act to minimize the occurrence of false-negative results, which also ultimately acts in the best interests of the patient and a more conservative assessment of metal hypersensitivity. This more conservative assessment may be particularly relevant to orthopaedic patients as the selection of available implant alloys grows for any given orthopaedic component (e.g., Ti alloy, Co alloy, and zirconium alloy).

- Several problems associated with contemporary LTT do remain unresolved.
  - Metal chloride solutions have been shown only to approximate soluble metal release from metal implant degradation products.
  - It is unclear what stimulation index number (i.e., threshold criteria) is appropriate for indicating the likelihood of a clinically relevant response.
- As the number of patients receiving implants grows and the clinical specialties expected to evaluate the phenomena of implant-related metal hypersensitivity widen, LTT may

provide an additional tool in the armamentarium of physicians.

Implant Debris Hypersensitivity: Summary

- It is unclear whether LTT-indicated hypersensitivity responses to metals affect orthopaedic implant performance in other than a few highly predisposed people.
- It is clear that some patients experience immune reactions directly associated with implanted metallic materials. LTT may be a useful test in those individuals who are highly susceptible (i.e., purportedly about 1% of joint replacement recipients) (Hallab et al. 2001), or LTT may be a practical alternative to detect subtle peri-implant bioreactivity phenomena that may not present dermally.
- Given the advantages and drawbacks of current LTT and the potential for erroneous testing and conclusions, is it very important that any facility conducting this testing fully disclose all testing parameters and that physicians be cognizant of some basic testing criteria such as follows:
  - All challenge agents should be identified and indicated as soluble or particulate (to date, no standard method exists for assessing an individual's reactivity to a particular particulate material challenge).
  - Culture medium, time of incubation, and method of proliferation detection should be indicated.
  - Autologous serum should be used to complex with challenge agents.
  - There should be some level of redundancy (e.g., triplicate, duplicate).
- It is likely that cases involving implant-related metal sensitivity have been underreported because of the difficulty of past diagnostic methods.
- Continuing improvements in LTT methods and accumulation of multicenter data will enhance any future assessment of patients particularly susceptible to implant hypersensitivity.
- The utility of LTT or LTT-like metal hypersensitivity testing methods will likely grow as the use of metallic implants increases and as expectations of implant durability and performance increase.

Conclusions

- Tremendous advances have been made in the past decade in the understanding of the biologic characteristics of particle-induced osteolysis and implant allergy, the biologic cascade involved in debris-induced responses, and the role of the individual host's immune system.
- During the next several years, it is anticipated that refined and new biologic testing will further characterize and predict the pathophysiologic features of debris-induced osteolysis.
- Carefully designed clinical studies will be required to define the role of hypersensitivity, genetic predisposition,

biologic variability, and prosthesis-related factors in the pathogenesis of nonspecific and specific biologic responses to implant debris.

References

Barranco VP, Solloman H (1972). Eczematous dermatitis from nickel. *JAMA* 220:1244.

> This is one of the earliest case studies implicating an orthopaedic implant as a source of metal sensitivity. A 20-year-old woman was examined for extensive eczematic dermatitis on her chest and back 5 months after she had received stainless steel screws to treat a chronic patellar dislocation. Treatment with topical corticosteroids abrogated her condition for 1 year, after which it worsened, with further generalized dermatitis. Additional topical corticosteroid application yielded poor results, and the stainless steel screws were removed. The day after screw removal, her eczema subsided and disappeared completely within 72 hours.

Blumenthal NC, Cosma V (1989). The effect of aluminum and gallium ions on the mineralization process. *Bull Hosp Jt Dis Orthop Inst* 49:192-204.

> This is a report of the effects of metal ions on various parts of the skeletal system determined by using in vitro systems that stimulate in vivo mineralization. The authors investigated the physical-chemical mechanisms of the actions of Al and gallium. Al accumulation in patients undergoing renal dialysis caused osteomalacia, whereas gallium was found to be an effective therapeutic agent for treating the hypercalcemia accompanying certain malignant diseases.

Campbell P, Ma S, Yeom B, et al. (1995). Isolation of predominantly submicron-sized UHMWPE wear particles from periprosthetic tissues. *J Biomed Mater Res* 29:127-131.

> In this investigation, a method of tissue digestion using sodium hydroxide was used to recover UHMWPE particles from tissues around failed THAs. Methods such as density gradient ultracentrifugation of the digested tissues were performed to separate the UHMWPE from cell debris and other particulates. Most of the particles counted were submicron in size.

Dorr LD, Bloebaum R, Emmanual J, Meldrum R (1990). Histologic, biochemical and ion analysis of tissue and fluids retrieved during total hip arthroplasty. *Clin Orthop Relat Res* 261:82-95.

> This investigation found large amounts of metal and polyethylene debris and high ion readings in capsule and fibrous membranes of both loose Ti and Co-Cr stems. Osteolysis-producing factors such as PGE_2, IL-1, and collagenase levels were found to be elevated when compared with control values. The authors reported that fixed stems were associated with less particulate debris in surrounding soft tissues and that failure of most metal hip stems was judged to be mechanical. This seminal study hypothesized that particulate debris and high ion readings are primarily a focal problem contained by the periprosthetic fibrous connective tissue encapsulation within the femoral canal and joint capsules.

Gautam S, Tebo JM, Hamilton TA (1992). IL-4 suppresses cytokine gene expression induced by IFN-gamma and/or IL-2 in murine peritoneal macrophages. *J Immunol* 148:1725-1730.

> This investigation using mouse macrophages stimulated with IFN-γ in combination with IL-2 examined the effect of IL-4 on inflammatory gene expression. The investigators showed that the IL-4–mediated suppression of IFN-γ/IL-2–driven TNF-α gene expression was mediated at the level of transcription. This study suggests that macrophage inflammatory function will depend on the precise stimulus composition.

Goldring SR, Schiller AL, Roelke M, et al. (1983). The synovial-like membrane at the bone-cement interface in loose total hip replacements and its proposed role in bone lysis. *J Bone Joint Surg Am* 65:575-584.

> This is a seminal study of the membrane present at the bone-cement interface. In this study, 20 patients with a loose, nonseptic failed THA at a site clearly remote from the pseudocapsule that reformed postoperatively were analyzed. This was the first study to show that this membrane could produce large amounts of PGE_2 and collagenase. Thus this capacity to generate PGE_2 and collagenase was postulated as an explanation for the progressive lysis of bone seen in some patients with loose cemented total joint implants. The investigators further suggested that loosening of the component may be a stimulus to the synthetic activity of this tissue, which leads to further resorption of bone, a cycle now accepted as fact.

Hallab NJ (2004). Lymphocyte transformation testing for quantifying metal–implant–related hypersensitivity responses. *Dermatitis* 15:82-90.

> This study examined the utility of LTT for predicting implant-related sensitivity in orthopaedic patients by contrasting LTT and patch testing protocols and examining original cohort LTT data of subjects with and without implants. The conclusion was that quantifiable lymphocyte reactivity, as exemplified by increased incidence and average reactivity levels in groups of subjects with implants, were metal implant specific (characteristic of adaptive immune responses), and it suggested that LTT may be useful in the determination of implant-specific sensitivity and may be an additional tool in the armamentarium of physicians.

Hallab N, Merritt K, Jacobs JJ (2001). Metal sensitivity in patients with orthopaedic implants. *J Bone Joint Surg Am* 83:428-436.

> In this review, we examined what was known of metal allergy and tried to consolidate all relevant studies to date. We showed that implant degradation products were associated with dermatitis, urticaria, and vasculitis and that if cutaneous signs of an allergic response appear after implantation of a metal device, metal sensitivity should be considered. We found that the prevalence of dermal sensitivity in patients with a joint replacement device, particularly those with a failed implant, is substantially higher than in the general population. We concluded that until the roles of delayed hypersensitivity and humoral immune responses to metallic orthopaedic implants are more clearly defined, the risk to patients may be considered.

Horowitz SM, Algan SA, Purdon MA (1996). Pharmacologic inhibition of particulate-induced bone resorption. *J Biomed Mater Res* 31:91-96.

> In this study, the authors used a rat calvaria/macrophage co-culture model to study the effects of various agents on bone resorption induced by macrophage exposure to bone cement particles (polymethylmethacrylate). They found that pamidronate was the only agent tested that suppressed the increase in bone resorption associated with macrophage exposure to bone cement particles to levels that were not significantly different from unexposed calvaria. They thus speculated that by "delaying or preventing bone resorption associated with macrophage exposure to bone cement particles, bisphosphonates may have a clinical role in cemented

joint arthroplasty by decreasing the rate or incidence of aseptic loosening and prolonging implant longevity."

Jacobs JJ, Gilbert JL, Urban RM (1998). Corrosion of metal orthopaedic implants. *J Bone Joint Surg Am* 80:268-282.

This extensive review focuses on electrochemical corrosion phenomena in alloys used for orthopaedic implants. A summary of basic electrochemistry is followed by a discussion of retrieval studies of the response of the implant to the host environment and the response of local tissue to implant corrosion products. We acknowledge the systemic implications of the release of metal particles.

Jacobs JJ, Roebuck KA, Archibeck M, et al. (2001). Osteolysis: Basic science. *Clin Orthop Relat Res* 393:71-77.

This is a review of the basic science of periprosthetic bone loss. It covers topics central to this chapter's discussion. Initially termed cement disease, it is now generally accepted that, in most instances, osteolysis is a manifestation of an adverse cellular response to phagocytosable particulate wear and corrosion debris, possibly facilitated by local hydrodynamic effects. The actions of the major chemical mediators responsible for the cellular responses and effects on bone are covered and include PGE_2, TNF-α, IL-1, and IL-6. This review also stresses that although initial animal studies are promising for possible pharmacologic treatment and prevention of osteolysis, well-controlled human trials are required before agents such as bisphosphonates can be recommended for general clinical use.

Jacobs JJ, Silverton C, Hallab NJ, et al. (1999). Metal release and excretion from cementless titanium alloy total knee replacements. *Clin Orthop Relat Res* 358:173-180.

This is an example of a metal ion analysis study of patients with total knee arthroplasty in which concentrations of Ti, Al, and V were measured in the serum and urine of patients. Here patients were categorized into one of five groups. In group 1, the patellar and tibial articulating surfaces were made of carbon fiber–reinforced UHMWPE. In group 2, the patellar and tibial surfaces were made of UHMWPE. In group 3, the femoral Ti alloy articulating surface was nitrogen ion implanted with UHMWPE patellar and tibial articulating surfaces. Patients in group 4 had failed patellar components, and group 5 was composed of age- and gender-matched control subjects without implants. Serum concentrations of Ti were approximately 50 times greater in patients with failed patellar components (group 4) and approximately 10 times greater in patients with carbon fiber-reinforced polyethylene bearing surfaces (group 1) when compared with groups 2 and 3 and the control subjects (group 5). For Al and V, no detectable differences were observed among any of the groups. In addition, analysis of 24-hour urine samples showed no significant differences in Ti, Al, or V concentrations among any of the groups. Elevated serum Ti levels may serve as a marker of patellar component failure or accelerated femoral component wear in total knee replacements with Ti alloy bearings. Again, we stressed that the toxicologic ramifications of these findings are unknown.

Jacobs JJ, Skipor AK, Urban RM, et al. (1994). Systemic distribution of metal degradation products from titanium alloy total hip replacements: An autopsy study. In: *Transactions of the Annual Meeting of the Orthopaedic Research Society.* New Orleans: Orthopaedic Research Society, p 838.

In this investigation, the serum concentrations and urinary excretion of Ti, Al, and V were measured in patients with cementless primary THAs. We found that serum concentrations of Ti were elevated approximately twofold in the patients who had a loose implant, compared with the values for the control subjects. No major differences were noted in terms of urine concentration of Ti, serum concentration of Al, or urine concentration of Al observed among any of the groups studied. V was found to be uniformly low in all groups.

Kerboull L, Hamadouche M, Courpied JP, Kerboull M (2004). Long-term results of Charnley-Kerboull hip arthroplasty in patients younger than 50 years. *Clin Orthop Relat Res* 418:112-118.

In this extensive review, the authors examined 287 Charnley-Kerboull low-friction THAs implanted between 1975 and 1990 in 222 patients younger than 50 years. The average age of the patients at the time of the index procedure was 40.1 years. The data for this series were as follows:
1. Mean follow-up was 14.5 ± 5.1 years.
2. Forty-five patients (52 hips) had a follow-up greater than 20 years.
3. The mean preoperative Merle d'Aubigne hip functional score was 9.6 ± 2.5 points versus 17.2 ± 0.8 points at the latest follow-up.
4. Twenty-five revisions were documented, 17 for aseptic loosening.
5. The mean wear rate was 0.12 ± 0.21 mm/year.
6. Considering 0.1 mm/year as the threshold for a normal wear rate, 196 hips had a normal or below normal wear rate (mean, 0.02 mm/year), whereas the remaining 91 hips had an abnormally high wear rate (mean, 0.28 mm/year).
7. The overall survival rate at 20 years was $85.4 \pm 5\%$ using revision of either component as the end point.
8. The only predictive factor of loosening was a wear rate higher than 0.1 mm/year.

Martell JM, Pierson RH, Jacobs JJ, et al. (1993). Primary total hip reconstruction with a titanium fiber-coated prosthesis inserted without cement. *J Bone Joint Surg Am* 75:554-571.

This is a large and prospective study of the intermediate-term clinical and radiographic results of 121 THAs (Harris-Galante porous Ti fiber–coated prosthesis) inserted without cement in 110 patients (average, age 49 years). Follow-up was 67 months (range, 55 to 79 months). The average preoperative Harris hip score was 55 points, and the average postoperative score was 93 points. Eleven femoral implants were unstable, and of these, 4 were revised. The authors found cortical erosion around the distal part of the femoral stem in 9 patients (8%) with stable implants. This study is one of the first to promulgate the use of cementless implants in which survivorship analysis at 5 years revealed a 97% chance of survival (95% confidence limit, 0.937 to 1.0).

Michel R, Nolte M, Reich M, Loer F (1991). Systemic effects of implanted prostheses made of cobalt-chromium alloys. *Arch Orthop Trauma Surg* 110:61-74.

In this investigation, the authors showed that by analyzing up to 16 elements from Co-Cr alloy/polyethylene hip joint prostheses using instrumental neutron activation, the analyses of organs revealed significant Co and Cr enrichment in several tissues and organs. Thus the authors concluded: "it can be seen that implant corrosion is not an occurrence of merely local significance, but one that affects the trace element status of the entire organism."

Rooker GD, Wilkinson JD (1980). Metal sensitivity in patients undergoing hip replacement: A prospective study. *J Bone Joint Surg Br* 62:502-505.

This is a prospective study of allergic contact dermatitis after metal-on-plastic THA in 69 patients, of whom 54 were available for review after operation. The investigators showed that before operation, 6 patients were metal sensitive, but only one remained so afterward. This is one of the only studies in which investigators did not find any increased sensitivity after metal-on-plastic hip replacement. In this early study, there was little evidence of a direct causal relationship between metal sensitivity and subsequent loosening. The results showing that cutaneous sensitivity may be the consequence of loosening, rather than its cause, and the conclusions that routine patch testing before hip replacement is no longer required are taken as established fact only in part. Many recent studies using newer analytic techniques have shown different results, and questions of metal allergy testing before TJA is currently revisited.

Schmalzried TP, Akizuki KH, Fedenko AN, Mirra J (1997). The role of access of joint fluid to bone in periarticular osteolysis: A report of four cases. *J Bone Joint Surg Am* 79:447-452.

This report of four case studies found that development of geodes in association with osteoarthrosis and of osteolysis in association with TJA was dependent on access of joint fluid to bone. These investigators also found that "the physical effect of pressure as seen with geodes, the fluid around prosthetic joints, also carries wear particles and increased levels of soluble factors that are capable of stimulating bone resorption at distant sites." They concluded that to prevent osteolysis there must be a limitation of access of joint fluid to bone.

Shanbhag AS, Hasselman CT, Rubash HE (1997). The John Charnley Award: Inhibition of wear debris mediated osteolysis in a canine total hip arthroplasty model. *Clin Orthop Relat Res* 344:33-43.

This study was among the first to investigate the efficacy of oral bisphosphonate therapy to inhibit wear debris–mediated bone resorption in a canine THA model. These investigators found that continuous administration of alendronate inhibited bone lysis for the 24-week duration of the study. Their conclusions that alendronate is incorporated in the mineralizing matrix, thus making it refractory to osteoclastic resorption, helped to induce interest in bisphosphonates in osteolysis in humans.

Silvennoinen-Kassinen S, Ikaheimo I, Karvonen J, et al. (1992). Mononuclear cell subsets in the nickel-allergic reaction in vitro and in vivo. *J Allergy Clin Immunol* 89:794-800.

This study describes Ni as a major cause of metal-induced contact allergy and purports that Ni-induced lymphoblast transformation occurred in vitro only in cells from Ni-allergic subjects. "CD4$^+$ cells and CD45RO$^+$ cells were overrepresented among the lymphoblasts of Ni-sensitive subjects, whereas CD8$^+$ and CD8$^+$CD11b$^+$ and CD4$^+$CD45R$^+$ cells were underrepresented." They found that Ni-reacting T cells used predominantly the TCR $\alpha\beta$ heterodimer. Other parts of the TCR were examined, but no preferential selection of Vβ5, Vβ6, or Vβ8 was observed.

Urban RM, Jacobs JJ, Tomlinson MJ, et al. (2000). Dissemination of wear particles to the liver, spleen, and abdominal lymph nodes of patients with hip or knee replacement. *J Bone Joint Surg Am* 82:457-476.

This is one of the few studies addressing the amount of metal implant products disseminated systemically in patients with THA and total knee replacement to determine the prevalence of and the histopathologic response to prosthetic wear debris in the liver, spleen, and abdominal para-aortic lymph nodes. The authors found that metallic wear particles in the liver or spleen were more prevalent in patients who had had a failed hip arthroplasty (7 of 8) than in patients who had had a primary hip replacement (2 of 11) or knee replacement (2 of 10). The main source of wear particles in most of these patients involved secondary nonbearing surfaces, rather than wear between the two primary bearing surfaces, as intended. In one living patient, dissemination of Ti alloy particles from a hip prosthesis with mechanical failure was associated with a visceral granulomatous reaction and hepatosplenomegaly that required operative and medical management. These investigators found metallic wear particles in the para-aortic lymph nodes in 68% of the 28 patients. In 38% (11) of all 29 patients with an implant who were studied post mortem, dissemination of metallic particles was noted in the liver or spleen, where they were found within small aggregates of macrophages as infiltrates without apparent pathologic significance. Polyethylene particles elicited a similar response. These investigators found on microscopic analysis that most of the disseminated wear particles were smaller than 1 μm. Not surprisingly, the authors concluded that the prevalence of particles in the liver or spleen was greater after reconstructions with mechanical failure.

Van der Vis HM, Aspenberg P, Marti RK, et al. (1998). Fluid pressure causes bone resorption in a rabbit model of prosthetic loosening. *Clin Orthop Relat Res* 350:201-208.

In this seminal study, high fluid pressures were found throughout the effective joint space after THA, and these high pressures were found to extend locally to the bone-implant interface. This study was the first to report that osteolysis can occur with only elevated fluid pressure in vivo in a rabbit model. This was the first direct proof that features of prosthetic loosening only ascribed to particle activation could be explained by the effects of fluid pressure.

Vollmer J, Weltzien HU, Moulon C (1999). TCR reactivity in human nickel allergy indicates contacts with complementarity-determining region 3 but excludes superantigen-like recognition. *J Immunol* 163:2723-2731.

This study investigated which parts of the TCRBV17 element are involved with Ni-induced activation of CD4$^+$ T-cell lines of Ni-allergic patients. The investigators found that amino acids in the CDR3B region of a VB17$^+$ TCR are critical for Ni recognition. CD4 independence implies a high affinity of receptor to the Ni/MHC complex.

Index

Note: Page numbers followed by b, f, and t indicate boxes, figures, and tables, respectively.

alloy